D0117283

Theory and Practice of Psychiatry

THEORY AND PRACTICE
OF PSYCHIATRY

Bruce J. Cohen, M.D.

OXFORD
UNIVERSITY PRESS
2003

OXFORD
UNIVERSITY PRESS

Oxford   New York
Auckland   Bangkok   Buenos Aires   Cape Town   Chennai
Dar es Salaam   Delhi   Hong Kong   Istanbul   Karachi   Kolkata
Kuala Lumpur   Madrid   Melbourne   Mexico City   Mumbai
Nairobi   São Paulo   Shanghai   Taipei   Tokyo   Toronto

Published by Oxford University Press, Inc.
198 Madison Avenue, New York, New York 10016
http://www.oup-usa.org

Oxford is a registered trademark of Oxford University Press

Library of Congress Cataloging-in-Publication Data
Cohen, Bruce J., 1938–
Theory and practice of psychiatry /
Bruce J. Cohen.
p. ; cm.   Includes bibliographical references and index.
ISBN 0-19-514937-8 (cloth)—ISBN 0-19-514938-6 (paper)
1. Psychiatry. I. Title.
[DNLM: 1. Mental Disorders.
2. Psychological Theory.
WM 140 C678t 2003]
RC435 .C59 2003   616.89—dc21   2002070409

2 3 4 5 6 7 8 9

Printed in the United States of America
on acid-free paper

Preface

This is a wonderful time in history to be practicing psychiatry. Neuroscientists are unearthing staggering amounts of information about the functioning of the brain at the anatomic, cellular, and subcellular level. An explosion of new pharmaceutical agents offers the prospect of safer and more effective treatments for mental illnesses that just a few decades ago were considered either purely "psychological" in origin, or untreatable, or both. The public is becoming more comfortable with the notion that mental illness is not synonymous with "moral weakness." Research in naturalistic settings (i.e., in typical clinical environments) is demonstrating to the insurance industry and to state and federal governments that psychiatric treatment not only can be efficacious; it can be cost-effective.

Further, we are learning more about which treatments are most effective for which psychiatric disorders. Ideally, the treatment that a clinician prescribes to a given patient should be dictated by that patient's particular needs, not by which residency program the treating clinician happened to attend or by the clinician's theoretical "orientation." This ideal increasingly is becoming a reality.

However, many things have remained the same. Stigma related to mental illness remains ubiquitous. Further, while the availability of a plethora of new pharmaceutical agents has encouraged even general physicians to familiarize themselves with recent advances in neuroreceptor subtyping (after all, why prescribe a $5HT_{1A}$ serotonin receptor partial agonist when you now can prescribe a $5HT_{2A}$ serotonin receptor antagonist?), it also has resulted in physicians being increasingly subjected to a bewildering array of confusing and often contradictory data. In addition, all of the new drugs in the world aren't especially useful if physicians fail to recognize that a mental disorder is present, or make the wrong diagnosis, or don't appropriately monitor for specific target symptoms through careful, serial mental status examinations. Many physicians report that they feel ill-equipped in these areas.

Finally, patients continue to present to physicians because their thoughts their emotions, their behaviors, and their *lives* are in a state of turmoil, not because they are worried that their brain chemistry is in a state of turmoil. The fact that some psychiatrists have come to see themselves as "psychopharmacologists" and are only meeting with patients for brief "medication checks" hardly represents a major advance in the history of psychiatry. Addressing patients' chemistry is not enough in many cases. The majority of patients currently referred to psychiatrists already have received several medication trials from their primary care physicians, often without having experienced significant benefits. If anything, the flood of new pharmaceuticals has brought into even greater relief the importance of being able to formulate a patient's case from more than just one perspective, particularly when the current treatment plan isn't working.

The dangers of biological reductionism are compounded by the fact that the bulk of care for the mentally ill is provided by nonpsychiatric physicians. For most general physicians, the process of asking about specific symptoms and then formulating a differential diagnosis is quite familiar. However, maladaptive personality traits, self-defeating behaviors, and crises that develop at particular developmental milestones in patients' lives don't lend themselves to traditional "disease" reasoning. Many physicians feel bewildered or frustrated when confronted with such cases. "Biological psychiatry," in holding out the hope that all conditions affecting mental life might one day be treated in the same manner as infectious diseases, often has promised more than it has delivered.

My goal, in the following chapters, is to present more than simply a description of each psychiatric disorder and of currently available treatment options; I describe an *approach* to psychiatry—its theory, its practice, and the relationship between the two. The major complaint I have heard from medical students and residents is that they lack a conceptual scaffolding on which they might hang the insights offered by mentors who approach the study of mental life from different clinical perspectives. Without this, they become frustrated. Lectures and journal articles appear to contradict each other. Sometimes, students of psychiatry resolve such conflicts either by aligning with one particular school of thought or by endorsing theoretical "eclecticism." Unfortunately, the former solution is unnecessarily narrow (even dogmatic), while latter solutions often involves applying various theoretical approaches in different cases without having a firm grasp of the relative strengths and weaknesses of each conceptual approach.

This text is intended for the person who wishes to learn how to "think psychiatrically." As such, the target audience includes medical students, general physicians, psychiatric residents, nurses, psychologists, and social workers. I wrote the first draft while teaching the second-year medical student course "Introduction to Psychological Medicine" at the University of Virginia School of Medicine. However, a genetic analysis of the text would reveal it also to be descended from the psychiatry program at the Johns Hopkins University School of Medicine, where Paul McHugh, M.D., and Phillip Slavney, M.D.—the authors of a slim, elegant treatise, *The Perspectives of Psychiatry*—introduced me to the theoretical approach that runs through this text.

I have attempted to maintain a conversational tone throughout, similar to what I might use when speaking to students after we have just interviewed a patient together. The goal is for students to have a psychiatry text that they might read from cover to cover. It's possible to dip into a particular chapter, but the reader who starts at the beginning and reads through to the end will note that later chapters build on discussions from earlier chapters. For example, there is some overlap between "normal" feelings of depression and anxiety, psychiatric diseases (such as major depressive disorder and generalized anxiety disorder) in which one's ability to regulate mood or anxiety becomes impaired, and personality disorders (such as histrionic personality disorder) that are characterized by excessive emotionality. Each of these conditions is discussed separately at appropriate points in the text. However, students who read through this textbook may gain a greater appreciation of the *relationships* between these different theoretical constructs than they would by reading either a large, multiauthored, "comprehensive" textbook of psychiatry or a short "pocket guide."

Chapter 1 attempts to address the fundamental questions that almost every intro-ductory student brings to the table. Is psychiatry a legitimate branch of medicine? How can clinicians reliably study something as vague as a person's thoughts or feel-ings? When a clinician applies a psychiatric diagnosis, is she just plastering an ar-tificial diagnostic label on what might simply be normal human experiences? Chap-ter 2 describes how psychiatrists address such questions as they perform the psychiatric history and mental status examination.

In Chapter 3, having discussed the strengths and limitations of the psychiatric method itself, we move on to the difficulties inherent in a field of inquiry where the practitioner simultaneously attempts to diagnose *clinical syndromes* that cut across individuals while also attempting to empathize with patients as *unique individuals*. Different schools of psychiatry and psychology have attempted to dodge these dif-ficulties by restricting their focus to one particular aspect of mental life. However, such circumscribed approaches offer clarity and internal consistency at the expense of intellectual breadth. Further, some disorders lend themselves more naturally to one conceptual approach than to another. Excessive reliance on just one approach therefore limits one's treatment options unnecessarily. Clinicians trained in only one conceptual approach may be forced to use a therapy that is suboptimal for particu-lar conditions. Given this, we will discuss the strengths and limitations of each the-oretical perspective. In discussing the major psychiatric schools of thought, we will condense them down to four primary theoretical approaches, or perspectives: dis-eases, dimensional variations, motivated behaviors, and life stories or narratives.

Some psychiatric illnesses are viewed most naturally from one perspective rather than from the others. For example, Alzheimer's disease is most commonly ap-proached from the disease perspective. Its occurrence in a particular individual can-not be explained solely based on that person's particular life story. However, the experience of *living* with Alzheimer's disease obviously varies from one individual to the next, and this experience clearly is shaped by each individual's dimensional personality traits and previous life history. A person with intense emotions who ear-lier in life witnessed his father's deterioration and demise due to Alzheimer's dis-ease may experience having the disease himself in a very different way than an emo-tionally bland person who has never had an earlier exposure to Alzheimer's disease. The latter individual may approach the illness in a more detached, stoical fashion.

In other words, these perspectives are not mutually exclusive. Given this, clini-cians are encouraged to shift between these four perspectives as they formulate a patient's case in order to overcome theoretical myopia. The view from any single perspective won't ever fully represent a patient's "reality," since the apparent clar-ity offered by individual perspectives is arrived at only by promoting certain ele-ments of mental life to the foreground while relegating other elements to the back-ground. However, by alternately viewing a patient from several different perspectives, the clinician may gain a more accurate panoramic view of the case. Having established this conceptual framework, we will move on in successive chap-ters to discuss specific mental disorders.

I'm indebted to my wife Hannah for her support—enduring with me the pains of authorship (including, on innumerable nights, sleeping with the bedside lamp on and somebody typing away next to her). I also would like to thank my children Madeline and Aaron both for their support and for helping me come to more fully appreciate the wide variety of thoughts, feelings, and behaviors that even a single, small person can experience over the course of a single day.

Charlottesville, Virginia   B.J.C.

Contents

Figures

Tables

Theory and Practice of Psychiatry

Chapter 1

Mental Life and Its Assessment

MENTAL LIFE

What is a psychiatrist? What conditions do psychiatrists treat? These apparently simple questions have proven to be sources of great contention. Various "schools of therapy" have offered different answers, typically based on quite different (even diametrically opposed) underlying premises. At the furthest extreme, some commentators have questioned the very existence of "mental illness." They have charged that psychiatrists apply "diagnostic labels" to any individuals who they consider to be "different" and therefore "in need of treatment." At the other extreme would be those who reply with what appears to be the obvious answer to both questions, that psychiatrists are physicians who specialize in the treatment of "mental illnesses" or "brain diseases," just as cardiologists are physicians who specialize in the treatment of cardiovascular diseases. But this definition is simply too narrow. Consider the following example:

An 18-year-old single male college freshman is brought to the emergency room by his dormitory supervisor after his roommate discovers him lying on the floor, somnolent and confused. The patient admits to having taken an overdose of sleeping pills. After treatment with gastric lavage and activated charcoal, a psychiatric consultation is requested.

The patient's father is an attorney and his mother is a realtor, both of whom have enjoyed success in their careers. His parents have always been proud of his academic achievements. In high school, he was a straight A student. However, college was proving to be much more difficult. A history major, the patient was having difficulty keeping up with the heavy reading load, in large part due to his spending hours taking copious notes. At the conclusion of his first semester, he received several B's, and this led him to become extremely anxious. His identity and self-esteem previously had been rooted in his academic successes. Over the past few weeks, he has felt like a "total failure." In addition, during orientation week the patient entered into an intense relationship with a female classmate. She broke up with him 1 week before the overdose, and this further contributed to him feeling lonely, helpless, like "a failure," and hopeless about his future. The patient is a fan of the late Kurt Cobain (who himself committed suicide), and over the past week he has listened repeatedly to Cobain songs while contemplating suicide.

On mental status examination, the patient initially appears withdrawn, but as the interview progresses he relaxes, makes better eye contact, and becomes more talkative. He speaks a normal amount, both spontaneously and in response to questions, without evidence of speech latency (long pauses) or disorganization of thought. His subjective mood is described as "sad." His observed facial expression and demeanor (his "affect") are consistent with his stated mood, and they are reactive (i.e., while he appears sad for most of the interview, at several points he is able to brighten appropriately). He denies experiencing hallucinations and no evidence is found of delusional thinking. Asked by the psychiatrist whether he wanted to die when he took the sleeping pills, the patient replies that he isn't sure, that perhaps he had "just wanted to sleep for a long time so that I wouldn't have to think about things." However, he does admit that he doesn't see much point in living, and he further states that if he had died from the overdose, "it wouldn't have been such a bad thing."

The psychiatrist assigns the diagnoses of adjustment disorder with mixed disturbance of emotions and conduct in the setting of an obsessive-compulsive personality disorder (more about these diagnoses later). He treats the patient with weekly psychotherapy sessions. Over the following 2 months, the patient's mood greatly improves and he gains insight into his personality vulnerabilities. For example, he ultimately comes to recognize that "failing" academically does not prove that he himself is "a failure," that there is a difference between not scoring 100% on an exam and "failing," and that his girlfriend's not loving him does not "prove" that he is an inherently "unlovable" person.

This patient demonstrates a personality style characterized by excessive perfectionism, self-criticism, and emotional dependency. These personality traits not only have contributed to his academic and interpersonal difficulties; they have also contributed to his having reacted to his current circumstances with such intense anxiety and sadness. His perfectionism and fastidious note-taking style have contributed not only to his failure to keep up with his academic reading load but also to his belief that any grade below an A constitutes failure. His personal background also likely has contributed to his holding such ingrained attitudes, particularly his having been raised in a family where academic and career successes were the norm. Finally, his identification with Kurt Cobain, who himself committed suicide, likely has contributed to his seeing suicide as a viable solution to his problems.

While this patient appears to have benefited from psychiatric treatment, he doesn't appear to have a "mental illness." His case demonstrates that psychiatrists don't only treat people with brain diseases. However, we wouldn't want to swing to the other extreme, concluding that "everyone should see a psychiatrist" or that psychiatrists are experts on all aspects of human nature. Psychiatrists treat a particular subset of humankind—psychiatric patients. To better understand just what defines a "psychiatric patient," let us return to our example of the college freshman. We'll assume that all details of his background history remain the same but that the mental status examination is very different:

On mental status examination, the patient makes no eye contact and displays a paucity of movement. He appears anxious and glances suspiciously around the room. He answers questions only after long pauses. His responses are brief and make little sense. Asked why he overdosed he replies, "The pawns are always the first to die . . . you can't trust the queen." He states that he read Thomas Kuhn during his first semester, and that after the breakup with his girlfriend he "experienced a paradigm shift." While he describes his mood as "low," his observed affect is neutral, with a restricted range of emotional responsiveness. Sometimes his affect is inappropriate; for example, he smiles while discussing mother's treatment for breast cancer the previous year.

He reports having had a low appetite over the past few weeks accompanied by a weight loss of several pounds. He hasn't slept for several days. He states that people in his dormitory are "tormenting" him by moving items in his room or replacing them with nearly identical items while he is asleep. He has felt obligated to stay awake to guard against such behavior. He believes that his former girlfriend, who he sometimes refers to as "the queen," is putting his classmates up to this. On occasion, he has overheard his classmates as they have talked about him. He has heard their voices through the walls, apparently coming from the hallway or the room next door to his own. They laugh at him, call him a failure, and comment on whatever he happens to be doing at that moment. When asked by the psychiatrist if the voices ever echo things that he himself is thinking, the patient raises his eyebrows and asks, "How did you know about that?" Asked by the psychiatrist whether he wanted to die when he took the sleeping pills, the patient replies that he isn't sure, that perhaps he had "just wanted to sleep for a long time so that I wouldn't have to think about things." However, he does admit that he doesn't see much point in living, and he further states that if he had died from the overdose, "it wouldn't have been such a bad thing."

How does this vignette differ from our first vignette? This time around, the patient is demonstrating delusions, auditory hallucinations, and extremely disorganized thinking and behavior. Such experiences are outside the realm of normal human experience, and therefore they are considered to be *symptoms* of a mental illness, most likely schizophrenia. We all have experienced sadness and anxiety, and we all can readily empathize with the sadness and anxiety expressed by the patient in the first example, even though his life story is not our own life story. However, in the second example, while we can empathize with how the patient's personality features and life story have placed him under stress, and while we even can empathize with the *content* of his persecutory delusions and hallucinations, empathic understanding alone doesn't help us to explain the occurrence of these symptoms.

By analogy, if this patient, while experiencing academic and interpersonal stress, had developed a high fever and chest pain and was now presenting to the emergency room coughing up green sputum, we would not respond by saying, "I can empathize with that. Sometimes when I'm under stress I get a high fever and cough up green sputum, too." Rather, we would recognize the patient as demonstrating changes in his bodily functioning that are outside the realm of what is considered to be "normal" or "healthy." Given this, we would consider him to be demonstrating symptoms of an *illness*, and we would likely give a label to his illness, such as pneumonia. Certainly, stress may have contributed to the patient having become more vulnerable to developing the pneumonia (through lowered immunity), but it can't in itself account for his pathologic symptoms.

This brings us back to one of our initial questions. What do psychiatrists treat? The answer lies not in how our two examples differ, but in how they resemble each other. In both cases, the psychiatrist's examination focused *on complaints arising in the realm of the patient's mental life* (such as thoughts, moods, and behaviors) as opposed to complaints arising out of the patient's skin, bones, and viscera. In other words, psychiatrists treat a wide range of disorders (some of which are diseases, many of which are not), but psychiatric evaluation always involves an exploration of the patient's mental life. This

book will delineate the various psychiatric conditions that arise in the realm of mental life.

OPERATIONALISM

The only way for a psychiatrist to study a patient's mental life is by asking the patient to describe what he or she is thinking and feeling. The psychiatrist then attempts to *classify* these descriptions into various categories. Therefore the methodology of psychiatry is based fundamentally on **phenomenology**, which is the study of mind in an indirect manner, through its public expression (i.e., through what the patient says or how the patient acts).

Put more simply, psychiatrists are not mind readers. In order to study the contents of patients' minds, they must ask these patients to introspect and then to describe their subjective mental experiences. In doing so, private mental events are made public. The **psychiatric interview and mental status examination** together consist of an interviewer first asking initial screening questions and then asking additional clarifying questions in order to obtain an increasingly refined phenomenologic description of the contents of the patient's mental life.

Psychiatrists then attempt to categorize mental experiences reported by the patient without embellishment or interpretation. Clearly one can't do this without explicit, previously agreed-upon, operational criteria as to what should "count" as constituting various pathological symptoms. For example, what experiences should be considered to constitute "hallucinations"? The operational definition of a hallucination is a "sensory perception without an external referent." During the interview, we must ask clarifying questions if we are to distinguish possible hallucinations from mere vivid thoughts:

> The psychiatrist is called to the emergency room to evaluate a man with no previous psychiatric history who presented with the chief complaint of "hearing voices." The emergency room physician is wondering if this is a case of first-break schizophrenia. The psychiatrist walks into the examination room and finds an anxious man in his thirties who reports that while driving his car he has been hearing a "voice" saying, "You should just kill yourself, you should just drive into a tree." When asked how long he has been hearing this "voice,"

the patient replies, "All night, ever since my wife walked out on me . . . I've just been driving, and I can't get this voice out of my head." The psychiatrist asks the patient, "Do you actually hear the voice through your ears, the way you're hearing my voice now, or is the voice more 'inside' your head." The patient replies that the latter is the case. The psychiatrist continues to ask clarifying questions. "Is it actually a 'voice,' or just a 'loud thought'?" The patient replies, "Well . . . it's like this thought, but it just won't go away! I can't stop thinking it. It's driving me crazy." The psychiatrist concludes that the patient is experiencing upsetting, vivid thoughts in the setting of severe emotional distress, but that the patient is not in fact experiencing hallucinations. The patient is admitted to the inpatient psychiatric unit but is administered no antipsychotic medication. By morning the "voice" has spontaneously resolved.

Obviously, there are limitations to this phenomenologic approach. First and foremost, the quality of the psychiatric interview depends upon the skill of the clinician. Unlike the case in a condition such as pneumonia, there are no laboratory studies that can detect hallucinations. (Standardized pencil and paper tests have proven to be useful supplements to, but not substitutes for, the clinical mental status examination.) The clinician also must enter the interview with a detailed knowledge base of the key phenomenologic signs and symptoms of a variety of mental disorders. Further, the clinician must have the capacity for empathy as she hones in on specific areas for further inquiry and continues to ask clarifying questions until she has a clear appreciation of the patient's subjective experience.

Another limitation of the operational approach is that it relies upon the abilities of the patient both to accurately introspect and to accurately convey information to the examiner. This may not be feasible for many patients. Examples include many children, patients who are mentally retarded or brain-damaged or delirious, patients who are not verbal (whether due to catatonia or aphasia), and patients who are paranoid and refuse to cooperate with the clinical endeavor entirely.

Therefore, in using the phenomenologic method, the accuracy of our conclusions will always be limited by the adequacy of the clinical interview. For example, if while interviewing a patient we notice that her gaze frequently darts around the room, or if we observe her talking to herself, we might infer that she currently is responding to auditory or visual hallucinations, even if she adamantly denies that this is the case. However, we can't conclude this to be the case with certainty. Perhaps she is simply very vigilant or likes to talk to herself. Collateral information from family members, acquaintances, or previous medical records often assumes a crucial role in such cases. Complicating matters, as we can see in the example presented above of the presumed first-break schizophrenic patient, the interviewer essentially has to teach the patient the operational criteria over the course of the interview in order for the patient to better assist the interviewer in making these distinctions. As noted by Sims (1988):

> The experienced physician palpates an enlarged kidney in his patient's abdomen. He invites the medical students to palpate the abdomen bimanually so that they too can learn to experience that barely perceptible, yet important, sensation. The phenomenological method of empathy employed in psychiatry is even more difficult to teach than this. It is like the doctor having to carry out his examination without hands. First, he has to train the patient to palpate his own abdomen bimanually in the required fashion and then, accurately describe what he feels. The doctor then interprets the patient's description to decide whether the kidney is enlarged without being able to put a hand on the abdomen himself. [pp. 7–8]

RELIABILITY AND VALIDITY

Given these limitations, is there a way to specify how certain we are when making a psychiatric diagnosis? In order to do so, we turn to the two most important elements of any operational classification scheme: reliability and validity. **Reliability** describes *the accuracy of our observational method and of our operational criteria*. In theory, this is a finite task, since if we ultimately could refine our diagnostic criteria to the point that they perfectly distinguished between all of the various psychiatric disorders, we would achieve 100% reliability. In contrast, **validity** describes *the accuracy of our presumptions*—that is, of the theories that we elaborate to explain the consistency (i.e., the reliability) of our observations. Achieving validity requires that we test the accuracy of a theoretical construct in as many different ways as possible (e.g., through psychological, biological, social, or historical methods). In contrast to reliability, validity can never be "100% achieved" or be considered "a given."

Clearly, reliability must come first. If every clinician or investigator used his or her own personal definition of schizophrenia, two clinicians would not be able to communicate about a case in the absence of an extremely detailed case history. Two researchers would not be able to compare the results their studies even if they each were ostensibly studying a series of patients with the diagnosis of schizophrenia. There also would be no way to study the natural course of schizophrenia, to compare it to the course of other psychiatric disorders, to search for biological markers that are not present in control subjects (i.e., people who do not meet the operational criteria for schizophrenia), or to rationally choose a treatment strategy based on what has been successful in treating other patients who carry the same diagnosis.

Granted, absent an understanding of the causes of schizophrenia, to study lists of symptoms or to debate taxonomic distinctions between schizophrenia and bipolar disorder appears a sterile academic exercise. Some have criticized current diagnostic criteria (which we will soon review in detail) for being nothing more than reductionistic "checklists." But how can we ever hope to understand the causes of schizophrenia unless we can assemble a relatively homogeneous group of patients, distinguish this group from another group of patients—the members of which we all can agree do *not* have schizophrenia—and then make comparisons between these groups (e.g., brain morphology, cerebral activity, cerebrospinal fluid content, etc.)?

One famous test of the reliability of psychiatric diagnosis took place in the 1960s after it was observed that the United States had a much larger percentage of patients diagnosed as having schizophrenia than did the United Kingdom while in the United Kingdom there was a much larger percentage of patients with a diagnosis of mood disorder than in the United States. Various theories might explain this difference—for example, differences in culture, in the racial makeup of the two populations, or even in climate (e.g., perhaps more people are depressed in England because it is so rainy there, etc.). A standardized interview was devised and clinicians from both countries interviewed patients from both countries. The dif-

ference in prevalence of illness in the two countries was found to be purely an artifact of international differences in diagnostic standards. At that time, the U.S. definition of schizophrenia was much broader than it is now. It subsumed cases that in Britain were classified as depression, mania, or personality disorder. When researchers from both countries adopted more reliable, standardized operational criteria, the international discrepancies disappeared.

A famous test of the validity of psychiatric diagnosis, the International Pilot Study of Schizophrenia, took place during that same time period. It was conducted by the World Health Organization and examined the diagnostic criteria for schizophrenia that were being used in nine countries: Colombia, Czechoslovakia, Denmark, India, Nigeria, Taiwan, the United Kingdom, the United States, and the U.S.S.R. The last two countries used broader criteria, while the other seven countries had independently developed similar, narrower criteria. As in the U.S.–U.K. study, a standardized, reliable diagnostic interview revealed that there was a group of patients with very similar symptoms in all of the countries. This finding argues for the validity of the diagnosis of schizophrenia itself. In other words, the diagnosis of schizophrenia isn't simply a "cultural label." Rather, schizophrenia occurs in every country studied to date, its symptoms are similar in each of these countries, and it is recognized as being an illness in every country. Again, reliability had to come first, but the establishment of reliable interview methods and diagnostic criteria then allowed for validation of the clinical syndrome.

HISTORY OF OPERATIONAL CRITERIA IN THE UNITED STATES

In the United States, psychiatric classification was first developed in response to a bureaucratic agenda, not a clinical or research agenda. The 1840 U.S. census contained one psychiatric diagnosis: "idiocy/insanity." By 1880, the census included seven diagnostic categories: mania, melancholia, monomania, paresis, dementia, dipsomania, and epilepsy.

In 1917, the American Psychiatric Association (APA) entered the picture. The APA collaborated with the Bureau of the Census to collect statistical data on people in mental hospitals. It still wasn't a clinical endeavor, however. During World War II, there was a need to classify mental disorders in servicemen. It therefore was the U.S. Army that had come up with the list of diagnoses this time. The Veterans Administration then adapted this list for clinical use. The World Health Organization then adapted these criteria when it published its sixth edition of the *International Classification of Diseases (ICD-6)*. This edition of the *ICD* was the first to even include a section on mental disorders. There were 10 categories for psychoses, nine for psychoneuroses, and seven for disorders of character, behavior, and intelligence.

In 1952, the APA adapted the *ICD-6* to create the first edition of the *Diagnostic and Statistical Manual of Mental Disorders (DSM-I)*. While this manual was the first to not only list diagnoses but also to emphasize clinical matters, it was still essentially only a glossary, offering only brief descriptions of each disorder. At the time, Adolph Meyer's "psychobiological" approach (in which mental disorders represented reactions of the personality to psychological, social, and biological factors) was in vogue; thus, every disorder is labeled a "reaction." In 1968, the *DSM-II* was published (mainly because the *ICD-8* was also coming out and the latter contained no definition of disorders), but beyond changing the word "reaction" to "neurosis," little had changed in 16 years.

In contrast, the publication of the *DSM-III* in 1980 was a watershed moment in psychiatry. Like the earlier editions, it was published concomitantly with the *ICD* (in this case the *ICD-9*). However, here the similarities ended. While the earlier editions provided brief, often single-paragraph descriptions of diagnoses, the *DSM-III* offered detailed operational criteria. The approach reflected the influence of a group of U.S. researchers—most notably those at Washington University in Saint Louis—who emphasized the need to develop explicit operational criteria for all of the mental disorders, to test the reliability of the criteria, and then to validate the disorders in multiple realms, including through studies of inheritance, of associated laboratory findings, and of the longitudinal course of illness.

The *DSM-III* also required clinicians to make a "multiaxial assessment" of the patient. In other words, clinicians were expected not only to as-

sign a primary psychiatric diagnosis but also to give consideration "in parallel" to lifelong traits, to comorbid medical problems, to the severity of current life stressors, and to the patient's overall current degree of functional impairment.

The *DSM-III* approach to diagnosis was *algorithmic*. For example, a patient could qualify for a disorder if he had three symptoms from category A, but he could also qualify if he had two symptoms from category B plus one symptom from category C. Some diagnoses were given priority over others. For example, if panic attacks occurred alone, the diagnosis of panic disorder would be made, but if they occurred along with significant symptoms of depression, the diagnosis would be major depression with panic attacks, as depression was considered to be a the broader diagnosis.

DSM-III was deliberately *atheoretical*. Diagnoses as disparate as nicotine dependence, sexual dysfunction, personality problems, schizophrenia, and delirious states were all referred to simply as "disorders." This is a key point: many clinicians and (also many attorneys) have assumed that simply because a condition is labeled a "disorder" and is treated by psychiatrists, it must be a "mental illness" or a "mental disease." However, this is not the case. Whether a "disorder" is a disease or simply a social construct is a question that goes to the *validity* of the diagnosis. The goal in *DSM-III* was simply to achieve a greater degree of *reliability*. The criteria presented were designed to promote further research, which in turn might better inform future decisions as to whether to modify (or even to eliminate) a disorder from subsequent editions of the manual.

That is just what occurred. In the years following the publication of *DSM-III*, research into all aspects of psychiatric disorders, including phenomenology, epidemiology, and pathophysiology, increased exponentially. In 1987, the APA issued a revised edition (*DSM-IIIR*) in response to concerns that some of the *DSM-III* criteria were ambiguous or inconsistent. Even at this point, a mere 7 years after the publication of *DSM-III*, there were plans for an even more substantial reassessment of the current criteria.

In 1994, the APA published *DSM-IV*. By then, a sizable empirical literature on the *DSM-III* criteria was available for most of the listed disorders. Committees of experts in each area were formed to review this literature and to determine if the current diagnostic criteria should be changed, if any disorders should be eliminated, and if any new disorders should be formally recognized. When an issue could be not be resolved through review of the published literature, unpublished data from researchers in that area were subjected to reanalysis to answer specific questions posed by the committee. In some cases, clinical field trials were conducted where alternative diagnostic criteria were used on the same patients to determine their relative sensitivity and specificity.

As could be expected, some compromises were necessary. While each committee's primary goal was to enhance the reliability and validity of psychiatric diagnostic criteria, thereby advancing the cause of psychiatric research, they also had to be mindful of clinicians who would be forced to utilize these criteria in their daily medical practice. Given this, traditional terminology and definitions were retained whenever possible, and criteria were kept as "streamlined" as possible. (For example, the *DSM-III* diagnostic criteria for somatization disorder required that 14 of 37 possible somatic complaints be present, but what good is this definition if clinicians can't remember all of the symptoms? In contrast, the *DSM-IV* criteria requires that patients have symptoms falling into four primary categories.) A final goal was to ensure compatibility with criteria published by the World Health Organization concomitantly in the *ICD-10*.

In an effort to balance the competing goals of keeping the *DSM* up to date and avoiding unnecessary overhauls in well-developed diagnostic criteria, the APA published the *DSM-IV Text Revision (DSM-IV-TR)* in 2000. This time around, text sections (e.g., prevalence, associated features, differential diagnosis) were updated to reflect research conducted since 1992, but no substantive changes in the criteria sets were considered. It is inevitable, though, that within the next decade clinicians will reference the diagnostic criteria from *DSM-V*.

FORM AND FUNCTION: CONCEPTUAL AMBIGUITY

Their unique focus on mental life forces psychiatrists to confront conceptual ambiguities not faced by other medical specialists. McHugh and

Slavney (1998) note that we do not begin the study of cardiology by asking, "What do cardiologists treat?" The answer is obvious. Cardiologists treat disorders of the cardiovascular system. Further, in the case of cardiology, the relationship between form and function is clear. What is the function of the heart? It is a pump. What is the form of the heart? Structurally, it has four chambers. The chambers contract, thereby forcing blood through one-way valves. Shifting our attention to the cellular level, form elucidates function even further. The cardiac chambers are comprised of myocardial muscle fibers, and these, too, contract when triggered. Zooming in further, even at the subcellular level form continues to elucidate function. The muscle fibers are composed of sarcomeres, they in turn are composed of interdigitating myofilaments that slide against each other when stimulated, and these in turn are composed of actin and myosin proteins. Even the chemical cascades that moderate and power the contractile process have been amenable to extensive study.

Unfortunately, in the study of mental life, a similar continuity between structure (brain) and function (mind) does not exist. This remains the case whether we try to "work our way up" from brain to mind or "work our way down" from mind to brain. For example, what are the functions of the human mind? They are many and varied. They include perceiving the world around us, experiencing emotions, experiencing appetites or drives, forming opinions, remembering the past, planning for the future, and communicating through language. Obviously, there is no mind without brain. However, regardless of whether we treat the mind as a mere epiphenomenon of brain activity (*materialism*) or cling to the Cartesian belief that mind and brain coexist "side by side" in some way (*dualism*), the precise nature of the relationship between mind and brain remains unclear. And despite major advances in the field of neuroscience, there remains no explanation for the most fundamental feature of mind—self-consciousness. In the words of McHugh and Slavney (1998):

For more than a century, clinicians have been able to *correlate* the occurrence of certain mental disorders, such as aphasia (the disruption of language capacity), with injury to particular parts of brain. This is helpful information, as it guides clinicians in understanding where damage in the brain may produce certain mental symptoms. . . . Even though they know that certain language impairments are associated with, emerge along with, and correlate in severity with injury to the temporal lobe, clinicians still are not able to explain how neural activity within this brain region produces our conscious sense of choosing our words and directing our conversations. . . . To put it in simple terms: correlation is not explanation. The mind is an experience; the brain is a physical structure. They are *not* identical. How the actions of brain elements evoke the personal experience of mental life and the intimate feelings of "minding" itself (grasped in such expressions as "myself," "my ideas," "my wishes," and especially "my choices") does not emerge from even the most advanced neuroscience. [p. 13]

This "gap" at the level of the mind–brain junction is of more than academic concern. For example, some critics have charged that psychiatrists seek merely to maintain the existing social order by labeling any individual differences as signs of pathology. Thomas Szasz (1970) goes so far as to state that the very construct "mental illness" is a myth:

In our scientific theories of behavior we have failed to accept the simple fact that human relations are inherently fraught with difficulties, and to make them even relatively harmonious requires much patience and hard work. I submit that the idea of mental illness is now being put to work to obscure certain difficulties that at present may be inherent—not that they need to be unmodifiable—in the social intercourse of persons. If this is true, the concept functions as a disguise: instead of calling attention to conflicting human needs, aspirations, and values, the concept of mental illness provides an amoral and impersonal "thing"—an "illness"—as an explanation for problems in living . . . The belief in mental illness, as something other than man's trouble in getting along with his fellow man, is the proper heir to the belief in demonology and witchcraft. [p. 20]

This so-called "antipsychiatry" approach is misguided. It postulates—simply because "mental illness" *can* be empathically understood using the language of mind (e.g., "conflicting human needs, aspirations, and values")—that we *should* reject any theories of mental illness that attribute symptoms of mental illness to abnormal brain activity. Rather than squarely address the conceptual ambiguity inherent in the mind–brain disjunction, it picks one side and then summarily rejects the other. Nonetheless, this "brainless"

conception has had great popular appeal and even appears to reflect the opinion of most members of the general public. For example, a recent survey revealed that 71% of the U.S. population thinks that mental illness is due to emotional weakness, 65% thinks it is caused by bad parenting, 45% believes that it is the victim's fault and that the victim can "will it away," 43% believes that mental illness is incurable, and 35% thinks that it is a consequence of "sinful behavior." Only 10% of the population believes that mental illness has a biological basis or involves the brain.

The diagnosis of major depressive disorder offers a dramatic case in point. Major depressive disorder affects more than 11 million Americans yearly and costs the economy about $44 billion per year in absenteeism, lost productivity and lifetime earnings, and health care. (This exceeds the estimated cost of other medical problems such as arthritis and hypertension.) Depressed patients experience as much or more limitation in their daily functioning and well-being as patients with diabetes, arthritis, gastrointestinal disorders, back problems, and hypertension. Up to 15% of people with major depressive disorder die by suicide. Unfortunately, while 80%–90% of individuals with depression can be successfully treated, only one-third of them seek treatment, and a recent survey by the National Mental Health Association found that most Americans know little about depression and that they typically see depression as a reflection of character weakness.

Similarly, physicians may fail to appreciate the presentation and associated morbidity of clinical depression. In the primary care setting, depression is routinely undiagnosed, untreated, or undertreated. Of 100 depressed patients who present in the primary care setting, only about 30 of them will be diagnosed. Of those 30 patients, only about 10 will be treated, and only about half of these 10 patients will comply with the prescribed course of treatment—that is, 5 of the original 100 patients.

Why do patients and even well-intentioned physicians miss the diagnosis? Dichotomous "mind–brain" thinking appears to play a major role. For example, if a patient presents to her primary care physician in the setting of some major life problems (such as significant medical illness or recent loss of a spouse), both the patient and the physician might find it readily "understandable" that the patient would feel sad. After all, who wouldn't feel sad under similar circumstances? Because the depressive symptoms can be "understood" empathically, an attempt is not made to "explain" them medically. Family members may fall into this same trap. Consider the following example:

A 69-year-old female nursing home resident is referred for psychiatric consultation by the nursing staff due after she makes several statements that she would like to kill herself. Two months before, she suffered a left frontal stroke, which left her with residual right-sided weakness and expressive aphasia. She initially appeared to be coping well. However, over the last 2 weeks she has become much more "anxious." She is sleeping about 2 hours per night, is eating poorly, and is no longer cooperating with her physical therapy regimen. Currently, she only takes her medications after great encouragement from the nursing staff and her family, and she says that she sees no point in taking her medications. She would rather that people, "Leave me to die." Her internist, noting her significant anxiety, initiated treatment with lorazepam (a benzodiazepine agent with anxiolytic but not antidepressant effects), which did lead to some improvement in her feelings of anxiety. Unfortunately, she now appears to be more sedated and she also has remained depressed and suicidal.

The patient's family describes the patient as having been strong-willed and independent throughout her life. They feel that, given this, the patient's current depressed and anxious state is an understandable psychological reaction to her new physical disability. The family is initially resistant to the idea of the psychiatrist prescribing an antidepressant medication. Her daughter asks, "Hasn't my mother already been through enough?"

The psychiatrist points out to her that the patient has all of the classic symptoms of major depressive disorder and that such depressions occur in the months following a stroke in up to 50% of patients. While the depressive symptoms often respond within several weeks to antidepressant therapy, if left untreated the symptoms might persist for over a year. Further, the degree of depression has been found to correspond more to stroke location than it does to the degree of physical impairment caused by the stroke, suggesting that the depression isn't solely a "psychological reaction" to stroke-related physical disability. The psychiatrist notes that lesions in the left frontal area have been particularly

associated with the development of poststroke depressive symptoms. Following this discussion, the patient and her daughter both consent to antidepressant treatment. Three weeks later, the patient's mood begins to improve, as does her intake of food and her cooperation with her physical rehabilitation program. She denies feeling suicidal and even says that she has "always been a fighter and I'm going to fight this, too." While she misses working in her garden and still reports feeling demoralized about having to be in a nursing home, as her acute depressive symptoms remit she gains the ability to engage in supportive psychotherapy aimed at helping her to cope with this transition.

As the above case demonstrates, in diagnosing a patient as having a mental illness, certain aspects of the patient's mental state are delineated as being abnormal in form and are then treated as symptoms of a disorder and not simply variations of ordinary human experience. In this case, the psychiatrist attempted to distinguish a major depressive episode from more common sadness in the face of painful life circumstances. In other cases, psychiatrists attempt to distinguish the clinical syndrome of dementia from ordinary forgetfulness or attempt to distinguish symptoms of generalized anxiety disorder from ordinary fear and apprehension.

Can psychiatrists accurately do this, or is "mental life" so nebulous a concept that it doesn't lend itself to such rigorous scientific scrutiny? One way of addressing this question would be to attempt to achieve greater scientific rigor by rejecting the notion of mental life outright. The "radical behaviorism" movement, exemplified by the psychologist B.F. Skinner, attempted to do this by postulating that since one can't actually observe "thoughts" or "feelings" one shouldn't presuppose that they even exist. All we can say with any certainty is that we are observing certain *behaviors*.

Skinner said he believed that the differences between any two individuals merely reflect their unique histories of selective behavioral reinforcement. In *About Behaviorism*, Skinner opined: "A self or personality is at best a repertoire of behavior imparted by an organized set of contingencies. The behavior a young person acquires in the bosom of his family composes one self; the behavior he acquires in, say, the armed services composes another." Given this, the construct "mental life" is chimerical, an artifact of our cultural tendency to take adverbs that describe certain types of behaviors and to replace them with nouns based on unfounded assumptions about what lies behind the behaviors. For example, if somebody acts "jealously," we infer the presence of an underlying "emotion" called "jealousy"; if someone acts "intelligently," we infer that they have "intelligence," and so on.

Currently, most behavioral scientists believe that the radical behaviorist approach is unnecessarily reductionistic and overly doctrinaire. It denies to us insights provided by other areas of study such as neurophysiology, genetics, personality theory, and psychoanalytic theory. For example, consider the two cases described above involving the college student and the elderly nursing home resident. In just a few sentences, we described their background and their current life circumstances, and in doing so, we immediately gained an empathic "sense" of their current desires, frustrations, and emotions. In contrast, we would be hard-pressed to achieve similar insight into their circumstances through the construction of a detailed list of observed sequential behaviors. While behavioral reinforcement of certain behaviors over others is clearly important (and is emphasized throughout this text), clinicians and researchers have found that thoughts and emotions *can* be studied. The remainder of this text will describe how this can be done in a scientifically valid way.

Interestingly, the appeal of radical behaviorism parallels the appeal of "antipsychiatry." Each approach avoids having to deal in a dialectical way with the fundamental discontinuity between mind and brain by simply declaring that mental life can be completely explained from one side of the chasm—that everything on the other side of the chasm is unimportant, irrelevant, or mistaken. The *DSM-IV* doesn't resolve these issues. In attempting to describe psychiatric disorders while avoiding endorsing any specific theories of causation, it also must remain silent about how to best treat these disorders.

In contrast, any truly comprehensive model of mental illness would have to be a synthetic one, incorporating data from a wide range of fields (such as sociology, biology, and psychology). In the absence of such a model, a wide variety of "schools" has evolved, each embracing its own theories, often while denigrating "competing" schools of thought. Therefore, the patient who seeks treatment for a mental disorder typically is forced to mull over whether to seek treatment from a psychiatrist, a clinical psychologist, a clinical social worker, or a licensed practical counselor, each of whom has received a greater or lesser degree of training in different specific theoretical approaches.

Further, even when speaking with a practitioner from one particular field—for example, psychiatry—the patient might begin the interview by inquiring into the psychiatrist's "orientation." Is the psychiatrist more "biological" or "psychological"? Even if the psychiatrist is more "psychological," the patient might wonder about the clinician's "school of therapy" (e.g., "psychoanalytic "cognitive," "existential," or one of the literally hundreds of other approaches to talk therapy).

One shudders to imagine encountering such a diversity of theoretical and treatment approaches in other fields of medicine—for example, when seeking treatment for congestive heart failure. The presence of such diversity in itself raises fundamental questions. Is one form of treatment "just as good" as any of the others? Are certain forms of treatment better only for some types of psychiatric disorder but not for others? Shouldn't the choice of treatment for a disorder be determined by what works best rather than by the patient's preference (for "drugs" versus "therapy") or by the theoretical orientation of the treatment provider?

However, within this host of theoretical approaches, two major ones can be discerned. Some approaches attempt to categorize certain mental phenomena as being abnormal in *form* and therefore in need of explanation, most commonly a biological explanation. Other approaches view all mental phenomena, whether "normal" or "abnormal" as being a *function*, or reflection, of certain underlying psychological processes. For example, they might reflect a conflict between certain conscious or unconscious beliefs. The major differences between these two approaches are highlighted in Table 1–1.

FORM AND FUNCTION CONTRASTED

The *form* of any particular mental experience can be delineated from the form of other mental experiences, and we can then judge whether that

Table 1–1. Approaches from Form and from Function Contrasted

Form	Function
Emphasizes brain	Emphasizes mind
Goal is scientific explanation	Goal is empathic understanding
Views patients as objects/organisms	Views patients as subjects/agents
Views patient "from outside"	Views patient "from inside"
Seeks causal connections	Seeks meaningful connections
Asks "What?" (i.e., what is the patient thinking, feeling, and doing?)	Asks "Why?" (i.e., why is the patient thinking, feeling, and behaving this way?)

Source: Adapted from material in McHugh PR, Slavney PR: *The Perspectives of Psychiatry*. Baltimore, Johns Hopkins University Press, 1986.

experience is "normal" or "abnormal" based on its phenomenological features (such as its characteristics, its frequency, or its association with other mental events).

For example, consider our second vignette, involving the college student who presented to the emergency room with what appeared to hallucinations and delusions. We could describe his hallucinations in more detail, noting that they appeared solely in the auditory realm rather than in any of the other four sensory modalities. We could also observe that his hallucinations were of voices that addressed him indirectly, commenting about him in the third person ("he") as opposed to directly addressing him in the second person ("you"). Similarly, in examining this patient's delusions, we could note that his delusions involved only persecutory themes, as opposed to somatic, grandiose, nihilistic, or jealous themes. His overall appearance also might be deemed relevant. For example, his facial expression was blunted, and at times inappropriate to the content of his speech. Also, the form of his speech was rambling and at times one thought didn't logically connect with the thought that preceded it. (We obviously have to use care in deciding whether his facial expression and speech were so different from normal that they should be considered a symptom of some underlying disease rather than simply a reflect of individual or cultural diversity. In more subtle cases, two different examiners might disagree. Such disagreement is rare in severe cases).

From the paradigm of "form," we view patients as biological organisms affected by particular types of illness with particular presentations. Our primary goal is to describe these illnesses and to describe how patients with the same illnesses resemble each other. Our goal is not to describe patients as unique individuals and how they differ from each other. The language used in written or verbal presentations of "psychiatric" patients' case histories therefore parallels the language used in "medical" case histories. While patients' subjective experiences clearly are relevant, they remain in the background, not in the foreground. Mostly, we view patients "from the outside" rather than "from the inside." For example, we might empathize with the patient who is currently having a heart attack, but we wouldn't suggest that this empathic understanding *explains* either his coronary artery disease or how he came to have these diseases. Nor would we suggest to the patient that helping him to understand how he is thinking or feeling should be the cornerstone of his treatment.

In contrast, from the perspective of *function*, this is precisely what we would be suggesting. Analogies between the mind and hearts can only be taken so far. For example, I *choose* whether or not to go to work each morning; I cannot choose to stop my heart from beating. People are not simply objects that sometimes break down and need to be repaired, like broken cars. Cars can't fix themselves—people often can. Our entire society—our laws, our social institutions, our interpersonal relationships—are premised on the notion that peoples' behavior is intentional and volitional. From the perspective of function, patients are viewed as subjects or agents, endowed with free will, with the capacity to get angry, to plan, to make decisions, to fall in love. The focus of this perspective is the empathic exploration of patients' mental experiences in order to better understand, "from within," why they have chosen to act the way that they do. In doing so, we hope to understand the *purpose or significance* of patients' symptoms. Sometimes, this requires us to postulate that their significance is unconscious or symbolic.

From this perspective, when we present a clinical case history, we are telling the story not of a disease but of a unique person (sometimes a person who happens to have a disease). The power of this model is self-evident. In our first vignette involving the college student who attempted suicide after facing significant failures for the first time both academically and romantically, the reasons for his despondency are clear. Were you interviewing him yourself in the emergency room, as the details spilled forth you might find yourself saying, "Well *now* I see why he's so depressed," or, "Of *course* he's depressed," or, "I myself would probably be depressed if I were in that situation."

Even after we modified our vignette such that the patient now presented with "pathological" symptoms (hallucinations, delusions, very disorganized thinking), we might try to empathically understand his behavior. We might interpret his psychotic symptoms as reflections of maladaptive coping strategies, of his using unconscious "defenses" against having to deal with emotions that are unacceptable to him. For example, according to classical Freudian psychoanalytic theory, patients with schizophrenia, being unable to deal with an unpleasant external reality, retreat ("regress") to an earlier developmental level. When they also can't accept various internal fantasies or impulses, they project these fantasies onto people in the outside world. As a result, they end up with difficulty being able to distinguish anymore between what is internal fantasy and what is external reality. For example, a patient with schizophrenia who can't accept that he is angry with his parents and that he has fears that he might hurt them ultimately might come to believe that it is "the other way around," that it is his parents who are angry with *him* and who even are conspiring to murder him.

Note how, when we are using the approach from form, we typically use passive verbs to describe the patient's experiences (for example, the patient "experiences" hallucinations or delusions). In contrast, when using the approach from function, we use active verbs (patients with

schizophrenia "regress to earlier developmental levels," "retreat from reality," or "project their internal conflicts onto other people"). This reflects how under the former approach emphasis is on the schizophrenia, which is seen as *causing* patients to have certain experiences, while under the latter approach the patients are seen as taking active roles, as *doing* things that account for their symptoms (even if they are doing these things unconsciously).

It would be a simple matter to view cases like the first vignette from the perspective of function and cases like the second one from the perspective of form. The rule of thumb might be, "If I can empathize with why the patient feels so bad, I'll view his symptoms as understandable expressions of a person in distress, but if he has more severe symptoms (for example, severe depressive symptoms or psychotic symptoms), I'll treat his symptoms as expressions of an underlying pathology." Perhaps we might refer the former group of patients for psychotherapy and refer the latter group of patients for pharmacotherapy. This strategy would clearly be inappropriate and misguided.

First, many conditions that appear to reflect biological illnesses can present with less severe symptoms. For example, there are patients who present with a chronic but less-severe form of clinical depression called dysthymic disorder. Should we use the approach from function and attempt to explore the psychological roots of their low self-esteem in an effort to help them to take responsibility for their feelings and to address underlying conflicts? Or should we use the approach from form, diagnosing them as "having" an illness, the result of a "chemical imbalance of the brain" for which they are not responsible and for which an antidepressant medication might be the most appropriate treatment?

Any patient, with any disorder, can be viewed from the vantage points of either form or function, from "within" or from "outside." Divvying up diagnoses between these two vantage points makes no more sense than always photographing some people from one angle and other people from a different angle. For example, in the case of our second vignette, the student presented with hallucinations, delusions, and disorganized thinking. From the vantage point of form, it is the *presence* of these abnormal experiences that allows us to "make the diagnosis" of schizophrenia. However, the *content* of our student's delusions can best be understood from the vantage point of function. For example, why does he call his girlfriend "the queen" and speaking of "paradigm shifts"? These references likely reflect not only the books that he has been reading (Machiavelli and Thomas Kuhn), but also his feelings of helplessness and inadequacy (feeling like "a pawn") compared to the girlfriend who broke off their relationship. Delusions obviously have to be about *something*, and each person who hallucinates hears *particular* voices or sees *particular* things.

Even psychoanalytic theorists have largely adopted such an approach, at least for patients with schizophrenia. While early psychoanalysts postulated that the cause of schizophrenic patients' "retreat from reality" was faulty mothering, leading to patients never gaining the capacity for trust, modern theorists usually do accept the research suggesting that underlying biological deficits in schizophrenia cause patients to inadequately "filter" external and internal stimuli, leading to the development of hallucinations and delusions. These theorists continue to emphasize, however, that interpretation of the content of patients' psychotic symptoms should play some role in their clinical treatment.

Second, many psychiatric disorders—alcoholism, for example—are characterized by patients engaging in some type of driven behavior that is considered to be excessive or aberrant. Patients with these disorders typically experience powerful cravings, cravings that often are influenced by biological factors. However, these patients also *choose* to engage in these behaviors. Given this, we can't simply assign such patients to one category or the other. For example, should society treat alcoholism as an "illness" that these individuals "have," that is beyond their ability to control? Or should we hold individuals who excessively consume alcohol fully accountable for their behavior, arresting them when they drink in public or when they drive while intoxicated? And if we do choose to arrest them, do we feel that the court should immediately divert them into treatment programs or do we feel that they are deserving of punishment? The ambivalence, the discomfort, that we tend to feel in contemplating

these issues relates directly to the conceptual ambiguity between form and function. Are these individuals passive objects or autonomous agents? Clearly they are both. For example, even if we adhere to the philosophy that addicted individuals will only be able to stop using alcohol or drugs when they acquire the genuine desire to quit, this should not prevent us from prescribing them medications designed to ease their biological cravings.

We all have minds as well as brains, and therefore mental life is something to be *both* understood and explained. In the absence of a synthetic model, clinicians must resist the temptation to engage in "mindless" biological determinism or "brainless" psychological interpretation.

In the wake of battles between "biological psychiatrists" and "psychotherapists," many commentators have advocated the "biopsychosocial" model described by George Engel. This model views all illnesses (including mental illnesses) as resulting from a wide variety of influences, which themselves fall along a hierarchy of natural systems, starting with "subatomic particles" at one end and "the biosphere" at the other. In between these two poles are atoms, molecules, organelles, cells, tissues, organ systems, the nervous system, the person, two persons, family, community, culture, and society. By placing "the person" right in the center, Engel emphasized how any theory of illness must include "psychological" factors (located within the person), "biological" factors (located "below" the person), and "social" factors (located "above" the person).

However, proposing that there is a "continuum" between biology, psychology, and sociology does not make it so. This model does not offer a synthetic theory of mental life in that it doesn't resolve the inherent tensions that exist between these different conceptual approaches. For example, placing "the nervous system" adjacent to "the person" with arrows pointing from one to the other hardly bridges the gap between mind and body.

More importantly, the biopsychosocial model doesn't offer guidance to the practicing clinician beyond suggesting that he "avoid reductionism" and "consider everything." When the distinctions are blurred between empirical, descriptive *observations* and psychological *interpretations*, or between *diseases* and *choices*, clinical formulations lose conceptual clarity. As a result, many clinicians in practice continue to emphasize one conceptual model over the other despite their avowals that they are "biopsychosocial" or (even worse) "eclectic" in orientation.

One goal of this text is to help the reader learn to formulate cases from the vantage points of *both* form and function, not by attempting to synthesize them "holistically," but by teaching the reader to *alternate* between them, while remaining mindful of the advantages and disadvantages of each approach. In this way, the reader can achieve a more comprehensive view of the patient.

Beginning students of psychiatry at this point likely are wondering, "Where is this all going? And what's with all the philosophical, theoretical, mumbo jumbo in the first chapter? Let's just get started already! In any case, will this be on the board exams?" To these students, my only response is the following: be patient, trust me, and quit whining.

Better yet, try the following experiment: Find a mental health clinician (psychiatrist, psychologist, social worker, etc.). Next, ask the clinician what his or her "orientation" is. Was the answer "eclectic"? Next, ask that clinician, "What do you mean by 'eclectic'?" Perhaps the answer was a mumbled, "A little of this, a little of that, it depends on the patient, it depends on the particular illness. . . . " Finally, ask the clinician if you can observe an actual patient interview and then discuss the clinician's diagnostic formulation. Does the clinician consider the patient's problems to reflect autonomous choices made by the patient, symptoms of an illness beyond the patient's control, or both? Or is this issue conveniently ignored? Finally, when the clinician makes such distinctions, is it based on scientific evidence, or is it in fact personal opinion (conservative or liberal attitudes) disguised as clinical judgment? These are hard questions, but they arise in every clinical encounter once you are attuned to them. The natural tendency for clinicians is to shrug such questions off, to move on to the next patient, to do what we feel most comfortable doing based on training and personal preference. But that approach is not "eclectic," and it's not "pragmatic." It's just intellectually lazy.

We can do better. Let us move on to considering what is gained and what is lost when we view patients from one or the other approach.

ADVANTAGES AND DISADVANTAGES OF REASONING FROM FORM

The first goal in reasoning from form is to observe the patient so that we can discern *what* the diagnosis is. The second goal is to explain how this diagnosis came to be present. In doing so, we attempt to distinguish which clinical variables are independent and which are dependent. Finally, we generate *testable hypotheses* and design studies aimed at testing the validity of these hypotheses. The "scientific method" is another way of describing the approach from form, and the remarkable achievements of modern Western medicine attest to its value.

The advantages of this approach are clear. First, our hypotheses are amenable to public testing. For example, we can make predictions about prognosis. If we suspect that, in our first clinical vignette, the student who feels suicidal because his girlfriend left him has a dependent personality disorder, that his personality reveals a tendency to feel helpless and suicidal whenever he is rejected, we might expect that if we followed up with this patient longitudinally over time we would see a similar pattern of similar episodes in situations where he feels abandoned. It's possible, however, that he might learn from these experiences and demonstrate improved coping skills over the course of time. In contrast, we might expect the student from our second vignette (the student that we diagnosed as having schizophrenia) to demonstrate a longitudinal course consistent with chronic, severe mental illness characterized by repeated hospitalizations and a failure to return to his premorbid level of functioning.

If our hypotheses ultimately turned out to be wrong, we simply would modify our hypotheses appropriately. For example, what if it turns out that *some* patients with schizophrenia *do* recover over time, rather than demonstrating a progressive decline in functioning? We would have to ask ourselves, why do these particular patients differ from other patients with schizophrenia who deteriorate? Similarly, what if some patients initially diagnosed with a "personality disorder" turned out to benefit from treatment with anti-depressant medications? Does this mean that they were "actually depressed," or might the neurotransmitters that these medications act upon also play a role in what we call "personality"? These in fact are questions that psychiatric researchers are currently asking, as we will see in subsequent chapters.

However, the *disadvantages* of reasoning from form are reflected in the disenchantment expressed by many patients (and many psychiatrists) toward the *DSM-IV*. With each progressive edition, the number of diagnostic entities has multiplied. While *DSM-I* had 132 pages and 106 categories, *DSM-IIIR* had 567 pages and 292 categories. The modern *DSM* favors "splitting" over "lumping" of mental phenomena. For example, a patient may be discharged from the hospital diagnosed with major depression, dysthymic disorder, bulimia nervosa, alcohol dependence, alcohol withdrawal, post-traumatic stress disorder, and borderline personality disorder. This seems like a lot of diagnoses for any one person to have, but such patients are commonly encountered.

In addition, scientific findings are often of limited generalizability and true advances made only slowly. This can be frustrating to clinicians who need to treat patients sitting in their office. Freud began his career as a neurologist and neuropathologist but found the science of his day inadequate to explain his patient's difficulties, and he shifted to a school of thought dominated by reasoning from function. This allowed him to offer more specific treatment recommendations.

In reasoning from form, there is a tendency toward doctrinaire reductionism. For example depressed patients are depressed because they "have a depression." Further, the treatment for depression is "antidepressant treatment." Not surprisingly, most patients currently admitted to psychiatric hospitals are prescribed a pharmacologic treatment within the first 24 hours, often after a cursory interview aimed at eliciting symptoms that might readily respond to medication. Pharmaceutical companies expend enormous sums of money each year attempting to persuade physicians to inquire about certain symptoms and to use their products if these symptoms are elicited. Many psychiatrists see four patients per hour for "medication management" visits, with

insurance plans or managed care organizations discouraging them from engaging the patient in psychotherapy. Of course, this problem is not unique to psychiatry. The modern medical marketplace requires that the clinician rapidly "make a diagnosis," prescribe the "indicated treatment," and move on to the next patient. Reasoning from form is not solely responsible for this state of affairs, but it provides a congenial means of perpetuating it. While physicians are trained as medical students to ask open-ended questions and to inquire into patients' personal backgrounds, when the ship is at risk of sinking, these are the first pieces of ballast to be cast overboard.

Finally, many patients resent being viewed as objects rather than as subjects. Many patients seen by psychiatrists are not mentally ill. They seek help because, for them, life is a predicament and they can't figure out why that is so. Certainly, using an analysis of form, they could be diagnosed as having an "adjustment disorder." (This condition is characterized by "difficulty adjusting to life circumstances.") However, an analysis from form has little else to offer. Even patients with psychotic illness—who stand to benefit the most from approach from form—often resent it. Psychiatric clinicians don't treat schizophrenia; they treat *patients* afflicted with schizophrenia. Psychiatrists who don't attend to this distinction tend to find themselves faced with patients who are "noncompliant" with treatment.

ADVANTAGES AND DISADVANTAGES OF REASONING FROM FUNCTION

Patients often derive great benefit from psychotherapy. While different schools of therapy emphasize different aspects of human experience, they all have a similar goal. They seek to give the patient an appreciation of his or her past and of the possibility of having a choice about the future. In the words of McHugh and Slavney (1986):

Psychotherapy thus functions on a very different level from physical treatments in psychiatry, which do not demand for their effectiveness that the patient reformulate his self-concept and life plans. Successful psychotherapy brings to patients a sense of mastery, personal accomplishment, and growth, which springs directly from the nature and intentions of the method itself. The patient and the physician share an achievement and a satisfaction that are special in medicine, for the enterprise is theirs and is built on communication and understanding. [p. 21]

But there also are disadvantages to this approach. Consider our vignette about the elderly woman is experiencing symptoms of major depressive disorder following a stroke. Were we to attempt to understand her suffering solely through interpretation, at the expense of recognizing that she is experiencing a pathologic disease state, we might not be able to treat her as effectively. More generally, when we view each patient only as a unique individual with a unique story we deny psychiatric patients the benefit of knowledge derived in other ways.

Also, in the approach from function, as less emphasis is placed on distinguishing various characteristics of the mental events themselves, there can be a blurring of diagnostic distinctions. While devotees of form tend to be "splitters," devotees of function are "lumpers." For example, whether a person has obsessive-compulsive disorder or an obsessive-compulsive personality disorder appears less relevant. However, these are different disorders with different treatment implications when analyzed in terms of their form. Similarly, rather than recognizing a patient as having a clinical depression *and* alcohol dependence that need be addressed separately, a therapist may see it as all "being part of the same underlying pathology" and in doing so may fail to address either condition effectively.

In the approach from function, theories may be advanced based on one or two case studies rather than based on having collected a large sample of patients and a control group. Even worse, generalizations may be made about the human condition in general based on experience with a relatively small group of self-selected clinic patients from a circumscribed geographic local. At it's worst, the approach from function can be as psychologically reductive as the approach from form is biologically reductive. Instead of all mental experiences being reduced to an imbalance of serotonin neurotransmission, in this case, "it's all sexual."

Another problem is that hypotheses cannot be proved or disproved. Imagine that a man presents because he repeatedly argues with his wife. Based on the patient's recollections of his relationship with his mother, the therapist suggests that the patient has unresolved sexual attractions to his mother and married a woman who resembled his mother for this reason. As these attractions are unacceptable to him, he takes any opportunity to insult his wife and picks fights over any minor matter. If the patient agrees with this interpretation, it is seen as being correct. If the patient becomes angry and disagrees with the interpretation, he might be seen as being in denial. If the patient denies any recall of ever having been sexually attracted to his mother, the attraction can still be there, at the level of the unconscious.

In addition, in the absence of testable hypotheses, there is no way to settle theoretical disputes between competing schools of therapy. Each school sees the others as "missing the boat," as having focused their attention on the "wrong" aspects of mental life. Many therapists, considering themselves to be of a certain "orientation" (such as psychodynamic, cognitive-behavioral, existential, or trauma-based), attend conferences only aimed at members of their own school, thereby discouraging cross-fertilization. The type of therapy a patient walking through the clinic door receives may have more to do with where and with whom a particular therapist trained than with the patient's particular clinical presentation.

SUMMARY

Psychiatry is the field of medicine that deals with complaints arising out of mental life. Psychiatrists' focus on mental events forces them to confront conceptual ambiguities that are less prominent in other branches of medicine. These difficulties directly relate to the chasm between mind and body.

In spite of these inherent limitations, mental life can be studied with a reasonable degree of reliability. Doing so requires that we adopt the method of clinical phenomenology, adopting specific operational criteria for phenomena such as perceptions (e.g., normal perceptions versus hallucinations), beliefs (e.g., normal beliefs versus delusions), various mood states (e.g., normal sadness versus clinical depression), and various behavior patterns (e.g., normal alcohol consumption versus alcohol dependence).

Patients are both biological organisms and unique agents who act in purposeful ways. These two fundamental aspects of mental life, form and function, comprise a dialectic. Theories proposing to integrate form and function have promised more than they could deliver, and clinicians therefore have tended to emphasize either one or the other aspect of mental life, sometimes to the detriment of their patients.

In the absence of a "unified field theory," psychiatric clinicians must learn to shift back and forth between these two conceptual models, remaining cognizant of the strengths and limitations of each model as they do so. The practical implications of using this approach will be emphasized throughout this text.

Chapter 2

The Psychiatric Evaluation

In taking the psychiatric history and performing the mental status examination, the goal of eliciting the key data necessary to generate a differential diagnosis must be balanced against the goal of establishing some rapport and an initial alliance with the patient, who may be quite distressed at the time. Sometimes the clinician has to take a step backward from one goal in order to step forward toward the other, especially in the case of patients who are cognitively impaired, agitated, or suspicious. A third goal is to achieve the first two goals in a timely manner. The less time that is available for the interview, the more structured and directive the interview must be. An evaluation in the emergency room setting may take 30–60 minutes, while a more comprehensive outpatient evaluation may last for over 90 minutes. Here is one version of the history and mental status examination. Where possible, I have indicated the *minimum requirements* for those situations where a briefer assessment is appropriate. The major sections of the psychiatric history are listed in Table 2–1, while the major elements of the psychiatric mental status examination are listed in Table 2–2. Following discussion of the history and mental status examination, we will discuss the physical examination and the use ancillary services such as psychological testing and clinical laboratory assessment.

THE PSYCHIATRIC HISTORY

Identification and Chief Complaint

The identification of the patient typically includes name, age, marital status, race, gender, occupation, and the concerns that precipitated the current evaluation. For example, "John Smith is a 32-year-old married, Caucasian male roofer with a history of alcohol dependence, who presents today requesting a referral for detoxification following a week-long drinking binge." Some clinicians prefer to record the patient's verbatim statement as to why he is here. This sometimes offers insight into the patient's current attitudes and expectations. For example: "My parents brought me in because they are worried that I want to hurt myself. I took some pills this morning, but I'm fine."

Informants

In the outpatient setting, the patient typically is the sole informant. However, in the emergency room or inpatient setting, information provided by collateral informants often proves to be invaluable and well worth the expenditure of extra effort. The clinician's degree of confidence in the accuracy of her final diagnostic impression hinges on her confidence in the reliability of her clinical data. Unfortunately, some patients are not reliable historians.

Table 2–1. Elements of the Psychiatric History

Identification and chief complaint
Informants
Present illness
Psychiatric history
Premorbid personality
Medical history, medications, drug allergies
Social history
   Birth
   Early development
   Education
   Occupational history
   Sexual marital history
   Children
   Current living situation
   Legal history
   Alcohol/substance history
Family history

Most commonly, patients are not deliberately attempting to deceive the clinician. For example, patients who are embarrassed by their current circumstances might minimize the severity of their symptoms. Similarly, patients who harbor delusions that are not patently "bizarre" might describe events leading up to the psychiatric referral that appear at first glance to be quite plausible, but with further investigation they turn out to have no basis in reality.

Sometimes, however, patients deliberately lie to the clinician. **Malingering** is the intentional production of false or grossly exaggerated physical or psychological symptoms. There are two major forms of malingering. *Simulation* (feigning) of psychiatric symptoms by people without illness most often is motivated by a desire to avoid military duty or work responsibilities, to obtain financial compensation, to evade criminal prosecution, or to obtain drugs. In contrast, in *dissimulation*, a person with a true psychiatric illness feigns wellness. For example, a patient with schizophrenia seen in the emergency room who seeks to avoid involuntary hospitalization might

Table 2–2. Elements of the Mental Status Examination

Appearance	Obsessions and compulsions
Speech	Phobias
Mood and affect	Cognition
Hallucinations	Insight and judgment
Delusions	

deny experiencing hallucinations when in actuality she has been hearing threatening voices throughout the interview. Similarly, a depressed patient with a strong desire to kill herself might not admit to the examining clinician that she has suicidal thoughts, given that the clinician, if apprised of this, would likely attempt to prevent the patient from acting on them.

In addition to bolstering the reliability of the diagnostic process, collateral informants can provide information that proves to be useful in gauging the risk posed by the patient to himself or others should he be discharged from the emergency room:

> A 37-year-old white male with schizophrenia presents to the emergency room for treatment of asthma but is noted by the emergency room physician to be actively psychotic. Psychiatric consultation is requested. The patient voices delusions that his parents are telepathically interfering with his thoughts and are poisoning his food. He says that he sometimes feels that he might have to kill them. The psychiatrist considers admitting the patient to the hospital. However, upon calling his parents, she learns that he is "at his baseline" in terms of his symptom severity, that he has made such threats for the past several years but has never acted on them, that he is seen weekly at the local community clinic, and that he is compliant with his medications (although he has shown an incomplete response to them). The patient is released without further psychiatric intervention.

Let us contrast the above example with the following example:

> A 37-year-old white male is dropped off at the emergency room by the police following an argument with his father, with whom he resides. He states that the argument followed the patient's refusal to pay his father money toward the rent. The patient states: "He tried to push me out the door, and so I pushed him back, but that was it." He describes one brief psychiatric hospitalization years ago, following an impulsive suicide attempt. He recounts how, after the police arrived at his house that night, his father took them aside and told them about the patient's "psychiatric history." The police then decided to bring the patient in for evaluation without even listening to his side of the story. On mental status examination, the patient is mildly disheveled but otherwise appears to be pleasant and cooperative. He displays no evidence of disorganized thinking, delusions, or hallucinations. The

psychiatrist decides that this is a domestic altercation and that to detain the patient on psychiatric grounds would be improper. She calls the father to let him know that the more appropriate response should the patient becomes assaultive in the future would be to press charges for assault and battery or to pursue eviction.

However, the father informs her that the patient has a long history of schizophrenia, with several past psychiatric admissions. Three months ago, the patient stopped taking his medication and refused any further outpatient treatment. He has been looking into neighbors' windows and taking mail from their mailboxes. The father has called the local clinic several times but has been informed that the patient's behavior wasn't severe enough to initiate civil commitment proceedings. Today, the patient escalated in suspiciousness and agitation, accused his father of conspiring with the neighbors against him, and finally pushed his father against the wall and threatened to kill him. Prior to becoming ill, the patient had been a physics graduate student. The father states that the patient is extremely intelligent and that "you can't believe a word he tells you." Following this discussion, the psychiatrist decides to pursue involuntary civil commitment.

In addition to family members, other useful sources of collateral information include previous hospital records (especially admission and discharge summaries) and previously treating clinicians. In more complex evaluations (e.g., disability or forensic evaluations), is isn't uncommon for school, military, or employment records to be reviewed as well.

Present Illness and Past Psychiatric History

At a *minimum*, the psychiatric history should include the age when symptoms of psychiatric illness first appeared, the patient's life situation at that time, whether the onset of symptoms was sudden or gradual, when the patient first received treatment for these symptoms, the number and duration of previous hospitalizations, and the course of the patient's symptoms over time (including the presence or absence of associated syndromal features for the major *DSM-IV* disorders, as will be discussed throughout the text). Life stressors commonly associated with exacerbations of illness (e.g., separations from family, occupational stress, arguments with friends, substance use) should be detailed, as should the severity of current symptoms and the current degree of social and occupational impairment.

When more time is available, a *more detailed history* would also include the dates of all outpatient and inpatient episodes of care, including the symptoms that precipitated the episode of care (e.g., worsening depression following divorce, suicide attempts, threats or acts of violence, delusions, or substance intoxication), a chronological summary of medications and psychotherapeutic interventions, and whether each treatment strategy was successful, partially successful, or ineffective. When medications have proven ineffective, attempt to determine whether this is due to the illness not improving despite an adequate dosage of medication and duration of treatment, due to the development of adverse side effects, or due to patient noncompliance.

Premorbid Personality

It is important to gain a sense of the patient's temperament prior to the onset of the present illness. Predispositions toward extroversion (e.g., tendencies to become bored easily, to prefer new or exciting activities, low frustration tolerance, poor impulse control) or introversion (enjoying the same daily routines, fearing change, perfectionism, self-criticism, pessimism) should be explored as well. This may require a collateral informant, as patients may have unrealistic self-appraisals. (For example, a narcissistic patient may insist that he always puts others before himself.)

Beware of labeling a patient's current psychiatric state as simply being a reflection of the patient's baseline temperament unless you have a clear history with regard to the latter, since acute mental illness can greatly distort the clinical picture. Without knowledge of the patient's baseline personality and functioning, you will be "flying blind," possibly unable to distinguish an acute, pathological state from the patient's baseline personality traits.

A 70-year-old widowed man presents as a patient with symptoms of depression, anxiety, difficulties sleeping, and difficulty leaving the house due to low energy and social withdrawal. The clinician diagnoses a major depressive disorder. The patient appears to be a needy, insecure man, leading the clinician to wonder if these premorbid traits might have predisposed the patient to become more depressed due to social isolation associated with aging. Following a 4-week course of medication therapy, the patient appears slightly less anxious but otherwise appears essentially the same. The clinician finds himself thinking, "He doesn't look all that depressed, just lonely." He postulates that perhaps the patient is now at his baseline state of functioning, and he calls the patient's son to obtain collateral information and also to discuss whether the patient might have more social support were he to move in with his son or into an adult home. The patient's son insists that—until 2 months ago—the patient was extremely independent. He walked 2 miles each day, did all of his own shopping, assisted infirm neighbors, and might drive on the spur of the moment to a neighboring state to visit friends. A similar episode 10 years earlier responded impressively to treatment with electroconvulsive therapy. The patient is referred for electroconvulsive therapy, and 2 weeks later, after six treatment sessions, he is much more outgoing and spontaneous. He reports that he feels about 90% back to his baseline state of functioning. In contrast, his son reports that his father is functioning at about "70% of his previous state." After three more treatment sessions, both the patient and his son agree that he is fully recovered. Nursing staff who witnessed the patient's course of recovery are impressed by the dramatic transformation.

Medical History, Medications, and Drug Allergies

The medical history should list all past and current medical problems and associated treatment interventions. Particular attention should be paid to medical conditions that have been associated with psychiatric syndromes, including head trauma (which patients often fail to report absent specific inquiry), and also any medications either previously or currently taken that have been associated with psychiatric symptoms such as mood lability or delirium. A full medical review of systems should be performed during initial evaluations.

Social History

A good social history provides a road map to understanding the patient from the vantage of point of function as it allows the clinician to make meaningful connections between various life events, thereby conveying the high points of the patient's life story in an efficient way. However, the social history also is essential from the vantage point of form. For example, only through the compilation of a sufficiently detailed life his-

tory is the clinician able to discern the presence of personality disorder. (By definition, a patient is only considered to have a personality disorder when she is determined to have demonstrated enduring, pervasive, inflexible traits that have an adversely effect on the way that she perceives the world and behaves and that are so extreme that they constitute a source of significant impairment or subjective distress. Clearly, one can only make such a diagnosis after having obtained a history that is sufficiently rich in detail for the clinician to have a sense of the patient's characteristic personality style.) Further, the impact of diseases such as major depressive disorder, schizophrenia, or dementia on the patient's interpersonal and occupational functioning also only become evident through the social history.

The clinician should note both the *information* provided by the patient and the patient's *attitude* while conveying it, since the latter also may provide insight into the patient's personality. For example, while interviewing a patient with histrionic personality disorder, the clinician might note the she has a style of speech that is very impressionistic, lacking in detail. Strong, dramatic opinions might be expressed, yet the underlying reasoning is vague and diffuse, without supporting facts and details. For example, she may describe her father as "just wonderful" but not provide any specific details. Similarly, while interviewing a patient with antisocial personality disorder, the clinician may note that he describes past episodes of severe violence or illegal behavior with a broad smile and that he does not demonstrate either remorse for his actions or empathy toward his victims.

At the *minimum*, the social history should include the following: level of education, current occupation, current marital status and the health of his or her children, an alcohol/substance history, and a legal history. However, when more time is available, a more detailed history typically includes the following.

Birth

While a patient may never have been informed of the details of her gestation or birth, briefly inquiring into whether there were any perinatal complications can prove useful, since a history of such complications has been associated with developmental learning or behavioral problems and with psychopathology in general. Schizophrenic patients are more likely to have experienced birth complications (especially perinatal hypoxia) than control subjects without mental illness. Schizophrenic patients who experienced such difficulties are more likely to demonstrate early age of onset of illness, more severe negative symptoms, and a poorer prognosis.

Early Development

Similarly, while many patients may not have knowledge of when they reached developmental milestones (such as the age of taking first steps or of first talking), patients or family members might report a history of developmental delays. The clinician also should inquire into childhood behavioral difficulties such as speech problems or phobias (e.g., school phobia, a fear of going to school), since these are associated with the development of childhood or adult anxiety disorders. Childhood conduct problems (such as bedwetting, cruelty to animals, fire-setting, oppositional behavior, lying, stealing, fighting, school suspensions or expulsions) are associated with the development of antisocial personality disorder. Did the patient experience any more severe or prolonged childhood illnesses? These can predispose to the later development of a somatoform disorder. Is there any history of physical, emotional, or sexual abuse? This can predispose to a variety of psychiatric difficulties, including personality disorder, mood disorder, anxiety disorder, and somatoform disorder.

Education

How far did the patient go in school? Was she at the top, middle, or bottom of the class? What were her typical grades? Did she have any best or worst subjects? If she left school prematurely, why did she do so? Is there any history of the patient having required special education? (Sometimes, a patient will have been raised in an area where special education wasn't available but will recall having been told that she was a "slow learner.") Did the patient have many friends in school? Was the patient involved in extracurricular activities?

Occupational History

List the various jobs the patient has held, how long he held them, and the circumstances under which he left. (For example, has he held many jobs, each for a few months, or has he worked at the same job for the past 30 years? When he left jobs, was this planned ahead in order to accept better jobs, or did he quit impulsively following argument with the boss or simply out of boredom?)

Is there a history of an inability to hold jobs due to exacerbations of illness? Alternatively, has job stress been a precipitant for relapses of illness? Has shift work interfered with the normal sleep–wake cycle and contributed to exacerbations of mood disorder? Is there a history of occupational decline (as can be seen in progressive illnesses such as schizophrenia and some forms of dementia)? If the patient has been in the military, was she honorably discharged or was she discharged due to disciplinary problems?

Sexual/Marital History

When did the patient enter puberty? Did this go smoothly? Does the patient experience physical or emotional problems associated with menstruation or menopause? How many relationships has the patient been in? How long have these relationships typically lasted? Have there been any particular recurring problems contributing to breakups? Is there a history of domestic violence? Note the dates of past marriages, along with the occupation of the current partner and the status of the current relationship.

In determining the level of detail of the sexual history, one obviously should use common sense. A very detailed history is essential when evaluating sexual dysfunction or paraphilia, but in other circumstances it can be intrusive. A *more detailed* sexual history should inquire into the patient's sexual fantasies and preferences, masturbatory habits, and into difficulties with hypoactive sexual desire, with achieving penile erection or vaginal lubrication, with premature ejaculation, and with anorgasmia. In assessing for the presence of a paraphilia, questioning should include inquiry into the use of pornography and into any paraphilic objects of sexual attraction, including fetishism (fantasies or practices with particular inanimate objects), transvestism (cross-dressing), sadism or masochism, exhibitionism, voyeurism, and frotteurism (rubbing against others).

Children

Record the ages of each child along with current grade in school or occupation and any history of health or behavioral problems. If the patient is a single parent currently being admitted to the hospital, remember to inquire into who will be looking after the patient's children.

Current Living Situation

Is the patient in a stable, supportive living situation, or is the living situation chaotic or stressful? For example, does the patient have supportive friends and family? If so, are they the "wrong kind of friends?" (For example, does an alcoholic patient's support system consist of his drinking partners?) If the patient is living with family, does the family have an appreciation of the patient's illness or do they repeatedly berate him for "just being lazy"? Do they help to monitor the compliance with treatment and medications or do they discourage him from seeing a doctor or taking medication?

Legal History

Inquire into any previous arrests and the sentences received. Is the patient currently facing legal charges? Does the patient appear to be seeking admission only to avoid the police? Is the patient currently on probation, and if so do the terms of her probation include a requirement that she participate in psychiatric or addictions treatment?

Alcohol/Substance History

Record current patterns of alcohol or drug use, including nicotine. A simple yet sensitive screening test for alcohol abuse (as well as substance abuse in general) is Ewing's four-question CAGE Questionnaire: (1) Have you ever felt you had to *cut down* on your drinking? (2) Have people *annoyed* you by criticizing your drinking? (3) Have you ever felt *guilty* about your drinking? (4) Have you ever needed a morning *eye-opener* (e.g., to calm your nerves or get rid of a hangover)? Any affirmative responses should trigger a more detailed inquiry.

If the patient has a history of alcohol use, inquire into any arrests for driving while intoxicated, amnestic episodes surrounding periods of intoxication ("blackouts"), and symptoms of complicated alcohol withdrawal (seizures, hallucinations, or delirium tremens). Explore when the patient first began drinking and the factors that contributed to the initiation of drinking, any current "triggers" that perpetuate the drinking, the patient's pattern of drinking (daily, continuous drinking versus episodic "binges"). Has the patient been "detoxed" before? Has he ever been through a rehabilitation program or gone to Alcoholics Anonymous? How long has the patient been able to remain abstinent?

When patients present with psychiatric symptoms such as depression or anxiety in the setting of ongoing substance abuse, the clinician should attempt to tease apart the extent to which the patient's symptoms appear to be secondary to the substance use versus the degree to which they are more independent of (or exacerbated by) the substance use. For example, has the patient continued to experience psychiatric symptoms even during periods of sobriety? However, if the patient's symptoms have routinely *preceded* relapses into substance use, perhaps the patient is "self-medicating" the psychiatric symptoms through illicit drug use. Also, inquire into when each substance was last used, since substance intoxication or withdrawal can present with psychiatric symptoms, with each drug demonstrating its own typical time course. Particularly for patients with a history of intravenous drug use, don't forget to inquire into whether the patient has been tested for infection with the human immunodeficiency (HIV) and hepatitis viruses.

Family History

At a *minimum*, inquire about any history of psychiatric illness, suicide attempts, substance abuse, or neurologic illness in the patient's immediate and extended family. Also ask whether any family members have experienced mood swings or bizarre symptoms that never reached clinical attention, and if any ever made suicide attempts.

Inquiry into the specific symptoms that other family members with psychiatric illness have experienced and even into what medications were useful in treating these symptoms also can be useful. Many psychiatric illnesses—for example, major depressive disorder and schizophrenia—are likely of heterogeneous etiology, and whether the symptoms respond better to one or another medication can vary significantly between patients. Given that genetic factors are often an important contributory factor, if the history reveals that one of the patient's family members who had a similar presentation of illness responded to one particular medication, the clinician might try this medication first with the current patient and potentially avoid having to ultimately "reinvent the wheel" following several failed trials of other agents.

A *more detailed* family history would describe each member of the patient's immediate family along with a brief description of that person's personality and occupation and his or her relationship with the patient.

THE MENTAL STATUS EXAMINATION

The mental status examination is a cross-sectional description of the patient's mental state at a single point in time. It includes both subjective descriptions by the patient and objective observations by the clinician. Some of this information can be obtained in the course of taking the patient's history; the remainder is elicited through direct questioning. The goal in conducting a thorough mental status examination is to assess for the presence of certain operationally defined forms that arise in mental life. While psychiatrists might quibble over the order or labeling of various elements of the mental status examination, the following elements, also listed in Table 2–2, are the most important: appearance, speech, mood and affect, hallucinations, delusions, obsessions and compulsions, phobias, cognition, and insight and judgment.

Some clinicians cluster some of these categories. Most notably, speech might be considered under Form of Thought while hallucinations, delusions, obsessions, compulsions, and phobias would be grouped into a category called Content of Thought. I've presented this more expanded format because it allows for a more systematic and thorough evaluation.

Appearance

Over the entire course of the evaluation, take note of the patient's *grooming and clothing*. Does she have tattoos or multiple scars (for example, parallel cuts in the forearm or thighs reflecting repetitive self-injury)? Is the patient neatly dressed

Table 2–3. Levels of Consciousness

Descriptor	Features
Alert and lucid	Normal level of consciousness with intact cognition
Clouding	Slight drowsiness (with or without agitation), with difficulty with attention and concentration
Drowsiness	Awake but sleepy, drifting into unconsciousness if no sensory stimulation provided, often dysarthric
Stupor	Sleeping but can be momentarily aroused with a strong or painful stimulus, demonstrating little or no movement even with painful stimulation
Coma	Deeply unconscious and completely unarousable

and groomed or is she disheveled? (The latter might reflect various conditions, such as dementia, schizophrenia, or substance intoxication.) Is she wearing brightly colored clothing (possibly indicating mania)? Is she wearing inappropriate clothing? Consider asking about this to determine if the patient's choice of dress reflects delusional thinking. (For example, the patient who wears a piece of tin foil on her head or wears a heavy hat even during the summer may be attempting to prevent "electromagnetic rays" from being beamed into her head.)

Also observe the patient's *behavior*. Does she appear anxious or uncomfortable? Is she withdrawn? Does she show a paucity of spontaneous movement and speech or "psychomotor retardation" (slowed mentation and movement)? Does she display inappropriate or agitated behavior? Does she appear to be responding to hallucinations (e.g., glancing all over the room)?

Observe the patient's *level of consciousness*. This can range along a continuum from alert and lucid at one pole through comatose at the other, as detailed in Table 2–3.

Some aspects of a patient's appearance will suggest an *underlying medical illness*. For example, dilated pupils in a delirious patient might indicate sedative-hypnotic or opiate withdrawal, marijuana intoxication, or anticholinergic intoxication. Argyll Robertson pupils (pupils that are bilaterally small, irregular, and reactive to accommodation but not to light) indicate underlying neurosyphilis. A Kayser-Fleischer ring (a brownish discoloration of the peripheral cornea due to abnormal copper deposition) is almost always present in Wilson's disease that has affected the brain, although it may be hard to see absent a slit-lamp examination in patients who have dark irises.

In this same vein, are there any signs of *motor abnormalities or movement disorder*? **Weakness** is a nonspecific sign that could reflect either a physical condition (such as malnutrition, stroke, delirium, or disuse atrophy) or a psychological one such as depression (where it typically accompanies feelings of anergia—i.e., a lack of drive).

Akinesia describes either a delay in the initiation of movements, or slowness in the execution of movements, or special difficulty in executing more complex movements. It most commonly is caused by either idiopathic Parkinson's disease or drug-induced parkinsonism occurring as a side effect of antipsychotic medication. While it is sometimes difficult to distinguish parkinsonian akinesia from depressive psychomotor retardation, the latter condition does not include the associated parkinsonian features of tremor, rigidity, and postural instability.

Akathisia is a subjective sense of uncomfortable motor restlessness. It most commonly occurs as a side effect of antipsychotic medication (also, more rarely, as a side effect of antidepressant medication). It may be difficult to obtain a history of akathisia from a psychotic patient. She may offer delusional interpretations of the akathisia—for example, complaining of snakes crawling under her skin or in her stomach. Sometimes akathisia and associated pacing are mistaken for psychotic agitation, leading the clinician to increase the dose of antipsychotic medication rather than to cut back the dose, thereby exacerbating rather than relieving the complaint. Similarly, it may be difficult to distinguish akathisia from somatic manifestations of anxiety. Complaints specifically referable to the legs are more characteristic of akathisia. Also, the objective signs of akathisia are quite typical: when patients with akathisia attempt to stand still, they shifts their weight from foot to foot, and when seated they may shuffle or tap their feet or repeatedly cross their legs.

Hypertonicity refers to increased muscle tone. There are three forms of hypertonicity: spasticity, rigidity, and paratonia. In **spasticity**, tone is increased in the flexors in the upper extremity and in the extensors in the lower extremity but not in the antagonist muscles. In attempting to move the patient's limb passively, one encounters an increase in resistance followed by an immediate decrease ("clasp-knife" phenomenon), and this is velocity dependent. Spasticity is commonly encountered in patients with hemiplegia due to lesions affecting the corticospinal tract.

In contrast, in **rigidity**, tone is increased throughout the entire of range of passive motion in both the agonists and antagonists, regardless of velocity, leading to a "lead-pipe" phenomenon. Rigidity is typically encountered in patients with lesions affecting the extrapyramidal motor system.

In **paratonia (Gegenhalten)**, the increased tone is erratic, with active resistance to passive movement in any direction at any velocity, such that the behavior appears almost deliberately "oppositional." This pattern is typically caused by extensive brain dysfunction as a motor release symptom similar to the grasp reflex.

Of note, **"cogwheel" rigidity** (intermittent resistance palpated along the tendon during passive movement) often accompanies hypertonicity in patients with parkinsonism regardless of whether the parkinsonism is idiopathic or medication-induced. However, this phenomenon is not an intrinsic feature of the hypertonicity. Rather, it reflects the presence of a postural tremor (a separate phenomenon from the parkinsonian resting tremor) superimposed upon the patient's rigidity.

Abnormal involuntary movements include dystonia, tremor, chorea, myoclonus, tics, stereotypies, and asterixis. **Dystonia** is a pattern of sustained muscle contraction, frequently causing twisting and repetitive movements or abnormal postures. As dystonia reflects pathology of the extrapyramidal, it can be suppressed (at least briefly) with some effort. The latter finding does not indicate that that patient's posturing is a "hysterical" (conversion) phenomenon. Dystonia can occur either due to neurological illness or as an acute side effect of antipsychotic medication.

Tremor is a pattern of rhythmic, regular, oscillating movements around a joint. The three types of tremor are resting tremor, intention tremor, and postural tremor. A *resting tremor* is maximal at rest and diminishes or disappears with activity. It is commonly seen with parkinsonism, along with bradykinesia and cogwheel rigidity. In contrast, an *intention tremor* is most prominent with activity (such as extending a finger to touch the examiner's finger). It is not present during either postural maintenance or at rest. It occurs in cerebellar disease. Finally, a *postural tremor* is minimal at rest or with motion and most prominent when a limb is being actively maintained against gravity—for example, with the patients' hands extended outward with fingers spread. It can result from a variety of conditions, including hyperthyroidism, side effects of medications (including lithium, carbamazepine, or valproic acid), alcohol or benzodiazepine withdrawal, or a progressive, idiopathic condition with an autosomal dominant inheritance pattern (familial tremor or benign essential tremor). Most commonly affected are one or both hands, the head, and the voice.

In contrast, **chorea** is a pattern of random, abrupt, irregular, involuntary "fidgeting" movements (**dyskinesia**) located throughout the patient's body, although most commonly in the face and distal limbs. When these involuntary movements are mild, the patient may unconsciously incorporate them into purposeful movements, distracting the casual observer or family member from recognizing its presence. Chorea occurs with gradual onset in progressive neurological disorders such as Wilson's disease, systemic lupus erythematosus, Huntington's disease, and Fahr's syndrome. It also can occur idiopathically. Acute dysknetic movements can occur as a reversible toxic side effect of dopamine excess induced by antiparkinsonian medications such as levodopa or dopamine receptor agonist medications. In psychiatric patients the most common cause of chorea is **tardive dyskinesia**, a potential long-term complication of antipsychotic medication therapy, discussed further in Chapter 8.

Myoclonus is a pattern of more complex, rapid, irregular jerking movements. It occurs in a variety of metabolic and neurologic disorders, including delirium (whether due to electrolyte disturbance, hypoxia, renal failure, hepatic failure, etc., as detailed in Chapter 5). It also can oc-

cur as a sequela of brain injury due to hypoxia, encephalitis, or Creutzfeldt-Jakob disease.

Tics are involuntary, sudden, rapid, recurrent, nonrhythmic, stereotyped motor movement (motor tics) or vocalizations (vocal tics). Motor or vocal tics can be *simple* (e.g., blinks or grunts) or *complex* (e.g., repeatedly touching a particular object or speaking a particular word). Motor and vocal tics can appear in isolation or together, the latter being the primary diagnostic feature of Tourette's disorder. They can be briefly controlled with conscious effort.

Asterixis is a flapping movement of the outstretched hands when the arms are extended with the wrists flexed (i.e., as if attempting to stop traffic). It represents the repeated momentary loss of postural tone rather than a tremor. Bilateral asterixis is a valuable sign in cases of altered mental status because it points unmistakably to a toxic-metabolic etiology (e.g., liver failure). It has never been described in the "functional" psychoses such as mood disorder or schizophrenia. The coarse tremor sometimes seen in delirium is a slower version of asterixis.

Stereotypies are purposeless, rhythmic, repetitive movements carried out at the expense of all other motor activity for long periods of time. Examples include repetitive hand clapping or banging of one's head against the wall. In contrast, *mannerisms* are purposeful movements that are carried out in a bizarre manner. For example, a patient with schizophrenia may repeatedly look at the examiner and rub his finger against his right ear lobe as a way of symbolically signaling to the examiner, "I can trust you."

Catatonia is an abnormality of movement or muscle tone associated with psychosis. Catatonia is diagnosed when the patient displays a combination of *motor signs* and signs of *psychomotor withdrawal or excitement*. The most common association with catatonia is mood disorder (25%–50% of cases), including both mania and depression; 10%–15% of cases are associated with schizophrenia, and the remainder occur in association with other mental disorders (including obsessive-compulsive disorder, personality disorders, and dissociative disorders). However, one must always be mindful that catatonia occurs in a wide variety of infectious, metabolic, and neurological conditions, can be due to a side effect of a medication, particularly antipsychotic and serotonergic antidepressant medications, and can be a feature of neuroleptic malignant syndrome (discussed in Chapter 8).

Motor signs of catatonia include **catalepsy** (holding an awkward position or posture for an extended period of time), **waxy flexibility** (partial passive resistance of a limb, often then followed by catalepsy), and **bizarre posturing**. Signs of catatonic withdrawal or excitement include **stupor** (a marked decrease in reactivity to and awareness of the environment), **mutism** (prolonged inhibition of speech), **negativism** (refusal to cooperate with even simple requests, e.g., standing up when asked to sit down), **impulsiveness, grimacing, stereotypies, mannerisms, echopraxia** (mirroring movements of the examiner), **echolalia** (echoing words of the examiner), and **verbigeration** (meaningless repetition of words or phrases).

Speech

Psychiatrists cannot read patients' thoughts (although some patients do hold this delusional belief). All that psychiatrists can do is examine what the patient says, distinguishing between what the patient says (the content of thought) and how she says it (the form of thought, as reflected in her speech). When the form of thought is abnormal, the patient is said to display a **formal thought disorder**. It is best to include a sample of the patient's speech in documenting formal thought disorder both because two clinicians listening to the same interview may disagree as to whether a patient "truly" displays thought disorder, and because thought-disordered speech—not conforming to the normal rules of syntax—can be extremely difficult to recall verbatim later on.

In order to understand pathological forms of thought, let us first examine the "normal" or "typical" procession of thoughts. In a typical pattern of thought process, thoughts can be seen as flowing from one thought to the next through a series of *associations*. Out of a constellation of possible associations that might potentially arise out of a preceding thought, one particular association ultimately is chosen. This is not a random, automatic, or reflexive event. Rather, normal thinking and speech are *goal-directed*. The goal is to get from thought A to thought Z in a linear and logical way—that is, via thoughts B, then C, etc., rather than from A to A′ to A″, etc.,

thus ending up off track, or on a tangent. Karl Jaspers, a German psychiatrist and early proponent of the careful phenomenologic approach, called flow of thought toward some particular end point the "determining tendency" of speech.

In describing a patient's speech, note the patient *flow of speech*. Does she speak spontaneously or only in response to questions? Does she answer at length or is she minimally responsive (e.g., answering yes or no with no further elaboration)? Are her replies appropriately prompt, or are there long **latencies of speech** prior to any reply? The latter often is exhibited by patients who are depressed and are experiencing psychomotor slowing. However, agitated patients (particularly manic or hypomanic patients, may display **pressured speech**.

As you listen to the patient's speech, consider also her *use of vocabulary*. Does the patient have a broad vocabulary and demonstrate the ability to engage in more abstract thought, or her vocabulary more rudimentary and her thinking more "concrete"? The latter findings suggest a lower level of intelligence. (This could later be confirmed by examination of the patient's occupational and social functioning and by formal intelligence testing, if indicated.)

Several pathological forms of associations are commonly exhibited by psychiatric patients. While they typically correlate with particular illnesses, none is pathognomonic. In **flight of ideas**, most often seen in manic patients, the speech is pressured and the speed at which associations are made is highly accelerated. (Patients often describe a subjective sensation of racing thoughts.) In flight of ideas, while the "determining tendency" of thought may be weakened, it remains present. In other words, associations are preserved, and the patient's speech would still be characterized as "goal-directed." However, because manic patients are so distractible, the goal keeps changing. For example, a manic patient might excitedly and rapidly relate the following:

I'm really hoping to be discharged soon. I'm getting better every day. I can see the light at the end of the tunnel. I love to drive. Do you have a driver's license? I hate the way I look on mine. It doesn't even look like me. I've been arrested for speeding a few times and had to go to court. I'm the court jester.

In contrast, in **retardation of speech** (often seen in major depressive disorder, in subcortical dementia, and in delirium), while associations remain preserved (although there may be an overall poverty of associations) and speech remains goal-directed, the speech proceeds at such a slow pace that in observing more extreme cases, the clinician might worry that the patient will never make it to the goal. Sometimes, the patient never does reach the goal, but due to an inability to sustain the concentration and effort necessary to do so rather than due to disorganization of thought.

In depressed patients, the content of this retarded speech typically is self-deprecating and nihilistic. For these patients, retardation of speech can be thought of as part of a larger syndrome of "psychomotor retardation." Other features of psychomotor retardation that tend to "keep company" with slowing of thought include: paucity of spontaneous movements; a slumped posture with downward gaze; a subjective sense of fatigue in which "everything is an effort" (loss of vital sense); a subjective feeling that time is moving more slowly; poor concentration and memory; narrowing of thought content with a tendency to ruminate on a few painful topics; and indecisiveness for even simple decisions. It can be helpful to look for these associated features in your mental status examination to help distinguish patients with true speech retardation from patients who simply are uncooperative or withdrawn.

Another form of speech that remains "goal-directed" but difficult to follow is **circumstantiality**. Here, the associations can be followed, but the speech is overinclusive and circumlocutious, full of unnecessary digressions and parenthetical clarifications, to the point where the patient "loses the forest for the trees." Typically, these patients do recall the initial question and apologize for digressing. This form of speech is most commonly noted in individuals with obsessional personalities who are anxious about the prospect of "leaving something out," but it does occur in some pathological states.

In contrast, let us now consider situations where the patient's speech demonstrates **loosening of associations**. In these cases, most commonly occurring in the setting of schizophrenia, the goal-directed quality of speech is lost. In the course of the interview, the patient may follow one statement with another that shows no discernible connection at all to the first. The clinician's first impulse might be to assume that she wasn't listening closely enough. It is as if a train were traveling along but suddenly jumped sideways, off the rails. This phenomenon has, appropriately enough, also been called "derailment" or (employing an equally vivid chess metaphor) "knight's move." When derailment occurs repeatedly, the entire coherence of speech is lost—hence the descriptor "word salad," or "verbigeration" in these more severe cases. For example, a woman with schizophrenia of the disorganized type was asked about her current mood and replied:

> I can't be happy because I'm taking pictures. I have a photographic memory. I copied a seventeen book around a hollow face and I have to presently band it against my religion, because my parents didn't teach me anything about sex, you know sterile and nonsterile, and I had to learn the hard way, Army style and Air Force style. It's dashing right now with a repeat performance. I'm at a halt, but I'm always thinking about blood and sterile and nonsterile and how a female feels in relation to a man. I thought it was bones because of my baby formula. My baby formula is chocolate milk and it's making a demander of sugar out of me.

In this example, we also can discern several other features of the thought disorder associated with schizophrenia. **Tangentiality** is one specific example of derailment in which a patient replies to the interviewer's question with a response that is irrelevant or makes no sense. In this case, the patient's reply to a question about her current mood was tangential.

Despite sometimes-colorful language, schizophrenic patients often are described as having **poverty of thought**, with a very restricted vocabulary. In order to fill this gap, the patient may include **neologisms**—words that are either made up or are used in a highly idiosyncratic way (e.g., "a seventeen book," or "band it"). The patient also may repetitively insert idiosyncratic **stock phrases** (e.g., "sterile and nonsterile") whose meaning may only become clear after a more extended interview.

Schizophrenic patients' speech also might be fragmented, with loss of normal syntax, so-called **telegraphic speech**. For example: "It's . . . unlikely I go . . . unlawful to keep me . . . unintentional behavior. . . . I will go home." Note that this sentence also demonstrates **clang associations**, where the association between words relies not on content but on words having similar first syllables (*un*likely, *un*lawful, *un*intentional). (Manic patients, however, may link the *last* syllables of words with **rhyme associations**, similar to playful verse or poetry.)

The most severe example of impoverished thought is **thought blocking**. In this case, the patient abruptly stops speaking in midsentence. This phenomenon differs from latency or retardation in that—when asked to describe his mental experience during the silence—the patient describes the subjective sense of his thoughts simply having "stopped" or "disappeared."

Mood

In inquiring into the patient's current emotional state, assess for feelings of sadness, elation, anxiety, anger, or apathy. Note that when patients are simply asked, "How do you feel?" they tend to offer vague responses related to their physical state, such as, "Not bad," or, "A little tired." It is therefore better to convey through a variety of more specific questions the type of information being sought. For example: "How is your mood?" "How are your spirits?" "How are you feeling inside yourself?"

If the patient reports feeling sad, clarify whether the patient still retains a normal degree of *emotional reactivity*. In other words, does the patient feel the same level of sadness throughout the day regardless of daily life events, or can her mood still be influenced (at least to some degree) by watching a comedy on television, going out with friends, or eating a good meal? In the most severe forms of mood disorder, the normal association between one's environment and one's emotional state (e.g., sad events making us feel sad, happy events making us feel happy) is severed. The emotional state becomes autonomous, persistent, and all-pervasive.

Also, assess how the patient's mood *varies over time*. Some depressed patients describe a **diurnal mood variation**, with the mood being lowest in the morning upon first awakening, with some improvement in mood as the day progresses. Diurnal mood variation may be subtle. For example, a high school student may notice that he doesn't seem to perform as well in his morning classes as in his afternoon classes. Diurnal mood variation also may be dramatic:

> A patient on the inpatient unit repeatedly refused a needed surgery each morning, tearfully stating, "I know I'm going to die," "It's hopeless," and "You doctors shouldn't waste your time on me." However, every afternoon she would brighten, consent to the procedure, and apologize for her comments earlier that day. She added, "You doctors shouldn't listen to me in the morning. I'm just not myself."

When patients appear to be sad or elated, assess the patient's *self-attitude*, which in mood disorder typically is altered in the same direction as mood. In other words, the changes tend to be *mood congruent*. Self-attitude may change so profoundly in depression that the patient may voice severe nihilistic or somatic delusions, such as delusions of profound poverty or of having extensive cancer that the tests have failed to reveal. In contrast, self-attitude is elevated in manic states, again sometimes to the point where a patient believes that she is a prophet or an angel of God. In milder, nonpsychotic depression or in lower-grade mania ("hypomania"), self-attitude changes can be subtle. For example, a depressed patient may feel that she isn't being as good a mother as she should be, or that she is letting down her coworkers because she isn't as productive as she should be. A hypomanic patient may feel more creative or may make impulsively make bad investment decisions out of a belief that "he can't lose." Since some patients are chronically self-deprecating and others have always been narcissistically self-important, try to gain some sense of what the patient's self-esteem is at baseline and of whether the current self-attitude represents a change.

Along with describing changes in both mood and self-attitude, patients with clinical depression often describe a change in "*vital sense*" (or "*vital self*"). This term describes the intimate relationship between a patient's mood and his perception of bodily health and function. While depressed patients may describe various somatic symptoms, upon further questioning it usually is found that, like the change in self-attitude, symptoms reflective of a change in vital sense are mood congruent. For example, while the depressed patient may complain of a "headache," she may describe it as more of "a sensation of heaviness . . . like a pressure." Similar feelings may be described in the abdomen or chest: "It's like a weight on my chest," or "It's a heavy feeling in my bowels, like there's a blockage." In severe cases, a patient may voice mood-congruent somatic delusions such as a belief that her "bowels are rotting inside" or that she "is completely empty inside."

In clinical depression (as opposed to ordinary sadness), patients report that their current mood and bodily state appear qualitatively "different" from how they would normally feel, even taking into account that they are currently in the midst of a stressful situation. "This just isn't the usual me . . . Of course I've been sad before, but I never felt like *this*," are common comments. Patients who previously have experienced episodes of clinical depression might relate that they feel "the same way that I felt back then." The patient may feel withdrawn and cut off from others, as if "I'm observing the world through a sheet of Plexiglas." He loses interest in his usual activities, including those that usually give him pleasure (**anhedonia**). Anhedonia may be linked to a change in bodily sensations. For example, patients may experience not only a loss of appetite but also have a feeling that the food "just doesn't taste good." Similarly, sounds may appear more muted, colors more bland. Sex drive (libido) is reduced or absent.

Closely linked to vital sense are the so-called **vegetative** (or **neurovegetative**) symptoms of mood disorder, a term used to describe the most common "somatic" manifestations of depression—that is, changes in sleep, energy, concentration and memory, and appetite. A helpful mnemonic for these symptoms involves imagining having to write a prescription for energy capsules, or "E CAPS" for the depressed patient, the prescription reading "SIG: E CAPS," as detailed in Table 2–4. The mnemonic also reminds one to ask about anhedonia ("interest"), diminished self-attitude ("guilt") and suicidal ideation.

We have already discussed decreased energy, loss of appetite, psychomotor retardation, and change in self-attitude (guilt) above. Patients with depression also may report either increased sleep (although some may be "taking to bed" without increased sleep, whether due to decreased energy, anhedonia, or social withdrawal,

Table 2–4. "SIG: E CAPS" Mnemonic for Symptoms of Major Depressive Episode

*S*leep (excessive increase or decrease)
*I*nterest (decreased interest in usual activities, i.e. anhedonia)
*G*uilt (decreased self-attitude)
*E*nergy (diminished energy or fatigue)
*C*oncentration (decreased, or indecisiveness)
*A*ppetite (decreased or increased, along with weight loss or gain)
*P*sychomotor agitation or retardation
*S*uicidal ideation (or recurrent thoughts of death)

i.e., an inability to face the world due to lowered self-attitude and hopelessness). Patients may also complain of initial insomnia (difficulty falling asleep), middle insomnia (restless sleep with frequent awakening), or terminal insomnia. The last, also called **early morning awakening**, is a classic symptom of depression. The patient typically describes waking earlier than planned and then being unable to fall back asleep. This symptom occurs in the melancholic form of major depressive disorder, often in association with diurnal mood variation (i.e., with mood being the lowest upon first awakening).

Inquire into the patient's *attitude toward the future*. Patients who are sad, with a lowered self-attitude, and with a loss of vitality and pleasure, not surprisingly also tend to have a bleak view of both the future and of their ability to alter it. These feelings of hopelessness and helplessness contribute to the patient developing **suicidal ideation**.

Always inquire into suicidal thoughts. You might begin in a more general way by commenting, "Sometimes patients in situations such as you've been describing feel hopeless, or even feel that they just can't go on. Has this been the case with you?" Then, ask more directly about suicidal thoughts and behaviors. Some patients have **passive death wishes**. They report a desire to die by natural causes in an accident, or might add, "I would never take my own life, but if I didn't wake up tomorrow morning, it wouldn't be such a bad thing." Other patients describe having an **active intent** to end their lives. When patients report suicidal ideation, inquire into whether the patient has formulated a specific suicide plan and into whether the patient has taken any steps to carry the plan out (for example, by hoarding medications, buying a gun, or putting his financial affairs in order). Also inquire into **thoughts of harming others** or **homicidal ideation**. These might be linked to the suicidal thoughts. For example, a man may decide to kill his family before killing himself, out of jealous concerns that, after his death, his wife and children might one day come to love another man in his place. A woman may decide to kill her children before taking her own life in order to spare them the pain of growing up without a mother.

The changes in self-attitude and vital sense that occur during manic states are the mirror images of the changes that occur during depressive states. The manic patient typically reports an elated mood (although in more severe mania the patient may be irritable and may even become assaultive). His self-attitude and vital sense are both elevated, sometimes to a delusional extent. He sleeps little (or not at all) but denies fatigue. In fact, his energy is increased, even to the point where he is "bursting" with energy. He feels that his creativity is heightened and that his concentration is wonderful (despite objective evidence of excessive distractibility). The patient may have lost the normal sense of social propriety going on spending sprees (even to the point of bankruptcy), making multiple long-distance phone calls, engaging in inappropriate sexual behavior, traveling long distances, or impulsively making major life changes (leaving his wife and children, quitting his job, etc.). Objectively, the patient's observed emotions may be very **labile**, rapidly fluctuating from elation to anger to tearfulness and back again, all in a brief span of time. He may demonstrate excessive motor activity, and in the most severe cases may become so disorganized and energized that he fails to eat and sleep and risks death due to malnutrition and exhaustion.

In **hypomania**, the patient's mood is elevated and expansive. Her self-attitude and vital sense are elevated, but not as severely as in full-blown mania. Delusions and hallucinations are absent. While the patient's behavior is not as extreme as that seen in mania, the most important finding is that it is out of character for the patient. One must also distinguish between the patient who has shifted from depression into hypomania and the patient who is finally feeling better and merely is "making up for lost time."

While inquiring into the patient's subjective mood, observe the patient's objective **affect**. Unfortunately, texts offer varying, contradictory definitions of these terms. The three most common definitions are:

Definition 1: *Emotions* are fleeting feeling states, *moods* are more persistent emotional states (e.g., persistent sadness or happiness), and *affects* are broader, more encompassing states that include not only the patient's mood but also the associated motivational states or drives (e.g., libido or appetite) and attitudes (e.g., hopefulness, pleasure, confidence, discouragement, etc.). Thus, "mood disorder" has historically been called "affective disorder," as the latter term describes a syndrome involving widespread bodily disturbances, with a change in mood being simply the most readily apparent and dramatic symptom.

Definition 2: *Mood* is the pervasive and sustained emotional state that colors one's perception of the world (e.g., depression, elation, anger, and anxiety), while *affect* refers to more transient, fluctuating changes in one's emotional state. If affect refers to today's emotional "weather," mood refers to this month's emotional "climate."

Definition 3: *Mood* refers to the patient's subjective feeling state, while *affect* describes the observable behavioral expression of his emotional state. Affect therefore includes facial expression, body habitus, eye contact, etc.

Currently, this last definition is the mostly commonly employed one and is therefore the recommended usage. In describing the patients, affect, note that it may be *consistent* with her subjective mood (e.g., she says that she feels sad and hopeless, appears sad, and frequently bursts into tears), or it may be *inconsistent, incongruent,* or *inappropriate* (e.g., she says that she feels sad but smiles and frequently bursts into laughter). The patient might display a *restricted range of affect* (or in more severe cases, a *blunted affect*). Blunting of affect occurs, for example, as a "negative symptom" of schizophrenia (see Chapter 8), in the "masked facial expression" of Parkinson's disease, or with the apathy that can accompany subcortical dementia (see Chapter 6). A manic or a histrionic patient may have a *labile* affect. Patients with bilateral hemispheric brain disease (e.g., due to head trauma, stroke, or multiple sclerosis) may display a form of affective dysregulation called **emotional inconti-**

nence. They inappropriately abruptly burst into tears or laughter, recognizing the excessiveness of their affective display but lacking an ability to control it.

Hallucinations

A **hallucination** is a true perception in the absence of an external stimulus. Hallucinations occur in any of the five sensory modalities, but the most common hallucinations experienced by psychiatric patients are auditory hallucinations. Sometimes, it isn't clear if a patient is hallucinating. If you ask the patient if he "hears voices," he likely will reply, "Well, I can hear your voice right now." Instead, try asking the patient if he "has ever heard voices when nobody else is around." Even when the question is clearly framed, the patient's response may be ambiguous, necessitating further corroboration:

> A depressed patient states to the psychiatrist on morning rounds, "I overheard some nurses talking about me from the hallway, telling each other that they're fed up with me and wish that I would just die already." Assuming that the nurses didn't in fact make these comments, the patient's experience could represent either auditory hallucinations or a *delusional misinterpretation* of voices that were actually overheard.
>
> A patient initially denies hallucinations when asked if he ever "hears voices." However, he does describe the delusion of his body being controlled by a computer, which transmits electrical signals to wires running throughout his body. When asked how he knows that such a machine actually exists, he replies that he can feel the surges of electricity running through his body and can hear a "pinging" sound when the machine is switched on and off. In this case, only further inquiry into the patient's delusional system revealed the presence of associated tactile and auditory hallucinations.

Auditory hallucinations can be *elementary* (e.g., machinery noises, rattles, whistles) or *complex* (e.g., voices that berate the patient). Elementary hallucinations are most commonly seen in acute delirious states, in which patients may be quite frightened of them.

Hallucinations of voices occur in several psychotic conditions, particularly schizophrenia, substance-induced psychotic disorders (such as alcoholic hallucinosis), and either depressive or manic episodes with psychotic features. The voices are often clear, but sometimes they are muffled or indistinct. In asking about hallucinations, clarify how many different voices there are, what the voices say, and whether they issue commands (so-called **command hallucinations**). If they do, ask the patient if she feels compelled to obey the commands and if the commands demand that the patient engage in potentially dangerous behavior.

When they occur in the setting of mood disorder, hallucinations often are mood congruent. For example, the depressed patient may hear voices berating him for being a failure and telling him that he deserves to die. (The patient might even *agree* with hallucinations—for example, agreeing that he is a failure and should just kill himself.) In contrast, the manic patient may hear voices telling him that he is gifted and loved by God. The depressed patient typically doesn't experience arguing voices, with one voice berating him and another voice praising him and rising to his defense.

In contrast, in schizophrenia, the patient often describes mood incongruent auditory hallucinations. For example, voices threaten the patient or tell her to kill herself. The patient is frightened of the voices, but she doesn't know why they are saying these things and disagrees with them. In schizophrenia, the content of the hallucinations may be more ambivalent, with hostile voices that insult the patient and friendly voices that defend her or even enter into an argument with the hostile voices, saying, "Leave her alone. She's a good person." In schizophrenia, the voices may echo the patient's thoughts (*thought echo*) or offer a *running commentary* about her behavior, such as, "Look at her. Now she's sitting down. Now she's turning on the television." For further description of the features of hallucinations typically seen in schizophrenia, see Chapter 8.

While *visual hallucinations* can be present in schizophrenia or psychotic mood disorders, they are much more commonly seen in delirium, dementia, or psychotic disorders due to a general medical condition (such as occipital lobe tumor, postconcussional state, epileptic twilight state, a drug-induced state from a hallucinogen such as LSD, or an encephalopathic state from renal failure, liver failure, or anticholinergic drug toxicity). Often the hallucinations are simple—for example, flashes of light. Delirious patients also commonly see small animals running around the room, deceased relatives who look at them but do not speak, or even very small people ("*Lilliputian" hallucinations*).

Tactile (or haptic) hallucinations can occur in schizophrenia or psychotic forms of mood disorder, where they often are associated with a delusion (as in the above example of the schizophrenic patient who could "feel" the electrical impulses from the machine that she believed was controlling her). In some cases it is difficult to determine with certainty whether a sensation is a tactile hallucination or a misinterpretation of true somatic sensation. (For example, the sensation of "bowels rotting" could be either a tactile hallucination or a delusional misinterpretation of normal peristalsis.) Tactile hallucinations commonly are associated with delirious states such as delirium tremens ("DTs") from alcohol withdrawal or delirium due to cocaine or amphetamine intoxication, where the sensation is often of something crawling on or under the skin (*formication*).

Olfactory hallucinations may occur in either schizophrenia or mood disorder, again often in association with a delusion. For example, a schizophrenic patient who believes that people are out to hurt her might also smell what appears to be poison gas coming from the air conditioner vents. A depressed patient may believe that he is emitting a foul odor, which he can also smell. Olfactory hallucinations can also occur in the setting of seizure activity, particularly in temporal lobe epilepsy, where the smell is usually unpleasant (e.g., burning rubber).

Gustatory hallucinations may accompany olfactory hallucinations. For example, food may be perceived has having both an unpleasant smell and and a foul taste. Note that while patients with depression may complain of food tasting bad (*taste aversion*), this often represents anhedonia rather than a true hallucination. Unpleasant tastes (especially metallic tastes) can also be experienced as a side effect of a variety of medications—for example, with the antibiotic metronidazole (Flagyl).

Some hallucinations are considered to be of no pathological significance. For example, **hypnagogic or hypnopompic hallucinations** occur when people are just falling asleep or are just waking up, respectively. When these hallucina-

tions are vivid or frightening and are accompanied by *sleep paralysis* (the inability to move or speak), the patient may have narcolepsy. Both phenomena are felt to represent elements of random eye movement (REM) sleep intruding into the waking state. (The other associated symptoms of narcolepsy to look for are *excessive daytime sleepiness* and *cataplexy*, the latter being a sudden loss of muscle tone bilaterally, often provoked by strong affect.)

Keep in mind that not all perceptual disturbances are hallucinations, as illustrated in Table 2–5. **Illusions** are sensory misperceptions of real external stimuli. Illusions can occur in healthy people—for example, when they hear the phone ringing or their name being called through the sound of running water while in the shower. Similarly, many people have awoken in the middle of the night in a darkened bedroom and seen a person standing there, only to find upon turning on the lights that they actually had seen a piece of clothing. Illusions can also be seen in pathological states. For example, the depressed patient who looks at his face and sees it "melting," or sees "the devil," is experiencing an illusion. While LSD is commonly called a "hallucinogen," it actually should be called an "illusionogen," since using it much more commonly leads to such illusions than to hallucinations.

Pseudohallucinations are perceptions that the patient recognizes as being internally generated (most commonly voices heard "inside of my head" rather than through the ears), often with preserved insight into the perception not being "real." The patient distinguishes the perception

Table 2–5. Differential Diagnoses of Hallucinations

Term	Definition
Hallucination	True perception in absence of external stimulus
Illusion	Sensory misperception of real external stimulus
Pseudohallucination	Perception generated from within but distinguished from one's own thoughts or from mental imagery
Vivid thoughts/imagery	Internally generated, seen or heard with one's "imagination" or "mind's eye"

from vivid thoughts or vivid mental imagery. Such experiences can occur along with true hallucinations in psychotic illnesses such as schizophrenia, but when they occur in the absence of other psychotic symptoms they likely represent a different pathologic phenomenon. For example, the perceptual abnormalities reported by patients with conversion disorder (see Chapter 13) and by patients with borderline personality disorder during so-called "micropsychotic episodes" (see Chapter 10) typically involve pseudohallucinations. In such cases, the patient typically retains insight, the perceptions are readily described to the examiner, and the perceptions may be psychologically meaningful to the patient (e.g., "I hear my mother and my ex-husband both telling me that I'm a loser and will never amount to anything.")

Vivid thoughts and **vivid mental imagery** are normal phenomena that shouldn't be confused with hallucinations or treated with antipsychotic medication. The patient described in Chapter 1 who "heard" a "voice in his head" telling him to kill himself following his wife having left him ultimately was found to be experiencing an intrusive, vivid thought rather than a hallucination or pseudohallucination. Similarly, when a patient states, "I see my deceased mother beckoning to me, calling my name," it is essential that the examiner further clarify the nature of this experience. For example, one could ask, "Do you literally see her, the same way you see me? Do you hear her voice the same way you are hearing my voice now? Or is it more in your 'mind's eye'?" The patient will often reply that it's "as if" she were right there, or that he can "practically" see her. A patient experiencing true hallucinations in the midst of a psychotic episode does not make such distinctions.

Delusions

Delusions are operationally defined as fixed, false, idiosyncratic beliefs. Obviously, before classifying a belief as delusional, we first must ensure that it is *false*. In the case of patently bizarre ideas—for example, that rays being beamed into the patient's head from outer space, or that family members are being replaced by identical-appearing imposters—the falsity of the beliefs can be presumed. In other cases, however, it might not be clear.

For example, when a patient on the psychiatry unit tells the staff that last night his roommate threatened to kill him, the staff should look into this prior to prescribing antipsychotic medication (since perhaps it is the patient's roommate who requires this medication). Similarly, a patient may report that her next-door neighbor has placed a voodoo curse on her and has told her through the fence that separates their property that she plans to have the patient committed to the psychiatric hospital and will then try to acquire her property. Are these delusions? Are these auditory hallucinations? Collateral information may prove to be essential in a case such as this, particularly if the patient comes from a culture that accepts the validity of voodoo curses.

Delusional beliefs should be *fixed*. This is not to say that delusional beliefs can't evolve over time. Rather, the patient isn't swayed from her belief by any amount of rational argument to the contrary.

A 43-year-old white male farmer with schizophrenia refuses to take antipsychotic medication to treat his delusions. He states that members of the Mafia are spying on him and are trying to kill him, although he has no idea why he has been targeted for this persecution. The psychiatrist attempts to reason with him. "Would it make any sense for the Mafia to be after a farmer who never did them any harm?" The patient agrees that this appears to make little sense. The psychiatrist next asks: "Haven't you had seven hospitalizations, during each of which you have been diagnosed with schizophrenia, a condition that presents with delusional thinking? Would you at least be willing to concede that—at least in theory—this belief of yours could be a delusion? This medication is used to treat delusions, and I think you could at least try taking it and giving me the benefit of the doubt." The patient concedes that this sounds reasonable. The psychiatrist is thrilled to have made some headway. However, an hour later the patient's nurse informs him that following their interchange the patient had stated to her: "That doctor sure was interested in talking me out of things and getting me to take that pill. Maybe he works for the Mafia, too. How do I know he didn't put poison in the pill?" In this case, the patient's delusional system did evolve over time, in that it came to include the psychiatrist as well. However, the belief that he is being persecuted is fixed—that is, not subject to dissuasion through rational argument.

Finally, delusional beliefs are *idiosyncratic*. If a patient states that he believes that Jesus was the son of God and died for our sins, and that when he takes the sacrament he is ingesting the blood and body of Jesus, we would not consider him to be delusional. Similarly, a member of an extreme right-wing militia group who states that the government is taking advantage of the populace and must be overthrown by force isn't necessarily delusional, even though his views are extreme and reflect a minority opinion. (Keep in mind, though, that some members of a cult or fringe group might in fact be delusional and might have been drawn by their beliefs to the group.) Again, the best way to distinguish between a cultural or religious belief and a delusion is through the use of a collateral informant, who can educate the psychiatrist as to the typical beliefs held by members of the group.

> A 23-year-old member of the Hare Krishna is brought to the emergency room by a friend, also a Hare Krishna member. The patient expresses multiple persecutory concerns. His friend informs the psychiatrist that the patient has always "seemed a bit odd," with difficulty getting along with others. He assures the psychiatrist that while the patient's thinking contains *themes* from Krishna teaching, it also is bizarre and highly idiosyncratic.

Patients with *systematized* delusions express multiple delusions comprising a broad, all-encompassing theme. For example, a patient might report an extensive belief system involving a government plot against him involving his supervisor at work, past employers, his wife, and the hospital staff. In contrast, delusions are considered *encapsulated* when the patient appears to function normally in all other areas outside of a single, discrete delusional belief.

> During an evaluation of a child with attention-deficit hyperactivity disorder, the child's mother indicates to the psychiatrist that it might be "useful" for him to speak with the child's father privately. The father is a successful professor of sociology with no previous history of psychiatric treatment. He reports that, for the past 20 years, he has been concerned about having venereal disease, despite his having been evaluated extensively by five different physicians, with all test results having been negative. One physician actually treated

him empirically with antibiotics for a week solely to allay his fears, but to no avail. He says that he has "learned to live with it" but tells the psychiatrist that his biggest fear now is that his child doesn't actually have attention-deficit hyperactivity disorder but actually has "inherited my venereal disease." The mental status examination is otherwise completely normal, and the father has had no history of social or occupational difficulties. The psychiatrist diagnoses delusional disorder, somatic type, as indicated by his single, encapsulated, somatic delusion.

The most common delusions encountered in clinical practice are listed in Table 2.6. These include *grandiose* delusions, *persecutory* delusions, *erotomanic* delusions (i.e., that another person, usually one of higher stature, is in love with the patient), delusions of *jealousy or infidelity*, delusions of *reference* (i.e., that incidental events have special significance for the patient, whether with persecutory or grandiose themes being prominent—e.g., that benign comments by television newscasters are in reality special messages designated for the patient), delusions of *passivity* (the patient's body is being physically or mentally controlled or influenced by outside forces), and *somatic* delusions (as in the example above). Delusions are considered *bizarre* when their content is implausible and outside the realm of normal human experience (e.g., the belief that the patient's thoughts are being inserted into his head by a supercomputer through a chip implanted in his tooth during a recent surgical procedure). They are considered *nonbizarre* if they are not obviously implausible (as was the case for the sociology professor's somatic delusions). Delusions are to be distinguished from **overvalued ideas**. The latter are unreasonable and sustained idiosyncratic beliefs that are maintained with less than delusional intensity, in that the patient can acknowledge the possibility that the beliefs may not be true. Many patients with personality disorders (i.e., with chronic, inflexible ways of be-

Table 2–6. Most Common Types of Delusions

Grandiose	Jealous (infidelity)	Passivity
Persecutory	Reference	Somatic
Erotomanic		

having and of perceiving the world) hold over-valued ideas.

> A 34-year-old couple are referred for evaluation by the family court in the setting of divorce proceedings. The husband is demanding full custody of the couple's 3-year-old child, asserting that his wife is "an unfit mother." The wife, however, claims that her husband is "paranoid." Throughout the evaluation, the husband is hostile toward the psychiatrist, claiming from the outset that he is "taking my wife's side." He also states that in his opinion the judge never even should have ordered him to undergo a psychiatric evaluation, and that the judge (a woman) likely was "biased against me from the outset" from "having seen too many custody cases where the husband was physically abusive."
>
> The husband's social history reveals a long-standing pattern of never having stayed with any job for more than a few months. He typically has quit jobs following disagreements with his supervisors over some minor matter. He describes his wife as being abusive toward their child. In support of this contention, he cites one instance where his wife firmly grabbed their child and yelled at the child as he was about to run into traffic in a busy parking lot. He describes another episode where she lost her temper and yelled at their child when the child refused to get out of the car at the supermarket. He misinterprets questions by the psychiatrist throughout the interview, accusing him of "trying to get me to incriminate myself." He also comments in an intimidating way, "If you know what's best for you, you'll grant me custody."
>
> The psychiatrist makes no diagnosis in the case of the wife, but he diagnoses the husband as having a paranoid personality disorder. He recommends that the wife receive custody and that visitation by the father be supervised. In the weeks that follow, the husband pursues a frivolous lawsuit against the psychiatrist and also files a complaint with the medical board and with the psychiatrist's hospital. He sends letters to local newspapers and makes harassing telephone calls to the psychiatrist's home late at night. He asserts that the psychiatrist has "ruined my life" and is "responsible for all of my current problems."

While patient in this example is irrational, rigid, and antagonistic, he does not appear to be delusional. His stories about his wife, about his former employers, and about the psychiatrist are not clearly false (although they appear to be misleading, heavily biased in his favor). He is suspicious ("paranoid" in the colloquial sense) in his way of perceiving the world, particularly his view of authority figures, but is not "psychotic."

This example also vividly demonstrates that "dangerous" is not synonymous with "psychotic." Most patients with delusions or hallucinations do not become violent as a result (although clearly some of them do), while many nonpsychotic individual acting in response to overvalued ideas can engage in extreme acts of violence. (Factors that increase the risk of individuals becoming violent, and how clinicians go about assessing this risk, are discussed in Chapter 17.)

Finally, this case illustrates the ambiguities that clinicians encounter in their daily work and how they sometimes must "draw lines" between two syndromes (in this case between paranoid personality disorder and delusional disorder, persecutory type). Whether such lines can or should be drawn is a subject for empirical study. For example, more of the family members of patients with delusional disorder of the persecutory type turn out to have paranoid personality disorder than would have been expected based on the latter condition's overall prevalence in the population. This finding suggests that the two disorders are genetically linked and that individuals who present with paranoid delusions may simply have inherited a more severe variant of a shared disposition.

Obsessions and Compulsions

Obsessions are persistent ideas, thoughts, impulses, or images that are experienced as intrusive and inappropriate and that cause marked anxiety or distress. These thoughts are not simply *ruminations* about real-life problems. Rather, the patient typically perceives them to be "senseless." Obsessions also are not *hallucinations*, since they are thoughts and not sensory perceptions of voices. And they are not *delusions*, since the patient acknowledges the irrationality of his ideas. (Since the patient recognizes obsessional thoughts as being products of his own mind, obsessions are different from the delusion of "thought insertion" seen in schizophrenia, where the patient believes that an outside force literally is inserting bizarre thoughts into his mind).

The patient with obsessive thoughts or images or urges tries to distract himself from them, but his anxiety level continues to build despite these efforts. **Compulsions** are repetitive behaviors or mental acts that the patient engages in (often involving rigid rules) in order to reduce the anxiety associated with the obsessions. After engaging in the compulsion, the obsessional anxiety does diminish, but only temporarily. Ultimately, it always returns, and the obsessive-compulsive cycle repeats itself. These two symptoms are the hallmark of obsessive-compulsive disorder (OCD).

Patients vary in their degree of insight into this process. For most of them, the obsessions are "ego-dystonic": they clearly recognize that their obsessions have little basis in reality. Most of them also realize that the compulsive behavior does little to decrease the likelihood that the thing that they most fear actually is coming to pass. However, a subset of patients don't retain this level of insight. Anther subset has "burned out," following repeated, failed attempts to resist engaging in their compulsions. They now simply attempt to incorporate the compulsions into their daily routine (sometimes in secret), even when doing so takes up several hours of their day and is mentally exhausting.

Most doctors neglect to ask about obsessions or compulsions, which is regrettable since they occur in the general population more commonly than one might imagine and because effective treatments for OCD are available. In the 1950s, it was estimated that OCD affected only 0.05% of the population. This view remained unchallenged until the early 1980s, when investigators from the Epidemiologic Catchment Area (ECA) survey interviewed members of the general public using a structured interview and found the 6-month prevalence of OCD to be 1.6% and the lifetime prevalence 2.5%. That makes OCD more common than either bipolar disorder or schizophrenia (each of which has a lifetime prevalence of 1%).

If these symptoms are so common, why are they so rarely mentioned, even to close friends? Many patients with OCD not only worry about being labeled "crazy" if their friends knew about their symptoms, but they secretly suspect that their friends would be right. Patients often are relieved simply to be told about the diagnosis, that they aren't losing their minds, and that many other people experience similar symptoms.

Gently inquire into obsessional thoughts and compulsive behaviors by asking: "Do you ever experience thoughts that repeat over and over like a broken record?" "Do you ever have to engage in certain behaviors or rituals over and over, almost like a superstition?" If answered in the affirmative, inquire into different specific types of obsessions and compulsions.

The most common obsession is a fear of *contamination by dirt or germs*—for example, when touching doorknobs or shaking hands with others. Compulsions associated with this obsessional fear include washing or bathing repeatedly (often to the point of injury to the skin) and phobic avoidance of any contact with feared objects such as sinks or toilets. Patients who avoid going out in public due to these fears ultimately may find themselves prisoners in their own homes.

Patients also may entertain *pathological doubt*. For example, a woman may be unable to shake the fear that she has left the oven on or the door unlocked. Such people may fear taking the subway, since "it's conceivable that a stranger just might push me onto the subway tracks." Patients may fear performing specific benign actions where there is a remote probability of initiating a "domino effect" or "chain reaction," with catastrophic results. For example, a patient may fear that flipping her bedroom light switch at night ultimately might lead to her daughter becoming injured. Such patients may be quite difficult to treat, as they may worry about every possible side effect or adverse outcome of treatment contained in a medication's package insert. Associated compulsions involve the patient repeatedly "checking"—for example, checking the oven, the coffee maker, or the door locks. They do so despite knowing that they have just checked only a brief while ago and that it's unlikely that things would be any different now.

The third most common obsessions involve resisted but intrusive *aggressive or sexual thoughts*. The patient typically finds these thoughts abhorrent and therefore is not only anxious but ashamed. For example, a dignified patient may experience repetitive images of shouting out curses while in church or images of hurting a child. Some patients who initially appear to have no compulsions associated with such thoughts do admit on further questioning to engaging in *mental* compulsions to allay their anxiety. For example, they might mentally repeat short prayers, such as, "God forgive me, God forgive me, God forgive me. . . . "

The fourth most common obsession involves having an *excessive need for order or symmetry*. Patients with this obsession experience extreme anxiety unless they arrange items a "specific way." Similarly, they may spend hours bathing or eating due to the need to adhere precisely to a particular routine. When they violate some aspect of the ritual, they may feel the need to repeat the entire routine from the beginning.

Other obsessions and compulsions include: the need to mentally count or spell items they encounter; somatic preoccupations about their behavior leading to acquiring some feared disease such as AIDS or cancer (although the preoccupation is not held with delusional conviction and is recognized at least at some points as being irrational); and fears of throwing anything away. This latter anxiety can lead to pathological hoarding or collecting behavior that can become so severe that it's degree of severity can be measured by how much room to ambulate through the piles of paper remains in the patient's home.

Phobias

Phobias are marked and persistent fears of specific objects or situations. There are three main types of phobias, as summarized in Table 2–7. A **specific phobia** is a fear of a clearly discernible, circumscribed object or situation. Exposure to the phobic stimulus almost invariably provokes an immediate anxiety response, sometimes even a panic attack. Adolescents and adults with this disorder generally recognize that the fear is excessive, but children may not.

Most often, the phobic stimulus is avoided. Sometimes, though, it is painfully endured. Specific phobias are common, and in many cases the phobia is mild enough so that it does not significantly interfere with the affected individual's functioning or cause her marked distress. In such cases, one wouldn't make a clinical diagnosis.

One focus of the fear commonly associated with specific phobias is *anticipated harm* from some aspect of that particular object or situation. For example, "fear of flying" typically is not so much a fear of airplanes as it is a fear of being in an airplane that crashes; similarly, a fear of dogs or spiders may actually be a fear of being bitten by a dog or a spider, and a fear of closed-in spaces may actually entail a fear of suffocation. Another focus of fear involves concerns about the possibility of *losing control*. For example, individuals afraid of blood and injury may also fear that they will faint, those afraid of heights may fear that they will become dizzy, and those afraid of closed-in spaces may fear that they will lose control, scream, or otherwise embarrass themselves.

The most common subtypes of specific phobias, in order of descending frequency, are as follows. **Situational type phobias** (e.g., fear of tunnels, bridges, heights, driving, flying, closed-in spaces, etc.), which have a bimodal distribution with regard to their age of onset, with one peak in childhood and a second peak in the mid-20s. Next are **natural environment type phobias** (e.g., fear of storms, heights, or water), which typically have a childhood onset, followed by **blood–injection–injury type phobias** (e.g., fear of seeing blood or an injury or fear of injections or medical procedures). This latter form of phobia typically runs in families and often is accompanied by a strong vasovagal response. Finally, there are **animal type phobias**, which also typically have a childhood onset. Having one type of phobia increases the likelihood of having another phobia of that same type (e.g., fear of cats *and* snakes), and some patients also have several types of phobias.

The second main type of phobia is **agoraphobia**. This refers to a fear of, or avoidance of, places or situations either where help may not be available or where escape might prove difficult or embarrassing. Patients most commonly fear leaving the safety of their home, especially in the absence of some companion (due to the first concern). They also may fear entering public places such as buses, theaters, supermarkets, or elevators (due to the second concern).

Table 2–7. Types of Phobias

Specific phobias
  Situational type
  Natural environment type
  Blood-injection-injury type
  Animal type
  Other type (e.g., fear of choking, vomiting, or contracting
    an illness; in children, fear of loud sounds or costumed
    characters)
Agoraphobia
Social phobia

Many patients with agoraphobia previously have experienced spontaneous **panic attacks**. They then have made a mental and behavioral association between the anxiety associated with the panic attack and the situation in which the panic attack occurred. For example, if a panic attack has occurred on an elevator, the patient may avoid elevators and only take the stairs. However, if an attack subsequently occurs on the stairwell, the patient might act as if the attacks now have "spread" to the stairs as well as the elevator. He will avoid both situations, although in actuality the attacks were not related causally to either situation. The patient's range of activities thus becomes increasingly restricted.

In such cases, patients develop agoraphobia due not only to the contribution of multiple-situational-type specific phobias but also due to the contribution of **anticipatory anxiety**. In the latter, the simple anticipation of anxiety potentially occurring in some feared situation triggers anxiety and further avoidance behavior. This "fear of fear itself" often persists even after the panic attacks themselves have been treated and have not occurred in some time.

The third type of phobia is **social phobia**. Here, patients experience marked and persistent fears of social or performance situations where they might be embarrassed. Typical situations include public speaking, eating in public places, using public restrooms, or attending parties or job interviews. In such situations, they tend experience autonomic symptoms such as sweating, blushing, and dry mouth. While some patients continue to function despite these fears, others become socially isolated and suffer from severe vocational and social disability, similar to what is seen in agoraphobia. As with agoraphobia or specific phobia, anticipatory anxiety often appears days or even weeks before some feared event. Ironically, anticipatory anxiety becomes a "self-fulfilling prophecy" when it contributes to actual or perceived poor performance once in the feared situation, leading to actual embarrassment and yet further anticipatory anxiety, and so on in a positive feedback loop.

One last example may help clarify some of the above distinctions. If a patient reports that he is afraid to eat alone in a public restaurant, try to clarify whether the patient *(1)* fears choking on the food (*specific phobia*), *(2)* fears that other restaurant patrons will notice him and laugh at the way that he eats (*social phobia*), or *(3)* fears having an anxiety attack while trapped in a public place without any assistance on hand (*agoraphobia*).

Cognition

Cognition involves several areas of cortical function, including orientation to place and time, memory (immediate and delayed recall as well as memory for facts and more remote events), attention and concentration, language functioning (comprehension, repetition, naming, reading, and writing), and visuospatial and constructional skills. One standardized and reliable tool for examining these areas is the Mini-Mental State Examination, or MMSE, illustrated in Figure 2–1.

In performing the cognitive examination, use of the MMSE rather than of a more informal approach is recommended for several reasons. First, the MMSE is a widely accepted neuropsychological screening tool familiar to most clinicians. Second, it is only through the use of a standardized assessment tool that one can track a patient's cognitive status reliably over time, regardless of who is performing subsequent examinations. Third, in the absence of a formal screening assessment, mild-to-moderate cognitive deficits may go unrecognized for months or years, especially since many mildly demented patients retain appropriate social skills and family members either are not present to give collateral history indicating cognitive difficulties or are present and answer most questions for the patient. Finally, poor performance on various cognitive tasks can reflect advanced age or limited education. In such cases, clinicians may inappropriately diagnose a dementing illness. The MMSE has been normed for the general population (Table 2–8) and therefore can help to decrease diagnostic bias.

The MMSE takes about 12 minutes on average to administer to patients with dementia. Patients with intact functioning require only a few minutes. The MMSE is both a quantitative and a qualitative screening tool. The best possible score is 30 points. Scores of 23 or below fall below the range of what would be expected for the average patient with at least a fifth-grade education and need to be explained. While many such

---

MMSE Sample Items

Orientation to Time
"What is the date?"

Registration
"Listen carefully, I am going to say three words. You say them back after I stop.
Ready? Here they are...
HOUSE (pause), CAR (pause), LAKE (pause). Now repeat those words back to me."
[Repeat up to 5 times, but score only the first trial.]

Naming
"What is this?" [Point to a pencil or pen.]

Reading
"Please read this and do what it says." [Show examinee the words on the stimulus form.]
CLOSE YOUR EYES

Figure 2–1. Sample items from the Mini-Mental State Examination. From Psychological Assessment Resources, Inc., with permission. Copyright 2001 by Psychological Assessment Resources, Inc., Odessa, FL 33556.

patients have delirium or dementia, this is not invariably the case. For example, a dyslexic patient may have difficulty spelling the word *world* backward or writing a sentence. A patient with a severe tremor may have difficulty writing a sentence or copying pentagons. An uncooperative or depressed patient may refuse to attempt to recall three objects. Therefore, in reporting MMSE scores, report not only the patient's total score, but also clarify *which items* the patient missed and why.

Keep in mind how advancing age and lower levels of education can negatively influence scores. As seen in Table 2–8, elderly individuals with lesser education are more likely to score below 24 even in the absence of demonstrable brain disease. For example, the mean MMSE score of individuals with 0 to 4 years of education ranges from 19 to 25 (declining with age), whereas mean scores of those with college education range from 27 to 29 (also declining with age). Using scores from the lower quartile of different levels of education in the normal population, Cummings suggested the clinical cutoff points listed in Table 2–9.

The MMSE is a screening tool and does not constitute a substitute for more detailed neuropsychological testing. For example, an alco-

holic patient might present with isolated difficulties with short-term memory. On the MMSE, she loses only 3 points out of the total of 30 because of an inability to recall any of three items presented to her after a brief delay. While her overall score of 27 is in the "normal" range and she does not appear to have a decline in multiple areas of cognition (i.e., a dementia), she still has a clinically significant memory disturbance, likely due to amnestic disorder (see Chapter 6). Similarly, a previously high-functioning patient may score 29, but loses his one point because of a total inability to accurately copy two interlocking pentagons. An isolated construction apraxia of this type may indicate significant brain dysfunction, possibly involving the right parietal area. In both cases, more detailed neuropsychological evaluation would be indicated.

Several other caveats should be kept in mind when using the MMSE. First, the memory test is relatively easy (i.e., only three objects need be recalled after only a brief delay), is insensitive to more subtle memory problems (making the test more specific but less sensitive in detecting early dementia), and doesn't adequately assess longer-term recall. (This last item can be assessed during the exam by asking patients to

Table 2–8. Median MMSE Scores by Age and Educational Level

Educational Level	18–24	25–29	30–34	35–39	40–44	45–49	50–54	55–59	60–64	65–70	70–74	75–79	80–84	≥85	Total
0–4 Years	22	25	25	23	23	23	23	22	23	22	22	21	20	19	22
5–8 years	27	27	26	26	27	26	27	26	26	26	26	25	26	23	26
9–12 years	29	29	29	28	28	28	28	28	28	28	27	27	25	26	28
College experience or higher degree	29	29	29	29	29	29	29	29	29	29	28	28	27	27	29
Total	29	29	29	29	28	28	28	28	28	27	27	26	25	24	28

Source: Data from the Epidemiologic Catchment Area household surveys between 1980 and 1984, weighted based on the 1980 U.S. population census by age, sex, and race. Adapted with permission from Crum RM et al.: "Population-Based Norms for the Mini-Mental State Examination by Age and Educational Level." *JAMA* 269:2386–2391, 1994. Copyrighted 1994, American Medical Association.

Table 2–9. Suggested Cutoffs for the MMSE Based on Years of Education

Years of Education	Cutoff
0–4	19
5–8	23
9–12	27
13 or more	29

Source: Adapted from Cummings JL: "Mini-Mental State Examination: Norms, Normals, and Numbers." *JAMA* 269:2420–2421, 1993. Copyrighted 1993, American Medical Association.

name past presidents in reverse chronological order.) There also is no testing of whether patients are better able to recall the items after they are offered cues or when asked to picked the items out of a list (i.e., "recognition" memory, as opposed to "recall" memory).

Second, the test is relatively insensitive to impairments of executive function and therefore is less useful in detecting dementing illness where the primary pathology affects the frontal lobe or subcortical structures (e.g., head trauma, Pick's disease, Huntington's disease, and Parkinson's disease; see Chapter 6). Also, as noted above, since the MMSE emphasizes language and memory functioning, it is more insensitive to isolated right hemisphere lesions.

Third, administration of the test isn't well standardized among clinicians (as opposed to researchers), leading to some degree of variability between testers. Most notably, one clinician might ask the patient to serially subtract 7 from 100 as the concentration task, while the next might ask the patient to spell *world* backward, which is an easier task. For patients with at least a high school education I recommend routinely using the serial 7s test, as this will increase sensitivity and also provide consistency over time. Otherwise, it won't be possible for you to follow a patient's cognitive status accurately over days (e.g., over a course of electroconvulsive therapy or during the course of a resolving delirium) or years (when following a patient with Alzheimer's disease).

Despite these caveats, the MMSE overall demonstrates good inter-rater reliability and can discriminate patients with Alzheimer's disease from normal, nondemented subjects with 87% sensitivity and 82% specificity. In dementia patients it correlates with a validating study, the elec-

troencephalogram (EEG). Forty-two percent of demented patients who demonstrate marginal impairment and 65% of patients with mild to moderate impairment as measured by the MMSE are found to have abnormal EEGs. While it may miss mild, early cases of Alzheimer's disease, MMSE scores predictably decline over time by 2–3 points per year. MMSE scores at time of entry into one study significantly correlated with change in living arrangement and mortality over the following year. The MMSE has also been found to reliably detect delirium in the intensive care unit setting and to have validity in delirium in that the magnitude of decline in MMSE score correlates with the magnitude of slowing observed on the EEG.

One can supplement the MMSE with ancillary bedside neuropsychiatric tests. For example, individuals with dementia may exhibit *ideomotor apraxia* (an impaired ability to execute motor activities despite intact motor abilities, sensory function, and comprehension of the required task). Ask the patient verbally (without demonstrating) to pantomime how he would use a comb to comb his hair or use a toothbrush to brush his teeth, or how he would wave goodbye. Patients may also exhibit *agnosia* (a failure to recognize or identify objects despite intact sensory function). For example, the patient, despite normal tactile sensation, may be unable to identify a coin or a key that is placed in her hand with her eyes closed. In more severe cases, she may be unable not only to name objects such as a pencil or a chair but to recognize what these objects are used for. In the most severe cases, a patient may be unable to recognize family members or even her own reflection in the mirror. Investigation through the history and cognitive examination into impairments of *executive functioning* is beyond the scope of the current discussion but is described in more detail in Chapters 4 and 6.

Beyond performing the MMSE and any supplemental cognitive tasks, estimate the patient's overall *level of intelligence*. The most useful gauge of intelligence at the bedside is patient's use of vocabulary. You can also gain a sense during the interview of how well the patient can *think abstractly*. Supplement these observations by asking the patient to explain *similarities and differences* and to *interpret proverbs*.

For example, the clinician might ask the patient how an apple and orange are alike. The replies, "They are both round," and "You bite into an apple and you peel an orange," are both examples of more concrete thinking than that demonstrated by the reply, "They are both fruit." Similarly, when asked how a table and chair are alike, replies such as, "You sit in a chair but next to the table," and "They both have legs," both reflect more concrete thinking. You can ask how a child and midget are different, or how a river and a canal are different. When asked to interpret proverbs—for example, "People in glasses shouldn't throw stones"—a concrete interpretation would be, "If you throw stones, you might break the glass."

Insight and Judgment

Between 25% and 60% of schizophrenic patients have moderately to severely impaired "insight" into their illness. While it might seem obvious that a delusional patient, by definition, wouldn't recognize that he is delusional, insight turns out to be a complex phenomenon in that it parallels the psychotic patient's view of the world and of himself. There is wide variability in how much insight a patient may have into being ill, and some patients retain *partial insight.*

For example, the patient with schizophrenia may deny having an illness but nonetheless may voluntarily agree to sign herself into the hospital and to take medication. When asked why she would do such a thing if she doesn't have an illness, she might reply that she agrees that she "has a problem with my nerves" and that she "needs to take medications for the rest of my life." However, she still might insist that she doesn't have a mental illness, and certainly not schizophrenia. In contrast, a different patient might agree that he carries the diagnosis of schizophrenia but will deny either being delusional or needing to take medications.

In other words, "insight" is a multidimensional rather than a unitary concept. In assessing for insight, ask several questions: Does the patient have an *awareness* of having specific pathological *symptoms*? If the patient has an awareness of these symptoms, to what does he *attribute* the symptoms? Does he believe that he has an *illness*? Does he agree that he needs *treatment* for the illness? Does he agree with the need for *medications* as part of the treatment?

Interestingly, studies have shown that a pa-tient's degree of insight isn't related in a simple way to the severity of psychotic symptoms. Further, a patient's insight might fail to improve even after his psychotic symptoms have improved. Rather, the patient may no longer be delusional or hallucinating at the time of hospital discharge but still will lack insight into the fact that the experiences he described at the time of admission were false.

A patient's degree of insight has important prognostic implications. Despite improvement in their symptoms, patients with poor insight at the time of hospital discharge have a poorer prognosis. Their hospital readmission rates are higher than those for patients with better insight, and they also have a greater likelihood of being unable to live independently in the community.

PHYSICAL EXAMINATION

In the inpatient psychiatric setting, the physical examination may be performed either by the admitting psychiatrist or by another physician. In the outpatient psychiatric setting, a full medical history should be taken in order to assess for the presence of medical conditions that are responsible for (or are exacerbating) the patient's psychiatric symptoms, or that might complicate the prescribed psychiatric treatment. While the outpatient psychiatrist also might perform a physical examination, more commonly the patient is referred to her primary care physician for this. Sometimes the psychiatrist does supplement another physician's physical examination—for example, by performing a focused neurological examination when consulting on a patient presenting with impaired memory. Physical examinations may be chaperoned, particularly when they involve patients who may become distressed by the examination (e.g., patients with histories of physical or sexual abuse, or patients assessed to be at greater risk of developing erotic or delusional beliefs about the psychiatrist).

PSYCHOLOGICAL TESTING

Psychological testing provides a useful adjunct to the psychiatric history and mental status examination in selected cases. It offers several advantages, including standardization of assessment (with defined norms for different patient populations and uniformity of scoring), objectivity (quantifiable validity and reliability), and the ability to assess a broad range of attitudes and aptitudes over a relatively short period of time.

Psychological testing provides particular assistance in difficult diagnostic situations (e.g., distinguishing cognitive complaints due to Alzheimer's disease from those due to clinical depression, distinguishing emotional immaturity from mild mental retardation, distinguishing dementia due to closed head injury sustained during a motor vehicle accident from feigned cognitive complaints motivated by hopes of winning a large financial settlement). It also provides assistance in describing the patient's psychological functioning, in assisting in treatment planning and monitoring, and in psychiatric research. The two major categories of psychological tests are listed in Table 2–10, along with the most tests within each category.

Cognitive tests measure particular skills, aptitudes, and academic achievements. They are designed to measure the patient's best performance (although in the clinical setting, one must take into account the adverse impact on peformance of a negative test-taking attitude, fatigue, an illness-like depression, or sedating medications). The patient's performance is then compared to results obtained from a normative sample. The Wechsler Intelligence Scales are comprised of a range of subtests that are divided into verbal tasks and performance tasks. Verbal tasks measure the fund of general information, word knowledge, verbal rea-

soning, social judgment, arithmetic skills, and number recall, while performance tasks measure visual recognition, temporal sequencing, visual–constructive skills for both familiar objects and abstract designs, and speed of visual–motor coordination. The performance of the general population as a whole on these tests falls along a normal distribution (or bell curve, as discussed in more detail in Chapter 3), with a mean intelligence quotient (I.Q.) score of 100. The patient's overall performance relative to the general population can therefore be numerically summarized by reporting the verbal I.Q., performance I.Q., and full-scale I.Q. scores.

While intelligence is closely correlated with academic performance, **achievement tests** more specifically assess academic skills such as reading, mathematics, and written expression. When these skills fall substantially below what would be expected for the patient's age group, level of schooling, and level of intelligence, a learning disorder (e.g., a reading disorder or mathematics disorder) might be diagnosed. These disorders are discussed in greater detail in Chapter 19.

Neuropsychological tests assess more specifically for impairments in specific areas of cognitive functioning (such as attention, concentration, verbal fluency, memory, abstract reasoning and problem solving, mental flexibility, speed of information processing, and sensory and motor functioning), most commonly in the setting of brain injury. Such information can aid the clinician both in clarifying the patient's diagnosis and

Table 2–10. Commonly Employed Psychological Tests

Cognitive and Neuropsychological Measures	*Personality and Symptom Severity Measures*
INTELLIGENCE TESTS	OBJECTIVE TESTS
Wechsler Adult Intelligence Scale-III (WAIS-III) (ages 16–adult)	Minnesota Multiphasic Personality Inventory–2 (MMPI-2)
Wechsler Intelligence Scale for Children (WISC-III) (ages 6–16)	Millon Clinical Multiaxial Inventory–II (MCMI-II) Revised NEO Personality Inventory (NEO-PI-R) Beck Depression Inventory–2 (BDI-2)
ACHIEVEMENT TESTS	PROJECTIVE TESTS
Wide Range Achievement Test–3 (WRAT-3) Woodcock–Johnson Psycho-Educational Battery—Revised (W-J) Kaufman Test of Educational Achievement (K-TEA)	Rorschach Inkblot Test Thematic Apperception Test Sentence Completion Test
NEUROPSYCHOLOGICAL TESTS	SEMISTRUCTURED INTERVIEW MEASURES
Halstead-Reitan Neuropsychological Test Battery Luria–Nebraska Neuropsychological Battery	Structured Clinical Interview for *DSM-IV* (SCID) Hamilton Depression Rating Scale (HDRS) Brief Psychiatric Rating Scale (BPRS)

in identifying areas of relative strength and vulnerability, thereby facilitating treatment planning and assessment of the patient's need for additional community or educational supports. Serial testing also allows the clinician to track whether the patient's performance is improving, declining, or remaining the same over time.

Neuropsychological testing is typically conducted by a psychologist with advanced training in the administration and interpretation of these tests. While some examiners prefer to perform a standardized battery of tests (the most common being the Halstead-Reitan Battery, which can require up to 10 hours to administer), many neuropsychologists prefer to tailor the testing by selecting a variety of measures designed to address the clinical questions raised in the patient's particular case.

Personality and symptom severity measures are designed to measure longstanding personality characteristics (traits) such as histrionic, hypochondriacal, or antisocial tendencies, or current psychological symptoms (states) such as depression, anxiety, or anger. The most commonly employed test is the Minnesota Multiphasic Personality Inventory–2 (MMPI-2). It is the best-studied and most commonly performed psychological measure and is available in over 100 languages. It measures both traits and states. It is self-administered and includes a standard set of 567 true/false questions. Examples include: "I wish I could be as happy as others seem to be," "I have used alcohol excessively," and "Evil spirits possess me at times."

The tester then sorts the responses (often with the assistance of a computer) into 10 clinical scales and three "validity" scales. The latter measure the patient's test-taking attitude (e.g., exaggerating pathological symptoms, minimizing pathological symptoms, or giving responses that are socially desirable but less than candid—e.g., "I have never failed to tell the truth."). The patient's score on each scale is based on how many questions he answered a particular way (yes or no) relative to the general population. Therefore, patients reveal something about their areas of psychological strength and vulnerability relative to the general population, based upon their degree of variation along each scale. In addition, the overall pattern of responses (high scores on one or two scales relative to lower scores on the other scales) provides valuable information, as the patient's overall "profile" can be compared to typical profiles of subjects who are members of various comparison groups (such as subjects drawn from the general population, chronic pain patients, patients with schizophrenia, patients pursuing personal injury litigation, etc.) Similarly, the Revised NEO Personality Inventory (NEO-PI-R) and Millon Clinical Multiaxial Inventory II (MCMI-II) ask a variety of true/false questions, with the former test dividing responses into five major domains of personality (neuroticism, extroversion, openness, agreeableness, and conscientiousness) and the latter dividing them into symptom scales consistent with *DSM* personality disorders and clinical syndromes.

Symptom severity scales ask patients to endorse the presence (or absence) and severity of symptoms of psychiatric illness. Some measures are designed to assign *DSM* diagnoses, but these tests do not constitute a substitute for a personal diagnostic interview. Many patients with psychiatric illness have subtle forms of illness (leading to low test scores and therefore underdiagnosis) while other patients without psychiatric illness endorse nonspecific symptoms such as decreased sleep or appetite when experiencing acute distress (leading to higher test scores and an overdiagnosis of illness). Still, these tests are useful both to screen for the presence of psychiatric illness in other populations (e.g., in a medical clinic) and to rate the severity of psychiatric symptoms over time (e.g., to track improvement during psychotherapy or pharmacotherapy, or to assess the efficacy of different interventions in a research trial).

An example of a symptom inventory is the Beck Depression Inventory–2 (BDI-2). This is a self-report measure with 21 questions about cognitive, affective, and vegetative symptoms of depression. Each question has four possible answers, scored from 0 to 4, with increasing numbers indicating an increased severity of symptoms. The total score can range from 0 to 84. Scores of 0 to 9 are considered to indicate no or minimal depression; 10 to 16, mild depression; 17 to 29, moderate depression; and 30 to 63, severe depression. For example, one question asks about failure:

0: I do not feel like a failure.
1: I have failed more than I should have.
2: As I look back, I see a lot of failures.
3: I feel I am a total failure as a person.

In contrast to objective tests, **projective tests** are unstructured (i.e., patients are asked to describe what they see, rather than indicate "true" or "false." They often focus on unconscious aspects of personality. Typically patients are presented with deliberately ambiguous images. For example, in the Rorschach Test, patients are shown cards with pictures of symmetric inkblots and asked to describe what the inkblot resembles. In the Thematic Apperception Test, patients are shown cards with depictions of various scenes (for example, a boy sitting at a table looking at a violin, or an older woman standing next to a younger woman, neither looking at each other) and they are asked to create a story about the scene. In the Incomplete Sentences Test, patients are given sentence stems and asked to complete a sentence (e.g., "My greatest fear is . . . ") Two different individuals will choose to structure such unstructured stimuli in their own characteristic ways; How they do so often reveals something about their self-image, their affective style, their prominent areas of concern, how organized they are in their thinking, and how they perceive interpersonal relationships.

Semistructured interview measures are designed to parallel a clinical interview, but the questions (and follow-up questions) are standardized and the clinician uses his or her judgment to determine whether a symptom is present or absent and how severe it is along the specified rating scale. These measures are most commonly used to ensure reliable diagnostic practice in research studies, although occasionally they are used in the clinic setting. The Structured Clinical Interview for *DSM-IV* (SCID) is extensively used in psychiatric research to confirm the presence of a particular *DSM* diagnosis. When patients endorse screening questions in the affirmative, more specific follow-up questions are asked, but the latter questions otherwise can be skipped, allowing for greater efficiency. The Hamilton Depression Rating Scale (HDRS) is the most commonly used measure of the severity of depressive symptoms in research studies. Again, in contrast to the self-administered Beck Depression Inventory, the scale is designed to require professional judgment over the course of a careful interview, including observation of the patient and requests for symptom clarification.

For example, the "Depressed mood (sadness, hopeless, helpless, worthless)" item is rated as follows:

0: Absent
1: These feeling states indicated only on questioning
2: These feeling states spontaneously reported verbally
3: Communicates feeling states nonverbally—that is, through facial expression, posture, voice, and tendency to weep
4: Patient reports virtually only these feeling states in his spontaneous verbal and nonverbal communication

The Brief Psychiatric Rating Scale (BPRS) also is used to rate the severity of psychiatric symptoms, in this case following the completion of a detailed mental status examination. The clinician rates the patient's presentation in 18 areas including anxiety, emotional withdrawal, conceptual disorganization, guilt feelings, tension, motor retardation, depression, and presence and severity of psychotic symptoms. Each area is rated from 0 ("not present") to 6 ("extremely severe"). The BPRS has principally been used to rate illness severity in schizophrenia research.

Laboratory Assessment

As with the physical examination, the major goal of the laboratory assessment is to assess for the presence and the severity of medical conditions that might present with psychiatric symptoms or complicate the treatment of a "primary" psychiatric disorder. Some laboratory tests are performed as general screens for medical illness. Other more specific tests are only ordered when particular "red flags" are noted in the history, mental status examination, physical examination, or initial laboratory assessment.

Laboratory tests also are ordered prior to and during the course of treatment with some biological therapies used to treat mental illness (e.g., electroconvulsive therapy and medications such as tricyclic antidepressants, lithium, or anticonvulsant agents) and to monitor serum drug levels (to ensure that the level is high enough to be of potential therapeutic benefit but not so high as to pose a greater risk of undue toxicity).

Finally, psychiatric researchers are attempting to elucidate **biological markers** ("biomarkers") associated with various mental illnesses. Bio-markers are physiological measures that allow for making a more accurate diagnosis (equivalent to clinicians using glucose tolerance tests to diagnose occult diabetes or cardiac enzyme assays to confirm the presence of myocardial infarction), or for predicting whether a patient might respond better to one particular treatment than to another, or for identifying patients at greater risk developing a psychiatric disorder in the future (similar to genetic tests currently available to family members of patients with Huntington's disease who carry a genetic risk of developing the disease but do not current demonstrate any of the identifying clinical symptoms).

Some authors advocate obtaining ancillary laboratory studies only when the patient's psychiatric presentation is "atypical" or particularly suggestive of a possible medical etiology. Examples of the latter type of presentation include: later onset of symptoms (e.g. after age 40); symptoms consistent with a possible Delirium (e.g., waxing and waning level of consciousness, impaired attention, visual or tactile hallucinations) or of possible Dementia (evidence of cognitive impairment); a medical history notable for med-

Table 2–11. Common Psychiatric Screening Tests

Serum electrolytes, glucose, blood urea nitrogen (BUN), creatinine
Serum chemistry panel (including hepatic enzymes)
Complete blood count (CBC)
Thyroid-stimulating hormone (TSH) assay, or full thyroid panel
Serum vitamin B_{12} level
Urine toxicology screen

ical illnesses associated with psychiatric symptoms or of medications associated with psychiatric side-effects; a history of alcohol or drug abuse; a family history of degenerative neurologic illness or of metabolic diseases associated with psychiatric symptoms; or an abnormal neurologic exam. Other authors have advocated that certain screening tests routinely be performed whenever patients present with the first onset of psychiatric symptoms (e.g., depression, anxiety, or psychotic symptoms), since these may be the earliest appearing manifestations (or even the only manifestations) of an otherwise occult medical condition. The most commonly performed laboratory screening tests are listed in Table 2–11. Some commonly performed supplemental tests are listed in Table 2–12.

Table 2–12. Common Supplemental Laboratory Tests

Test	Typical Indications
Urinalysis	Assesses for renal failure, urinary tract infection, diabetes, and dehydration, which can be associated with delirium and worsening of cognition or behavioral disturbance in dementia
Pulse oximetry	Assesses for hypoxia, which can contribute to delirium or dementia; oximetry performed during sleep assesses for sleep apnea
Neuroimaging (computerized tomography [CT] or magnetic resonance imaging [MRI] scan)	Assess for cerebrovascular disease, tumor, brain trauma, bleeding in delirium, dementia, and atypical psychiatric presentation. CT is less expensive, more rapid (useful for claustrophobic patients), and useful for detecting acute bleeding. MRI offers absence of exposure to radiation and contrast dye, superior resolution, and better visualization of small ischemic lesions, demyelinating lesions, and vascular malformations. Contraindicated in patients with pacemakers or ferromagnetic foreign bodies. Magnetic Resonance angiography (MRA), often performed with MRI, is useful in assessing for presence of aneurysm, vascular malformations or occlusions, or changes suggestive of vasculitis
Electroencephalogram (EEG)	Assesses for seizure activity, focal slowing associated with brain lesion, diffuse slowing associated with hypoactive delirium or advanced dementia, low-voltage fast activity associated with hyperactive delirium, and other specific patterns suggestive of particular diseases (e.g., diffuse, periodic, symmetric, sharp or triphasic slow waves in Creutzfeldt-Jakob disease). EEG during sleep (polysomnography) useful in assessment of sleep disorders *(continued)*

Table 2–12. Common Supplemental Laboratory Tests (*Continued*)

Test	Typical Indications
Screening test for syphilis (RPR or VDRL)	Syphilis can present with psychosis, mood lability, and dementia. A positive serum rapid plasma reagin (RPR) test should be followed by the more specific fluorescent treponemal antibody absorption (FTA-ABS) test. A CSF venereal disease research laboratory (VDRL) test is used to diagnose tertiary or CNS syphilis
Erythrocyte sedimentation rate (ESR)	Nonspecific sign of inflammation, elevated in autoimmune disease, infection. Decreased in anorexia nervosa, and so potentially useful in distinguishing this from wasting illness)
Antinuclear antibodies (ANA)	Seen in systemic lupus erythematosus (SLE), sometimes associated with cognitive decline, psychotic symptoms, or mood changes. Positive test confirmed with more specific antinuclear and anti-DNA antibody assays
Human immunodeficiency virus serology (HIV)	HIV can present with mood changes, psychotic symptoms, or dementia, even preceding other manifestations. Positive enzyme-linked immunoabsorbent assay (ELISA), because of risk of false-positive, must be confirmed by Western blot analysis
Urine heavy metal screen	Lead, mercury, manganese, aluminum, and arsenic toxicity can present with cognitive symptoms, fatigue, psychotic symptoms
Screening for acute intermittent porphyria	Autosomal dominant disorder of heme synthesis that can cause depression, panic attacks, or psychotic symptoms, even in the absence of "classic" symptoms (abdominal pain with nausea and headache, polyneuropathy, autonomic dysfunction, seizures, delirium). Attacks may be precipitated by barbiturates or tricyclic antidepressants. During acute attacks, urine uroporphyrin, porphobilinogen (PBG), and aminolevulinic acid (ALA) concentrations may be elevated
Screening for Wilson's disease	Autosomal recessive disorder of impaired copper clearance, leading to progressive accumulation of copper in brain, liver, heart, bone, eyes. First presents in teens and 20s with mood and personality changes and extrapyramidal movement disorder. Urine and serum copper are elevated and serum ceruloplasmin (which binds copper) is low
Screening for cardiac and pulmonary disease (electrocardiogram [ECG] and chest X-ray [CXR])	Cardiac and pulmonary disease can present with fatigue or anxiety, but they also can complicate psychiatric treatment with tricyclic antidepressants, lithium, antipsychotic agents, or electroconvulsive therapy (all of which can precipitate cardiac arrhythmia)
Single photon emission tomography (SPECT) or positron emission tomography (PET) studies	Rarely used in clinical settings. Findings noted in populations of patients with many psychiatric disorders neither sensitive nor specific enough to allow for confirmation or diagnosis. Some clinicians use to assess etiology of dementia. (On SPECT and and PET scans, focal or patchy hypoperfusion suggests vascular dementia; bilateral temporoparietal hypoperfusion suggests Alzheimer's disease)
Lumbar puncture	Used when psychiatric symptoms are accompanied by signs of meningeal inflammation or other symptoms suggestive of meningitis

SUMMARY

The study of psychopathology involves the delineation of specific types of thoughts, feelings, and behaviors out of the multitude of thoughts, feelings, and behaviors that comprise mental life. These then are labeled as "symptoms." If symptoms are the ingredients, clinical syndromes are the recipes. One can't cook without understanding how to obtain the best ingredients. Therefore, the goal of the current discussion has been to provide guidelines for conducting the clinical evaluation while also offering a basic lexicon of the most common symptoms of psychopathology.

A rich description of the patient's presentation

should always precede any attempt at explanation. The deeper you delve into the phenomenology of your patients' inner worlds, and the clearer you can be in describing what you find there, the deeper will be your empathic understanding (from the point of view of function) and the more accurately you can assign an appropriate clinical diagnosis (from the point of view of form).

At this point you now have the tools necessary to interview a psychiatric patient. However, once you have interviewed the patient and elicited a variety of different symptoms, you will find that these symptoms are a mixed bag. There appear to be different *types* of symptoms. Now that we have described the phenomenon, can we explain it? It is here, in the realm of the clinical formulation, that psychiatry becomes confusing for most students, and even for many seasoned clinicians. The psychiatric formulation is the subject of the next chapter.

Chapter 3

Psychiatric Formulation from Multiple Perspectives

We have interviewed a patient and have obtained a wide array of data: historical information, evidence of the patient's interpersonal style of functioning, current symptoms and signs suggesting a possible superimposed illness. How do we *use* this data to formulate the case? The *DSM-IV*, being atheoretical, offers guidelines for description but not for explanation. Here is an example of one patient encountered in clinical practice:

Chief complaint: A 14-year-old female is brought in for evaluation by her parents, who are concerned about her social withdrawal and lack of weight gain. After initial consultation, she is admitted to an inpatient eating disorders unit, where the following history is obtained.

Psychiatric history: She has no previous psychiatric history. The present symptoms had their onset about 1 year prior to admission, when the patient received braces and her orthodontist recommended that she avoid eating candy. At that point she became more anxious about her diet and began to exclude a variety of foods. During the present school year, she has become interested in vegetarianism and has avoided any red meat or "fatty" foods. After she lost several pounds, friends initially complimented her on her appearance and she appeared to be happy about this. However, over the past few months, her parents have noted her to appear less happy than usual, more withdrawn, and more tired. She has lost even more weight over the

past few months and has told her parents that she "feels fat." During the current evaluation, she states that she tries to eat less than 1000 calories per day. She denies having used laxatives, diuretics, or diet pills and denies engaging in binging behavior. Over the past few months, she has increased her amount of aerobic exercise to 2 hours daily. She thinks about food "all of the time," feels that her ideal weight would be 65 pounds, and notes that the thinner she gets the better she feels about herself. Later in the interview, though, she admits to having felt increasingly sad over the past several months. She often becomes tearful, has experienced more difficulty falling and staying asleep, has lower energy, and has more difficulty concentrating in class. (Her grades in school have declined from A's to C's.) She also takes less pleasure in activities that she formerly enjoyed, such as going to the movies with friends.

Premorbid personality: Her parents describe her as hard working and conscientious, a "perfectionist" about her schoolwork. As a small child she always preferred to do things "her own way." She has gotten along well with other children but has tended to associate with a small circle of friends. Until this past year, she has tended to be a happy child, but over the past school year her parents have noted a clear change in her temperament. She has been more sad, more of a worrier, and more irritable.

Social history: The patient is the product of a normal delivery and had normal developmental milestones. She and her parents deny any history of childhood behavioral problems, and she denies any history of having experienced physical or emotional abuse. She is currently in the seventh grade. She has been a straight A student in a program for gifted students until this year, when she became so concerned about maintaining her A average that her mother requested that she be returned to regular classes. She has been active in ballet and is an officer in several school clubs. She is not sexually active and has never dated. She has not reached menarche, and she describes herself as "not looking forward" to this. She denies having used nicotine, alcohol, or illicit drugs and she has no legal history.

Medical history: She denies any history of medical problems. She is taking no medications. She has no history of drug allergies.

Family history: Both parents are in their mid-40s. Her father is a university professor and her mother is an office manager in a medical practice Her father drank heavily for about 20 years but has been abstinent for the past 5 years. Her mother has a history of having become more depressed several years ago and she was treated at that time with antidepressant medication to good effect. Her parents divorced when she was 5 years old, in large part because of her father's drinking. Both parents have remarried. They still sometimes argue about child support and visitation issues. The patient lives with her mother and stepfather. She describes a good relationship with both parents and stepparents. Her mother describes their relationship as a very close one, and the patient describes how after her parent's divorce she felt that she had to "take care of" her mother. The family history is otherwise notable for alcoholism in two paternal uncles and possible depression in her maternal grandmother.

Mental Status Examination: The patient appears extremely thin and younger than her age. Despite it being warm outside, she is wearing a bulky sweatshirt. She speaks quietly and demonstrates a paucity of spontaneous speech and movement. There is no evidence of formal thought disorder. She describes her mood as "bored." Her observed affect is one of sadness. She describes a lowered self-attitude, including worries that she is being "too hard on my parents" and is a "burden on them." She describes a change in vital sense, including lowered energy and a feeling of detachment from other people. She denies suicidal ideation. She denies having experienced hallucinations or delusions. While she also denies obsessions or compulsions, she does describe constant thoughts about food and constant fears of becoming overweight as well as a compulsive need to strictly monitor her caloric intake. She believes herself to be "fat," and when the examiner holds her very skinny wrist next to his own wrist (which she does not believe to be "fat") and asks her whether her wrist looks "fat" in comparison to his, she says that it does. Her score on the Mini-Mental State Examination score is 29, due to her forgetting one of three items upon delayed recall. She had no insight into her problems, and she states that her career goal is to become either a nutritionist or a physician.

Physical exam: She is 5'2" and weighs 70 pounds. Heart rate is 52 and blood pressure is 90/40. She is at Tanner stage 2–3 for breast development, axillary hair, and genital development.

Laboratory studies: Her complete blood count is notable for microcytic anemia, while her chemistry panel demonstrates hypokalemia, decreased serum protein and albumin levels, and low serum iron.

Consistent with our discussion of form and function in Chapter 1, one can see how this patient presents as both a unique individual who is in a state of distress and as a person who demonstrates the symptoms of several operationally defined conditions. Using *DSM-IV* operational criteria, this patient can be described as follows:

Axis I: Anorexia nervosa
         Major depressive disorder, single episode, moderate
Axis II: Obsessive–compulsive personality disorder
Axis III: Malnutrition; amenorrhea; hypokalemia; iron-deficiency anemia
Axis IV: Problems with primary support group; educational problems
Axis V: GAF 35

While these criteria allow us to reliably *describe* this patient's symptoms and life difficulties, how are we to *explain* them? For this, we require an *explanatory conceptual framework.* Take, for example, the diagnosis of anorexia nervosa. The patient's symptoms fulfill the diagnostic criteria for this condition because she *(1)* is refusing to maintain a body weight that is at or above the minimally normal weight for her age and height; *(2)* has an intense fear of gaining weight or becoming fat, despite being underweight; *(3)* has a distorted image of her body's weight and shape; and *(4)* is amenorrheic.

But *why* is this patient thinking and acting this way? Should we view her symptoms through the prism of her *life story*, as the expressions of a person in distress, best understood by her past and current life experiences? Or should we view her as having a *biological disease*—that is, a breakdown in the structure or function of some bodily part? Or do eating problems reflect a difficulty in *regulating her behavior*, leading to an "addictive" behavior pattern similar to that seen in patients who have difficulty regulating their intake of alcohol? Finally, should we perhaps view her symptoms as the reflection of several underlying *personality vulnerabilities*, such as her chronic tendency toward excessive perfectionism and self-criticism?

Each of these four conceptual approaches to case formulation requires us to view the patient from a particular theoretical *perspective*. Each perspective brings some aspects of her presentation to the foreground but does so at the expense of relegating other aspects to the background. Unfortunately, some clinicians, due to varying personal backgrounds and professional training experiences, approach patients from only one or the other of these vantage points. Since each perspective is grounded in a different fundamental logic, clinicians from different theoretical schools can end up disagreeing with each other as to which form of treatment is the "best" for a given patient.

For example, if we view this patient's self-starvation primarily as a pathological, addictive *behavioral disturbance*, our primary treatment intervention will be to attempt to discourage her from engaging in this behavior and to encourage more appropriate eating behavior. (This is the way that we approach severe alcoholism. Exploratory psychotherapy tends to be ineffective for patients in the midst of severe alcohol dependence. The primary initial intervention is to offer "detoxification" and to encourage abstinence, thereby interrupting the cycle of inappropriate drinking behavior. Subsequent treatment then focuses on helping the patient to maintain abstinence behavior.)

In contrast, if we view this patient's self-starvation as a reflection of an underlying *disease process*, we will be less concerned with preventing her from engaging in starvation behavior than with addressing the underlying bio-

logical factors that have brought about her pathologic behaviors. An adherent to a pure disease perspective would consider the behavioral approach to be superficial in that it attempts to address the surface phenomena while failing to address the underlying biological pathology.

In contrast, a pure behaviorist would consider the patient's behavior to be the pathology, and would add that—even if biological factors do *contribute* to her aberrant behavior—a variety of other factors such as personality traits or culture may be equally if not more important contributors. Therefore, the behavioral theorist would view the disease approach as superficial, reductionistic, and naïve.

Now into this debate enters the psychoanalytically oriented psychotherapist, who views the patient from the perspective of her life story. The therapist sees the patient's eating behavior as the conscious behavioral expression of, or defense against, underlying unconscious psychological conflicts. Given this, the psychotherapist might view both the disease and behavioral approaches as superficial, Band-Aid fixes, prescribing pills or restricting behaviors while minimizing or even ignoring these deeper psychological issues.

Can we simply integrate these competing viewpoints into one, "holistic," "biopsychosocial" formulation? Unfortunately, this is easier said than done. As the above example demonstrates, one can't truly integrate approaches that rely on completely different causal assumptions. A better approach is to study each approach separately, to learn about their underlying *logics* (or rules) and to remain mindful of their respective advantages and liabilities in applying them to a given patient. The savvy clinician, in formulating a case, doesn't attempt to integrate these perspective. Rather, she shifts back and forth between them and does so *consciously* rather than haphazardly, recognizing that in doing so she is removing one pair of conceptual "colored lenses" and replacing them with a pair of a different color.

Following the approach of McHugh and Slavney, this text utilizes four conceptual perspectives as the "conceptual scaffolding" for patient formulation. These are (1) the *disease perspective*, (2) the *dimensional perspective*, (3) the *behavior perspective*, and (4) the *life-story perspective*. This chapter explores the logic of each perspective. In doing so, it also offers an introduction to the most commonly encountered psychiatric syndromes. Note that while any psychiatric illness is capable of being viewed from any of the perspectives, some conditions lend themselves more naturally to being viewed primarily from one particular perspective.

THE DISEASE PERSPECTIVE

Underlying Logic

The disease perspective proposes that—despite individual variation—there are categories, or classes, of patients who have symptoms that distinguish them from the general population. This view stands in contrast to our everyday assumption that "people are basically all the same."

Medical writers have disagreed about the definition of "disease." Some have used the term synonymously with the term "clinical syndrome." When used this way, the clinical syndrome alcoholism could be called a disease since alcoholism is associated with a typical pattern of symptoms, progression over time, and prognosis. Here, however, we will define disease more narrowly as *a breakdown in the structure or function of a bodily part.*

When using this definition, it is readily apparent that not all clinical syndromes are diseases. Virtually everything we treat in psychiatry is a "syndrome" (or, to use *DSM* terminology, a "disorder"). In Chapter 1, we began with the example of an 18-year-old student who became depressed following a breakup with his girlfriend, who was diagnosed by the psychiatrist as having an adjustment disorder. The *DSM-IV* operationally defines the syndrome of adjustment disorder as the development of emotional or behavioral symptoms in response to an identifiable stressor (or stressors), occurring within 3 months of the onset of the stressor(s), with the symptoms or behaviors being "clinically significant" (as evidenced by either marked distress in excess of what would be expected from exposure to the stressor or by significant impairment in social or occupational or academic functioning). Adjustment disorder also is a "diagnosis of exclusion"; in other words, patients only are diagnosed as having adjustment disorder if they don't also meet the diagnostic criteria for another primary

disorder such as major depressive disorder or schizophrenia.

This doesn't sound like the definition of a biological disease. Note that denying that patients with adjustment disorder have a disease is not equivalent to concluding that they do not suffer. For example, the student described in Chapter 1 does appear to be suffering and likely even has a higher risk of dying by suicide than the average person. This patient also benefited from psychiatric treatment (in this case, psychotherapy). Disorders don't have to be diseases to benefit from treatment. Given this, if the only perspective psychiatrists used were the disease perspective, we would have little to offer many patients.

Using the disease perspective, our understanding of the pathophysiology of any disease advances in three stages. First, a *clinical syndrome* is identified. In other words, a group of patients with similar subjective symptoms or objective clinical signs is distinguished from the unaffected or "normal" population. Second, the affected group is compared to the unaffected group, using tools such as epidemiologic information, bacterial cultures, serologic tests, and radiographic studies in an attempt to identify an underlying *pathological disease entity*. Finally, once the pathological disease entity has been identified, it becomes the object of further study aimed at identifying its *etiology* (i.e., the agent responsible for causing this particular pathology).

While the approach from function is not irrelevant from the disease perspective (obviously, it is important to empathize with patients who are affected by a disease), the disease perspective relies *primarily* on the approach from form. As discussed in Chapter 1, when using the approach from form, observation and classification always precede attempts at explanation. Clinicians engage in the process of *differential diagnosis*, whereby they generate a list of potential etiologies for a patient's clinical presentation, remaining mindful that similar clinical syndromes can be caused by more than one pathology and that a given pathology can have more than one possible etiology.

For example, consider the clinical syndrome of "congestive heart failure" (Fig. 3–1). Common symptoms include dyspnea, fatigue, and cachexia and common clinical signs include jugular venous distension, pulmonary rales, dull-

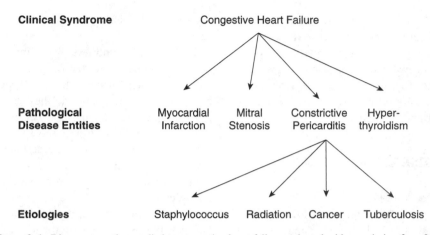

Figure 3–1. Disease reasoning applied to congestive heart failure. Adapted with permission from McHugh PR, Slavney PR: *The Perspectives of Psychiatry*, 2nd edition. Baltimore, Johns Hopkins University Press, 1998.

ness to percussion over the lung bases, and dependent edema. Findings on chest X-ray include an enlarged cardiac silhouette, distention of pulmonary veins with redistribution to the apices, and pulmonary effusion. The same syndrome can be caused by multiple forms of pathology, including myocardial infarction, mitral stenosis, constrictive pericarditis, and hyperthyroidism. The prognosis and treatment plan for congestive heart failure will vary based upon the underlying pathology that is discovered through the diagnostic workup. For a given pathology, further investigation may reveal the etiology. For example, constrictive pericarditis can be caused by inflammation due to an infectious agent (such as staphylococcus, meningococcus, or tuberculosis), radiation, trauma, metastatic cancer, or connective tissue disease. When no etiology is discernable, the etiology is deemed to be idiopathic.

Modern disease reasoning dates back to the seventeenth century when Thomas Sydenham argued that theories of disease etiology based on "vital energies," excesses or deficiencies of "nervous energy," and the like (which led to treatments such as blood-letting and cathartics), were unsupported and that bedside observation and distinguishing between various syndromes must precede attempts at explanation. He offered detailed descriptions of syndromes such as malaria, scarlet fever, chorea, gout, and congestive failure (dropsy) and demonstrated that malaria could be treated with quinine obtained from cinchona bark.

The power of this model in the modern day is dramatically demonstrated by the case of the acquired immune deficiency syndrome (AIDS). In 1981, a clinical syndrome was identified among homosexual males. It consisted of life-threatening opportunistic infection, or Kaposi's sarcoma, or both. The syndrome developed in previously healthy individuals and was accompanied by laboratory evidence of cellular immunodeficiency. Once the clinical syndrome was identified epidemiologic studies were conducted, which demonstrated that the syndrome appeared to be propagated through the exchange of blood or bodily fluids and also demonstrated that recipients of blood and blood products (including hemophiliacs) and intravenous drug abusers were also at higher risk of contracting the disease. The eventual pathology was determined to be a loss of T4 cells. By 1984 (only 3 years later), it was discovered that the etiology for this syndrome was a retrovirus later called the human immunodeficiency virus (HIV). By the end of that year an assay had been developed to detect the presence of the virus, thereby confirming the clinical diagnosis and allowing for screening of blood transfusion products. Since then, clinical treatment of patients infected with the HIV virus has shifted from merely treating the complications of the virus to rational therapy—that is, the use of drugs that target the virus itself.

Psychiatric Applications

Most physicians are comfortable applying disease reasoning to psychiatric conditions because it is so familiar from their medical training. Several psychiatric conditions clearly are diseases. Not only have the clinical syndromes been identified but the process of clinicopathologic correlation has progressed to the point where their clinical presentations have been linked to known pathologies (although their ultimate etiologies may remain uncertain). These syndromes include delirium and dementia. Both of these clinical syndromes are characterized by a *loss of normal mental capacities* (such as consciousness or memory), sometimes accompanied by the *appearance of new forms of mental phenomena* (such as hallucinations or delusions).

For example, the syndrome of **delirium** is characterized by a *change in the level of consciousness and in the ability to sustain attention*. The deficits tend to wax and wane, ranging from normal (or even hypervigilant) through drowsiness, stupor, or coma. While delirious patients may exhibit other clinical symptoms such as a decline in cognition (as in dementia), changes in mood (as in mood disorder), or hallucinations and delusions (as in schizophrenia), the changes in the level of consciousness and attention are the hallmark features.

As might be imagined, given these patients' global impairments, the *pathology* in delirium involves widespread decreases in cerebral metabolic activity. As was the case for congestive heart failure, the pathological state is a "final common pathway" that can be caused by multiple *etiologies*, including infection, substance intoxication or withdrawal, endogenous or exogenous toxins, brain trauma, stroke, hypoxia, liver failure, renal failure, or dehydration. As was the case for heart failure, sometimes the etiology is idiopathic, but this does not change the fact that the patient has a delirium, since the diagnosis is made on clinical grounds. (In other words one shouldn't change the diagnosis from delirium to schizophrenia upon finding that the results of various clinical studies were all "normal." The presence of some underlying deliriogenic process can still be inferred.)

The theory that delirium is a disease has been *validated* in multiple domains. The electroencephalogram (EEG), which measures regional cerebral activity, usually demonstrates global slowing of activity in a degree proportional to the extent of the observed decline in the patient's level of consciousness. This is demonstrated in Figure 3–2. Further, laboratory findings characteristic of the underlying medical etiology typically are present, such as a CAT scan of the brain indicating the presence of a stroke or serologic testing confirming the presence of liver or renal failure. Delirium is discussed in greater detail in the Chapter 5.

A second psychiatric syndrome that clearly appears to be a disease is **dementia**. The clinical syndrome of dementia is operationally defined as a *global decline in cognition from a previous level, in clear consciousness*. Again, one can see associated changes in mood or hallucinations in patients with dementia, but the defining disturbance is the decline in cognition. The cognitive decline is a *global* one, which distinguishes dementia from isolated neuropsychological deficit syndromes such as isolated amnesia (memory deficit, which in isolation would constitute an amnestic syndrome), aphasia (language deficit), or agnosia (recognition deficit). In dementia, the cognitive disturbance represents a *decline* from a previously higher level, which distinguishes dementia from **mental retardation**, which is lifelong and is not progressive. (Note that patients with mental retardation can develop a superimposed dementia later in life, as occurs in Down's syndrome, where patients develop Alzheimer's disease at an earlier age than is typical in the general population.)

As with delirium, dementia can be caused by a variety of *pathologies*. These include Alzheimer's Disease, cerebrovascular disease, brain tumor, subdural hematoma, vitamin deficiencies (such as with vitamin B_{12}), endocrine conditions (such as hypothyroidism), infection of the brain or meninges (for example, with HIV virus or syphilis), and other, less common, pathologies. The syndrome therefore is validated through serologic studies, radiographic studies, and even (although rarely) brain biopsy.

The *etiology* of these various pathologies is the subject of active investigation. For example, postmortem studies of the brains of patients who have died with Alzheimer's disease reveal characteristic plaques and neurofibrillary tangles, but the etiology of these lesions remains uncertain. As was the case with delirium, the treatment that a patient with dementia receives depends upon the pathology and etiology of his illness. For example, dementia due to hypothyroidism is treated

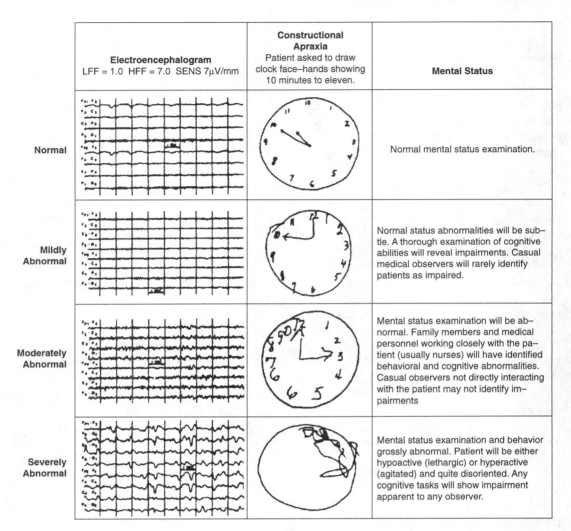

	Electroencephalogram LFF = 1.0 HFF = 7.0 SENS 7μV/mm	Constructional Apraxia Patient asked to draw clock face–hands showing 10 minutes to eleven.	Mental Status
Normal			Normal mental status examination.
Mildly Abnormal			Normal status abnormalities will be sub-tle. A thorough examination of cognitive abilities will reveal impairments. Casual medical observers will rarely identify patients as impaired.
Moderately Abnormal			Mental status examination will be ab-normal. Family members and medical personnel working closely with the pa-tient (usually nurses) will have identified behavioral and cognitive abnormalities. Casual observers not directly interacting with the patient may not identify im-pairments
Severely Abnormal			Mental status examination and behavior grossly abnormal. Patient will be either hypoactive (lethargic) or hyperactive (agitated) and quite disoriented. Any cognitive tasks will show impairment apparent to any observer.

Figure 3–2. Correlation between EEG, cognition, and level of consciousness in delirium. Reproduced with with permission from Trzepacz PT, Wise MG: "Neuropsychiatric Aspects of Delirium." *American Psychiatric Press Textbook of Neuropsychiatry*, 3rd edition. Washington, DC, American Psychiatric Press, 1997.

by providing supplemental synthetic thyroid hormone. In contrast, this treatment is not effective for the patient with dementia due to Alzheimer's disease.

Disorders such as delirium and dementia demonstrate the greatest strength of the disease method, which is the potential for discovering *rational therapies*—that is, treatments designed specifically to redress an underlying etiology. For example, the primary goal of research into the etiology of Alzheimer's disease is to discover a therapy that doesn't simply treat the behavioral or emotional symptoms of the illness but that arrests or reverses the disease process itself, or

even offers primary prevention against ever developing Alzheimer's disease (through vaccination, for example.)

In contrast to rational therapy, most of the currently available treatments in psychiatry are *empirical therapies*—that is, therapies serendipitously discovered to be useful despite an unclear mechanism of action. For example, in 1957, patients treated for tuberculosis with iproniazid were noted to experience improvement in their mood, particularly in the case of patients suffering from clinical depression. Not surprisingly, when iproniazid and related agents were discovered to elevate brain levels of serotonin through the inhibition of monoamine oxidase, the theory that clinical depression might reflect a serotonin deficiency state quickly followed, and the role of serotonin in psychiatric illness remains the subject of extensive investigation even a half century later.

For several other syndromes encountered in psychiatry, the disease perspective appears apt, despite continued uncertainty about their underlying pathology and etiology. These include the **mood disorders** and **schizophrenia**. The clearest evidence that these conditions are diseases is the fact that in their most severe forms they include symptoms that are beyond the realm of normal human experience. These symptoms, called **psychotic symptoms**, include **hallucinations, delusions**, and **thought disorder**. Further validating evidence includes family and twin studies (which suggest that genetic factors likely play a contributory role) and endocrine, neurotransmitter, and neuroimaging studies (which suggest the presence of associated biological abnormalities).

While these findings are tantalizing, definitive pathologic findings remain elusive. Given this, there are no "gold standard" ancillary tests available to confirm or refute the presence of these conditions. The clinician determines them to be present almost entirely on clinical grounds (i.e., through the history and mental status examination).

Mood disorder (bipolar disorder, major depressive disorder, or dysthymic disorder) is defined by the presence of a *pathological change in mood* (either depressed or elevated). The change in mood generally occurs in clear consciousness (distinguishing it from delirium) and without a significant change in cognition (distinguishing it from dementia). While psychotic symptoms (hallucinations, delusions, or thought disorder) also might be seen, the change in mood is the hallmark feature.

Patients in the midst of a mood disorder often describe mood fluctuations that feel qualitatively different from those that occur in the course of everyday life. Mood states tends to be excessive, pervasive, and unrelated to recent life events. The changes in mood are accompanied by changes in one's self-attitude and by vegetative symptoms. (These symptoms are described in greater detail in Chapter 2; theories of pathology and etiology are discussed further in Chapter 7.)

Schizophrenia is defined operationally as the presence of psychotic symptoms, in clear consciousness, without a prominent decline in cognition and without a significant change in mood. Thus, schizophrenia is a diagnosis of exclusion made when psychotic symptoms occur in the absence of delirium, dementia, or mood disorder. While some particular psychotic symptoms (e.g., bizarre delusions involving one's body being controlled by alien forces) are more *suggestive* of schizophrenia than of delirium, dementia, or mood disorder, none of these symptoms is *pathognomonic* of schizophrenia.

In summary, certain conditions in psychiatry present with symptoms that are outside the realm of normal human experience that therefore constitute presumptive evidence of underlying disease processes. These symptoms include impaired consciousness, impaired cognition, impaired regulation of mood, and psychotic symptoms. Clinicians faced with patients who demonstrate such symptoms employ a diagnostic hierarchy. Any of these symptoms can be seen in delirium, but the hallmark feature of delirium is a change in the patient's level of consciousness and attention. When these features aren't present, consider next the diagnosis of dementia. The hallmark feature of dementia is a global decline in cognition from a previous level. When cognition is relatively unaffected, consider mood disorder, where the hallmark feature is a pathologic change in mood, typically accompanied by changes in self-attitude and vital sense. When impaired consciousness, cognition, and regulation of mood are not the primary features but the patient still presents with psychotic symptoms, consider schizophrenia.

Delirium is considered the *supraordinate* diagnosis since a delirious patient can exhibit symptoms of any of the other conditions. Dementia comes next, followed by mood disorder, and then schizophrenia. Why not reverse this order? For example, why not decree that delirium should only be diagnosed in the absence of all of the other conditions and make schizophrenia the supraordinate diagnosis? The rationale for the present diagnostic hierarchy is grounded in both theoretical and practical considerations. In addition to delirium being associated with the greatest degree of overall cortical dysfunction, it also is associated with significant, acute morbidity such that the implications of overlooking it are the greatest. Also, the presence of delirium always reflects some underlying medical pathology, but this pathology will only be addressed through rational therapy if delirium is recognized.

Similarly, why diagnose mood disorder more broadly than schizophrenia? Again, specific treatments available for the treatment of mood disorder that usually aren't given to patients with schizophrenia. For example, major depressive disorder with psychotic features usually is treated with the combination of an antipsychotic medication and an antidepressant medication, while a psychotic manic episode due to bipolar disorder usually is treated with the combination of an antipsychotic medication and a mood-stabilizing medication such as lithium carbonate. In contrast, when schizophrenia is diagnosed, most commonly an antipsychotic drug alone is prescribed.

Given this, while placing mood disorder above schizophrenia in the diagnostic hierarchy may lead to some patients who actually have schizophrenia mistakenly being diagnosed with mood disorder and being placed on an antidepressant drug or lithium, it is probably better to err on this side than to deprive patients who actually have mood disorder but are mistakenly diagnosed with schizophrenia from receiving potentially useful treatment interventions.

This algorithm obviously represents an oversimplification. Here are some caveats, to be elaborated upon further in future chapters as we discuss specific disorders.

First, patients with *dementia, mood disorders, or schizophrenia* certainly are not "immune" from also developing a superimposed *delirium*. For example, a patient with bipolar disorder who has become depressed might overdose on lithium and then become delirious due to lithium toxicity. How does the clinician determine if a delirious patient also has another psychiatric condition, such as mood disorder or schizophrenia? Sometimes he can do so based on a through review of the patient's longitudinal history; a single, cross-sectional mental status examination is less useful since acutely delirious patients may display symptoms commonly seen in these other conditions. In any case, the first goal is to treat the delirium. Following this, assess for whether other psychiatric symptoms remain.

Second, patients with *dementia* are particularly prone to developing a superimposed *delirium* since they can be particularly sensitive to even minor pathological insults. A history of pre-existing cognitive decline in the patient with delirium suggests that this is the case. Again when delirium is present, treat this first and then assess for the present of an underlying, predisposing dementia.

Third, patients with *dementia* often experience not only cognitive deficits but impairments in their ability to regulate mood, leading to *major depressive episodes*. Since clinical depression can exacerbate cognitive and behavioral impairments, one should address the depression first (at least as best as one can) and then assess the severity of any remaining cognitive deficits.

Fourth, patients with *major depressive disorder* demonstrate characteristic cognitive difficulties that—in more severe cases—can become so disabling that the depressed patient meets the diagnostic criteria for having *dementia*. This condition was previously termed "pseudodementia of depression." However, a more appropriate term is "dementia of depression." The term "pseudodementia" implies that these patients don't have a "real" dementia, simply because the cognitive deficits result from a "psychiatric" disturbance rather than from a "neurologic," or "organic," disturbance such as vascular disease. However, this artificial distinction places explanation before observation. If such patients meet the diagnostic criteria for dementia, they have a dementia. In fact, research is revealing that, at the biochemical level, cognitive disruption in depressed patients, stroke patients, and Alzheimer's disease patients may reflect disruption of similar neural pathways. Given this, when diagnosing dementia, always assess for depressive symptoms, and consider major depressive disorder in the differential diagnosis of dementia. When a major depressive disorder is present, treat this first and then assess whether evidence for another dementing process still remains.

Fifth, patients with *schizophrenia* can have periods of superimposed mood changes that are similar to those observed in patients with *mood disorders*. When these symptoms are relatively transient and don't play a significant role in the overall course of illness, the diagnosis of schizophrenia is retained. However, if the patient does appear to have displayed prominent features of both illnesses over time, the diagnosis would be amended to *schizoaffective disorder*. While the latter diagnosis constitutes a mixed bag that includes atypical cases of psychotic depression, bipolar illness, and schizophrenia, it also appears that some patients are unfortunate enough to have overlapping features of more than one disorder. (Consider, for example, the patient whose father had schizophrenia and whose mother had bipolar disorder.)

Sixth, for simplicity's sake, at this stage I have omitted several other conditions from the diagnostic hierarchy. I will flesh them out later in the text. For example, there are the mood disorders that resemble depression or mania and the psychotic disorders that resemble schizophrenia but appear to be etiologically related to an underlying *general medical conditions* or *substance abuse*. I've also left out the diagnosis of *delusional disorder*, a psychotic illness distinguished from schizophrenia by the presence of circumscribed and nonbizarre delusions, by the absence of thought disorder, and by the absence of prominent hallucinations. Finally, I have left out the *anxiety disorders* despite the fact that these also demonstrate evidence for contributory biological factors.

THE DIMENSIONAL PERSPECTIVE

Underlying Logic

In contrast to the disease perspective, which emphasizes some condition that a person *has*, the dimensional perspective focuses on what people *are*. For example, we do not ask whether a person "has" height or "has" weight, we ask what the person's height or weight *is*. Similarly, just as people can vary in their physical characteristics, they also can vary in their psychological characteristics.

For a physical characteristic such as weight, individual variation along a dimensional continuum reflects the combined influence of genes and environment. The same applies to variation along a dimension for psychological characteristics. When a person's physical characteristics fall into the outer extremes in one direction or the other, this confers both advantages and vulnerabilities, depending on the situation. (For example, a very tall person might be successful at basketball but

also have difficulty fitting into small cars and be prone to banging his head on door frames.) This rule also applies to more extreme variations along psychological dimensions.

In everyday life we frequently think about our peers in dimensional terms. When we gossip or joke or complain about our coworkers, we typically take note of their personal idiosyncrasies and might even speculate about how a particular person would likely act were she to be placed in a particular situation. What we are taking note of in such cases is that individual's *personality*, or *temperament*. These terms refer to the totality of one individual's differences from other individuals. However, while one person might resemble another person in some ways, she might differ in other ways. Given this, it is useful to break up the concept of "personality" into smaller elements, called *attributes*, *aptitudes*, or *traits*. Put more simply, "personality" represents the total of a person's individual traits.

Psychiatric Applications

As was the case with the disease perspective, our goal in using the dimensional perspective is to move beyond intuition and personal acumen and to discuss patients more precisely, followed by attempts at explanation. In the words of Francis Galton, the nineteenth-century founder of psychometric personality testing: "An ordinary generalization is nothing more than a muddle of vague memories of inexact observations. It is an easy vice to generalize. We want lists of facts, every one of which may be separately verified, valued and revalued, and the whole accurately summed."

An example of psychological variation along a dimensional continuum is **intelligence**. We don't ask if a person *has* an intelligence quotient (I.Q.); rather, we ask "how high" or "how low" that person's I.Q. *is*. Everyone agrees that there *is* such a thing as intelligence and most agree that it can measured with a high degree of reliability. However, theorists disagree over what lies *behind* this construct (i.e., over whether the construct of "intelligence" is valid). We measure intelligence with I.Q. tests, which determine a person's aptitudes in performing a variety of tasks, with different tasks measuring different aspects of the more global construct of intelligence. Our reliability, and our confidence in the

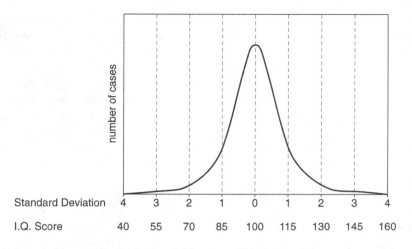

Figure 3–3. Bell curve demonstrating distribution of I.Q. scores within the population.

overall score, increases along with the number of different types of tasks that we have asked an individual to perform.

If we perform I.Q. tests on an entire population, we would expect the scores to fall along a normal distribution in a bell-shaped, or gaussian, curve (Fig. 3–3). In such a distribution, about 68% of the population falls within 1 standard deviation of the mean, about 95% of the population falls within 2 standard deviations, and about 2.5% falls above or below these margins. A test such as the Weschler Adult Intelligence Scale (WAIS) has been standardized over a wide range of normal subjects, thereby allowing the test-makers to convert raw test scores into standardized scores, with the mean score being 100.

As one can see, we can operationally define the level of a person's intelligence as being "abnormal" in relation to the general population, be it "subnormal" or "superior," by drawing *demarcations* at the standard deviation boundaries. A score below 70, which by definition falls at least 2 standard deviations below the mean, represents **mental subnormality**. We can further subdivide this group of "subnormal" individuals, based upon how far they lie from the mean score, as illustrated in Table 3–1.

Obviously, these demarcations are artificial, even arbitrary. This is most obvious at the margins: Is the person with an I.Q. of 74 really all that different from the person with an I.Q. of 68? Given this, in diagnosing mental subnormality, clinicians consider not only the individual's raw

score on an intelligence test but also the individual's level of adaptive functioning (i.e., his effectiveness in meeting various age-appropriate standards of social or occupation functioning, as defined by other members of his cultural group).

The *DSM-IV* follows the American Association on Mental Retardation in requiring that for individuals to be diagnosed with Mental Retardation (MR), they not only should have an I.Q. score below 70 but should also demonstrate impairments in at least two of the following areas of adaptive functioning: communication, self-care, home living, social/interpersonal skills, use of community resources, self-direction, functional academic skills, work, leisure, health, and safety. Further, the deficit should have begun before the age of 17 (thereby distinguishing mental retardation from dementia).

It can be stigmatizing to saddle individuals with categorical labels such as mental retardation or personality disorder based on where they fall along a dimensional continuum. Given this, why do it? Measurements and diagnostic labels, when applied appropriately, are useful. They al-

Table 3–1. Categories of Mental Retardation

Category	I.Q.
Mild mental retardation	50–55 to about 70
Moderate mental retardation	35–45 to 50–55
Severe mental retardation	20–25 to 35–40
Profound mental retardation	Less than 20–25

low us to understand a patient's strengths and vulnerabilities relative to other people. This in turn allows us to realistically assess whether her goals for the future are viable and to assist her to utilize her strengths and to compensate for her vulnerabilities as she attempts to achieve these goals.

"Intelligence" was recognized as constituting an important predictor of success in life centuries before the advent of intelligence testing. While investigators may disagree as to the *cause* of variations in intelligence, it is hard to argue with the fact that one's intelligence (as measured by I.Q. tests) highly correlates with a variety of other independent measures of life success, such as academic advancement, occupational status, and socioeconomic status. Similarly, placing individuals with MR into subcategories based upon their I.Q. scores helps to predict and to meet their educational, vocational, and social needs.

For example, individuals with *mild MR* (about 85% of the MR population) demonstrate minimal impairment in sensorimotor areas. They often are not distinguishable from children without mental retardation until a later age. By their late teens, they can acquire academic skills commensurate with the sixth-grade level. By their adult years, they usually have achieved social and vocational skills adequate to support themselves in the community. They may never have received a diagnosis of MR and in fact they may be indistinguishable from the general population much of the time. However, they may require supervision or guidance during times of social or economic stress. Clinicians working in emergency rooms or outpatient clinics frequently overlook the possibility that patients presenting in crisis following an interpersonal or financial setback might have mild MR, despite their having noted that the patient has "limited coping skills."

Individuals with *moderate MR* (about 10% of the MR population) also benefit from vocational training and with moderate supervision they, too, can attend to their personal care. However, in school they are unlikely to progress beyond the second-grade achievement level. During adolescence, their difficulties recognizing social conventions may impede their ability to sustain peer relationships. In their adult years, most are able to perform unskilled or semiskilled work under supervision either in sheltered workshops or in the general workforce. They adapt well to life in the community, although usually in supervised settings.

Individuals with *severe MR* (about 3%–4% of the MR population) acquire little or no communicative speech in early childhood, but during their school years they may learn to talk. They are unable to perform vocational work but can be trained to perform simple tasks in a closely supervised setting. They often can live in the community either with family or in a group home, and they can be trained to perform basic self-care. Individuals with *profound MR* (about 1%–2% of the MR population) are minimally able to care for themselves and require constant supervision.

The example of mental retardation also illustrates some other aspects of dimensional perspective. First, to say that a quality varies along a dimensional gradient says little about what lies *behind* that variation. For example, height is influenced by heredity but also by environmental factors such as nutrition. Similarly, while I.Q. clearly has hereditary components, environmental factors (such as childhood social deprivation) and diseases also play a role. In reality, when careful epidemiological studies are done (which include *all* members of the population, including those who are institutionalized) it turns out that distribution along the bell curve isn't symmetric. There are more impaired individuals than there are gifted ones, reflecting a greater prevalence of impaired individuals than is predicted by the normal distribution. This is particularly the case for the severe and profound MR groups. Individuals in these subcategories are more likely to have been affected by diseases or environmental insults that have contributed to their impaired intelligence. The following factors have been causally associated with MR:

Heredity conditions (approximately 5%): These include inborn errors of metabolism inherited mostly through autosomal recessive mechanisms (such as Tay-Sachs disease), other single-gene abnormalities with Mendelian inheritance and variable expression (such as tuberous sclerosis), and chromosomal aberrations (such as Down's syndrome and fragile X syndrome).

Early alterations of embryonic development (approximately 30%): These include chromosomal changes (e.g., Down's syndrome due to trisomy 21) or prenatal damage due to toxins (e.g., maternal alcohol consumption, infections).

Pregnancy and perinatal problems (approximately 10%): For example, fetal malnutrition, prematurity, hypoxia, viral and other infections, and trauma.

General medical conditions acquired in infancy or childhood (approximately 5%): For example, infections, traumas, and poisoning such as lead toxicity.

Environmental influences and other mental disorders (approximately 15%–20%): For example, deprivation of nurturance and of social, linguistic, and other stimulation, and severe mental disorders (e.g., autistic disorder).

Idiopathic (approximately 30%–40%): This leaves the largest group, for whom the cause of the mental retardation remains unknown even after extensive investigation. Many members of this group likely are "physiologically subnormal" rather than "pathologically subnormal." The former individuals are more likely to fall in the mild MR group.

This is not to say that one's success in life depends solely on intelligence. For the population as a whole, intelligence plays an important role, but for specific individuals in specific situations, intelligence is but one factor. For example, the association between intelligence and the social prestige of one's chosen profession is a statistical one; demonstration of the association is only possible because the ranges for intelligence and of career prestige scores are wide. In contrast, there is only a modest correlation between I.Q. score and job success (with intelligence accounting for only 4% of the variance) or between I.Q. and socioeconomic status (with intelligence accounting for only 16% of the variance). Members of a given occupation demonstrate a narrower range of intellectual variation; given this, within an occupation, other variables such as motivation, personality, and access to advancement opportunities play a greater role than intelligence in determining job success.

The example of intelligence illustrates several points about the dimensional perspective. First, while the validity of the construct of intelligence may be debated, the idea that individuals can vary along this dimension is readily appreciated. Second, we can identify categories of individuals by using a continuous dimensional measure, but only by making artificial demarcations. Third, where one finds oneself along a dimension can reflect the contribution of multiple factors, including genetics, diseases, and environmental factors. Fourth, deviation along a dimension of variation can place an individual at risk for becoming emotional distressed when the individual finds himself or herself in a situation that taxes an area of vulnerability.

We can apply this same line of reasoning to the dimension of **personality**. As with intelligence, the notion that personality varies within the general population dates back to long before the advent of personality testing, at least as far back as ancient Greece. The humoral theory proposed four personality types: melancholic, choleric (irritable), sanguine (optimistic), and phlegmatic (apathetic). These four types were believed to reflect the relative proportion of four bodily humors: black bile, yellow bile, blood, and phlegm, respectively. Each type represents a particular constellation of personality traits.

While current physiologic thinking has rejected the humoral theory, these constellations of personality types still ring true. For example, people who are very neat often (although not invariably) are perfectionists and self-doubting as well; those who are self-dramatizing may also be emotionally labile. Today we would label these personality types obsessive-compulsive personality disorder and histrionic personality disorder, respectively.

Personality types represent *ideals*. In actuality, individuals may demonstrate prominent characteristics of several types. Further, at the categorical demarcation points, it can be debated whether an individual should be included within the category or not. But, as was the case with intelligence, it often is useful to think about individuals in this way, since it helps us to understand their particular strengths and vulnerabilities. Everybody experiences life stress, but only some people end up seeking professional help in the face of stress. Further, one person may become distraught in the face of one particular type of situation but not another type of situation, while the opposite may be the case for another person. Ernst Kretschmer described the type of events that elicit characteristic responses from particular types of people as "key experiences." He analogized these experiences to "keys" that fit a given person's "lock," thereby releasing powerful emotional responses.

For example, a man who is very *dependent* may be content in his everyday life, without difficulty tolerating occupational or financial difficulties. However, he may become hopeless, even suicidal, following his wife leaving him. However, a man who is very *perfectionistic* might have no difficulties following a romantic rejection but might become extremely anxious when asked to cover for a vacationing colleague due to his desire to perform 80 hours of work in a 40-hour work week while also refusing to "cut any corners" or to prioritize these tasks. In further contrast, a very *narcissistic* person may have no difficulties covering for a vacationing colleague but might be thrown into a state of depression, anxiety, or rage by a meeting with a supervisor where his job performance is criticized.

As was the case with intelligence, there are pitfalls to typological reasoning about personality. First, at what degree of severity do we label a person as having a "pathological" personality type? Second, these personality categories tend to be awkward: while we can sense the "central concepts," the boundaries between them tend to overlap. For example, the construct of *borderline personality disorder* (discussed in detail in Chapter 10) has been used by different clinicians in different ways, sometimes to refer to characteristic types of behaviors, at other times to refer to a characteristic volatile temperament, and at still other times to refer to characteristic ways of perceiving the world even in the absence of the first two features. Scales designed to diagnose borderline personality disorder, even when reliable, don't always diagnose the same patients as having this disorder as do other scales that also were designed to diagnose borderline personality disorder. In other words, while personality types can be operationally defined and are clinically useful, validity remains a major concern.

Another danger inherent in describing people as being of certain personality types is that these labels can come to be seen as explanations in themselves, especially when they are applied thoughtlessly. Once the clinician has come up with a label, she can distance herself from the clinical phenomenon, as if the label explains everything. For example, faced with a patient who repeatedly cuts her forearms with a razor

and then presents to the emergency room asking for help, the clinician might comment, "She's just a borderline" (referring to the diagnosis of borderline personality disorder). But saying this really doesn't explain much. It's just a convenient description of the patient's presentation. The tautology—"borderlines" are people who repeatedly cut on themselves; the patient repeatedly cuts on herself; the patient is a borderline"—tells us nothing about *why* patients like this one act the way that they do, nor does it tell us how we can help them to stop.

However, a diagnostic category such as borderline personality disorder, applied appropriately, can be invaluable. The recognition that a patient demonstrates features of borderline personality disorder syndrome helps to guide a clinician's questioning during the diagnostic interview such that associated features that otherwise might have been missed can be explored. Further, making a diagnosis of borderline personality disorder has important therapeutic implications since it offers some guidance as to which psychotherapeutic interventions or pharmacologic agents are most likely to be helpful (and also as to which interventions might make things worse).

Whether personality disorders are best approached dimensionally or categorically is a subject of ongoing discussion. *DSM-IV* uses a categorical approach, listing descriptive criteria for each personality disorder. Clinicians are asked to apply these criteria in order to determine, for example, whether a patient "has" a borderline personality disorder or not, "has" a histrionic personality disorder or not, or even meets enough criteria from both categories to be diagnosed as having *both* personality disorders. According to the categorical approach, people with a personality disorder are presumed to be *qualitatively* and not simply quantitatively different from people without them. For example, the *DSM-IV* defines a personality trait as being a "pathological" trait when it is maladaptive, inflexible, and a source of distress either to the patient or to the people around the patient.

The *DSM* definition of a pathological trait stands in contrast to a dimensional model, which asks the more *quantitative* question, "While we all have some histrionic traits, just *how* histrionic is this person relative to the general population?"

From the dimensional perspective, a person would be considered to have a personality disorder when specific traits are so excessive that they render the person excessively vulnerable to difficulties in settings or situations that tax those traits. (Note the similarity between this formulation and the requirement in the case of mental retardation that MR only be diagnosed when the patient both has low intelligence as measured by an I.Q. test and demonstrates evidence of impaired social, academic, or occupational functioning due to low intelligence.)

As was the case with intelligence, whether a trait is *apparent* at a given point in time depends upon the current circumstances. One may not appreciate how sensitive to rejection a person is until the person has been rejected. Further, a trait that can be an asset in one setting may prove to be a liability in a different setting. For example, traits such as aggressiveness or "workaholism" may be assets at work but liabilities in one's personal life.

Given this, the psychiatric diagnostic assessment should include a detailed social history that elicits examples of how the patient acted at various points in his or her life under a variety of different circumstances. Another source of such data is *collateral informants*, who—when asked to describe the patient's personality—typically offer anecdotes that provide a window into the patient's typical cognitive, emotional, and behavioral "style." The psychiatrist also can rely upon her observations of the patient's behavior during the current evaluation and upon her "gut" reactions to the patient.

Finally, the clinician can turn to standardized *psychological tests*. These are not a substitute for the clinical interview, and they can be influenced by the patient's current emotional state (especially when the patient is in the midst of an acute psychiatric disease such as depression). What psychological tests offer is a standardized method of comparing the patient's intensity of traits and pattern of different traits to findings from members of other groups.

As was the case for intelligence, to say that a particular personality trait varies along a bell curve in the general population says little about the cause of this variation in a given individual. Variation in traits likely reflects multiple factors, including genetic influence (which accounts for

about half of the variation), environmental factors, and disease or other biological factors. For example, one biological model, proposed by Larry Siever (1991) proposes that variations along four dimensions of personality reflect variations in brain activity within four neurotransmitter systems. In this model, *cognitive organization* is related to dopamine activity, *affect regulation* is related to norepinephrine activity, *impulse control* is related to serotonin and norepinephrine activity, and *anxiety modulation* is related to one's degree of cortical (GABA—γ-aminobutyric acid) or sympathetic (norepinephrine) arousal. (This example also demonstrates that while the presumed *physiology* of personality variation has changed since antiquity—we now speak of four "neurotransmitter systems" rather than of four "humors"—the conceptual approach remains remarkably similar.)

The *DSM* multiaxial coding scheme was designed to encourage clinicians to diagnose both state-related disorders (such as major depressive disorder, schizophrenia, substance abuse) and lifelong trait-related disorders (personality disorders and mental retardation) rather than viewing these two types of conditions in a mutually exclusive fashion. The former are coded on *Axis I*, the latter on *Axis II*. In other words, the issue is not whether a particular patient has a major depressive disorder *or* has a personality disorder. Patients with personality disorder are more prone to develop a major depressive disorder, and an early onset of depression may so substantially affect personality development that it predisposes the patient to develop a personality disorder. Similarly, medical conditions that predispose to the development of psychiatric symptoms should not be overlooked and are coded on *Axis III*. Current life stressors are listed on *Axis IV* (Table 3–2), and the patient's current degree of social and occupational impairment in occupational and social functioning is coded on *Axis V* (Table 3–3).

My goal at this point is to introduce the concept of personality as consisting of multiple traits, each of which varies continuously along a dimension in the general population, and to demonstrate how the logic of dimensional reasoning varies from the logic of disease reasoning. Dimensional reasoning emphasizes individual variations in disposition rather than cat-

Table 3–2. *DSM-IV-TR* Psychosocial and Environmental Problems: These Are Listed on Axis IV Using the Multiaxial Classification Scheme

Problem	Examples
Problems with primary support group	Death of a family member; health problems in family; disruption of family by separation, divorce, or estrangement; removal from the home; remarriage of parent; sexual or physical abuse; parental overprotection; neglect of child; inadequate discipline; discord with siblings; birth of a sibling
Problems related to the social environment	Death or loss of friend; inadequate social support; living alone; difficulty with acculturation; discrimination; adjustment to life-cycle transition (such as retirement)
Educational problems	Illiteracy; academic problems; discord with teachers or classmates; inadequate school environment
Occupational problems	Unemployment; threat of job loss; stressful work schedule; difficult work conditions; job dissatisfaction; job change; discord with boss or coworkers
Housing problems	Homelessness; inadequate housing; unsafe neighborhood; discord with neighbors or landlord
Economic problems	Extreme poverty; inadequate finances; insufficient welfare support
Problems with access to health-care services	Inadequate health-care services; transportation to health-care facilities unavailable; inadequate health insurance
Problems related to interaction with the legal system/crime	Arrest; incarceration; litigation; victim of crime
Other psychosocial and environmental problems	Exposure to disasters, war, other hostilities; discord with nonfamily caregivers such as counselor, social worker, or physician; unavailability of social service agencies

Source: Reprinted with permission from the *Diagnostic and Statistical Manual of Mental Disorders, Fourth Edition, Text Revision.* Copyright 2000 American Psychiatric Association.

egorical differences that distinguish the "normal" from the "pathological," and it stresses the implications of these variations based on one's current circumstances. Personality and personality disorders are discussed in greater detail in Chapter 10.

THE BEHAVIOR PERSPECTIVE

Underlying Logic

If the disease perspective focuses on conditions that a person has while the dimensional perspective focuses on what a person is, the behavior perspective focuses on what a person *does.*

Behavioral disorders may appear to be quite disparate, as they involve a wide variety of behaviors. These disorders include *eating disorders* (including anorexia nervosa and bulimia nervosa), *substance-related disorders* (such as alcohol dependence or cocaine dependence), *sex-*

ual disorders (such as paraphilia), and *impulse control disorders* (such as compulsive shopping, compulsive shoplifting, self-injurious acts, and firesetting). What all of these disorders have in common is that they involve **behaviors**—that is, *activities designated by their consequences.*

We engage in many behaviors that are internally or biologically motivated but that also are shaped by factors such as personality and environment. These include eating, sleeping, and sexual activity. We don't always engage in these activities exactly the same way, and superficially disparate behaviors can only be understood when one is mindful of the goal of the behavior. For example, one might wolf down a hamburger at lunchtime while driving across town but eat in a very different manner later the day at a formal dinner party. While individual actions in these two settings might appear very different, the behavior in both situations is still "eating." Simi-

Table 3–3. *DSM-IV-TR* Global Assessment of Functioning (GAF) Scale: The Score Is Listed on Axis V Using the Multiaxial Classification Scheme

Code	
(Note: Use intermediate codes when appropriate, e.g., 45, 68, 72)	
91–100	Superior functioning in a wide range of activities; life's problems never seem to get out of hand; is sought out by others because of his or her many positive qualities. No symptoms
81–90	Absent or minimal symptoms (e.g., mild anxiety before an exam), good functioning in all areas, interested and involved in a wide range of activities, socially effective, generally satisfied with life, no more than everyday problems or concerns (e.g., an occasional argument with family members)
71–80	If symptoms are present, they are transient and expectable reactions to psychosocial stressors (e.g., difficulty concentrating after family argument); no more than slight impairment in social, occupational, or school functioning (e.g., temporarily falling behind in schoolwork)
61–70	Some mild symptoms (e.g., depressed mood and mild insomnia) OR some difficulty in social, occupational, or school functioning (e.g., occasional truancy, or theft within the household), but generally functioning pretty well, has some meaningful interpersonal relationships
51–60	Moderate symptoms (e.g., flat affect and circumstantial speech, occasional panic attacks) OR moderate difficulty in social, occupational, or school functioning (e.g., few friends, conflicts with peers or coworkers)
41–50	Serious symptoms (e.g., suicidal ideation, severe obsessional rituals, frequent shoplifting) OR any serious impairment in social, occupational, or school functioning (e.g., no friends, unable to keep a job)
31–40	Some impairment in reality testing or communication (e.g., speech is at times illogical, obscure, or irrelevant) OR major impairment in several areas, such as work or school, family relations, judgment, thinking, or mood (e.g., depressed man avoids friends, neglects family, and is unable to work; child frequently beats up younger children, is defiant at home, and is failing at school)
21–30	Behavior is considerably influenced by delusions or hallucinations OR serious impairment in communication or judgment (e.g., sometimes incoherent, acts grossly inappropriately, suicidal preoccupation) OR inability to function in almost all areas (e.g., stays in bed all day; no job, home, or friends)
11–20	Some danger of hurting self or others (e.g., suicide attempts without clear expectation of death; frequently violent; manic excitement) OR occasionally fails to maintain minimal personal hygiene (e.g., smears feces) OR gross impairment in communication (e.g., largely incoherent or mute)
1–10	Persistent danger of severely hurting self or others (e.g., recurrent violence) OR persistent inability to maintain minimal personal hygiene OR serious suicidal act with clear expectation of death
0	Inadequate information

Source: Reprinted with permission from the *Diagnostic and Statistical Manual of Mental Disorders, Fourth Edition, Text Revision.* Copyright 2000 American Psychiatric Association.

larly, while many factors shape the behavior—culture, social custom, the current availability of certain types of food—the behavior of eating can only be understood fully once one appreciates the primary underlying goal of the behavior—that is, to ingest food either for pleasure or to relieve uncomfortable feelings of hunger.

This *goal-oriented nature* is one of the features shared by biologically driven behaviors. Other features include: that these behaviors *occur intermittently*, that they are *selectively provoked by stimuli that are later ignored* and that *the drives to engage in these behaviors vary in intensity and can be voluntarily suppressed.*

For example, while at a restaurant, a person initially may not feel very hungry. However, his feelings of hunger may increase upon reading through the menu or seeing other diners' entrees being carried past his. Even after he has eaten a large meal and feels so distended that he "can't imagine ever feeling hungry again," new cravings may be triggered after the waiter brings around the dessert cart. In this case, an even more enticing, specific gustatory stimulus was presented to him (sweets), which triggered cravings that wouldn't have been evoked had the waiter brought some other type of food (e.g., a tray of baked potatoes). After eating dessert, the person again may feel that he will "never be hungry again," only to find that he again feels hungry the very next morning. Similarly, the person who has not engaged in sexual intercourse for some time may note increased sexual cravings, only to find that this appetite decreases or disappears following intercourse and then increases again after some period of delay. The intensity of sexual drive may vary from one individual to another, as may the circumstances or stimuli that trigger sexual cravings.

Individuals engage in motivated behaviors to satisfy **cravings**. Cravings have two complementary characteristics: a *search for pleasure* (such as satiety or orgasm), and also a *desire for release from a state of tension* (hunger or sexual arousal). Thus, motivated behaviors follow a typical cycle: craving, consummation, decreased craving and the replacement of the motivated behavior by other activities, and increased craving at a later point in time. However, this cycle is subject to the *influence of both internal factors and external factors*. For example, an alcoholic patient may experience increased cravings for alcohol due either to being in a state of alcohol withdrawal (an internal factor) or to feeling angry and guilty after an argument with his wife (an external factor).

Motivated behaviors are *biologically driven* and *preoccupying*. They aren't simply casual choices. However, they also aren't simply "hardwired" reflexes. For example, the drives associated with motivated behaviors tend to become more intense and preoccupying the longer that they are suppressed. A student who skipped breakfast and lunch before an afternoon lecture might have trouble paying attention to the lecture, so preoccupying is her hunger. This would not be the case for a reflex, since a reflex is the same all of the time. Similarly, the food that appeared so preoccupying just before a meal might hold no interest once the meal is completed, which also wouldn't be the case for a simple reflex.

Another difference between motivated behaviors and biological reflexes is that motivated behaviors, while biologically driven, still involve an element of *choice and volitional control*. Even when we are powerfully *influenced* by intense biological drives, we still can elect to *suppress* these drives. For example, we may wish to have

sexual intercourse more often than we do, or may wish to have intercourse in inappropriate places, but most of us strike a balance between our personal drives and societal norms. Individuals may abstain from eating for religious reasons (e.g., Yom Kippur, Lent, or Ramadan) or as a political protest, while priests or nun may elect to eschew sexual activity completely.

Similarly, while individuals with anorexia or bulimia nervosa or with alcohol or cocaine dependence experience very strong cravings to engage in pathological behavior, they typically have some degree of voluntary control over their behaviors. The bulimic individual may only vomit when she is alone, while the cocaine-dependent individual may abstain from drug use if she suspects that a police officer is nearby. Similarly, while medications may play a useful ancillary role in treating behavioral disorders due to their ability to modify underlying biological factors, the most effective treatment interventions are cognitive and behavioral therapies that attempt to educate patients about the nature of their pathological behaviors, the negative impact of these behaviors on their lives, situations where they at greater risk of losing control, and ways that they might gain control over the behavior.

Psychiatric Applications

When should we consider an individual's behaviors to constitute a *pathological syndrome*? This question has engendered a great deal of confusion and debate mainly because it raises the related questions of when (if ever) we should consider an individual's behavioral a "disease" outside of his control and when (if ever) we should consider the individual to not be responsible for aberrant behavior.

Behaviors take place within the context of the larger society. Given this, societal attitudes about specific behaviors play a greater role than they would for a syndrome such as diabetes in deciding whether the behaviors are "symptoms" of a "disease." For example, from the behavior perspective, it is clear that *homosexuality* isn't a disease—it is a pattern of behavior. (For that matter, so is heterosexuality.) As societal attitudes toward homosexuality have changed over the past two decades, so have diagnostic classifications. Homosexuality has become progressively "demedicalized." While homosexuality was classified as a pathological "sexual deviation" in the *DSM-II*, it is not even listed in the *DSM-IV*. Homosexual behavior has not changed—societal attitudes have. In contrast, *alcohol dependence* has been increasingly "medicalized" over the past several decades. While it has traditionally been viewed as a moral failing, it more often is viewed today as an "illness."

Social judgments about personal accountability also play a role in whether we consider a behavioral problem to be a pathological disorder. For instance, we might agree that the alcoholic has an "illness" when he is seen on the medical unit, but when he appears in court after having hit a person with his car while driving in an intoxicated state, society holds him accountable for his behavior. He is seen as having failed to exercise sufficient control. Similarly, we might consider the pedophile to have powerful aberrant urges to have sex with children when he is seen in the clinic, but we still find him deserving of punishment when he appears in court on child molestation charges.

Two stumbling blocks hinder any resolution of this debate: *semantic confusion* (a behavior is labeled a "disease" simply because a clinical syndrome can be discerned and because some of the reinforcing factors are biological in nature) and *conceptual uncertainty* as to the nature of biological drives in general. This brings us back yet again to issues of reliability and validity. At present, we have neither reliable nor valid ways of measuring how "strong" an individual's biological drives are, and certainly not of measuring whether they are so strong that they are "irresistible." How are we to distinguish whether the pedophile who illegally engaged in sexual behavior with children or the substance abuser who illegally used cocaine had urges to engage in these behaviors that they *could not* resist or whether they had "normal" (or perhaps "moderately increased") urges that they *chose* not to resist?

Granted, we don't have any laboratory test to determine whether a patient is or is not "actually" hallucinating. However, we tend to feel more confident in our decisions about this latter issue. Hallucinations are either present or they are not present. In contrast, the difference between an "irresistible impulse" and an "impulse not resisted" appears to be more a matter of degree and—in the words of psychiatrist Loren

Roth—is "as clear as the line between twilight and dusk."

Even if we could reliably measure the intensity of these underlying drives, the behaviors themselves vary in the population along a continuum. While some people clearly have more difficulty modulating their intake of alcohol than other people, there are no bright lines demarcating the "social drinkers" from the "problem drinkers" or from the "alcoholics." This is also the case for behaviors such as dieting, gambling, shopping, and repetitive lying. Where we draw these lines unavoidably will be somewhat arbitrary and will unavoidably be influenced by societal values. The man who enjoys walking around naked in the privacy of his own home may not require any treatment; however, if he repeatedly exposes himself in public, he may be referred for treatment (typically by the court, following an arrest for indecent exposure).

The diagnostic criteria for behavioral disorders categories are often disjunctive. *Disjunctive diagnoses* contain symptoms linked by "or" rather than "and." For example, myocardial infarction is a conjunctive diagnosis characterized by certain clinical symptoms along with changes in the electrocardiogram and elevation of cardiac enzymes. In contrast, systemic lupus erythematosus is a disjunctive diagnosis since it is diagnosed based on the presence of any four out of 11 disparate types of symptoms (e.g., skin rash, *or* arthritis, *or* renal disease, *or* seizures).

Disjunctive diagnoses most often exist when we know less about the underlying pathology and don't have a gold standard pathognomonic clinical sign or test that confirms the diagnosis. For example, myocardial infarction would be a disjunctive diagnosis were it not for the confirmatory laboratory tests. Even in the absence of "classic" cardiac symptoms, we can use laboratory tests to determine if the patient has had a "clinically silent" myocardial infarction. In contrast, behavioral disorders are diagnosed disjunctively. An individual can be diagnosed as being "an alcoholic" for a variety of disparate reasons: if using alcohol has led to signs of physiologic tolerance or withdrawal, *or* if it has led to a drunk driving arrest, *or* if it has led to marital problems, *or* if it has led to occupational problems, *or* if it has led to cirrhosis, *or* if the person only drinks rarely but on one those occasions the alcohol caused delirium or severe disinhibition.

Overall, we typically consider behaviors to be "pathological" either when *the object of the drive is socially unacceptable* or when the *strength of a normal drive is so intense that it causes suffering or injury to the patient or to the people around him*. Examples of the former include pedophilia, repetitive self-injury, and factitious disorder. (The last condition, also called Munchausen's syndrome, is characterized by the repetitive feigning of illness in order to obtain medical attention, especially hospitalization or surgery.) Examples of facititious disorder include the patient who goes beyond normal dieting behavior to the point of being diagnosed with anorexia nervosa and the one who goes beyond everyday social drinking to the point of being diagnosed with alcohol dependence.

Further, behaviors are considered pathological when they have become *self-sustaining*. In other words, the individual continues to engage in the behavior long after the initial motivating is gone. For example, the patient with alcohol dependence may have *initiated* his drinking behavior for a variety of reasons (peer pressure, the example of parents who drank, loneliness) but in most cases he drinks today largely because he drank yesterday. To spend hours in psychotherapy addressing "why" the patient began drinking may be helpful in motivating him to stop drinking, but it doesn't address the *current reinforcers* of his pathological behavior, be they *internal reinforcers* (drinking to avoid going into alcohol withdrawal) or *external reinforcers* (passing the liquor store every day on the way home from work, thereby triggering a craving for alcohol). Similarly, the anorexic patient starves herself today because she starved herself yesterday: exploratory psychotherapy in the absence of behavioral interventions aimed at combating her worsening malnutrition and establishing more normal eating patterns can end in tragedy

Alcohol dependence is listed in the *DSM-IV* as a "disorder" (as is every other condition.) But is it also a "disease"? If so, what is the broken bodily part? A key difference between the behavioral perspective and the disease perspective is that the disease perspective emphasizes categorical differences between people while the behavioral perspective emphasizes universal behaviors that become a source of disability for the subset of people who engage in the behaviors to an extreme extent. Again, because of these different logics, the goals of the two perspectives are different.

The goal of the disease perspective is to discover what lies "behind" the clinical phenomenon and then to treat it. Following this, pathological symptoms should improve. For example, making the correct diagnosis of bipolar disorder with a current manic episode guides our decision to administer a mood-stabilizing medication such as lithium carbonate, and the manic state typically improves shortly afterward.

However, from the behavior perspective, the *behavior itself* always must be addressed, since the key feature of behavioral disorders that they tend to become self-sustaining. Biological factors play a role as internal reinforcers of the behavior, and addressing these factors can be an important adjunct to treatment aimed at helping the patient learn to resist his urges. However, the track record of "biological psychiatry" in "curing" behavioral conditions has been disappointing. Taking the drug naltrexone can help decrease the craving for alcohol, and wearing a nicotine patch can help decrease the craving for a cigarette, but most patients find that such interventions, used in isolation, are a far cry from a "cure."

Because they are so powerfully driven and because they are reinforced by a wide variety of environmental and psychological factors, behavioral disorders are among the most difficult conditions that clinicians encounter. The object of treatment is to help the patient achieve control rather than to "prescribe a cure." However, in many cases the patient has little desire to achieve greater control, whether due to lack of insight into the behavior being problematic ("denial") or due to a fear of anticipated physical and psychological symptoms that might accompany attempts to break the behavioral cycle. Involuntary treatment is less likely to be successful than elective treatment, confirming the relevance of the joke about the number of psychiatrists that it takes to change a light bulb. (The answer is, "Only one, but the lightbulb has to really want to change.")

Sometimes, patients initially coerced into involuntary treatment (whether by family members, employers, or the court) are able to achieve greater insight over the course of therapy. Given this, an *initial* lack of insight or lack of motivation to change isn't an absolute bar to accepting the patient into a treatment program. However, one must always consider factors such as the patient's motivation for seeking treatment and the context of the treatment, since patients coerced into involuntary treatment for a behavioral disorder may readily learn to "talk the talk" in order to achieve discharge from the program while failing to truly accept the importance of "walking the walk.")

The misguided belief that the mental health system can (or should) "cure" people with behavioral disorders has led to public skepticism about the efficacy of mental health treatment in general. When substance abusers, child abusers, or sex offenders referred for court-ordered treatment are later rearrested for similar offenses despite having been "treated," the field of psychiatry is seen as having naïvely promised more than it could deliver. This is unfortunate, since mental health treatment clearly benefits many patients with behavioral disorders. Greater public appreciation of the differences between behavioral disorders and pure "diseases" might help the public see the role of clinical treatment in a more appropriate light.

THE LIFE-STORY PERSPECTIVE

Underlying Logic

The final perspective—and perhaps the perspective most associated with psychiatry—is the life-story perspective. This perspective views the patient as a *particular individual with a unique life story*. Understanding the story allows us to understand the patient's current state of emotional distress.

This perspective comes naturally to all of us since we routinely use it in our daily lives. The emphasis here is not on the symptoms a person *has* (as in the disease perspective), on the way the person is (as in the dimensional perspective), or on the things the person *does* (as in the behavioral perspective). Rather, it is on the *meaning* of the patient's thoughts, feelings, and behaviors.

However, there are as many stories as there are lives; in fact, each life contains many stories. How do we go about choosing the *relevant* ones? An internal logic does guide this perspective, but it is not the logic of the natural sciences. Rather, it is the *logic of narrative*. It is very different from the logics of diseases, dimensions, and behaviors. A failure to appreciate the rules of the logic of narrative has led to "wars" between various schools of psychotherapy, each laying some claim to having discovered the "truth" about human nature and human suffering.

The essence of this logic is that *narratives are stories that are constructed, generally by the patient with the assistance of the therapist, using the clinical data at hand*. A story is considered "correct" if it illuminates the clinical issue at hand and if it proves to be helpful to the patient.

Stories are not data. Rather, they connect the data and attempt to "make sense" of the data, through *narrative interpretations*. Just as they are not data, stories are not facts. They are "true" only to the extent that they are accepted and useful to both the therapist and the patient. When a patient describes an incident to a therapist, the therapist does not have access to the actual *historical truth* (the truth as it would have been recorded by a hidden video camera)—only to the *narrative truth*, (the patient's subjective perception of the truth). Consider the following two examples:

Example 1. A patient presents seeking help with "controlling my temper." His wife has threatened to take the children and leave him unless he learns to do so. In the course of describing his social history, he describes a pattern of repeated past insults by authority figures, including his father (who was verbally, although not sexually, abusive) and his current supervisor at work. According to the patient, his supervisor harps on even minor work deficiencies, causing the patient to then "take my anger home with me." The therapist suspects that perhaps the patient has paranoid and narcissistic personality features that influence his world view, but can't conclude this with certainty. She recognizes that at this point she just doesn't know the "historical truth." Fortunately, her primary goal isn't to discover the historical truth but to help the patient learn to better cope in the world as he sees it. Over the course of psychotherapy, the therapist suggests that perhaps the patient's father wasn't as "abusive" as he now recalls; it sounds as if perhaps his father didn't know how to handle his anger well and tended to "explode" out of frustration, much as the patient does. The patient ultimately comes to see both his father and his supervisor in a more sympathetic light. He recognizes that, while his view of the world as a hostile place has been shaped by his father's behavior toward him during childhood, this view isn't always accurate now that he is an adult. He decides that in many circumstances "it just isn't worth getting so angry," and he resolves to control his temper more around his children, especially given the detrimental effect of his own father's anger. Despite this positive outcome, the psychiatrist never really knows with certainty how the patient's father "really" treated him. She only knows how the patient, an adult attempting to reconstruct events from childhood from fallible memory, *perceives* his father as having treated him.

Example 2. A patient presents for treatment of depression, panic attacks, repetitive relationship difficulties, and bulimic behavior. In recounting the social history, she recalls her father as having been verbally, although not sexually, abusive. Based on the patient's current symptoms, the therapist comes to suspect that she was sexually abused as child, perhaps by her father. He suggests this possibility to the patient. At first the patient rejects the theory, but over the next few weeks she begins to experience recurrent, vivid dreams. Her first dreams involve being chased by an unknown person. These give way to dreams of being sexually abused by person "whose face remains in the shadows." Finally, she recognizes the face as her father's face. She later "recovers" a memory of her father having sexually abused her when she was 5 years old. In discussing this with her therapist, she comes to realize that she has "repressed" the awareness of this abuse until now. She subsequently breaks off all contact with her parents and decides to press criminal charges against her father. The therapist testifies in court—based solely upon his sessions with the patient and without having reviewed outside data or interviewed collateral informants—that he knows "for a fact" that his patient was abused, based both on "what she told me" and on "the nature of her clinical symptoms." This therapist has confused "narrative truth" with "historical truth" and has overstated the degree of certainty to which he can reach his conclusions under such circumstances.

The German psychiatrist and philosopher Karl Jaspers explored the logic of narrative in great detail. He called interpretations between points of data *meaningful connections* and described their essential properties.

First, meaningful connections are interpretations. As such, the listener imposes the pattern. There is no single "correct" interpretation, and different listeners will make different connections and therefore construct different stories. This is particularly likely to be the case when the listeners come from different theoretical backgrounds.

Second, meaningful connections follow the "hermeneutic round." Hermeneutics is the science of interpretation. It was originally applied to biblical studies and emphasized how readers' interpretations of the "meaning" of biblical passages are shaped as much by their own personal and cultural background as by the content of the text. One can apply the same analysis to attempts by readers to discern the "original intent" of the founding fathers as they wrote the United States Constitution, or the intent of James Joyce as he sat down to write *Ulysses*.

The major difference between psychotherapy and literary interpretation is that patients aren't passive texts: they themselves play an active role in the interpretive endeavor. This leads to the "hermeneutic round." The patient presents selected historical data to the therapist, who listens attentively and then suggests an interpretation (shaped by his own background and experience) involving certain themes. The patient listens to the interpretation and then presents the therapist with yet more historical data, the choice of which has been influenced by the therapist's interpretation. The therapist interprets this new data, and so on. In this way, patient and therapist collaborate in a process whereby interpretations beget further interpretations.

This process often invokes the feeling that the therapy is "really getting somewhere." This sense of "finally understanding" may motivate the patient to change preconceived attitudes and self-destructive behaviors, as in the first example cited above. However, the process also may focus disproportionate emphasis on one particular piece of data to the exclusion of other relevant data. Therapists may be led astray by an overzealous commitment to one particular theory or agenda. The two examples cited above illustrate the "hermeneutic round" at work. In both cases, the therapist's contributions were reciprocated by the patient and vice versa, but with two very different outcomes depending on the therapist's approach.

Third, in making meaningful connections *opposite interpretations can be equally meaningful.* The following example (obviously exaggerated) presents two opposite interpretations for the same phenomenon, each of which is plausible:

A patient presents to a psychiatrist for psychoanalytic psychotherapy because he is always yelling at his wife and can't figure out why. At one point over the course of therapy, the psychiatrist asks him to describe his childhood feelings toward his mother. The patient replies that he didn't have either positive or negative feelings toward her and that he doesn't think much about her in general. The therapist finds it hard to believe that the patient could be so indifferent toward such an important figure in his life. Of note, in describing his mother, the patient uses very similar terms to those he initially used to describe his wife. The therapist suggests that perhaps the patient married a woman who resembles his mother because—despite his avowals of indifference—he "actually" has always, unconsciously, *hated* his mother. He has refused to acknowledge this hate *consciously,* since such feelings are unacceptable. As a result he has *repressed* these feelings of hate. However, marrying a woman who is so like her has allowed him to recreate his relationship with his mother, including his anger toward her.

However, what if the therapist had suggested that perhaps the patient acts so indifferently toward his mother because he has always unconsciously *loved* his mother to the point of having experienced sexual longings for her. Again, he couldn't acknowledge such feelings because they are taboo and unacceptable, and as a result he has repressed them. Marrying a woman who is so like her has allowed him to fulfill his incestuous fantasies, but because of his guilt over symbolically acting on his childhood incestuous longings, he has used the defense of *reaction formation.* In other words, he has dealt with unacceptable thoughts and feelings by substituting diametrically opposed thoughts and feelings. In this case, rather than accept that he wants to have sex with his wife/mother, thereby engendering extreme anxiety and self-loathing, he tells himself that he is *furious* at his wife and *refuses* to have sex with her. He may even come to blame his wife for this problem, in which case he is displacing his anger at himself by *projecting* it onto his wife, another pathologic defense mechanism.

Fourth, meaningful connections are inconclusive. As they are based on interpretations, meaningful connections can't ever be conclusively "proven" or "disproved." There is no external source of validation. Consider the example given above. If the therapist presents to the patient the interpretation that he has sexual longings for his mother and the patient replies, "Perhaps you're right," the therapist might take this as "confirmation" that his interpretation is "correct." However, if the patient angrily replies that the therapist is *crazy* to interpret his current problems with his wife in such a way and even hurls *invectives* at the therapist, the therapist might conclude that the patient "protests too much." Perhaps the patient has become angry as a defense—a form of "resistance"—because he "can't handle the truth." In other words, no reaction by the patient conclusively disproves the therapist's theory.

Meaningful connections are inconclusive not only because they cannot be externally validated but also because we are working with living patients and not with static texts. Patients' lives continue to proceed as we work with them. Our interpretations remain inconclusive because patients are "moving targets."

Fifth, meaningful connections are unlimited in number. There are literally hundreds of different schools of psychotherapy. The above example involved psychoanalytic interpretations. However, an existential therapist, or a cognitive-behavioral therapist, or even a different psychoanalytic therapist might have made different (but equally plausible) interpretations.

Sixth, to understand is both to illuminate and to expose aspects of the patient's life. As the above examples illustrate, interpretations can enlighten the patient or can demean the patient by treating the patient as an object. Sometimes interpretations convey to the patient that the therapist thinks that she understands the patient better than the patient understands himself and this can elicit significant hostility. For example, therapists learn early in their training that to try to end an argument with one's spouse by making an interpretation as to the spouse's unconscious motivations is generally a bad idea.

Finally, meaningful connections tend to become inappropriately generalized from a small number of individual cases into more general facts about human nature. This can be useful, but it can also lead therapists to assume that they know the "answers" to life's problems, to the point of reductionism or caricature. For example, Sigmund Freud commented that "Hysterics suffer mainly from reminiscences," while Harry Stack Sullivan commented that "The hysteric might be said in principle to be a person who has a happy thought as to a way by which he can be respectable even though not living up to his standards." These aren't so much "laws" as they are maxims or proverbs, similar to "Absence makes the heart grow fonder." And does absence make the heart grow fonder? Or is the rule, "Out of sight, out of mind"? In fact, both are true—for different people, in different situations, at different times. The same can be said of why hysterics act the ways that do.

Psychiatric Applications

We shouldn't reject the whole psychotherapy enterprise just because of the protean and inclusive nature of interpretations. We also shouldn't demean the life-story perspective as being "softer" than the disease perspective. It's just that the "rules" of these two perspectives are different. The life-story perspective doesn't adhere to the scientific method. Patients benefit from psychotherapy, though, and psychotherapy cannot proceed without therapists formulating clinical cases through the use of interpretation. However, good therapists separate their observations from their interpretations and, when making interpretations, remain mindful of the fact that they are doing so.

Further, despite these caveats, the life-story perspective may be the most powerful of the four perspectives. Psychotherapy, in addition to being employed as monotherapy for "problems of living," is also routinely used in *conjunction* with the other three perspectives. After all, patients don't present for treatment because they are "depressed" or are "having panic attacks" or are "alcoholic." They present because they are demoralized and confused about difficulties that they are experiencing in their *lives*. Even a pure "psychopharmacologist" (i.e., a psychiatrist who attempts to avoid getting caught up in psychotherapy by dedicating herself to the motto, "Better living through chemistry") cannot avoid using the life-story method. When she treats patients who present with symptoms of major depressive disorder, she can't simply prescribe an antidepressant medication. She first must explain how her patient's difficulties appear to reflect the presence of a psychiatric illness and how the illness might respond to treatment with medication. Many patients will benefit

just from having received such information, even before they begin taking any medication. They have been offered an explanation that "makes sense" of their suffering and they have been offered the hope that with treatment they might regain control over their lives.

In other words, all treatment involves a component of psychotherapy. This is why clinical drug trials require a comparison group of subjects receiving a pharmacologically inert "placebo" tablet. Regardless of whether a research subject is given the active agent or the placebo, he or she encounters concerned clinicians who listen to their difficulties and offer them help. In actuality, placebo-controlled drug studies are comparing medication *plus* a nonspecific form of supportive psychotherapy to placebo plus supportive psychotherapy. When the active agent doesn't perform significantly better than placebo (for example, when 40% of subjects with peptic ulcer disease improve with active medication while 30% improve with placebo treatment), we tend to discount the effectiveness of the agent, since it's "not much better than placebo." However, the more interesting question raised by these studies is this: *why* is this "placebo effect" so powerful? After all, a treatment that is effective for 30% of subjects is quite impressive.

Sometimes, cases of "placebo response" actually reflect the natural course of the patient's illness. (After all, sometime an illness improves without any medical intervention.) However, in many cases, the mere *knowledge* that one is receiving treatment from skilled, concerned professionals constitutes powerful therapy in itself. The nature of the placebo effect remains an area of active investigation. For example, *how* do placebo responders differ from placebo nonresponders? Can we parse out which particular *elements* of treatment are responsible for this therapeutic effect? One also can apply such reasoning when designing research protocols aimed at determining the mechanism of action of formal psychotherapy, as discussed in Chapter 18.

"PERSPECTIVES" VERSUS "MULTIAXIAL CLASSIFICATION"

How can we apply of these perspectives to the clinical formulation in a particular patient's case? At this point, let us return to the clinical example presented at the beginning of this chapter. This 14-year-old patient presented with anorexia nervosa, major depressive disorder, and obsessive-compulsive personality disorder, all in the setting of multiple life stressors.

Where does one begin in a complex case like this? The patient's anorexia nervosa and major depressive disorder, both being state-related disorders, are both coded on Axis I, while her obsessive-compulsive personality disorder, being a lifelong trait-related disorder, is coded on Axis II. Her physical conditions (malnutrition, amenorrhea, hypokalemia, and iron-deficiency anemia), while all reflecting the self-starvation associated with anorexia, are also physical conditions that require clinical intervention and are listed on Axis III. Note, however, that formulating the case using the four perspectives and not simply the multiaxial scheme allows us to make further distinctions.

For example, both major depressive disorder and anorexia nervosa are coded on Axis I. However, we might approach the former primarily from the disease perspective and prescribe a combination of medication and psychotherapy. We could approach the latter primarily from the behavior perspective and initiate weight restoration and treatment of her medical complications followed by cognitive-behavioral psychotherapy aimed at examining her dieting behavior and attitudes and exploring internal triggers (such as low self-esteem and perfectionism) and external triggers (such as the extreme anxiety she experiences when her scale informs her that she has gained even a single pound). We would treat her obsessive-compulsive personality disorder primarily from the dimensional perspective while also keeping in mind through the life-story perspective the role that her symptoms may play in perpetuating a maladaptive relationship with her parents or in preventing her from having to deal with conflicts associated with puberty.

A tempting approach would be to focus primarily on the patient's clinical depression (since a medication might help with this) while hoping that once she is less depressed her other problems will "take care of themselves." Unfortunately, in severe cases of anorexia nervosa, antidepressants aren't very helpful (although *following* weight restoration they can play an important adjunctive role as part of a more comprehensive treatment plan).

Further, to focus on only one perspective (in this case, the disease perspective) at the expense of the other perspectives would lead us to overlook important features of her case. Scan this patient's case history several times, each time with a different perspective in mind. The same information assumes a different role from each different perspective. For example, a particular life stressor can be meaningful to the patient (life-story perspective), it can be a "stressor" that contributes to or triggers a biological depression (disease perspective), it can be a behavioral reinforcer (behavior perspective), or it can contribute to emotional disturbance by acting as a "key experience" that stresses particular personality vulnerabilities (dimensional perspective). The patient's case can also be appreciated from the paradigms of both form and function in that her symptoms are both symptoms of psychopathology and are "understandable" expressions of an individual in distress.

This case also demonstrates how important it is for the clinician to "shift gears" in formulating a case if he or she is to utilize *multiple* treatment strategies simultaneously, each tailored to address different aspects of the patient's presentation. Here is another example:

> A 50-year-old man is admitted with a history of periods of severe depression which also are associated with heavy drinking. He is now feeling suicidal following his wife just having left him. Following admission to the inpatient psychiatric unit, he goes into alcohol withdrawal, complicated by several medical problems. In addition, he has a history of severe personality problems; he is very self-centered and reacts with excessive rage and sadness to virtually any perceived slights. His son reports that, as a result, he has few friends and his coworkers have difficulty getting along with him. Following a complete history, physical examination, and laboratory assessment, the case is formulated as follows:
>
> Axis I: Major depressive disorder, recurrent, moderate
> Alcohol dependence
> Alcohol withdrawal
> Axis II: Narcissistic personality disorder
> Axis III: Obesity, type 2 diabetes, alcoholic hepatitis
> Axis IV: Occupational problems (unemployment); housing problems (homelessness); problems in primary support group (separated from wife)
> Axis V: GAF score of 50

Again, using the "perspectives" scheme, we would distinguish between this patient's depression and his substance dependence. Using the *DSM-IV* coding strategy we would list both conditions under Axis I, but we might still approach the patient's depression primarily from the disease perspective and his alcohol dependence primarily from the behavior perspective.

Treatment of his major depressive disorder might include a combination of psychotherapy and antidepressant medication, while treatment of his substance abuse would include detoxification followed by behavioral interventions aimed at helping him to recognize provoking factors (both environmental and internal) that contribute to his cravings for alcohol. We would encourage him to explore how he might interrupt his usual cycle of substance use (for example, going to AA meetings each night instead of to bars, avoiding walking past the liquor store, and avoiding his usual drinking partners). Psychotherapy also would take into account his personality vulnerabilities (e.g., we would try to avoid getting into confrontations with him when he complains that we are "talking down to him"), while also trying to help him gain greater insight into the way that perceived threats to his self-esteem act as important triggers for relapses into depressive episodes or alcohol use.

Finally, we would be attentive to his unique life story and the way that might shed light on his current difficulties. (For example, in this case the patient's father had been physically and verbally abusive toward the patient's mother and toward the patient himself. This may have contributed to the patient's propensity to engage in similar behaviors toward his own wife and children. It may also have contributed to his tendency to distrust other people and to feel helpless and depressed when it appears that he is "failing" at something.)

SUMMARY

In this chapter, we have discussed psychiatric formulation from four clinical perspectives: diseases, dimensions, behaviors, and life stories. Each perspective hews to a different internal logic and each carries different treatment implications. Clinicians who routinely rely on just one or another of these four perspectives fail to appreciate the complexity of mental life itself and the complexity of how different types of psychiatric disorders alter mental life. Like the blind men in the famous parable, each feeling an isolated part of an elephant but failing to recognize the elephant for what it is (thinking instead that the trunk is a snake, the leg a tree trunk, etc.) they run the risk of "missing the elephant."

Unfortunately, this is not to say that—even using all four of these perspectives—we will be able to identify the "the whole elephant." While research continues to bring us closer to understanding the links between heredity, personality, life stress, and illness, we still do not have a "unified field theory."

A better metaphor for psychiatry, proposed by McHugh and Slavney, is that of a tapestry, made up of distinct yet interwoven themes. As illustrated in Figure 3–4, the warp of *constructs* (the

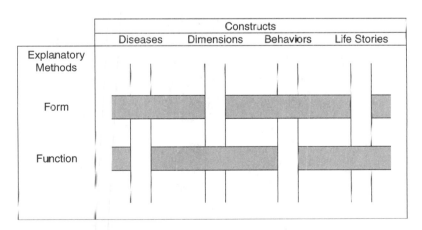

Figure 3–4. The interlocking nature of explanatory methods and explanatory constructs. Reproduced with permission from McHugh PR, Slavney PR: *The Perspectives of Psychiatry.* Baltimore, Johns Hopkins University Press, 1986

four perspectives) is interwoven with the woof of *explanatory methods* (form and function). Each construct and explanatory method have their own distinct set of premises, strengths, and liabilities. In formulating each unique case, we weave these disparate strands together.

In the chapters that follow, we will explore different classes of psychiatric disorders. Using primarily the disease perspective, we will discuss delirium, dementia, the mood disorders, the anxiety disorders, and the psychotic disorders. Next, using primarily the dimensional perspective, we will discuss the various personality disorders. We then will focus on the behavior perspective as we discuss eating disorders, substance-related disorders, somatoform disorders, dissociative disorders, and sexual and gender identity disorders. We also will use the behavior perspective as we discuss two particular behaviors that cut across diagnostic categories and that are of particular concern to psychiatrists—suicide and interpersonal violence. We then will discuss psychotherapy and how all physicians can maximize the therapeutic benefit of doctor–patient encounters by using specific techniques derived from the life-story perspective.

Before doing so, however, we must spend a bit more time exploring the nature of the tapestry depicted in Figure 3–4. While the strands of the tapestry appear clear in a schematic drawing, the conceptual distinctions between these different perspectives begin to blur as we shift our attention from thoughts, moods, and behaviors to neuroanatomy, hormones, and neurotransmitters. Since a primary goal of this text is to help the reader actually *use* psychiatric theory as the basis for sound psychiatric practice, we must first explore some of the known neurobiological underpinnings of diseases, dimensions, and behaviors. We will also examine how life events exert an influence on brain activity (for better and for worse) and vice versa.

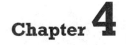

Chapter 4

Clinical Neurobiology
from Multiple Perspectives

If you press your face up against a television screen, ostensibly sharp images break down into a jumble of colored dots. This is the case regardless of the current *content* being displayed on the screen. Similarly, the four perspectives presented in Chapter 3 appear to break down the more one "zooms in" from the level of clinical phenomena to the level of neuroanatomy and neurochemistry.

This phenomenon occurs for several reasons. First, our limited understanding of the neurophysiology of everyday mental experience, to say nothing of the pathophysiology of psychiatric illness, makes it difficult to trace backward from specific clinical symptoms to specific types of brain pathology. Second, each psychiatric disorder likely contains contributory elements from each of the four perspectives, such that there are few "pure" conditions. Third, it is probable that each perspective shares underlying neurobiological processes with the other three perspectives. Finally, since neural networks interact so closely with other, any correlation between a given illness and a given neurotransmitter system or given brain region will be simplistic and excessively reductionistic.

In this chapter, we will discuss some of the neurophysiologic contributors to mental life in general and to psychiatric illness in particular Our discussion will emphasize how diseases, extremes of dimensional variation, and aberrant behaviors—when viewed at the neurobiological level—tend to boil down to a single common theme. The theme is that physiologic and behavioral responses that are *adaptive* and that enhance the survival of an organism under most circumstances also have the propensity to become *maladaptive* under other circumstances, thereby becoming sources of psychiatric morbidity.

Given this, it might be tempting to employ just one overarching perspective, a "neurobiological perspective." However, neurobiological theories offer little utility in themselves as one is formulating a clinical case and establishing a treatment plan. Rather, within each clinical perspective, they inform our thinking and help us achieve greater insight into the underlying etiologies of psychiatric disorders.

DIMENSIONAL VARIATIONS OR DISEASES?

Are disorders such as major depressive disorder, generalized anxiety disorder, and obsessive-compulsive disorder best viewed from the disease perspective or from the dimensional perspective? For example, an individual might present with a "milder" or "subclinical" form of these disorders, but couldn't such an individual simply have a sad or anxious "personality," or "temperament"?

At the neurobiological level, such distinctions tend to break down. Biological temperaments such as mild-to-moderate sadness or anxiety may even be conserved through the generations because, at "lower doses," they confer particular advantages. For example, the tendency toward "modest" obsessive-compulsiveness can be an asset for an individual working in the field of research. In the research setting, traits such as organization, precision, and the ability to repeatedly perform an experimental protocol in exactly the same way are highly valued.

Unfortunately, a subset of individuals appear to be endowed with obsessive-compulsive traits that are *so* severe that they become a source of disability. Given this, severe cases (i.e., major depressive disorder as opposed to a sad personality, obsessive-compulsive disorder as opposed to temperamental anxiety and perfectionism) may reflect more severe variation along a dimensional continuum. In other cases, it may reflect milder genetic variation *plus* a superimposed disease process. Variation along these dimensions may also predispose individuals to developing superimposed disease processes, much like deficient immunity predisposes one to develop superimposed infections.

The dimensional perspective and the disease perspective are, after all, both rooted in biology. For example, dimensional variations in temperament likely reflect underlying dimensional variations in neurochemistry. Concentrations in the brain of the various neurotransmitters etiologically implicated in the mood and anxiety disorders—dopamine, norepinephrine, serotonin, and others—likely vary among members of the general population along dimensional continuums.

Further, the extent to which individuals' neuroreceptors are "receptive" to binding with these neurotransmitters also appears to vary along a continuum. In other words, the configurations of two individuals' serotonin receptors are not exactly the same. Slightly different protein configurations of serotonin receptor confer a greater or lesser degree of "fit" with serotonin molecules. These phenotypic variations probably reflect underlying genotypic variations in the genes that code for serotonin receptors.

If it weren't for such genotypic variation, all of us would basically be the same at birth. (We still might differ to some degree due to the im-

pact of life experience, but research suggests that genetic contributions to personality are quite substantial, accounting for at least half of the variation between individuals.) The overall pattern of these variations—in neurotransmitter concentration, in neuroreceptor density, in neuroreceptor configuration—confers upon each of us at birth a unique "neurochemical identity," or "neurochemical fingerprint."

A relatively small number of relatively minor genetic variations likely account for a substantial degree of phenotypic variation. However, the unfortunate corollary of this rule is that even small degrees of genetic variation may confer upon an individual a significantly increased risk of developing an Axis I (state-related) or Axis II (trait-related) psychiatric disorder.

Given this, delineations that we have made between diseases and dimensions break down at the neurochemical level. Overlap between Axis I and Axis II illnesses at the neurobiological level may explain findings from longitudinal studies of children and adolescents followed into adulthood. Children and adolescents who have Axis II personality disorders are more likely than their nonaffected peers to be diagnosed with Axis I illnesses during adulthood. Conversely, children and adolescents with Axis I disorders such as major depressive disorder are more likely than their nonaffected peers to be diagnosed with personality disorders in adulthood.

Of course, other theories also might account for this phenomenon. For example, having an Axis I psychiatric illness throughout childhood may impede normal personality development, contributing to the development of an Axis II personality disorder. Similarly, children with Axis II personality vulnerabilities have greater difficulty coping with stressful life events, and therefore they probably are particularly vulnerable to developing Axis I mental illnesses later in life.

However, it still appears likely that the predisposition to develop either an Axis I or Axis II disorder reflects underlying neurobiological vulnerability, and that at least some Axis II personality disorders might better be viewed as "subsyndromal variants" of Axis I disorders and vice versa. Given the substantial degree of overlap between Axis I and Axis II disorders and between "normal" "abnormal" traits, some researchers seeking to work backward from disordered emotions to disordered brain physiology have adopted a broadly construed dimensional approach that emphasizes "symptom clusters" and "degrees" to which symptoms are present rather than emphasizing the "presence" or "absence" of discrete Axis I or Axis II diagnostic entities.

STRESSFUL LIFE EVENTS OR DISEASES?

Just as distinctions between the disease and the dimensional perspectives become blurred at the cellular level, so too do distinctions between these two perspectives and the life-story perspective. Subjectively, we can readily appreciate events in our lives as being psychologically meaningful. However, at the cellular level, life events obviously must be translated into changes in brain neurochemistry, or even brain neuroanatomy. Were this not the case, we would not be able to emotionally respond to external events, would not be able to recall these events later on, and would not be able to adapt our behavior on the basis of past experience.

Our understanding of how the brain's "hardware" (neural pathways) and "software" (chemistry and synaptic connections) transcribe life experience remains rudimentary. Research suggests that exposure to life experiences can encourage or suppress the activity of specific genes located within neurons.

These genes in turn influence neuronal functioning in several ways. For example, they affect the production of neurotransmitters and surface neuroreceptors, the number and complexity of dendritic branches, and the relative strength or weakness of synaptic connections formed between a neuron and its neighboring neurons. They also influence whether neurons (and their surrounding glial cells) express neurotrophic and neurotoxic substances. These latter substances "fertilize" some dendritic branches and synaptic connections and "prune away" others, thereby helping the brain to "remodel" its own neuroanatomy, a process called **neuronal plasticity**.

To appreciate the complexity of neuronal plasticity, consider two neurons facing each other such that the thick tangle of arborizing dendritic branches of one neuron intermingles with a tangle of dentritic branches from the other neuron.

Note that a single dendrite from one neuron is capable of forming synaptic connections with multiple dendrites from the adjacent neuron and also that each neuron is capable of releasing not just one neurotransmitter but multiple neurotransmitters. To untangle the pattern of connections between just these two neurons would be a formidable task. Now consider that the brain contains an estimated 100 billion neurons and over 100 trillion synaptic connections.

Brain changes in response to life events are typically adaptive, enabling the organism to interact with and adapt to the surrounding environment. However, in the face of more severe, adverse life experiences (be they single, highly traumatic events or less severe but chronic stressors) the brain's response can become a source of psychopathology. Apparently, the various components of the body's "stress thermostat," normally adaptive in nature, become maladaptive when the "temperature" is set too high for too long.

One component of this "stress thermostat" is the **glucocorticoid system**. Glucocorticoids are secreted by the adrenal system as part of the "fight or flight response" that occurs in response to brief, stressful circumstances. When secreted *transiently*, glucocorticoids *aid survival*. They help us to mobilize energy stores, increase our cardiac output, stimulate our immunity, and suppress nonessential biological activities such as growth, tissue repair, and sexual functioning. In contrast, when secreted *chronically and excessively* (as in Cushing's syndrome), glucocorticoids contribute to the *development of systemic diseases*, including hypertension, diabetes, amenorrhea, impotence, ulcers, and immune system suppression.

Excessive glucocorticoid secretion also appears to be bad for the brain, causing dendritic atrophy, impaired neurogenesis, even neuronal death (**neurotoxicity**). In particular, neurons located in the *hippocampus*, known to play a major role in the consolidation of short-term memories into long-term memories, contain a high concentration of glucocorticoid receptors. The hippocampus is known to be particularly sensitive to neurotoxicity, perhaps because of this. Also of note is that two psychiatric illnesses known to be associated with both stressful life events and with memory complaints—major depressive disorder and post-traumatic stress disorder—are associated with a significant loss of hippocampal volume when the brains of affected patients are compared to those of control subjects by using volumetric magnetic resonance brain imaging.

A second component of the "stress thermostat" is a complex balance between excitatory synapses (mostly mediated by the amino acid *glutamate*) and *inhibitory synapses* (mostly mediated by *γ-aminobutryric acid, GABA*). Glutamate appears to be the brain's major excitatory neurotransmitter. Virtually every neuron in the brain has glutamate receptors and these receptors are triggered by even minute amounts of glutamate. There are three major subtypes of glutamate receptor, with the N-methyl-D-aspartate (NMDA) receptor being perhaps the most important one. This receptor includes a ligand-gated calcium ion channel. When glutamate binds to the NMDA receptor, this calcium channel opens and calcium flows into the neuron. Intracellular calcium concentrations are tightly regulated, and even mild increases in the intracellular calcium concentration activate several calcium-dependent enzymes (protein kinases and phosphorylases).

The balance between excitation and inhibition also appears to be an essential contributor to neuronal plasticity. However, as was the case with the glucocorticoid system, excessive neuronal excitation in the face of stress can result in the brain being exposed to "too much of a good thing"; neuropathology may be the result. Excessive calcium influx causes neurons to be "excited to death" since excessive enzymatic activity produces too high a concentration of free radicals, which in turn are toxic to neuronal membranes. This **excitotoxicity** has been implicated in brain damage associated with a variety of neurologic diseases, whether they involve acute ischemic injury (as in *stroke*) or chronic degeneration (as in *Parkinson's disease, Huntington's disease, Alzheimer's disease*, and *amyotrophic lateral sclerosis*). Again this process has been best studied in the hippocampus.

These first two elements of the "stress thermostat" also appear to interact with each other. For example, excessive glucocorticoid activity can cause neurotoxicity, both directly (through excessive glucocorticoid receptor stimulation) and indirectly (by elevating hippocampal concentrations of glutamate and by increasing hippocampal neurons' sensitivity to glutamate's toxic effects).

A third component of the "stress thermostat" is the contribution of **neurotrophic factors**. These are proteins that promote the growth, differentiation, and survival of neurons and their supporting glia. If neurons are "trees," neurotrophic factors are "fertilizer." Neurotrophic factors play an important role early in life in nervous system development, when they influence neuronal migration and synaptogenesis. Neurons exposed to neurotrophic factors are protected while neurons that aren't exposed to them experience "programmed cell death," also called **apoptosis**. In the course of normal brain maturation, somewhere between 50% and 90% of the nearly 1 trillion neurons initially present in the immature human brain "self-destruct" through apoptosis. This enables only the "fittest" neurons and synaptic connections to survive, a process that has been called "neural Darwinism." This process also demonstrates the importance role of early life experience in helping to shape brain development.

Neurotrophic factors continue to play an important role in the adult brain. They help to mediate synaptic plasticity by favoring the growth of some dendritic connections over others. They also share some characteristics of "traditional" neurotransmitters. For example, they are synthesized by neurons in order to influence the activity of neighboring neurons. Also, their release appears to be influenced by the activity of traditional neurotransmitters and vice versa.

Like the first two components of the stress thermostat, this third component appears to be adaptive under most circumstances but maladaptive and a source of pathology under other circumstances. When the degree of neurotrophic activity is inadequate, or when the degree of activity fails to adequately compensate for competing glutamate-mediated excitotoxicity, excessive neurotoxicity can occur.

This third component of the stress thermostat also interacts with the first two components. In the hippocampus, excessive glucocorticoid activity appears to inhibit the release of neurotrophic factors and also appears to interfere with the effectiveness of neurotrophic factors. Given this, the administration of exogenous neurotrophic factors might offer a novel treatment strategy, not only for neurodegenerative disorders but for mood or anxiety disorders as well. (While this is theoretically possible, whether it will prove to be the case in practice remains to be seen. Exogenously administered neurotrophic factors also might encourage the random or inappropriate growth of the *wrong* neurons or glia, perhaps even increasing the risk of developing a brain tumor.)

Overall then, heritable variations in personality may be linked at the neurobiological level to heritable vulnerabilities to disease. Genetic predispositions, life stressors, learned behaviors, comorbid medical conditions, and previous episodes of psychiatric illness all contribute to changes in gene expression. These changes in turn mediate dendritic branching patterns and the strength of different synaptic connections, thereby influencing regional brain neurophysiology.

As the resolution of anatomic and functional neuroimaging technology improves, and as more potential "biomarkers" of psychiatric illness are identified, researchers may reach the point where they are able to demonstrate that patients who improve following psychiatric treatment (whether with psychotherapy or with psychotropic medication) do so as a result of corrective changes to these modulatory systems. Should such tests become available in the treatment setting, they might allow clinicians not only to reliably confirm and to validate the presence of specific types and subtypes of psychiatric disorders but also to rationally choose treatment interventions that have been rationally designed to target specific areas of impairment.

MALADAPTIVE BEHAVIORS OR DISEASES?

As with dimensions of personality and as for stressful life events, behavior can be studied at the level of brain neuroanatomy and neurophysiology. At this level, distinctions between the disease perspective and the behavior perspective also become blurred. We even can approach many psychiatric diseases from the behavioral perspective—that is, by thinking of them as maladaptive responses of systems normally intended to modulate animal behavior in response to changing environments.

Table 4–1. Some Internal Factors That Modify Human Behavior

Memory	Mood
Anxiety	Executive function and attention
Pleasure	

Animal behavior is not random and it also does not consist simply of reflex responses to the current external environment. An animal's behavior in a given situation is influenced by a variety of factors, some of which are listed in Table 4–1. These factors include our *sensory perceptions* of the outside world, our current internal physiologic state (hunger, fatigue, libido, etc.), our current *emotional state* (happiness, sadness, fear of present harm, or anxiety about the potential for future harm), our *memories* of earlier, similar situations, and our overall *cognitive assessment* of the current situation (e.g., "safe," "dangerous," "pleasant," "unpleasant," "boring," or "novel").

These factors don't simply "converge" at the end point of behavior. They interact with each other. For example, our memories of a past event are linked to memories of the emotions that we felt at the time of that event. When past behaviors or circumstances have been associated with pleasurable emotional states, we are more likely to repeat these behaviors or place ourselves into similar circumstances. (In the language of animal research, we are more likely to engage in *approach behaviors*.) When past behaviors or circumstances have been associated with aversive emotional states (such as pain or anxiety), we are more likely to avoid similar behaviors or circumstances in the future. (We are more likely to engage in *avoidance behaviors*.)

Therefore, emotions don't simply add spice to life. They are essential ingredients of life. Through their associations—with internal physiologic states, with external life events—emotions better allow us to modify our future behavior based on our past experiences. They also affect our performance as we engage in these behaviors. For example, mild anxiety usually improves one's performance, but severe anxiety usually impairs performance.

How do brain states and behavior affect each other? The modulating influences listed in Table 4–1 appear to influence our behavior through independent but interconnected *neural circuits* (also called *neural networks*). These circuits can be studied in a variety of ways.

In laboratory animals, these circuits can be elucidated by lesioning or stimulating various regions of the brain and observing the resultant behavioral changes. Similarly, human subjects who have had strokes that involve specific brain regions or who have neurologic illnesses known to affect specific neural circuits can be assessed for associated cognitive, emotional, and behavioral changes.

We also can study healthy human subjects by using noninvasive *structural neuroimaging techniques* such as computerized tomography (CT) or magnetic resonance imaging (MRI), or by using *functional neuroimaging techniques* such as functional magnetic resonance imaging (fMRI), positron emission tomography (PET), or single photon emission tomography (SPECT). Some creative research protocols have asked subjects to submit to functional neuroimaging while simultaneously engaged in various behavioral tasks or exposed to stimuli designed to arouse specific emotions.

Patients affected by psychiatric illnesses such as dementia, mood disorders, anxiety disorders, schizophrenia, and substance use disorders also have been studied with functional neuroimaging. Typically, resting-state scans are compared to the resting-state scans of non-ill control subjects. Also, scans can be obtained from both patients and control subjects either while the patients are experiencing active symptoms (such as hallucinations) or while they are performing tasks or given medications designed to provoke their symptoms. (For example, a patient with obsessive-compulsive disorder who has severe fears of dirt or contamination might be scanned at rest and then after a wet Kleenex has been placed into his outstretched hand. A patient with schizophrenia might be scanned at rest and then while performing a task that demands advance planning and mental flexibility.) Patients' scans can be compared to the scans of nonaffected control subjects both at rest and when exposed to the same stimuli. This allows researchers to identify particular brain regions in psychiatric illnesses that demonstrate either excessive activity or insufficient activity and the relationship between brain activity and symptoms of the illness.

In another paradigm, functional neuroimaging is obtained during a period of active illness, followed by another scan once the patient has received treatment and has achieved symptomatic improvement. This allows researchers to determine both whether specific regions of the brain are hypoactive or hyperactive during periods of illness and also whether symptomatic recovery is associated with normalization of this activity. (One might expect this to be the case for psychiatric disorders caused by reversible pathological states, but not for psychiatric disorders caused by persistent trait vulnerabilities.)

Results from these converging approaches to elucidating brain structure–function relationships suggest that the various mental disorders cannot simply be divvied up between various brain regions. Rather, *constellations* of brain regions, dynamically interacting with each other, work in concert to regulate sensory perceptions of the outside world, emotions (such as anger, anxiety, and sadness), basic cognitive abilities (such as memory and language), and higher-level cognitive abilities (such as the exercise of attention, the suppression of reflex emotional or behavioral responses, and the use of judgment and advance planning).

While a precise understanding of just how activity along these circuits "translates" into a person experiencing a specific mood state or experiencing cravings to engage in particular behaviors continues to elude us, these models are useful both to scientists and to practicing clinicians. They draw our attention to particular *aspects* of clinical phenomena, thereby providing suggestions as to where one might intervene to interrupt feedback loops that have become either abnormally entrenched (as in the case of the intrusive anxiety and traumatic memories that occur in post-traumatic stress disorder) or pathologically self-reinforcing (as in the case of the craving, pleasure, and driven behaviors that occur in the substance use disorders). What follows is a brief overview of these circuits, emphasizing their presumed roles as neurobiological substrates of pathologic behaviors.

Memory

Memory allows us to modify our behavior over time since behavior is influenced not only by our immediate circumstances but also by our recollection of past experiences. **Short-term memory** and **long-term memory** are dependent on the intact functioning of related but distinct brain pathways. Further, the encoding of new memories is a separate process from the retrieval of stored memories.

For example, patients with **amnestic disorder** due to a brain injury (discussed further in Chapter 5) can retrieve information from long-term memory and also can retain information in short-term memory. However, they are impaired in their ability to *consolidate* new information so that it moves from short-term memory into long-term memory. For example, they can remember a short list of numbers in their heads if they focus attention on the task and continually repeat the numbers. (This is what we all do when trying to retain a new telephone number for a period of time just long enough to dial it.) After a brief delay, though, this information is forgotten. This is called an *anterograde memory deficit*. Amnestic patients also usually demonstrate a *retrograde memory deficit* for some period of time preceding the onset of their disorder. The densest retrograde deficit involves the period of time immediately preceding the brain injury, while memory for events occurring long before the injury is usually unaffected.)

There are two major forms of long-term memory, as displayed in Figure 4–1. **Declarative memory** (also called explicit memory) is memory for consciously recalled facts. There are two types of declarative memory: episodic memory and semantic memory. **Episodic memory** is a memory for events, whether personal (autobiographical) or impersonal (public). Examples of episodic memories include memories of one's wedding, of having eaten a Big Mac for lunch yesterday, or of needing to buy milk today on the

way home from work. **Semantic memory** is memory for general facts. An example of semantic memory is knowing the date of one's birthday. One doesn't recall the event of having been born, just a date on the calendar. The second form of long-term memory is **nondeclarative memory** (also called implicit, or procedural memory). This refers to a memory of learned behaviors. Examples include the memory of how to ride a bicycle and of how to play tennis.

The contents of declarative memory can be verbalized, and because of this declarative memory can be assessed directly using psychological measures. For example, a list of words can be presented to the patient and the percentage of words that the patient later spontaneously recalls or recognizes from a list can be calculated. In contrast, nondeclarative memory can be studied only indirectly, by asking the patient to engage in various tasks over time and assessing whether their performance improves over time or remains the same.

Typically, we rely on all of these forms of memory, seamlessly integrating them. We recall the brand of car that we own (semantic memory), where we parked it this morning (episodic memory), and how to drive it (procedural memory). In dementia, a disease that affects the brain diffusely, all three forms of memory are impaired. For example, patients in later stages of dementia have naming difficulties, can't recall recent events, and have trouble learning new skills and utilizing previously learned skills. In the more limited amnestic disorder, both aspects of declarative memory are impaired, but nondeclarative memory remains intact. For example, patients with amnestic disorder still can be classically conditioned. Further, their performance

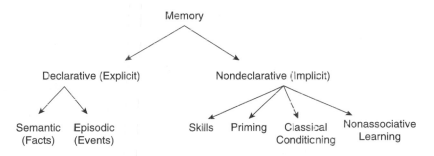

Figure 4–1. A taxonomy of memory. Adapted from Squire LR, Zola-Morgan S: "Memory: Brain Systems and Behavior." *Trends Neurosci* 22:170–175, 1988.

on complex tasks such as solving puzzles or reading words backward in a mirror improves over repeated testing sessions, despite their demonstrating no declarative memory of having ever previously performed these tasks.

The fact that individuals with amnestic disorder retain nondeclarative memory despite such profound losses in the realm of declarative memory suggests that neuroanatomically distinct systems mediate these two types of memory. Brain-lesioning studies in lab animals confirm this hypothesis. A **medial temporal lobe circuit** (mediated primarily by *acetylcholine*) appears to be particularly important for explicit memory, while a **basal ganglia/frontal lobe circuit** (mediated primarily by *dopamine*) appears to be most important for implicit memory. The medial temporal lobe circuit (discussed in more detail in Chapter 5) includes the hippocampus, fornix, the mammillary bodies of the hypothalamus, and the medial thalamic nuclei. Brain lesions involving any of these sites along the circuit (such as those listed in Table 6–2) can cause an amnestic disorder to occur.

However, the medial temporal lobe circuit does not appear to be the actual storage site for long-term memories. For example, patients with amnestic disorder don't lose previously stored long-term memories, with the exception of memories for events just proximate to their brain in-

jury. Their primary deficit lies in their ability to *consolidate* short-term memories into longer-term memories. By analogy, if the brain is thought of as a computer, what is lost is the ability to move data from RAM (short-term memory) onto the hard drive (long-term memory), but not the ability to access information previously stored on the hard drive. The relatively brief retrograde amnesia (days to weeks) suggests that this is the period of time required for movement from short-term to long-term memory. Long-term memories likely are stored across a broad swath of cerebral cortex. As a result, severe dementing diseases associated with diffuse cortical damage (such as Alzheimer's disease, multiple strokes, severe traumatic brain injury, CNS infection, and vitamin deficiency) *are* capable of erasing long-term memories.

Anxiety and Pleasure

Our present behavior is influenced by more than just our declarative memories of similar past circumstances. Along with remembering the details of past events, we remember whether these events were painful or pleasurable. We are drawn to situations that—based on previous experience—we expect to be pleasurable, and we try to avoid situations that we expect to be unpleasant.

Separate but related neuronal circuits mediate

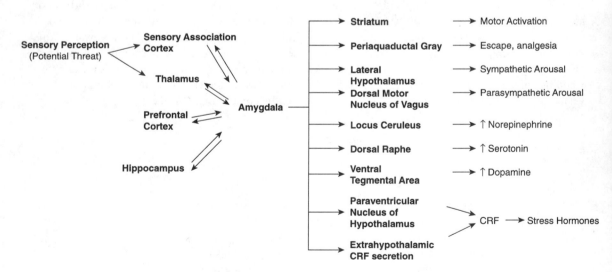

Figure 4–2. The fear circuit, centering on the amygdala. Adapted with permission from Charney DS, Bremner JD: The Neurobiology of Anxiety Disorders." *Neurobiology of Mental Illness.* Edited by Charney DS, Nestler EJ, Bunney BS. New York, Oxford University Press, 1999.

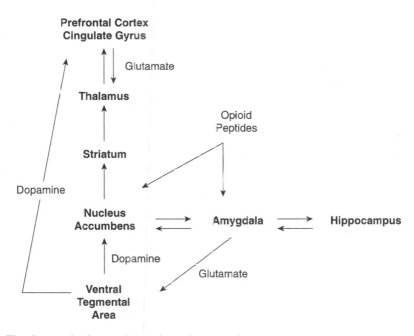

Figure 4–3. The pleasure circuit, centering on the nucleus accumbens.

these two types of emotional responses. Noxious or dangerous experiences trigger a **fear response**, mediated by a circuit centering on the *amygdala*. This circuit is described (in simplified form) in Figure 4–2. Positive experiences trigger a **pleasure response**, mediated by a circuit centering cn the *nucleus accumbens*. This circuit is described (again in simplified form) in Figure 4–3.

Both of these circuits are integrated nct only with each other but also with the above-described memory circuits. The relationship between emotion and memory is a complex two-way street. Emotionally arousing stimuli are strong inducers of declarative and nondeclarative memory formation. (One example is the large number of people who can remember exactly where they were and what they were doing when they first heard that President Kennedy had been shot or that the World Trade Center towers had been destroyed.) Further, our declarative memory of past situations helps us to cognitively appraise our current situation, thereby better modulating our present emotional responses.

While the medial temporal lobe circuit mediates the consolidation of "cognitive" aspects of memory, the amygdala and nucleus accumbens appear to mediate the consolidation of "emotional" aspects of memory. These different types

of memory for a given past event are *subjectively* experienced as being seamlessly integrated, but neuropathological studies in both animals and humans reveal evidence of distinct systems.

For example, animals whose amygdala has been lesioned demonstrate attenuated fear responses. Similarly, some humans with strokes involving the amygdala report having an intact "cognitive memory" that certain situations should be considered "dangerous," but their emotional and visceral *sensation* of fear when placed in such situations is greatly attenuated. In contrast, stimulating the amygdala in animals elicits fear-like behaviors and autonomic arousal, while electrical stimulation of the amygdala in conscious humans elicits a classic fear response (including sensations of anxiety and depersonalization, visceral sensations in the chest and epigastrium, and changes in autonomic activity).

Normally, the circuits mediating memory, fear, and pleasure are adaptive: they help us to appraise the significance of both internal and external stimuli and then, through their efferent pathways, help us to respond appropriately. For example, in the face of sensory perceptions of an external stimulus interpreted as "dangerous," the acute fear response literally "takes over" the body. It overrides ongoing biologic activities and diverts the body's resources almost exclusively toward self-protection. (In most cases, sensory perceptions are first filtered through a longer pathway that includes sensory association cortex. However, in acute emergencies a second, even more direct afferent pathway allows the sensory perception to bypass association cortex and proceed straight though the thalamus to the amygdala, thereby allowing preprogrammed behavioral responses to occur within milliseconds. For example, notice how quickly your fear response kicks in if you are driving and experience a near collision or suddenly see a police car with lights flashing in your rear-view mirror.)

Consistent with this central role, the amygdala sends efferent output to every major part of the brain. The amygdala triggers the *hypothalamus* to release corticotropin-releasing factor (CRF), which in turn triggers the pituitary gland to release adrenocorticotropin hormone (ACTH), which ultimately stimulates the adrenal gland to release cortisol, a glucocorticoid stress hormone. (As discussed above, glucocorticoids play an essential role in the stress thermostat. While cortisol feeds back on almost all of these brain pathways, CRF itself also acts as a neurotransmitter for neurons within the amygdala, possibly mediating some aspects of the fear response as well as other negative emotional responses.)

The amygdala also activates both the *sympathetic and parasympathetic nervous systems* (producing increased blood pressure and heart rate, sweating, piloerection, pupillary dilatation, suppression of nonessential visceral activity, activation of key motor systems, and increased alertness). In addition, it activates *endogenous opioid peptide release*, thereby suppressing pain. Finally, projections from the amygdala to the *locus ceruleus*, the *raphe nuclei*, and the *ventral tegmental area* increase the release of norepinephrine, serotonin, and dopamine, respectively. These neurotransmitters also contribute to a state of increased arousal and vigilance, help the organism to focus attention on the perceived threat, and enhance the formation of declarative and nondeclarative memories of the situation.

In the wake of this initial fear response, an **anxiety response** can occur at a later point in time. Because memories of the dangerous stimulus and the circumstances surrounding it have been encoded, future stimuli or circumstances that suffi-ciently resemble the original ones can trigger a similar (but usually less intense) physiologic response. This latter anxiety response appears to be mediated less by the amygdala than by a related region, the *bed nucleus of the stria terminalis*. (Of note, this brain region so resembles the amygdala in its cellular organization that it, the nucleus accumbens, and the basal forebrain are sometimes called the "extended amygdala.")

In contrast to the fear and anxiety responses, the pleasure response occurs in the setting of pleasurable stimuli or situations, such as eating or sexual activity. The pleasure, or reward, pathways include the nucleus accumbens (the major component of the ventral striatum), the basal forebrain, and regions of the medial prefrontal cortex. While the fear and anxiety responses encourage "fight or flight" behaviors, the pleasure response encourages "approach behaviors." (Stimuli that are associated with a sense of pleasure and that encourage approach behaviors are termed *rewards*. When a rewarding stimulus increases the probability that an animal will repeatedly engage in behaviors that have been paired with administration of the pleasurable stimulus, it s considered to be a *reinforcing* stimulus.)

Clearly, the *memory* of pleasure or of positive emotions is a necessary component of this pleasure system. Positive "emotional" memories might be stored within the nucleus accumbens and associated structures, while the system also has reciprocal connections to both the fear circuit and to the hippocampal circuit, again allowing for a subjective sense of seamless integration of these different types of memory and behavioral responses. The interdependent nature of the functional circuits governing declarative memory, fear, and pleasure is underscored by the finding that all three circuits are modulated by the same neurotrophic factors, utilize similar intracellular signaling cascades, and demonstrate similar adaptations in dendritic morphology in response to life experience.

All of the structures in the reward pathway are richly innervated by *dopamine*, supplied by the *ventral tegmental area (VTA)* in the midbrain. Generally speaking, rewarding and reinforcing stimuli appear to exert their affects either *(1)* by enhancing *dopamine release* from the VTA or *(2)* by potentiating the *effects* of dopamine release within the pleasure system, or *3)* by producing effects *similar* to dopamine release.

While the emotional and behavioral responses associated with the memory, anxiety, and pleasure circuits are usually adaptive, even necessary for the organism to survive, *excessive* activity along these circuits may account for the severe emotional and behavioral symptoms that characterize many psychiatric disorders.

For example, excessive activity along the *anxiety circuit* may account for the fear, anxiety, and anxiety-laden memories that are the primary feature of all of the various anxiety disorders. In **panic disorder**, an acute fear response occurs spontaneously and inappropriately. In the **phobic disorders**, relatively benign stimuli become associated with severe fear responses, usually leading to individuals developing compensatory avoidance behaviors. In **obsessive-compulsive disorder**, fears of specific situations become unduly amplified (obsessions) leading to the development of excessive and irrational compensatory behaviors (compulsions).

In **generalized anxiety disorder**, both the physiologic manifestations of the anxiety response and cognitive expectations of future harm become exaggerated, leading affected individuals to experience significant subjective distress even in the face of relatively minor objective stress. Finally, in **post-traumatic stress disorder**, exposure to a severe, fear-inducing stimulus leads to the development of intense, pervasive anxiety and intrusive "emotional memories." Typical symptoms include anxiety, autonomic hyperarousal, intrusive reexperiencing of the traumatic event (through recollections, dreams, or flashbacks), excessive psychological distress or physiologic reactivity upon exposure to internal or external cues that symbolize or resemble some aspect of the traumatic event, and phobic avoidance of stimuli associated with the trauma.

Similarly, the *pleasure circuit*, while normally adaptive, appears to play a prominent role in psychiatric conditions associated with "addictive" behaviors. Most notably, while the presumed purpose of this circuit is to provide a connection between *natural* reinforcers (such as eating or sexual activity) and feelings of pleasure, **drugs of abuse** *directly* activate neurons in this circuit through chemical means. Chemical reinforcers

such as nicotine, cocaine, and heroin tend to be more powerful than natural reinforcers; they also allow an individual to achieve the pleasure response more reliably than do natural reinforcers. These factors encourage repetitive use of the drug of abuse, even in individuals who are aware of the social, psychological, and physical problems that are being caused or exacerbated by their substance use (i.e., **substance dependence**).

Further, the brain *adapts* to this repeated, excessive stimulation, such that the normal compensatory mechanisms are no longer sufficient to return the pleasure circuit to its default state of homeostasis. The drug of abuse no longer achieves the desired effect, and increased amounts of the drug are required (a phenomenon called **tolerance**). In addition, reduction or discontinuation of the drug is associated with acute physiological and psychological symptoms, including autonomic arousal, anxiety, depression, and craving for the drug (a phenomenon called **withdrawal**).

Longer-term abstinence symptoms can persist even for weeks to months. These include lower-grade anxiety, dysphoria, anhedonia, and insomnia. Several circuits, all interlinked, likely contribute to these symptoms, including: persistent decreases in dopamine and opioid peptides along the pleasure circuit, similar decreases in dopamine and opioid peptides along the frontal attention–motivation circuit (as described below), reduced activity along the serotonergic mood-regulatory circuit (also described below), and excessive activity along the anxiety circuit (including excessive CRF and glucocorticoid release).

Even months to years after the cessation of drug use, some individuals continue to experience cravings for the drug, particularly when exposed to stimuli previously associated with their drug use. (For example, cravings may occur when the individuals are around friends who have used alcohol or drugs with them, when they pass a liquor store, or when they witness drug use in a film.) Perhaps these persistent, intrusive, visceral memories of the intoxication experience are the equivalent of the "flashbacks" that occur in post-traumatic stress disorder. In this case, however, the intrusive emotional memories are associated with rewarding stimuli and pleasurable sensations rather than aversive stimuli and anxious sensations. Further, it is likely that dopaminergic activity along this circuit is not associated with the pleasure of consummatory reward per se, but with the appetitive motivation, the *drive*, to engage in effortful behaviors to obtain that reward.

Behavioral disorders also can involve natural rather than chemical reinforcers. Examples include **anorexia** and **bulimia nervosa**, **sexual paraphilia**, and **compulsive overeating, shopping, gambling**, or **weightlifting**. These disorders also may involve the pleasure circuit and might be thought of as instances of "addiction without the drug." Unfortunately, disorders of motivated behavior that involve natural rather than chemical reinforcers likely also are sustained by a variety of social and psychological reinforcers, such that it has been difficult to devise animal models.

An alternative theory suggests that these latter disorders might be variants of obsessive–compulsive disorder rather than variants of addiction. However, as the above discussion suggests, these two theories are not mutually exclusive, since substance dependence and obsessive-compulsive disorder may themselves be related. (A core feature of both disorders is the repetitive performance of a particular group of behaviors to the exclusion of other important life activities and despite adverse consequences.)

Attention and Executive Function

We have discussed how the memory, fear, and pleasure circuits overlap with each other through shared connections at the level of the hippocampus and amygdala. They also overlap with each other through shared connections with a fourth circuit. This last circuit includes the frontal lobes and their associated cortical and subcortical regions, including the parietal lobes, the cingulate gyrus, and the basal ganglia. It mediates the ability to focus attention on salient stimuli while simultaneously filtering out extraneous stimuli.

The brain is bombarded at any given moment by a multitude of stimuli generated both from within the organism and from the external environment. Since the brain has limited processing power, it is crucial that it have the ability to selectively attend to specific stimuli while ignoring others, while also retaining the ability to read-

ily shift attention back to these ignored stimuli should the situation demand it.

For example, let us imagine that you are trying to read a book in the park while your child plays on the swings. To accomplish this, you obviously must have the ability to focus your attention (and to sustain that attention over time) on your book. Next, you also must be able to filter out a wide variety of extraneous stimuli: the sounds of children and their parents talking to each other, the visual images of people on bicycles riding past, the feel of the breeze on your face, the sensations of your lungs moving air in and out, the sensation of gastric distension as you digest your breakfast. Then, you must be able to intermittently shift your attention from your book to your child and then back to your book. Each time you look up, you have to be able to rapidly locate your child in space and to distinguish her from the other children. What's more, even if you are deeply absorbed in your book, the sound of your child's voice crying out is capable of "breaking through" your state of absorption, immediately drawing your full attention in your child.

As the above example demonstrates, "attention" is not a unitary phenomenon. It includes the abilities to: *(1) focus attention* on a particular location in space (such as your daughter's position on the playground) *(2) sustain attention* over time to a particular stimulus (such as your book) or to only one aspect of a stimulus (such as the words printed in the book but not the color or shape of the book), and *(3) filter out competing stimuli* (such as extraneous noises, visual perceptions and somatic sensations).

The first phenomenon, orientation of attention, involves *the frontal lobes, the thalamus, and parietal association cortex*. The importance of this circuit becomes most evident in examining patients who have suffered a stroke involving the posterior parietal cortex (particularly if it was a right hemisphere stroke). Such patients often demonstrate a **neglect syndrome**. They fail to attend to relevant stimuli that appear in the contralateral world.

Visuospatial neglect is the most easily demonstrated phenomenon. For example, when asked to copy a picture of a clock face, patients with a neglect syndrome may only draw the right side of the clock face or may cram all of the numbers into the right-hand side. (Typically, one can direct the patient's attention to the left side of the picture, thereby illustrating that this phenomenon is not simply the result of a co-occurring left visual field deficit.) Patients with a neglect syndrome also may fail to respond to auditory or tactile stimuli presenting from the contralateral world, particularly when presented simultaneously with a *competing* stimulus delivered to the ipsilateral side. For example, they may be able to recognize each time the examiner taps on either the left or right thigh separately, but they may only perceive the right thigh to have been touched when both thighs are tapped at the same time. In severe cases, patients with neglect syndromes can demonstrate complex cognitive and behavioral manifestations extending beyond simple inattention, including a complete lack of insight into the very fact that the contralateral side of their body is paralyzed (termed *anosognosia*).

The second attention phenomenon, sustained attention over time to a selected stimulus or aspect of a stimulus, appears to involve the *anterior cingulate gyrus and adjacent areas of the frontal cortex*. This region is richly innervated by terminals from dopamine neurons projecting from the VTA.

In contrast, the third and related attention phenomenon, the dampening of potentially distracting sensory stimuli, requires the *thalamus*, which acts in a "gatekeeper" role. For example, during functional neuroimaging studies where subjects are asked to sustain attention on one type of stimulus while trying to ignore various distracting stimuli that are introduced throughout the task, the pulvinar region of the thalamus demonstrates increased activity.

Together, these circuits mediate **executive function**. Executive function subsumes multiple "upper-level" aspects of motivated behavior including motivation, planning, judgment, working memory, sustained attention, filtering of extraneous stimuli, shifting readily from one aspect of a task to another and back again, monitoring for any difficulties as they arise, and generating new strategies when necessary. Impairments in executive function contribute to the morbidity associated with several psychiatric disorders, including attention-deficit hyperactivity disorder, dementia, schizophrenia, and major depressive disorder.

Attention-deficit hyperactivity disorder, or ADHD (discussed in Chapter 18) includes two types of symptoms—those involving *inattention* and those involving *impaired impulse control*. While the cause of ADHD is unknown, the condition appears to have a strong genetic component and neuroimaging studies also suggest that individuals diagnosed with ADHD demonstrate less activity in their *frontal and cingulate cortex* when compared to control subjects. In these two regions, *dopamine* plays an important role as a mediator of memory and sustained attention, and it is notable that stimulant medications (which increase dopamine transmission) also are effective in treating both of the types of symptoms seen in ADHD.

In those cases of **dementia** where the frontal lobes or their associated subcortical structures are affected (described in Chapter 5), typical symptoms include impaired memory and mental flexibility, loss of normal social judgment, apathy, irritability, and personality changes. Similar symptoms also characterize the cluster of "negative" symptoms seen in **schizophrenia**. These symptoms are as much a source of disability as are the "positive" symptoms of schizophrenia such as hallucinations and delusions.

Patients with **major depressive disorder** often complain of impaired concentration and memory and these patients also have difficulty performing tasks requiring sustained attention. A greater severity of depression is associated with a greater degree of cognitive and attentional impairment. The latter deficits typically improve substantially once remission from the depressive episode is achieved, although more subtle deficits may remain even in the euthymic state.

Mood

"Mood" is a complex subjective phenomenon. It affects animal behavior more indirectly than do fear and pleasure. Because of this, behavioral scientists have had difficulty devising animal models of depressive and manic states. While this chapter emphasizes the neurobiology of mood, theories of depression in general (along with associated treatment implications) are discussed in Chapter 6.

Psychological Theories of Depression

In the early twentieth century, psychological theories of depression predominated, especially psychoanalytic theories that postulated that loss or trauma early in an individual's life could make her vulnerable to developing depression later on, especially when faced with stressors that echo the original stressor. (While these theories emphasized "pure" psychological processes, they would not be incompatible with the neurobiological theories discussed above that suggest that trauma can lead to lasting, detrimental effects on neuronal systems.)

Monoamine Theories of Depression

In the late 1950s, two classes of medications, the *monoamine oxidase inhibitors (MAOIs)* and the *tricyclic antidepressants (TCAs)*, were discovered to have clinical efficacy in treating depression. Both discoveries occurred only as a result of serendipity. The first MAOI, iproniazid, was an antituberculosis agent that was found to improve the moods of tuberculosis patients, leading clinicians to study it in depressed patients. Imipramine, the first TCA, was originally studied as an antipsychotic drug. While it offered little relief from psychotic symptoms, it fortunately was recognized for its antidepressant effects.

By the 1960s, researchers had determined that both classes of medication increased brain levels of the biogenic amines *norepinephrine (NE)* and *serotonin (5-hydroxytryptamine, or 5-HT)*. Further, it was noted that *reserpine*, an antihypertensive drug that depletes biogenic amines, could cause depression in about 15% of individuals. These two findings paved the way for the **biogenic amine hypothesis of depression**, which posited that clinical depression is the result of a monoamine deficiency. Monoamine oxidase (MAO) is the enzyme that degrades both NE and 5HT. Thus, MAOIs, by inhibiting the *breakdown* of these neurotransmitters, increase their levels. In contrast, TCAs inhibit their neuronal *reuptake* from the synaptic cleft. Like MAOIs, they therefore raise the levels of both NE and 5HT, but by a different mechanism. However, subsequent research has failed to fully validate the biogenic amine hypothesis.

First, studies of monoamine metabolite concentrations in patients with mood disorders have yielded confusing, even contradictory, results. Some studies indicate that levels of monoamine metabolites are decreased in the cerebrospinal fluid of depressed patients compared to levels seen in nondepressed control subjects, but other investigators have found no differences or even increases. Second, most research subjects who are given agents that deplete biogenic amines do not become depressed. Third, while antidepressant medications raise monoamine levels in all depressed patients, they only provide effective relief from depressive symptoms for about 60% of patients. Fourth, synaptic monoamine levels rise rapidly with the initiation of antidepressant therapy, but the clinical response doesn't occur for up to several weeks.

Taken together, these findings suggests that the clinical response to antidepressant medication isn't caused by increases in monoamine levels per se but by later-onset adaptations in brain functioning that occur *in response* to this shift in monoamine homeostasis. (It also is noteworthy that more recently introduced agents, while offering the benefit of having fewer side effects, have not proven to be any more efficacious, nor have they been found to act any more rapidly, than the tricyclic antidepressants and monoamine oxidase inhibitors introduced a half-century earlier.)

Given these difficulties, researchers shifted their attention in the 1980s from monoamines to their respective presynaptic and postsynaptic receptors, leading to the **neuroreceptor hypothesis of depression**. Antidepressants that inhibit monoamine degradation or reuptake affect these receptors indirectly, while other agents also have direct receptor agonist or antagonist properties. Animal research indicates that *downregulation of both the β-adrenergic norepinephrine receptor and the 5-HT$_{2A}$ serotonin receptor* occurs after several weeks of treatment with most antidepressants. The fact that this receptor downregulation correlates temporally with the observed delay in clinical response in the treatment setting doesn't prove causality, but it tantalizingly suggests that some relationship between these two events exists.

However, the neuroreceptor hypothesis of depression, like the monoamine hypothesis of depression before it, remains imperfect. A plethora of research into neuroreceptors and how they respond to various types of pharmacologic and nonpharmacologic challenges raises as many questions as it answers.

For example, **electroconvulsive therapy (ECT)** is the most effective treatment currently available for mood disorder. Like the TCAs and MAOIs, ECT causes downregulation of the β-adrenergic receptor. However, unlike TCAs and MAOIs, it causes upregulation of the 5-HT$_{2A}$ receptor. Meanwhile, the antidepressant *bupropion* effectively treats depression but has no appreciable effects on either the serotonin or norepinephrine systems and doesn't downregulate the β-receptor. *Thyroid hormone* is an effective adjunctive treatment for depression despite the fact that it augments β-adrenergic receptor function. Finally, *propranolol*, a β-adrenergic receptor antagonist, has no antidepressant effects (and may even cause depression in some individuals).

Just as the fact that monoamine modulators are efficacious in treating depression doesn't provide conclusive evidence that abnormalities of monoamine metabolism are the "cause" of major depressive disorder, neither does that fact provide conclusive evidence that monoamine receptors constitute the "cause." It may simply be that these agents initiate a "domino effect" that ultimately improves the patient's depressive state through effects even further "downstream" than the monoamine receptor.

Non-monoamine Theories of Depression

Recent research suggests that non-monoamine systems also play a significant role in the etiology of depression. We already have touched upon several such non-monoamine systems, including the neurotrophic system, the glucocorticoid system, and the excitatory amino acid system. We also have discussed how major depressive disorder is more than just changes in mood. It also includes alterations in memory, attention, executive function, and biological drives such as sleep, appetite, and libido. Each of these elements may involve distinct but interrelated alterations in regional pathophysiology.

These "non-mood" aspects of mood disorder are not simply epiphenomena of the depressive state. In other words, depressed patients don't simply perform poorly on cognitive tests because they are sad and lack the motivation or energy to apply themselves fully to the testing. Rather, these associated symptoms are important phenomena in themselves. The cognitive features in particular are significant since they can persist in attenuated form even following "recovery" from the depressive episode. As noted above, structural neuroimaging studies in humans reveals that hippocampal atrophy is present in the more severe cases. In other words, clinical depression appears to be "bad for the brain" and may even turn out to be a subtle, chronic neurodegenerative disorder.

Animal research suggests that a wide range of antidepressants and mood stabilizers also act on these non-monoamine systems. They may even bolster the activity or the effects of neuroprotective factors, thereby helping to "heal the brain" when they are taken over a period of months to years.

Monoamine and non-monoamine systems appear to be closely related. The persistent increase in brain monoamine levels that occurs in the setting of regular administration of antidepressant medications stimulates postsynaptic monoamine receptors. These in turn trigger *second messenger transduction systems*, which induce the phosphorylation of various *transcription factors* that regulate neuronal *gene expression*.

One such transcription factor is **cyclic adenosine monophosphate (cAMP) response-element binding protein (CREB)**. CREB activates genes that code for neurotrophic proteins (such as **brain-derived neurotrophic factor, BDNF**) as well as for receptors for neurotrophic factors. Given this, it likely is significant that in animals, hippocampal levels of both CREB and of the messenger RNA that codes for CREB increase in response to the chronic administration of a variety of different antidepressants. This increase even occurs over a period of time that parallels the delayed onset of effect noted in depressed humans who are treated with antidepressant medication.

Similarly, a series of repeated electrically induced seizures (i.e., a course of electroconvulsive therapy) has been found to promote both hippocampal BDNF expression and even sprouting of hippocampal neurons in animals. This effect (which occurs only after a *series* of such seizures are induced) occurs over a period of time that parallels the onset of clinical effect seen in depressed humans receiving a series of ECT treatments.

Several *endocrine abnormalities* also are associated with major depressive disorder, including dysregulation of the **hypothalamic-**

pituitary-adrenal (HPA) axis, the **hypothalamic-pituitary-thyroid (HPT) axis**, and the **hypothalamic-growth hormone axis**. These abnormalities likely are centrally mediated and reflect both neurotransmitter dysfunction and the body's response to chronic stress. (Unfortunately, none of these findings has proven to be of sufficient sensitivity or specificity to confirm the diagnosis of major depressive disorder in individual patients.)

We have touched on the relationship between stress, psychiatric illness, and the glucocorticoid system. Given this, it is noteworthy that major depressive disorder is associated with hyperactivity along the HPA axis. Depressed patients, as a group, have higher levels of corticotropin-releasing factor (CRF) and of cortisol.

Hyperactivity of the HPA axis can be assessed in the clinical or research setting using the *dexamethasone suppression test*. Dexamethasone is a synthetic analogue of cortisol. Subjects administered dexamethasone therefore experience feedback inhibition of the HPA system, with a resultant decrease in their serum cortisol level. The latter is assessed through blood draws performed at standardized intervals following dexamethasone administration. However, 50% of patients with major depressive disorder *don't* suppress their cortisol secretion following dexamethasone administration.

Interestingly, this abnormality usually remits when the depressive episode has resolved, but those recovered patients who remain "nonsuppressors" demonstrate a much higher rate of relapse into depression. This suggests that glucocorticoid hyperactivity is both a "state" phenomenon and in some cases an underlying biological vulnerability. While this finding has important theoretical implications, the test is too nonspecific to offer great utility in the clinical setting. In addition to major depressive disorder, "nonsuppression" also has been noted in patients

with schizophrenia, alcohol abuse, eating disorders, malnutrition, fever, hypertension, cardiac or renal failure, advanced age, and pregnancy.

Some patients with depression turn out to have *hypothyroidism* and their depression improves when this is addressed. Thyroid hormone also is useful as an adjunctive treatment in cases of refractory depression, even in patients who are not hypothyroid. The hypothyroidism associated with depression can be subtle. Table 4–2 describes the different "grades" of hypothyroidism.

Grade 1 hypothyroidism, the most severe and obvious form of hypothyroidism, is associated with a decrease in the serum thyroxine (T4) level. Grade 2 hypothyroidism is milder. It is associated with a normal peripheral thyroxine but with elevated thyroid-stimulating hormone (TSH) levels. Grade 3 hypothyroidism is associated with a "sluggish" thyroid. While the serum TSH level is normal, but the pituitary demonstrates an exaggerated degree of TSH release in response to infusion of thyrotropin releasing hormone (TRH) during a *TRH stimulation test*.

While grade 3 hypothyroidism isn't diagnosed on routine thyroid screening tests, about 15% of depressed patients have this condition. It has been associated with the presence of more treatment-refractory depression and with rapidly cycling bipolar disorder. Depressed patients also have a higher than expected rate of grade 4 hypothyroidism, which is characterized by autoimmune thyroiditis (i.e., by the presence of circulating antithyroid antibodies, despite currently normal levels of T3, T4, and TSH and a normal TRH Stimulation Test).

Unfortunately, as with the adrenal axis and Dexamethasone Stimulation Test, the TRH Stimulation Test is neither sensitive nor specific enough to be of much utility in the clinical setting. In fact, while depression can be a symptom of subtle ("subclinical") hypothyroidism (which is associated with an exaggerated TSH response

Table 4–2. Grades of Hypothyroidism

Grade	T3, T4	Basal TSH	TSH after TRH Stim.	Antithyroid Antibodies
I	Decreased	Increased	Increased	Often present
II	Normal	Normal	Increased	Often present
III	Normal	Normal	Increased	Often present
IV	Normal	Normal	Normal	Present

to TRH infusion), about 25%–30% of depressed patients demonstrate a *blunted* TSH response to TRH infusion. These patients turn out to have high levels of central nervous system TRH despite having normal peripheral thyroid indices.

Given this finding, one theory is that these depressed patients are experiencing *hypersecretion of TRH*, similar to the hypersecretion of CRF discussed earlier. The TRH hypersecretion leads to downregulation of the anterior pituitary's TRH receptors and therefore to a blunted TSH release in response to exogenously administered TRH. Perhaps this TRH hypersecretion represents yet another example of the normally adaptive "stress response" becoming a source of pathology when it is excessive in degree or in duration. Consistent with this hypothesis, as was the case with the Dexamethasone Suppression Test, those depressed patients who have responded to antidepressant therapy but who continue to display a blunted response on the TRH Stimulation Test have a higher rate of relapse than those patients whose test results have normalized.

Finally, activity along the growth hormone axis demonstrates a similar picture. Clonidine infusion normally increases growth hormone secretion. However, in depressed patients this response tends to be blunted. Depressed patients also demonstrate blunting of the growth hormone surge that normally occurs during the first few hours of sleep.

Global Neurophysiologic Theories of Depression

Neurophysiologic theories exploring the etiology of depression have focused on both *global* and *regional* brain abnormalities in depressed subjects. For example, radioisotope studies have shown an *excess of residual sodium* in both manic and depressed patients, and this finding is consistent with the finding of decreased activity of the enzyme *Na–K–ATPase* in many patients with bipolar disorder. This enzyme is responsible for transporting sodium out of and potassium into neurons, thereby maintaining an electrical gradient across the resting neuronal membrane. Excessive sodium leaking into neurons could contribute to an unstable state of neuronal hyperexcitability. Patients who have recovered from an episode of illness demonstrate a restoration of the normal electrolyte balance.

The extent of sodium leakage may be greater in manic than in depressive states, and this may explain the greater degree of agitation and excitement in the manic states. (The notion that mania is a more severe state in the "same direction" as depression, while apparently contradicting the notion that depression and mania are "polar opposites," is nonetheless compatible with the observation that some patients present in "mixed states," simultaneously demonstrating features of both mania and depression.) Further, since monoamine reupake across the presynaptic membrane also is an energy-dependent process requiring Na–K–ATPase, a "sluggish enzyme" also might contribute to a state of intraneuronal monoamine depletion. Also consistent with this theory is the fact that lithium (which is effective in treating both mania and depression) is known to substitute for intraneuronal sodium, thereby hyperpolarizing the cell membrane and decreasing neuronal excitability.

Other researchers have examined *abnormalities in circadian rhythms* in patients with mood disorders. Depressed patients are "phase advanced" in many of their biological rhythms. A classic finding is that *REM latency*, the time between falling asleep and the first period of rapid eye movement activity, is shorter in depressed patients. (The degree of shortening correlates with the severity of depression, and patients who require inpatient treatment or who have a psychotic depression demonstrate the greatest degree of shortening.) Another finding is a shifting of REM sleep. Rather than the usual pattern, where the bulk of REM sleep occurs in the early morning hours, in depressed patients the bulk occurs in the first half of the night. Some depressed patients also display an increased density of REM sleep. It is notable that both sleep deprivation and early morning exposure to bright light have antidepressant effects. Perhaps this is because they help correct this state of being "phase advanced."

These sleep abnormalities often resolve with treatment, suggesting that they are state-related phenomena. However, like the abnormalities in neuroendocrine function described above, these abnormalities appear to also be "biological markers" of some underlying trait vulnerability. For example, depressed patients who demonstrate decreased REM latency are more likely than patients without a change in REM latency to later relapse back into depression. Similarly, depressed relatives of patients who have decreased REM latency are more likely to themselves demonstrate REM latency. Even more noteworthy, relatives of depressed patients who have no history of having been depressed but who demonstrate decreased REM latency appear to be at greater risk of becoming depressed at some point in the future.

Regional Neurophysiologic Theories of Depression

Functional neuroimaging techniques have allowed researchers to study *regional brain activity* in depressed patients while they still are in the midst of a depressive episode. These scans most commonly have been obtained "at rest" (i.e., in the absence of physiologic or cognitive stimuli designed to exacerbate depressive symptoms). While findings from different investigators have varied, the most consistent finding has been *reduced metabolic activity in the dorsolateral prefrontal cortex*. Greater magnitudes of reduced activity have been associated with a greater severity of depressive symptoms. One theory is that this reduced frontal activity contributes to symptoms of depression such as psychomotor retardation and impaired executive function.

In contrast, some studies also have demonstrated *increased activity in the ventral prefrontal cortex*. Less consistent findings have included reduced activity in the anterior cingulate gyrus, in the basal ganglia (particularly the caudate), and in the parietal and temporal lobes. (As discussed above, these areas, along with dorsolateral frontal lobe, appear to comprise a circuit, such that reduced activity at one node along the circuit causes other nodes to demonstrate a similar decrease.)

Some studies have gone one step further. They attempt to determine whether changes in brain activity that are associated with depression *resolve* following treatment of the depression, regardless of whether the treatment consisted of antidepressant medication or psychotherapy. While findings have varied between different studies, treatment with either modality has been associated with changes in the brain metabolic activity. These changes include normalization of the decreased metabolism in prefrontal and left anterior cingulate gyrus regions as well as increases in metabolic activity above that seen in control subjects in the left temporal and the right basal ganglia regions.

These changes in brain activity conceivably reflect the brain's response to treatment of the underlying depressive state. Some of the changes have been noted regardless of whether treatment consisted of medication or psychotherapy, while other changes have been more specifically associated with the use of a particular treatment modality. It is tempting to speculate that the former changes reflect shared mechanisms of therapeutic action while the latter changes reflect modality-specific effects. (As of this writing, no study has included a third group that received the combination of medication and psychotherapy.)

At this point, however, it would be premature for us to reach such conclusions, for several reasons. First, we don't know enough about the variability of the functional neuroimaging techniques themselves to determine whether or not some of these changes would have occurred in the absence of treatment. We also do not currently know the effect of the psychotropic medications themselves on brain activity, regardless of whether or not they treated the patient's depressive symptoms. (To determine this would require the presence of control subjects who had no psychiatric illness but who were administered antidepressant medications for at least several weeks.) In addition, we can't be sure that psychiatric treatments don't also cause other changes in brain metabolism that are so subtle that they are below the resolution of today's neuroimaging technology. It might be these changes that are responsible for the patient's improvement, not the changes described in the neuroimaging studies. Finally, it remains unclear at this point whether the abnormal brain activity noted in patients who are in the midst of a major depressive episode reflects changes due to the depressive episode or due to a predisposing trait disturbance. Similarly, the strategy of focusing on particular regions where abnormal activity has been described, in order to determine whether such abnormalities "resolve" with treatment might itself be flawed. Perhaps, for example, patients' symptomatic improvement actually reflects compensatory increases in activity in other distinct regions of the brain on which we aren't directing our attention.

Stress Diathesis Model of Depression

The **stress diathesis model** attempts to synthesize biological and psychological theories of mood disorder. Also applicable to other psychiatric disorders, including the anxiety disorders and psychotic disorders, this model suggests that while some individuals are constitutionally vulnerable to psychiatric illness, the phenotype only declares itself following exposure to a life stress such as a loss, a trauma, or a severe blow to one's self-esteem. In the case of mood disorder, individuals may be genetically endowed with a "depressive temperament" which makes one even more vulnerable to the detrimental effects of these subsequent life stressors. Ultimately limbic–diencephalic dysfunction is triggered, which in turn causes an acute affective episode to occur, as illustrated in Figure 4–4.

Once the affective episode occurs, the episode itself becomes yet another life stressor, further perpetuating the cycle. To make matters worse, it also likely triggers changes in the brain at the cellular level, and an individual who has experienced one episode becomes more predisposed to experience subsequent episodes. Robert Post has proposed a "kindling model" to help explain just how these changes might occur. He begins by noting that while early affective episodes of depression or mania are separated by relatively long intervals of remission, these intervals become progressively shorter as the disease progresses. Further, psychosocial stressors seem to play a more important role in triggering the early episodes than they do in triggering subsequent episodes.

Post then analogizes these changes to those that have been described in a rat model of epilepsy. In this model, repetitive electrical stimuli are delivered to the amygdala of a healthy rat. Each stimulation is too weak in itself to trigger a seizure. However, if one delivers enough of these subconvulsive stimulations in a row, the rat ultimately has a seizure. Then, if one triggers a sufficient number of such seizures, the rat begins to experience *spontaneous* seizures. The external stimulations have acted as "kindling": once the epileptic "fire" has begun to burn on its own, the kindling is no longer necessary.

Similarly, depressive or manic episodes initially may be triggered by one or more life stressors. While none of these stressors—in itself—may have been enough to trigger such an episode, genetically vulnerable individuals exposed to sufficient stress ultimately do become depressed or manic. Once the mood disorder has been "kindled," subsequent episodes could be triggered by much milder stressors or might even arise autonomously (i.e., in absence of any stress at all). (Note that the comparison to epilepsy is meant

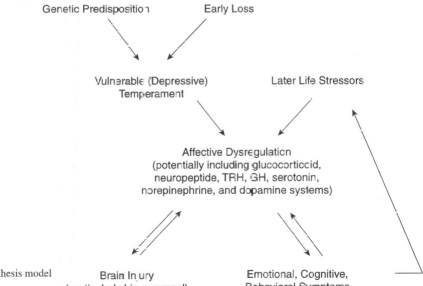

Figure 4–4. A stress-diathesis model of mood disorder.

to be an analogy. While bipolar disorder sometimes is treated with anticonvulsant medications, there is no evidence that mood disorders are epileptic in origin. However, sensitization at the level of gene transcription may take place in both epilepsy and kindled mood disorder.)

This model suggests that while early life experiences permanently alter our "hardwiring" (for better or for worse), some plasticity remains. Psychotherapy, by providing a "corrective emotional experience," may also promote neurophysiologic changes. Another implication of this model is that it is important to recognize mood disorder early in its course, initiate aggressive treatment, and continue prophylactic treatment in order to ensure that "the fire is put out and stays out."

For example, a 22-year-old patient who has achieved remission from a first episode of mania that was treated with lithium will likely ask whether he should remain on lithium indefinitely. The answer likely is "yes," since to discontinue prophylactic medication and take a "wait and see" approach might worsen his long-term prognosis. If he does have another manic or a depressive episode, he not only will have to deal with the immediate repercussions (embarrassing behavior, missing work days, hospital admission), but he might become even further predisposed to experience further episodes despite the resumption of lithium prophylaxis. In addition, his illness may become more refractory to treatment, analogous to a cancer that becomes more refractory to chemotherapy later in its course.

Overlap between Disease Categories

Overlap between Depressive and Anxiety Disorders

From a biological dimensional perspective, it is not surprising that having one Axis I disorder increases one's risk of developing another Axis I disorder from a different "category." For example, many patients with major depressive disorder also experience prominent anxiety symptoms, while anxiety disorders such as generalized anxiety disorder, panic disorder, and obsessive-compulsive disorder commonly are associated with co-occurring major depressive disorder.

Depressive and anxiety disorders are unique in some ways but share other features. Table 4–3 divides these differences and similarities into three categories: *cognitive aspects*, *motivational aspects*, and *somatic aspects*. (These distinctions are not pure ones. For example, mental slowing, anhedonia, and anergia, while in different categories, may all be related.) In both depressive and anxiety disorders, patients express a general sense of distress, demonstrate impaired attention and concentration, and complain of fatigue and sleep disturbances. However, depressed patients are more likely to complain of guilt, hopelessness, impaired motivation, and diminished neurovegetative functioning, while anxious patients

Table 4–3. Unique and Shared Features of Depressive and Anxiety Disorders

	Depression	Shared	Anxiety
Cognitive aspects	Sadness Hopelessness ↓ Self-esteem Social withdrawal Mental slowing	↓ Concentration Demoralization Rumination General distress Somatic concern	Apprehension Worry Irritability
Motivational aspects	Anhedonia ↓ Drive		↑ Drive (When anxiety not severe)
Somatic aspects	↓ Libido ↓ / ↑ Appetite Anergia	Fatigue Sleep disturbance	Palpitations Shortness of breath Chest pain GI discomfort Diaphoresis Restlessness ↑ Muscle tension

are more likely to complain of apprehension about the future, of excessive worry about minor matters, and of a variety of somatic symptoms consistent with excessive autonomic arousal.

These areas of overlap are of more than theoretical relevance. They carry important treatment implications. For example, about a third of patients with major depressive disorder also have panic attacks. When these patients are treated with benzodiazepines, their panic attacks are typically ameliorated but they remain depressed because benzodiazepines aren't effective antidepressants. Similarly, many patients with obsessive–compulsive disorder develop superimposed episodes of major depressive disorder. Nonserotonergic antidepressants (such as desipramine or electroconvulsive therapy) effectively treat their depressive symptoms but leave the obsessive-compulsive symptoms untouched. Patients who have both obsessive–compulsive disorder and bipolar disorder may require a serotonergic antidepressant to treat the obsessive-compulsive symptoms, but this could in turn trigger a manic episode.

The "art" of psychopharmacology, emphasized throughout this text, consists of attempts to delineate dimensional symptom complexes through specific clinical inquiry. This then allows for "educated guesses" as to which class of medication or type of psychotherapeutic interventions might ameliorate such symptoms *without* exacerbating other symptoms or causing new symptoms.

Monoamine dysregulation has been implicated in all of these disorders, and medications that alter monoamine transmission are the mainstay of pharmacologic treatment for all of them. Monoamines exert diverse effects throughout the brain and spinal cord, modulating many basic physiologic functions, and it is likely that when patients present with a "mixed" picture of anxiety and depression, they are experiencing dysregulation involving multiple neuronal pathways. These probably include the frontal–limbic–temporal "mood" circuit (Fig. 4–4, leading to sadness, guilt, and hopelessness), the "fear" circuit (Fig. 4–2, leading to apprehension, worry, and autonomic hyperarousal), and the "pleasure" circuit (Fig. 4–3, with deficits along this latter pathway leading to impaired motivation and anhedonia).

Monoaminergic medications (including antidepressants, stimulants, and antipsychotics) are "blunt instruments." They modulate the activity of serotonin, norepinephrine, and dopamine across all of these circuits simultaneously. A second class of medications, the benzodiazepines, works quite differently, by modulating the activity of γ-aminobutyric acid (GABA).

The GABA System

GABA and glutamate, the brain's major inhibitory and excitatory neurotransmitters, respectively, differ only by a single carboxyl group. In fact, the precursor to GABA is glutamate. GABA plays an important role in both the central and the peripheral nervous systems. In the cerebral cortex, it is released primarily by intrinsic inhibitory neurons, allowing them to achieve local tonic inhibition over cortical pyramidal neurons' excitatory activity. Loss of such inhibition may contribute to excessive cortical electrical activity, leading to anxiety or seizures.

There are two known subtypes of GABA receptors. The **GABA$_B$ receptor** is heavily concentrated in the dorsal horn of the spinal column. The antispasmodic muscle relaxant **baclofen** binds to this receptor. This receptor doesn't appear to be closely associated with anxiety, and benzodiazepines do not affect it. The **GABA$_A$ receptor**, however, appears to play a major role in mediating anxiety.

We have already discussed how it takes several weeks for serotonergic and noradrenergic antidepressants to exert their clinical effects. This delay is presumably due to serotonin and norepinephrine receptors exerting their effects on the postsynaptic neuron only indirectly, through second messenger systems. In contrast, the GABA$_A$ receptor has a completely different mechanism of action, one which allows for a rapid onset of pharmacologic effect.

The GABA$_A$ receptor is made up of several subunits, each of which is shaped like a helix or column. Several of these columns combine to form a transmembrane chloride channel called the **GABA receptor complex**. GABA is the chloride channel's primary "gatekeeper." When GABA attaches to the *GABA recognition site* on this complex, it causes an allosteric modification to the channel which leads the channel to assume an "open" configuration, allowing for an influx of chloride. This in turn causes hyperpolarization of the neuronal membrane, thereby decreasing neuronal excitability. While GABA is the *primary* gatekeeper, its ability to open the chloride channel can be *allosterically modulated* by a variety of other receptors, none of which in itself (i.e., in the absence of GABA) has the ability to open the chloride channel.

The α and β subunits of the $GABA_A$ receptor include the GABA recognition site while a third (γ) subunit includes a **benzodiazepine receptor**. Why the GABA receptor complex should contain a receptor for benzodiazepine medication is unclear. While the discovery and subsequent synthesis of this receptor led to a search for an "endogenous" or "natural" benzodiazepine, no such substance has been discovered.

Benzodiazepines are *positive allosteric modulators* of the GABA channel. In other words, when they occupy the benzodiazepine receptor site, the effect of GABA is amplified. Therefore, benzodiazepines have anticonvulsant, muscle relaxant, sedative-hypnotic, amnestic, and anxiolytic effects.

Benzodiazepines are useful in treating the cognitive and somatic symptoms listed in Table 4–3 that are unique to the anxiety disorders or that are shared across the anxiety and depressive disorders. However, benzodiazepines are not useful in treating the cognitive, motivational, and somatic symptoms that are unique to the depressive disorders and might even exacerbate these symptoms.

Several other positive allosteric receptor sites also have been identified, including receptor sites for **barbiturates** and for **alcohol**. Like the benzodiazepines, these agents also have anxiolytic (and potentially depressive) effects. Benzodiazepines and barbiturates have "substituted" for alcohol in the treatment of alcohol withdrawal states, ameliorating symptoms of alcohol withdrawal and allowing for a more controlled medication taper than might be accomplished with alcohol.

The anxiolytic, sedative, and anticonvulsant effects of alcohol, barbiturates, and benzodiazepines all stem from their ability to potentiate the effects of GABA on the chloride channel. Conversely, too rapid a withdrawal of any of these agents after a sufficient period of regular exposure can lead to the chloride channel "slamming shut," thereby causing a state of *withdrawal*. The symptoms of this withdrawal state are the exact opposite of these agents' agonist effects. Patients in the midst of alcohol, barbiturate, or benzodiazepine withdrawal typically experience anxiety, autonomic hyperarousal, and— in severe cases—delirium and seizures.

A *benzodiazepine receptor antagonist*, **flumazenil**, also is available. Flumazenil competes with benzodiazepines at the receptor site, blocking their clinical effect. When it is administered to subjects who haven't received benzodiazepines, it exerts little effect. However, when administered to subjects who either have overdosed on benzodiazepines or have received benzodiazepine anesthesia, it leads to a rapid increase in their level of consciousness. (An important caveat is that if flumazenil is administered to patients who have taken a benzodiazepine chronically before having overdosed and therefore have developed physiologic dependence, it precipitates an acute state of benzodiazepine withdrawal.)

There are two subtypes of benzodiazepine receptor. **BZ_1 receptors** are especially concentrated in the cerebellum. **BZ_2 receptors** are concentrated in the hippocampus, striatum, and spinal cord. It is believed that the BZ_1 receptors are more responsible for the sedative effects of benzodiazepines, while the BZ_2 receptors are more responsible for their anticonvulsant and muscle relaxant effects. For example, the hypnotic agents **zolpidem (Ambien)** and **Zaleplon (Sonata)** have chemically distinct structures from the benzodiazepines. They bind to the BZ_1 receptor but not to the BZ_2 receptor. They have a sedative effect and cause little disruption to the normal REM sleep pattern. They lack muscle relaxant and anticonvulsant effects. Their sedative effects are reversed with flumazenil.

The Serotonin System

Serotonin is present even in phylogenetically ancient organisms with simple nervous systems. It modulates a wide variety of essential physiologic functions, including feeding, sexual activity, and aggressive behavior (Table 4–4). In humans, serotonergic neurons are located along the midline (or raphe) of the brain stem and send projections throughout the brain and spinal cord.

Table 4–4. Physiologic Functions Influenced
by Serotonin

Aggression/impulse control	Endocrine regulation
Anxiety/affect	Gastrointestinal functions
Appetite/satiety	Motor activity
Cardiovascular functions	Pain
Circadian rhythms/sleep	Reproductive functions
Cognitive functions	Sensory functions

Source: Adapted from Murphy DL, Andrews AM, et al:
"Brain Serotonin Neurotransmission: An Overview and Update With an Emphasis on Serotonin Subsystem Heterogeneity, Multiple Receptors, Interactions With Other Neurotransmitter Systems, and Consequent Implications for Understanding the Actions of Serotonergic Drugs." *J Clin Psychiatry*, 59(suppl 15):4–12, 1998. Copyright 1998, Physicians Postgraduate Press. Adapted by permission.

The diversity of nuclei innervated by serotonin likely explains the heterogeneity of the biological effects that it mediates. Another factor contributing to its broad spectrum of activity is the heterogeneity of serotonin receptor subtypes. To date, 15 different serotonin receptors have been identified, each of which has different properties, as detailed in Table 4–5. Therefore, serotonin can even have one effect in one brain region and the opposite effect in a different region.

Medications that increase synaptic serotonin levels have proven to be effective antidepressants. Serotonin also appears to play a signifi-

Table 4–5. Identified Serotonin Receptors and
Their Signal Transduction Methods

Receptor	Signal Transduction
5-HT$_{1A,B, D\alpha,D\beta,E,F}$	$\downarrow$ cAMP, $\uparrow$ K$^+$ channel
5-HT$_{2A,B,C}$	IP-3, DAG, cGMP
5-HT$_3$	Ligand-gated ion channel, IP-3
5-HT$_4$	$\uparrow$ cAMP
5-HT$_{5\alpha,5\beta}$	Unknown
5-HT$_6$	$\uparrow$ cAMP
5-HT$_7$	$\uparrow$ cAMP

Abbreviations: cAMP, cyclic adenosine monophosphate; DAG, diacylglycerol; cGMP, cyclic guanosine monophosphate; IP-3, phosphatidyl inositol.
Source: Adapted from Murphy DL, Andrews AM, et al: "Brain Serotonin Neurotransmission: An Overview and Update With an Emphasis on Serotonin Subsystem Heterogeneity, Multiple Receptors, Interactions With Other Neurotransmitter Systems, and Consequent Implications for Understanding the Actions of Serotonergic Drugs." *J Clin Psychiatry* 59(suppl 15):4–12, 1998. Copyright 1998, Physicians Postgraduate Press. Adapted by permission.

cant role in the anxiety disorders. The best evidence for this is that anxiety disorders such as panic disorder and obsessive–compulsive disorder (OCD) respond to treatment with selective serotonin reuptake inhibitors (SSRIs), agents whose direct effect lies almost entirely within the serotonin system. As noted above, in the case of OCD, the illness appears to respond preferentially to serotonergic antidepressants, while noradrenergic antidepressants and GABAergic benzodiazepines have little effect.

Similarly, β-adrenergic receptor antagonists such as propranolol attenuate *peripheral* manifestations of anxiety mediated by norepinephrine, such as tremulousness, tachycardia, hypertension, and diaphoresis, but they have little direct effect on *cognitive* aspects of anxiety such as obsessional rumination, worry, and irritability. In contrast, the SSRIs appear to treat these cognitive manifestations despite having little effect on the autonomic features of anxiety. Therefore, the serotonin system seems to be tied up with the subjective emotional distress associated with depression and anxiety.

When an antidepressant medication raises serotonin levels, it likely affects all 15 receptors. This may account for *side effects* associated with serotonergic antidepressants. For example, while the decreased libido and anergia associated with clinical depression may respond to treatment with antidepressant medications, there also are patients who complain of lowered libido or affective "flattening" as side effects of taking serotonergic medications. Patients treated with selective dopaminergic or noradrenergic medications rarely complain of these side effects (although these latter agents tend to be less effective in treating anxiety and some people even complain of increased anxiety as a side effect).

Given this, patients who present primarily with cognitive and physiologic symptoms of anxiety, worry, irritability, aggression, or impaired impulse control, whether in the setting of a mood disorder or anxiety disorder, may particularly benefit from serotonergic medications. Patients presenting predominantly with anhedonia and anergia are perhaps less likely to respond to these agents, and in some cases these complaints may be exacerbated by selective serotonergic medications.

This latter group of patients may show a better response to treatment with either selective noradrenergic or dopaminergic medications or with agents that demonstrate a "mixed" monoaminergic profile (such as tricyclic antidepressants, monoamine oxidase inhibitors, or venlafaxine). Alternatively, pharmacologic researchers are attempting to synthesize serotonin receptor agonist and antagonist agents that are even more selective—that is, that target a given serotonin receptor *subtype*. Such agents might be used alone or might be used in combination with currently available "broad-spectrum" serotonin reuptake inhibitors. In the latter case, they might be employed to block the adverse effects associated with stimulation of a particular receptor subtype while still leaving those serotonin receptor subtypes associated with positive effects "open" to pharmacologic stimulation. However, such agents still may prove to be less effective in combating anergia and anhedonia than medications with noradrenergic or dopaminergic effects.

The Norepinephrine System

Like neurons that contain serotonin, those that contain norepinephrine project throughout the brain and spinal cord. In the brain, norepinephrine is released primarily from noradrenergic neurons whose cells bodies are located in the pons in the locus ceruleus and lateral tegmental areas. When laboratory animals' locus ceruleus is electrically stimulated, they display behaviors consistent with anxiety.

Autonomic arousal plays an important role in behavior, mediating wakefulness, arousal, stamina, motivation, attention, learning, and memory. However, excessive norepinephrine activity is associated with symptoms of autonomic hyperarousal such as tachycardia, dilated pupils, tremor, and sweating. Once people experiencing such physical symptoms become aware of them, they may become even *more anxious*, thereby creating an anxiogenic positive feedback loop.

For example, during a public speaking engagement, an individual may experience *performance anxiety* (i.e., stage fright), associated with sweats, tremor, a pounding heart, a cracking voice, and a sensation of one's mind "going blank." As the individual perceives these symptoms, he or she may then experience cognitive aspects of anxiety, such as a fear of public humiliation, which serves to even further increase the state of autonomic hyperarousal.

Cognitive interventions (such as relaxation techniques) and medications both can help to break this cycle. Noradrenergic agents modulate the autonomic response by acting either at presynaptic or postsynaptic noradrenergic receptors. At the postsynaptic terminal are *α-1 and β-adrenergic receptors* that, when stimulated by norepinephrine, *facilitate* the anxiety response. In contrast, the noradrenergic neurons themselves contain presynaptic *α-2 adrenergic autoreceptors* both on their cell bodies and at their presynaptic nerve terminals. These provide negative feedback inhibition, similar to a "thermostat." Stimulation of these autoreceptors by norepinephrine *decreases* presynaptic neuronal, thereby preventing adrenergic arousal from becoming excessive.

Beta-adrenergic blocking agents, such as propranolol, blunt peripheral autonomic arousal. These drugs therefore are most useful in cases of social phobia or performance anxiety. However, while these agents decrease the *autonomic manifestations* of anxiety, they aren't as useful in treating *psychological symptoms* of anxiety such as worry and apprehensive expectation. Serotonergic and GABAergic medications are more useful in addressing these psychological symptoms. Further, and consistent with the postulated role of norepinephrine as a mediator of positive affect and motivation, some patients treated with β-blockers experience depressive symptoms such as anergia and anhedonia as a side effect.

Clonidine is an *α-2* agonist. By stimulating the autoreceptor, clonidine "turns down" norepinephrine release. Clonidine commonly is used to treat autonomic hyperarousal that occurs during opiate withdrawal. It also has been used to treat Tourette's syndrome and attention-deficit hyperactivity disorder. It may be mildly effective in all of the anxiety disorders, although it isn't considered the drug of first choice for any of them. Like the β-blockers, clonidine's major limitation is that it has little direct effect on the psychological symptoms associated with anxiety.

The Dopamine System

Dopamine also is active throughout the brain, but predominantly in four circuits: the *mesocortical*, *mesolimbic*, *nigrostriatal*, and *tuberoinfundibular* circuits. These are discussed in greater detail in Chapter 8 and are illustrated in Figure 8–2.

There are at least five different dopamine receptors, each of which is associated with different intracellular second messenger effects, and each of which is more prevalent in different locations.

Dopaminergic activity along these different circuits mediates very different effects. Mesocortical dopamine activity is an important mediator of motivation, reward-seeking behavior, and sustained attention. *Deficient dopaminergic activity along the mesocortical circuit* may be associated with the cognitive and volitional complaints associated with attention-deficit hyperactivity disorder, major depressive disorder, and schizophrenia.

However, *excessive dopaminergic activity along the mesolimbic tract* has been associated with psychotic symptoms such as those occurring in schizophrenia. The traditional antipsychotic agents used to treat schizophrenia block dopamine receptors along *all* of the dopaminergic circuits. While patients treated with these agents usually experience a lessening of psychotic symptoms, they also may complain of an exacerbation of cognitive symptoms such as apathy and impaired memory and executive function. In contrast, agents that increase dopamine release, such as methylphenidate and dextroamphetamine, may lessen these complaints but also can exacerbate psychotic symptoms. The newest group of "atypical" antipsychotic agents appears to allow patients to "have their cake and eat it, too," as they block dopamine activity along the mesolimbic circuit while boosting dopamine activity along the mesocortical circuit, thereby allowing for improvement in both types of symptoms.

Complicating matters further, there is significant "crosstalk" between these three monoamines. *First*, each neurotransmitter influences the release of all of the other neurotransmitters. For example, serotonin-containing neurons from the brain-stem raphe nuclei project to both the locus ceruleus and the ventral tegmental area, thereby influencing norepinephrine and dopamine secretion, respectively. The complexity of serotonin's influence is suggested by Table 4–6, which lists the effects of stimulating serotonin receptors attached to neurons containing other neurotransmitters. To give but one example, when serotonin stimulates a dopamine neuron's $5HT_{1A}$ serotonin receptor, it *inhibits* dopamine release, but when

Table 4–6. Examples of Serotonin Activity on Other Neurotransmitter Systems

Neurotransmitter System	Effect	Serotonin Receptor
Dopamine	↓ Release	$5\text{-}HT_{1A}$
	↑ Release	$5\text{-}HT_3$
Acetylcholine	↓ Release	$5\text{-}HT_3$
	↑ Release	$5\text{-}HT_{1A}$
Glutamate	↓ Release	$5\text{-}HT_{1A}$
	Potentiation	$5\text{-}HT_2$
Norepinephrine	↓ Release	$5\text{-}HT_1$
Cholecystokinin	↑ Release	$5\text{-}HT_3$

Source: Adapted from Murphy DL, Andrews AM, et al: "Brain Serotonin Neurotransmission: An Overview and Update With an Emphasis on Serotonin Subsystem Heterogeneity, Multiple Receptors, Interactions With Other Neurotransmitter Systems, and Consequent Implications for Understanding the Actions of Serotonergic Drugs." *J Clin Psychiatry* 59(suppl 15):4–12, 1998. Copyright 1998, Physicians Postgraduate Press. Adapted by permission.

serotonin acts on a dopamine neuron's $5HT_3$ receptor, it *stimulates* dopamine release.

Second, serotonergic and noradrenergic neurons project in parallel to the cortex and striatum, where they synapse on the same neurons. It therefore is likely that they regulate the activity of each other through summative or competitive effects on these postsynaptic neurons.

Third, these are not completely separate circuits. In fact, some neurons release serotonin, norepinephrine, and dopamine. For example, the antidepressant drug mirtazapine antagonizes the α-2 norepinephrine autoreceptors. As described above, this receptor inhibits the neuronal release of norepinephrine, such that a receptor antagonist triggers the *increased* release of norepinephrine. However, this drug also appears to enhance serotonin transmission, again apparently through stimulation of α-2 receptors located on the cell bodies and dendrites of serotonergic neurons. In addition, the norepinephrine reuptake protein also has a high affinity not only for norepinephrine but for dopamine, such that norepinephrine reuptake inhibitors also appear to act as dopamine reuptake inhibitors.

Given the extent of this monoamine "crosstalk," and also given the possibility that antidepressants with very different pharmacologic profiles may have similar "downstream" effects at the level of postsynaptic neuronal modulation, it would be overly simplistic to assume that one could simply "target" a specific symptom with specific pharmacologic agent. This being said, though, the above distinctions provide a useful heuristic for the clinician attempting to design a rational pharmacologic treatment regimen based on a patient's current symptom profile, response (or lack of response) to previous medication trials, and side effects experienced during previous medication trials.

SUMMARY

Neurobiological theories do not resolve the mind–brain ambiguities, since ascribing different properties to various brain regions tells us little about *how* nerve activity is translated into the subjective experience of having thoughts and feelings. They don't even explain how this activity is translated into basic animal behaviors.

While these theories do not close the gap between mind and brain, they do help us better understand what is taking place on either side of the gap. In this chapter, we have discussed how our behavior is influenced by memory, by emotions such as anxiety, pleasure, and sadness, and by the application of selective attention and executive function.

We also have discussed how these processes are normally adaptive and help to enhance survival, but how under some circumstances they can become maladaptive and sources of morbidity.

For example, normal processes such as genetic variations in neurotransmitter production and neuroreceptor binding properties, while likely helping to assure survival for many of us, also can become a source of morbidity for those of us who vary to greater degrees along particular psychological dimensions, such as the tendency to experience sadness or anxiety.

Similarly, biological defenses mobilized in response to stress, while typically adaptive, apparently can become sources of pathology when they excessively tax dormant biological vulnerabilities or when stressors are traumatic in nature, or are prolonged or repetitive. Normal physiologic processes—such as the glucocorticoid stress response, excitatory neurotransmission, and apoptosis—come to be turned against the brain. Synaptic plasticity—which normally allows individuals to form memories and to alter future behavior in response to past life experiences—may play a role in allowing psychiatric symptoms to become entrenched, to become chronic or recurrent in nature or even to progress to the point of neurodegenerative decline.

Viewed from this vantage point, *DSM-IV* categorical distinctions tend to blur, as do the careful distinctions laid out in the last chapter between the four clinical perspectives. However, the current diagnostic nomenclature is essential for the treatment of *patients* and not just for the treatment of their neurons. Neurobiological models are instructive but reductionistic. They fail to offer a *clinical* framework that allows us to formulate a differential diagnosis or to design a comprehensive treatment plan tailored to the patient's specific symptoms and circumstances.

For example, both a hug from a friend and a visit to a 12-step program such as Alcoholics Anonymous likely have an impact on brain neurophysiology. However, an alcoholic patient who is experiencing difficulty achieving abstinence from alcohol is much more likely to benefit from the 12-step program than from the hug. It undoubtedly is true that all psychological experiences—be they diseases, dimensions, behaviors, or life stories—"ultimately reside in the realm of brain neurobiology." However, this is tantamount to stating that all human beings "ultimately reside on the Earth." The statement undoubtedly is true, but this knowledge isn't particularly useful when one is trying to figure out how to get from New York to Chicago, or even when trying to figure out how to get across town.

For that, one needs a *road map*. By necessity, a good map *simplifies* what it purports to represent, highlighting some elements and completely dispensing with others. Obviously, if a map faithfully reproduced every detail of what it purported to represent, it would be of little utility.

Each theoretical perspective presented here offers a different road map of the same city. While each map includes the same phenomenologic landmarks, the maps vary in which landmarks they choose to highlight. In the following chapters, we will use these perspectives to structure our discussion, to provide us with a sense of direction as we attempt to navigate through the hurly-burly of psychiatric symptoms, theory, and practice.

Chapter 5

Delirium

Delirium is one of the most common psychiatric diagnoses and is perhaps the most lethal one. Despite often being iatrogenic in nature, clinicians frequently ignore or misdiagnose it. Delirium also provides us with an excellent example of a syndrome best discussed using the disease perspective. Given this, we first will consider the *clinical syndrome* of delirium—its bedside phenomenology, prevalence, and associated morbidity and mortality. Then, we will move one level "deeper," to the *pathology* of delirium. As was discussed in the last chapter, a variety of pathologic insults can be responsible for causing the same final clinical picture. After this, we will move even deeper, examining some *etiologies* associated with these various forms of pathology.

Lastly, we will move "upward" again to the bedside in order to discuss the various ways that delirium is treated. As will prove to be the case for all diseases, some treatment strategies are *nonspecific* and provide only symptomatic relief. For example, agitated or disorganized behavior and psychotic symptoms can be treated through appropriate monitoring, behavioral interventions, or the prescription of psychotropic medications. In contrast, other strategies are *specific*, designed to address the underlying etiology of the delirium. For example, delirium due to infection is best treated by prescribing an appropriate antibiotic.

THE CLINICAL SYNDROME

Phenomenology

In the last chapter, we defined delirium as a syndrome characterized by a pathological *change in the level of consciousness*, which typically waxes and wanes from normal (or even hypervigilant) through drowsiness, stupor, or coma. We noted that while patients who are delirious can display changes in cognition (as in dementia), changes in mood (as in mood disorder), or hallucinations and delusions (as in schizophrenia), the change in consciousness is the hallmark feature of delirium.

This basic definition comports with the earlier *DSM-IIIR* definition shown in Table 5–1 as well as with the currently used *DSM-IV* definition shown in Table 5–2. As demonstrated in Table 5–3, *DSM-IV* also allows the clinician to subcategorize delirium in a particular case based upon the presumed etiology (although this may not be known with certainty at the time of the initial evaluation).

The diagnosis of delirium offers a good example of how expert committees struggle to

Table 5–1. *DSM-III-R* Criteria for Delirium

A. Reduced ability to maintain attention to external stimuli (e.g., have to repeat questions) and to appropriately shift attention to new external stimuli.
B. Disorganized thinking, as indicated by rambling, irrelevant, or incoherent speech
C. At least two of the following:
  1. Reduced level of consciousness—for example, difficulty keeping awake during examination
  2. Perceptual disturbances: misinterpretations, illusions, or hallucinations
  3. Disturbance of sleep–wake cycle with insomnia or daytime sleepiness
  4. Increased or decreased psychomotor activity
  5. Disorientation to time, place, or person
  6. Memory impairment—for example, inability to learn new material, such as the names of several unrelated objects after 5 minutes, or to remember past events, such as history of current episode of illness
D. Clinical features develop over a short period of time (usually hours to days) and tend to fluctuate over the course of a day
E. Either:
  1. Evidence from the history, physical examination, or laboratory tests of a specific organic factor (or factors) judged to be etiologically related to the disturbance, or
  2. In the absence of such evidence, an etiologic organic factor can be presumed if the disturbance cannot be accounted for by a nonorganic mental disorder—for example, manic episode accounting for agitation and sleep disturbance

Table 5–2. *DSM-IV-TR* Criteria for Delirium

A. Disturbance of consciousness (i.e., reduced clarity of awareness of the environment) with reduced ability to focus, sustain, or shift attention
B. A change in cognition (such as memory deficit, disorientation, language disturbance) or the development of a perceptual disturbance that is not better accounted for by a preexisting, established, or evolving dementia
C. The disturbance develops over a short period of time (usually hours to days) and tends to fluctuate during the course of the day

Source: Reprinted with permission from the *Diagnostic and Statistical Manual of Mental Disorders, Fourth Edition, Text Revision.* Copyright 2000 American Psychiatric Association.

Table 5–3. Types of Delirium in *DSM-IV-TR*

DELIRIUM DUE TO . . . [GENERAL MEDICAL CONDITION]

There is evidence from the history, physical examination, or laboratory findings that the disturbance is caused by the direct physiological consequences of a general medical condition

SUBSTANCE-INDUCED DELIRIUM

There is evidence from the history, physical examination, or laboratory findings that either:
  —The symptoms developed during substance intoxication, or
  —Medication use is etiologically related to the disturbance

SUBSTANCE-WITHDRAWAL DELIRIUM

There is evidence from the history, physical examination, or laboratory findings that the symptoms developed during, or shortly after, a withdrawal syndrome

DELIRIUM DUE TO MULTIPLE ETIOLOGIES

There is evidence . . . that the delirium has more than one etiology

DELIRIUM NOT OTHERWISE SPECIFIED

Doesn't meet the criteria for any of the more specific types—for example:
  —Insufficient evidence to establish a specific etiology
  —Due to causes not listed above—for example, sensory deprivation

Source: Reprinted with permission from the *Diagnostic and Statistical Manual of Mental Disorders, Fourth Edition, Text Revision.* Copyright 2000 American Psychiatric Association.

come up with workable disease definitions. As can be seen, the *DSM-III-R* definition is long and lists a wide variety of associated symptoms. It also emphasizes attention deficit rather than level of consciousness, since the former may be a more sensitive indicator in subtle cases. However, impaired attention is a nonspecific finding that is observed in many medical and psychiatric disorders. It also can be hard to assess in uncooperative patients. The *DSM-IV* task group, after some debate as to whether impaired attention or impaired level of consciousness should be considered "primary," decided to award *both* symptoms equal status as part of a single criterion.

Another problem with the *DSM-III-R* criteria was that "disorganized thinking" is often difficult to assess in those patients with sparse speech. This criterion was therefore eliminated. Finally, as they did with many of the other *DSM-III-R* criteria sets, the *DSM-IV* delirium work group attempted to "streamline" the criteria, provided that they could do so without adversely affecting diagnostic sensitivity and specificity.

I haven't emphasized the "short period of time" criterion in my definition. The major goal of this criterion is to help distinguish delirium from dementia, since the latter diagnosis typically presents with more insidious onset (sometimes even over a period of years). However, many patients are chronically delirious, whether due to having a chronic medical illness or because they are chronically taking deliriogenic medications. This is particularly the case for elderly patients and nursing home residents. Also, some types of dementia do have an acute onset (especially those due to acute cerebrovascular events or acute brain trauma). Given this, keep an eye out for delirium even in patients who haven't demonstrated an "acute" decline in functioning. (This having been said, when you are faced with a patient without any previous psychiatric history who demonstrates a rapid decline in mental status, think delirium first.)

> The psychiatrist is called to the surgical OR recovery room to evaluate a 65-year-old man who—1 day after cardiac bypass surgery—is anxious, tearful, hallucinating (seeing cats running around the room and attempting to drink from an imaginary cup), and voicing suicidal ideation. The consultant is asked "to assess for acute-onset, psychotic major depression and recommend appropriate antidepressant therapy."

The psychiatrist diagnoses postoperative delirium. The patient's agitation and psychotic symptoms are treated acutely with low doses of the antipsychotic drug haloperidol. He is frequently reoriented and a sitter or family members stay in the room with him. The physical exam is unremarkable, and a CAT scan of the brain reveals no evidence of a stroke or intracranial bleeding. The next day, the patient develops a low-grade fever and an elevated white blood cell count. While he does not demonstrate a cough and is not short of breath, a chest X-ray reveals new bibasilar infiltrates consistent with a diagnosis of aspiration pneumonia. Antibiotic therapy is initiated. Several days later the patient is feeling much better, denies any symptoms of depression, and has no recollection of any of the events of the past week.

Some clinicians would label chronic cases of delirium as "reversible dementia." For some reason, semantic debates about what to call delirium are common. Despite the relative simplicity of the *DSM-IV* criteria, clinicians have had difficulty figuring out how to label acutely confused patients. Table 5–4 lists some of the terms his-

Table 5–4. Synonyms for Delirium

Acute brain failure
Acute brain syndrome
Acute brain syndrome with psychosis
Acute confusional state
Acute dementia
Acute organic psychosis
Acute organic reaction
Acute organic syndrome
Acute reversible psychosis
Acute secondary psychosis
Cerebral insufficiency
Confusional state
Dysergastic reaction
Exogenous psychosis
Infective-exhaustive psychosis
Intensive care unit psychosis
Metabolic encephalopathy
Oneiric state
Organic brain syndrome
Reversible cerebral dysfunction
Reversible cognitive dysfunction
Reversible dementia
Reversible toxic psychosis
Toxic confusion state
Toxic encephalopathy

Source: Adapted with permission from Trzepacz PT, Wise MG: "Neuropsychiatric Aspects of Delirium." *American Psychiatric Press Textbook of Neuropsychiatry*, Third edition. Washington, DC, American Psychiatric Press, 1997.

torically used to describe confused patients. All are essentially synonyms for delirium.

Consider the term "ICU psychosis." Obviously, the fact that a patient's hospital bed happens to be in an ICU should not be enough to make that person become psychotic. The ICU does not contain unique vapors that would cause patients to enter such a state. Many ICU patients become delirious because they have multiple risk factors for doing so. Wise and Brandt (1992) comment:

These terms are sometimes used synonymously and at other times are used as though they describe different clinical syndromes. For example, Peura and Johnson (1985), who described the side effects of intravenous cimetidine in patients who had gastroduodenal mucosal lesions, stated that one patient developed delirium, one patient had hallucinations, and a third patient had mental confusion. These three patients did not have different disorders. All three had a delirium. It would sometimes appear that confusion describes both delirium and its literature.

Not uncommonly, clinicians also tend to argue over whether a patient in fact is delirious. The most common request posed to psychiatrists who consult on medical and surgical units is, "Please assess for depression." The most common psychiatric diagnosis that they make is delirium. Often, the delirium hasn't been recognized because it has been subtle, or because it has been waxing and waning over the course of the day. For example, while the primary physician may have been prompted to seek psychiatric consultation when the patient burst into tears during morning medical rounds, the patient may have been "quietly confused" for several days before this more dramatic incident. Similarly, a "change in mental status" may only be noted once the patient exhibits a change in *behavioral* status, most notably aggressive behavior or refusal of medical care.

The consultant may diagnose delirium based on the nursing staff reporting that the patient's postoperative confusion worsens every evening (*sundowning*). In contrast, the surgical team has been interviewing an alert, coherent patient every morning, during their 6 AM walk rounds. Or, the consultant may be called in to examine a patient who has become "acutely paranoid." This paranoia typically represents an effort by the confused patient to make sense of distorted percep-

tions. For example, a nurse may have dropped a tray outside of the patient's room, and the resultant "bang" sounded like a gunshot to the delirious patient. He then expresses concerns that "there are people outside the room, trying to kill me."

These distinctions are of more than academic importance. Not uncommonly, the primary physician has just initiated antidepressant or anxiolytic medication therapy for a presumed mood or anxiety disorder at the time of psychiatric consultation. The psychiatrist then recommends that these medications be discontinued out of concern that they could exacerbate the patient's delirium.

Sometimes debate centers on the role of laboratory testing in "confirming" or "disconfirming" the diagnosis of delirium. For example, an emergency room psychiatrist might diagnose delirium, but the emergency room attending physician might opine that the patient "isn't delirious" since "her lab studies are fine." The key point here is that the *mental status examination* is sometimes a more sensitive indicator of an underlying metabolic disturbance than are routine laboratory tests. In the example cited above, a patient became delirious prior to his white blood cell count increasing or his chest X-ray demonstrating signs of aspiration pneumonia.

Surprisingly, while "level of consciousness" sounds like a nebulous thing to assess, when two evaluators standing at the bedside are asked to rate a patient's level of consciousness on a scale of 0 to 10, the interrater reliability is very good. (Try this on walk rounds some time; you'll be amazed.) The best way to assess for impaired attention, memory, and other cognitive functions at the bedside is by performing a Mini-Mental State Examination, as discussed in Chapter 2. Keep in mind that at one given point in time, the Mini-Mental score may be in the "normal" range but that *serial* examinations often reveal waxing and waning deficits.

Prevalence

While the point prevalence of delirium in the general population is relatively low (0.4% in adults age 18 years and older, 1.1% in those age 55 and older), the prevalence is much higher in the general hospital setting. Studies that have screened for delirium in patients at the time of admission to a medical or surgical unit have found that about 10%–15% of all patients are delirious on admission. Patients may also become delirious during their hospital stay, and studies using somewhat different screening tools to assess for delirium in medical and surgical patients in the midst of treatment have found prevalences of between 10 and 40%.

Certain classes of hospitalized patients are at greater risk of developing delirium, including the elderly (30%–40% of those in the hospital, up to 60% of those residing in nursing homes), postoperative patients (40%–50%), AIDS patients, burn patients (20%), patients with brain injury or dementia, and patients in drug withdrawal. Studies in the hospice setting have found that up to 80% of patients with terminal illness become delirious as they near death.

Morbidity and Mortality

The morbidity from delirium is considerable. It poses a clear short-term physical danger to both the staff (whom the patient may strike) and the patient (who may require restraints in order to ensure safety or to prevent the patient from pulling out nasogastric and intravenous lines, thereby resulting in decubitus ulcers and aspiration pneumonia).

Delirium is also associated with an increased likelihood of longer-term functional decline and need for discharge to an institution rather than to home. For example, inpatients who are 65 years or older who are delirious are three times more likely to be discharged to a nursing home than those who are not delirious.

Delirium prolongs hospitalization, especially for postoperative patients. Even worse, it may bode poorly for recovery, and many delirious patients even fail to derive any benefit from having received the operation. For example, one study assessed the status of orthopedic patients at their 6-month postoperative follow-up visit. Those patients who had developed a postoperative delirium following their surgery were much less likely to have derived any functional benefit from the surgery. Another study focused specifically on patients who had been treated for femoral neck fractures. Patients who became postoperatively delirious spent twice as long in the hospital as their peers who hadn't become delirious. They were more likely to die, to be bedridden, to require walking aids, and to require

discharge into a rehabilitation program. Among patients discharged into the latter setting, delirious patients required four times longer to recuperate to the point where they could be discharged than nondelirious patients.

While most patients with delirium fully recover, some patients do not. After the acute delirium resolves, residual neurologic signs or persisting symptoms of dementia may be noted in some patients. For example, this course of illness has been described in postcardiotomy patients.

This is not to say that the delirium itself *caused* the persisting deficits. More likely, some acute pathological insult to the brain—for example, ischemia, infection, or trauma—results in *both* acute, severe deficits and chronic, more subtle deficits that become apparent only after delirium has resolved. However, delirium may be a "red flag," indicating the presence of some underlying medical illness. If this turns out to be an illness responsive to clinical intervention (sepsis, for example), recognizing the need for treatment and intervening early may improve the patient's longer-term prognosis.

The mortality associated with delirium is also significant. Again, while these deaths are not always the direct result of the delirium itself, clearly the diagnosis of delirium is a clinical marker indicating a much greater risk of dying. One study compared the rate of death in the hospital between elderly delirious patients and demented patients. Of the patients who had been diagnosed with delirium, 22% died during that hospitalization, a rate 5.5 times greater than for members of the dementia group. Studies of elderly hospitalized patients diagnosed with delirium have noted death rates during that hospital stay of as high as 75%. Six months after hospital discharge, another study followed up on 77 elderly patients who had been diagnosed with delirium by a consultation psychiatrist during their stay. By that time, 25% of the patients had died.

PATHOLOGY

The clinical syndrome of delirium can be caused by multiple pathological processes. While a severe enough insult might make anybody delirious, in clinical practice some populations are clearly at greater risk. One way to conceptualize this relationship is as follows:

Predisposing Factor + Pathologic Insult
$$\longrightarrow \text{Delirium}$$

Predisposing Factors

One such group is *the elderly*. As noted above, up to 40% of hospitalized elderly patients are delirious. The elderly are more susceptible to experiencing adverse effects of their medical problems, such as anemia or infection. They are also more susceptible to medication side effects. The latter is the case due to three major ways in which medications interact with the older patients' bodies differently than they do with younger patients' bodies.

The first difference involves *pharmacodynamic factors*. This term refers to differences in the physiologic effects of a drug at a given blood level. Since elderly patients have decreased neuronal mass, they experience heightened central nervous system sensitivity to the sedative and cognitive side effects of medications. This problem is further exacerbated by declines in neurotransmitters such as acetylcholine (especially in Alzheimer's disease), and dopamine (especially in Parkinson's disease).

The second difference involves *pharmacokinetic factors*. This term refers to differences in the amount of a drug that is available at a given dose. For example, older patients have decreased lean body mass (i.e., muscle and water). This in turn leads to increased serum concentrations of most drugs. Even when a patient's weight has remained unchanged with aging, he or she has experienced an increase in body fat and a decrease in muscle mass. This in turn contributes to a wider distribution and slower clearance of drugs that are fat-soluble, such as benzodiazepines, sedative-hypnotics, neuroleptics, and tricyclic antidepressants. Also, older patients have decreased hepatic metabolism (phase I oxidation) of drugs. This leads to the drugs having both an increased half-life and delayed appearance of active intermediate metabolites. (The latter is an issue particularly with many benzodiazepine agents.)

The third difference involves the *coexistence of other diseases*. Older patients have more illnesses. Not only do these diseases place the patient at greater risk of developing a delirium in themselves, but they typically create the need for polypharmacy, which in turn increases the likelihood of the patient experiencing cumulative medication toxicity. Malnutrition and chronic inflammatory diseases also lead to decreased synthesis of plasma-binding proteins and therefore higher bioavailability of drugs to the brain. Renal disease can cause decreased glomerular filtration rate, thereby leading to decreased renal clearance of drugs. Similarly, hepatic disease can lead to decreased metabolism of many drugs.

Postoperative patients are also at high risk for becoming delirious. For example, the prevalence of delirium in postcardiotomy patients ranges from 15% to 75%. Risk factors in this population for becoming delirious include: age, duration of time spent on the bypass pump, severity of postoperative illnesses, serum level of anticholinergic drugs, increased levels of CNS adenylate kinase, decreased cardiac output, the complexity of the surgical procedure, complement activation, embolism, and nutritional status (as assessed by serum albumin levels).

While one might assume from this long list that postoperative delirium in such patients is a near inevitability, this is not the case. Preoperative interviews by a consultation psychiatrist have been found to reduce the risk of developing a postoperative delirium by 50%. In fact, a factor analysis of 28 risk factors from 44 studies over 25 years showed that despite improved technology, the rate of postcardiotomy delirium hadn't declined. Of all of these factors, only preoperative psychiatric evaluation correlated (negatively) with the occurrence of postcardiotomy delirium. Presumably, the psychiatrist helped to identify risk factors that were amenable to clinical intervention, such as potentially deliriogenic medications that could be discontinued prior to surgery.

Delirium occurs in up to 30% of *burn patients*. Not surprisingly, older patients and patients with a greater severity of burn are more at risk of becoming delirious.

Another group of patients at greater risk of becoming delirious are patients with *brain injury*, including patients with stroke, head trauma, neurodegenerative disorders, dementia, and HIV. During an acute consultation, it can be difficult to determine if a delirious patient has an underlying dementing illness acting as a predisposing factor until after resolution of the delirium. At this later stage, it may remain difficult to determine if any residual cognitive deficits are due to the persisting low-grade delirium, to a preexisting but previously undiagnosed dementia, or to a new brain injury resulting from the same pathological insult that caused the delirium.

A 72-year-old white female presents in acute delirium with combativeness, anxiety, and visual hallucinations alternating with periods of somnolence. She is afebrile. Laboratory workup is notable for a urinary tract infection being noted on urinalysis, along with a slight leukocytosis. The rest of her workup (which includes a head CT, electrolyte and chemistry panels, B₁₂, RPR, and thyroid studies) is unremarkable. She is symptomatically treated with behavioral redirection by the nursing staff and with low doses of haloperidol for her psychotic symptoms and agitation. Following the initiation of antibiotic treatment, she becomes alert and behaviorally appropriate. However, she remains disoriented to date and continues to demonstrate short-term memory and attention deficits. Additional history reveals that while she for decades had managed the household finances for herself and her husband, her daughter has been performing this task for the past several years, as both the patient and her husband have experienced difficulty "keeping track of bills." Her daughter also more recently has been overseeing the patient's medications, filling a pill box for her each week. The patient has continued to dress herself, bathe, and cook appropriately. Based upon the clinical history and workup, a diagnosis is made of probable dementia of the Alzheimer's type, along with a resolved, superimposed delirium due to urinary tract infection.

The *human immunodeficiency virus (HIV)* is highly associated with delirium. The delirium can be caused by the *direct effects* of the virus on the brain, by *secondary complications* (opportunistic infections and/or CNS or systemic tumors), and by *medications*. HIV invades the brain shortly after infection, and the virus itself causes a meningoencephalitis that can become chronic. Subcortical brain regions are the most affected (including the periventricular white matter, basal ganglia, thalamus, and brain stem), while the cortex is relatively spared. Therefore, these patients can develop subtle neuropsychological deficits, and ultimately a *subcortical dementia* (discussed in more detail in the next chapter). In summary, the HIV virus both *causes* delirium and renders the HIV-infected patient more *vulnerable* to delirium.

Patients in *drug or alcohol withdrawal* are also at greater risk for developing delirium, either directly (due to the withdrawal itself) or indirectly (due to comorbid medical conditions).

A patient hospitalized for a hip replacement develops a postoperative delirium 3 days into her hospital stay. Contributing factors are found to include hyponatremia, postoperative anemia from blood loss, the use of narcotic analgesia, and amitriptyline (a highly anticholinergic agent) given for sleep. In addition, discussion with her family reveals that she has taken the benzodiazepine drug lorazepam on a daily basis for at least the past year, "for nervousness." Her pulse and blood pressure are noted to be slightly elevated, and she is slightly tremulous with her hands outstretched, although she is not diaphoretic. While clinicians often avoid giving benzodiazepines to calm delirious patients out of concern that they might sometimes exacerbate delirium, in this case the psychiatrist recommends that lorazepam be restarted to treat possible benzodiazepine withdrawal. He also recommends discontinuing both the amitriptyline and the narcotic analgesia. The patient receives a blood transfusion to treat her anemia. Her confusion gradually resolves over the following 3 days.

Pathologic Insults

As the above example demonstrates, a variety of pathologic insults can cause delirium in a vulnerable patient. There may be clues to the cause of delirium based on the clinical presentation. To cite just a few examples, new symptoms of dysuria and urinary urgency may lead the clinician to check a urinalysis for signs of a urinary tract infection; asterixis may lead the clinician to suspect liver disease; elevated vital signs, tremor, or diaphoresis may lead the clinician to suspect alcohol or sedative-hypnotic withdrawal. However, in many cases the history and physical exam are unrevealing and the clinician must "cast a wide net" using ancillary tests. One useful mnemonic (and also a reminder of the morbidity and mortality associated with delirium) is "I WATCH DEATH," as outlined in Table 5–5.

One of the first places to look in assessing delirium is the patient's *medications*. Table 5–6 is a partial list of some of the classes of medications most commonly associated with delirium. Many of these medications have *anticholinergic effects*, even if they are not categorized as such. Table 5–7 lists cholinergic

Table 5–5. "I WATCH DEATH" Mnemonic for Delirium

*I*nfectious	Sepsis, encephalitis, meningitis, syphilis, urinary tract infection, pneumonia
*W*ithdrawal	Alcohol, barbiturates, sedative-hypnotics
*A*cute metabolic	Acidosis, electrolyte disturbance, hepatic and renal failure, other metabolic disturbances (Glc, Mg, Ca)
*T*rauma	Head trauma, burns
*C*NS disease	Hemorrhage, CVA, vasculitis, seizures, tumor
*H*ypoxia	Acute hypoxia, chronic lung disease, hypotension
*D*eficiencies	B_{12}, hypovitaminosis, niacin, thiamin
*E*nvironmental	Hypothermia, hyperthermia, endocrinopathies (diabetes, adrenal, thyroid)
*A*cute vascular	Hypertensive emergency, subarachnoid hemorrhage, sagittal vein thrombosis
*T*oxins/drugs	Medications, street drugs, alcohol, pesticides, industrial poisons (carbon monoxide, cyanide, solvents, etc.)
*H*eavy metals	Lead, mercury

Source: Adapted with permission from Wise MG, Gray KF, Seltzer B: "Delirium, Dementia, and Amnestic Disorders." *American Psychiatric Press Textbook of Psychiatry*, third edition. Washington, DC, American Psychiatric Press, 1999.

receptor affinities for various commonly prescribed drugs. While the anticholinergic effects for a particular medication may be modest, many elderly and medically frail patients take three or more such medications, and the anticholinergic effects are cumulative.

Drugs especially likely to cause delirium are benzodiazepines, centrally acting antihypertensives, opioids, digitalis, antiparkinsonian agents, tricyclic antidepressants, and corticosteroids. Patients and physicians might overlook over-the-counter drugs, especially salicylates and anticholinergics. Also, do not forget about topical ophthalmic medications. While only small amounts of such medications are given, they are applied to the eye, which itself is a direct extension of the brain.

Etiology

The disease perspective posits that the same clinical syndrome can be caused by multiple pathologies, while the same pathology can be caused by multiple etiologies. Delirium is an excellent example. The pathology underlying the clinical syndrome of delirium is *widespread alteration in cerebral metabolic activity* affecting both cortical and subcortical structures. This alteration affects the patient's arousal, attention, information processing, and sleep–wake cycle. It also can lead to *secondary dysregulation of neurotransmitter synthesis and metabolism*. For example, there can be a deficiency of substrates for oxidative metabolism (glucose, oxygen), disturbed passage of ions through cell membranes, disturbed homeostasis of neurotransmitters (serotonin, norepinephrine, acetylcholine), or (in the case of some drugs) false neurotransmitters.

Table 5–8 lists some proposed mechanisms by which different etiologies may have their pathological effects. Of note, sensory deprivation (e.g., in elderly patients who have vision

Table 5–6. Potentially Deliriogenic Medications (a Partial List)

Antimicrobials (especially penicillins, cephalosporins, quinolones)	Barbiturates
	Benzodiazepines
Antiarrhythmics	Corticosteroids
Anticholinergics (and psychotropic medications with anticholinergic properties)	Gastrointestinal agents
	Immunosuppressive agents
Anticonvulsants	Lithium
Antihistamines (including H_2-blockers in antacids and H_1-blockers in allergy and sleep aids)	Muscle relaxants
	Opiates
Antihypertensive agents (including β-blockers, clonidine)	Salicylates
Antineoplastic agents	Sympathomimetic agents (including amphetamines, phenylpropanolamine)
Antiparkinsonian agents (both anticholinergic and dopaminergic)	Theophylline
Antituberculous agents	

Table 5–7. Anticholinergic Drug Levels for 25 Medications (in ng/mL of Atropine Equivalents), Ranked by the Frequency of Their Prescription to Elderly Patients

1. Furosemide	0.22
2. Digoxin	0.25
3. Dyazide	0.08
4. Lanoxin	0.25
5. Hydrochlorothiazide	0.00
6. Propranolol	0.00
7. Salicylic acid	0.00
8. Dipyridamole	0.11
9. Theophylline	0.44
10. Nitroglycerin	0.00
11. Insulin	0.00
12. Warfarin	0.12
13. Prednisolone	0.55
14. α-methyldopa	0.00
15. Nifedipine	0.22
16. Isosorbide dinitrate	0.15
17. Ibuprofen	0.00
18. Codeine	0.11
19. Cimetidine	0.86
20. Diltiazem hydrochloride	0.00
21. Captopril	0.02
22. Atenolol	0.00
23. Metoprolol	0.00
24. Timolol	0.00
25. Ranitidine	0.22

Source: Adapted with permission from Tune L et al: "Anticholinergic Effects of Drugs Commonly Prescribed for the Elderly: Potential Means for Assessing Risk of Delirium." *Am J Psychiatry* 149:1393–1394, 1992.

and hearing deficits) can contribute to decreased cortical activity and slowing of the EEG and can also contribute to delirious patients misinterpreting environmental stimuli since they are poorly perceived to begin with. Further, loss of visual or auditory input to their respective cortical sensory association areas may disinhibit these areas and has been described as a cause of hallucinations even in nondelirious patients (Given this, make sure that hospitalized patients still wear their glasses and hearing aids. Not uncommonly, when patients are asked if they have a hearing aid, they reply, "Yes, it's over there in the drawer.")

However, sensory loss in itself has not been shown to cause delirium and shouldn't be used to "explain away" the presence of delirium in an elderly patient. Nor should it be assumed that a patient's confusion is due to being in an unfamiliar hospital environment and that it will resolve "once he's back in his own home."

Treatment

Delirium is a medical emergency. The ultimate outcome of treatment depends upon the cause of the delirium, the patient's underlying health, and the timeliness of treatment intervention.

The initial focus of treatment is on diagnosing and treating those conditions that might lead to increased morbidity and mortality. At this stage, medications prescribed for symptomatic treatment are sometimes helpful but sometimes make the situation worse. For example, *benzodiazepines* can calm an anxious patient but also may potentially further confuse or behaviorally disinhibit the patient. *Antipsychotic drugs*, if used in delirium tremens (DTs), could lower the seizure threshold and precipitate seizures. Antidepressants, when prescribed to treat sadness, anxiety, or sleep disturbance due to delirium, might exacerbate delirium due to anticholinergic or serotonergic toxicity. In general, then, the goal should be to taper or discontinue all nonessential medications.

In addition to the *history and physical exam,* *ancillary tests* should be ordered. These typically include a complete chemistry panel (including electrolytes, BUN and creatinine, glucose, calcium, albumin, ammonia level, and liver function studies), complete blood count, erythrocyte sedimentation rate (ESR), toxicology screen (along with blood levels of relevant medications), urinalysis, electrocardiogram, chest X-ray, and pulse oximetry or arterial blood gas. If the cause of delirium remains unclear, frequent (even daily) laboratory tests and physical examination may be required, as delirium may precede the clinical or laboratory findings that indicate its cause.

Based on the clinical situation, additional ancillary tests could include thiamine and folate levels (see discussion in the next chapter on Wernicke's syndrome), thyroid studies, antinuclear antibodies, heavy metal screen, and urinary porphobilinogen (to test for acute intermittent porphyria). *Neuroimaging* (by CAT or MRI scan) can help to rule out a mass lesion, stroke, tumor, or normal-pressure hydrocephalus. If one suspects a possible CNS infection (due to the presence of fever or meningeal signs), a *lumbar puncture* would be indicated.

Table 5–8. Proposed Mechanisms by Which Different Etiologies Can Lead to the Same Pathology in Delirium

Etiology	Mechanism
Tricyclic antidepressants	Cholinergic and histaminergic receptor blockade; serotonin, norepinephrine, dopamine reuptake inhibition
Opiates	Direct opioid receptor agonist effects; indirect dopaminergic and glutaminergic effects, inhibition of Na–K–ATPase
Low-potency antipsychotics	Cholinergic and histaminergic receptor blockade
Benzodiazepines and barbiturate intoxication	Enhanced GABA activity (suppressing neuronal transmission)
Benzodiazepine and barbiturate withdrawal	Deficient GABA activity (increasing neuronal irritability)
Hallucinogens	Serotonin agonist effects; increased cortical and limbic neuronal activity
PCP	Inhibition of the PCP–NMDA receptor; norepinephrine and serotonin reuptake inhibition, blockade of sodium and potassium channels, anticholinergic effects
Fever/hyperthermia	Toxic effects of cytokines, increased peripheral and cerebral metabolic demands
Head injury	Direct cortical and axonal injury, indirect anticholinergic effects due to injury of cholinergic neurons
Metabolic abnormalities	Altered cerebral metabolic rate; altered neuronal membrane potentials; altered neuronal morphology
Hepatic failure	Failure of liver to detoxify intestinal substances including ammonia, mercaptans, fatty acids, phenol, GABA; also increased blood–brain barrier permeability. In brain, ammonia and other toxins may interfere with Na–K–ATPase pump, inhibit cholinergic activity, act at GABA receptor, and/or act as false transmitters
Renal failure	Secondary metabolic derangements; increased permeability of blood–brain barrier to toxins (e.g., organic acids), increased brain calcium and CSF phosphate
Diabetic ketoacidosis or hyperosmolar state, hyponatremia	Decreased brain water volume, altered neuronal membrane potentials

The *electroencephalogram (EEG)* can be particularly useful in the evaluation of suspected delirium. Most delirious patients have reduced cerebral metabolic activity, reflected in slowing of background brainwave activity (see Chapter 3, Fig. 3–2). Since patients with major depressive disorder or schizophrenia don't show these changes, the EEG can help both to confirm the diagnosis of delirium and to distinguish it from other psychiatric illnesses. Further, the EEG can help in identifying some neurologic etiologies of delirium, such as complex-partial seizures (where one may see focal ictal activity, particularly in the temporal region), or a discrete lesion such as a cortical infarct or tumor (where one can see focal slowing).

However, the absence of EEG findings does not eliminate the possibility of delirium. The EEG is sensitive, but not 100% sensitive. For example, in the absence of a previous EEG in a normal waking state, one can't be completely certain that the patient didn't start out with a fast baseline rhythm, which then slowed to a state that is in fact slower than baseline but still interpreted as being "within the normal range." In addition, there are some *hyperactive* forms of delirium (particularly delirium associated with DTs, hyperthermia, and PCP intoxication). In these cases, cerebral metabolism is either *normal or increased*, and this is reflected in the EEG by background low-voltage fast activity rather than background slowing. In addition, since the degree of slowing correlates with the degree of decline in the patient's level of consciousness, the EEG may be less sensitive in more subtle cases of delirium (although *serial EEGs* still may be useful in such cases). Finally, the EEG is not 100% specific, either. For example, patients with advanced dementia due to Alzheimer's disease also may present with EEG slowing, even in the absence of delirium.

In terms of *symptomatic* management, the goal is *to keep the delirious patient comfortable and to keep the patient and hospital staff safe*. Family members or staff should be on hand to help reorient the patient. Try to place the patient near the nursing station to help minimize agitation or falls. Familiar objects in the room are often helpful, and a large calendar and clock can help the patient remain oriented. Adequate lighting at night can help minimize illusions, as can having a window in the room. If the patient has a hearing aid or glasses, try to ensure that he is actually wearing them.

Staff should closely frequently assess the patient for any signs of clinical deterioration. Vital signs, fluid and nutritional intake, and urine output should be monitored. Ensure that oxygen prongs remain in the patient's nostrils (and not on the patient's forehead), that the patient isn't pulling out her intravenous lines, and that she isn't crawling over the bedrails. Restraints may be required, especially at night. During the daytime, a "geri-chair" with a locking front tray is one useful way to help keep the patient safe but also out of the bed, thereby decreasing the risk of aspiration and decubitus ulcers.

In cases of agitation not due to substance withdrawal, the medication of choice is likely oral, intravenous, or intramuscular administration of the antipsychotic agents haloperidol or droperidol. (The latter is related chemically to haloperidol and is used in anesthesia. It is more sedating, has a more rapid onset, and carries a slightly greater risk of causing hypotension.) These drugs aren't associated with respiratory depression (as benzodiazepines can be), carry little risk of hypotension, and aren't significantly anticholinergic.

However, antipsychotic drugs can cause extrapyramidal reactions including akathisia, parkinsonism, and acute dystonic reactions (see Chapter 7 for further discussion), and the neurologic exam should be monitored. For unclear reasons, extrapyramidal reactions appears to be less common when these agents are administered intravenously, and very high doses of haloperidol (up to 1 or 1.5 g) have been administered intravenously in the ICU setting without precipitating extrapyramidal reactions. (If haloperidol is administered intravenously, the IV line should be cleared with saline first, since heparin can precipitate intravenous haloperidol.) Because intravenous administration bypasses first-pass hepatic metabolism, intravenous doses are often administered at half the oral dose. The haloperidol can be administered frequently, especially if hemodynamic monitoring is in place. However, very high dosages rarely have been associated with cardiac arrhythmias, including torsade de pointes.

In cases where agitation is mild or where the patient is elderly or infirm, a single intravenous 0.5–2 mg dose of haloperidol first could be administered. In moderate to severe cases of agitation, 5–10 mg would be the starting dose. The patient should be observed for a half hour. If there is no response, one then might administer a second dose that is twice the initial dose. If there is no response to this after 30 minutes, one then might administer a third dose that is twice the second dose. Once the patient is calm, one should calculate the total milligrams administered that have been administered and give this amount divided over the following 24 hour period. Try giving two-thirds of the dose at night (to help treat "sundowning" and restore a normal sleep–wake cycle) and one-third either in the morning or subdivided between morning and afternoon.

Sometimes, a severely agitated patient won't respond to haloperidol and coadministration of oral or intravenous lorazepam allows for a synergistic anxiolytic and sedating effect. Once the patient is calm, attempt to gradually taper the haloperidol over the next several days. Since the antipsychotic medication may be masking a persisting delirium, a gradual taper along with behavioral observation for worsening of clinical status may be more prudent than abrupt discontinuation.

SUMMARY

Delirium is a syndrome that presents with psychiatric manifestations but always reflects underlying biological disarray. The hallmark feature of delirium is a change in the patient's level of consciousness along with attention difficulties. Regardless of their medical specialty, all physicians will encounter delirious patients. The most important element in the treatment of delirium is recognizing that it is present. Psychiatric consultation may prove helpful in the process of diagnosing the condition, discerning likely causes, and providing symptomatic management. Consultation may also be helpful for primary prevention. In the psychiatric setting, disorders such as dementia, mood disorder, and schizophrenia shouldn't be diagnosed until delirium has been excluded. Delirium also can complicate the treatment of these other conditions. The Mini-Mental State Examination is a useful bedside tool to help in diagnosing this condition, and the EEG can be a useful confirmatory test. However, as with all psychiatric disorders, the diagnosis ultimately is an empirical one, based on a careful history and mental status examination.

Chapter 6

Dementia

A recent study estimated that the annual cost of all forms of dementia in the United States was somewhere between $20 billion and $38 billion and that the annual cost of caring for Alzheimer's disease patients was as high as $47,000 per patient per year. The cost is expected to increase as the number of patients with dementia increases. In 1985 there were 2.4 million Americans with moderate to severe dementia, and this number is expected to increase to between 6.1 and 9.8 million by 2040; the care of these persons will cost up to $149 billion annually.

This projected increase is due to the aging of the U.S. population since the prevalence of dementia increases with advancing age. Five percent of Americans over age 65 have a severe dementia. The prevalence doubles every 5 years through about age 80, reaching about 50% by age 85. However, dementia is not an inevitable part of the aging process, and most elderly patients are not demented.

In this chapter, we will discuss dementia primarily from the disease perspective, exploring its phenomenology, the various pathologies associated with dementia, and the etiologies associated with these pathologies. Along the way, we'll distinguish dementia from two less severe conditions, mild cognitive impairment and amnestic syndrome.

Finally, we will focus on dementia due to Alzheimer's disease, since this is the most common cause of dementia. While the underlying etiology of Alzheimer's disease is not fully understood, it is the object of intense research. While currently available behavioral and somatic treatments for dementia often provide significant relief to patients and their families, they still only treat symptoms. No treatments are available that are capable of reversing or arresting the progression of this disease.

The ultimate goal of the disease perspective, however, is to move from bedside phenomenology to bench research as to etiology, apply what is learned from this to the prospective design of theoretically effective treatment strategies, and then to move back to the bedside to subject these treatments to empiric study. Given this, as we discuss Alzheimer's disease, we will explore not only *currently* available symptomatic treatments but also aspects of the disease that may one day be susceptible to intervention, based on current etiologic theories.

PHENOMENOLOGY

Dementia

The clinical syndrome of dementia is characterized by a *global decline in cognitive functioning in clear consciousness*. The decline is global in that the patient with dementia has impaired memory along with impairments in several other cognitive domains, such as visuospatial skills, language, praxis, judgment, personality, and abstract thinking. The impairment represents a decline from a previous level (which distinguishes dementia from mental retardation) and takes place in clear consciousness (which distinguishes dementia from delirium). Multiple pathologies can cause dementia, and several etiologies can cause these pathologies. The overwhelming majority of dementia is attributable to either **Alzheimer's disease** or **vascular dementia**. However, a large number of other medical disorders can cause dementia, including neurodegenerative disorders, space-occupying lesions such as tumor or subdural hematoma, hydrocephalus, metabolic–endocrine disorders, nutritional deficiencies, toxins (including alcohol), infections, collagen–vascular disease, and other conditions. Table 6–1 summarizes a basic differential diagnosis of Dementia.

The first goal in treating dementia is to *establish the diagnosis of dementia* (and especially rule out the patient actually having a reversible delirium). The second goal is to determine as best as one can the *cause of the dementia*. We are especially interested here in uncovering causes of dementia that are amenable to clinical intervention that could arrest or reverse disease progression if caught early on. Examples include *metabolic or nutritional factors* (such as *vitamin B12 deficiency* or *hypothyroidism*), *subdural hematoma*, *neurosyphilis*, and *normal-pressure hydrocephalus*. We particularly need to assess for the presence of a *major depressive disorder*, since this can cause significant cognitive dysfunction but is amenable to treatment via antidepressant therapies. (This syndrome once was called **pseudodementia.** However, given that the cognitive dysfunction associated with major depression is as "real" as that caused by so-called "organic" diseases, the syndrome is now more-often labeled **dementia of depression.**)

The third goal is to *establish a treatment plan*. Components of such a plan might include *symptomatic and behavioral management* (including treatment of delusions, agitation, or sleep disturbance through behavioral or pharmacologic

Table 6–1. Differential Diagnosis of Dementia

ALZHEIMER'S DISEASE

VASCULAR DEMENTIA

FRONTAL LOBE DEGENERATION
(e.g., Pick's disease)

HEAD TRAUMA

EXTRAPYRAMIDAL/SUBCORTICAL DISORDERS
(e.g., Parkinson's disease, Huntington's disease, progressive supranuclear palsy, multisystem atrophy, Lewy body disease, cortical–basal ganglionic degeneration)

SYSTEMIC DISEASE
(e.g., chronic renal disease, cardiac failure, vasculitis)

METABOLIC, NUTRITIONAL, AND ENDOCRINE DISTURBANCES
(e.g., thyroid or B12 deficiency)

INTRACRANIAL MASS LESIONS
(e.g., tumor, subdural hematoma)

INFECTION
(e.g., syphilis; Creutzfeldt-Jakob, HIV)

TOXINS
(e.g., mercury, aluminum, chronic alcohol)

GENETIC DISORDERS

HYDROCEPHALUS

measures), *family education and support*, and *treatment of any comorbid conditions* that might exacerbate cognitive or behavioral symptoms. The last can include medical problems (such as urinary tract infection, heart failure, and medication side effects) and other psychiatric problems (such as depression, anxiety, psychotic symptoms, and aggression). A more recent goal, as our understanding of the etiology of dementia has expanded, has been to initiate pharmacologic treatments that might *slow disease progression*.

Not all cognitive disturbances meet the full criteria for dementia. Isolated neuropsychological deficits short of dementia exist—for example, an isolated aphasia due to stroke. However, two especially important disturbances that can be difficult to distinguish from dementia, especially early dementia, are mild cognitive impairment and amnestic syndrome.

Mild Cognitive Impairment

Mild cognitive impairment (MCI) has gone by a variety of names over the years, including age-associated memory impairment, age-related cognitive decline, and benign senescent forgetfulness. As can be inferred from these other terms, for years it has been considered to be a "normal part of aging," important primarily because it is to be distinguished from dementia. Patients typically present stating that they have difficulty coming up with the right word or recalling a name (with the words being "on the tip of the tongue"); are absentminded, misplacing things more than they used to; and have some increased difficulty concentrating. The primary intervention has been to screen for the possibility of dementia and—should dementia fail to be discovered—offer reassurance.

However, this condition is not necessarily so "benign" after all: several recent prospective studies following individuals with MCI over a period of from 2 to 4 years have found that about 12% per year progress to a diagnosis of Alzheimer's disease. In contrast, the conversion rate for the general population ranges from 0.2% in the 65–69 year age range to 4% in the 85–89-year age range. Given this, there has been some debate among clinicians as to whether primary care clinicians should routinely be screening for such impairment, just as they screen for early signs of other diseases.

On the other hand, not all individuals with MCI have progressed to Alzheimer's disease. This even was the case in one prospective study that tracked patients for 7 years after they were diagnosed with MCI. This finding indicates either that the progression from MCI to Alzheimer's disease is not inevitable or that the rate of progression is quite variable. Given this, and given that there are no early clinical interventions available that impede the progression from MCI to Alzheimer's disease, the benefits of early screening remain uncertain.

If a therapy were to become available that could slow or halt disease progression, routine cognitive screenings likely would become the norm. Proposed therapies, such as vitamin E, ginkgo biloba, cholinesterase inhibitors, and Cox-2 anti-inflammatory agents have mostly been studied in cases of overt Alzheimer's disease. There, they have provided only slight benefit. Would such agents be more effective in MCI, and could they alter the progression from MCI to Alzheimer's disease? Multiyear prospective controlled trials designed to addressed these questions are currently in progress.

Amnestic Disorder

Patients with **amnestic syndrome** experience an *isolated* deficit in memory without other cognitive impairment. They don't demonstrate a decline in multiple aspects of cognition, as seen in dementia, and they don't demonstrate a change in consciousness as would be seen in delirium. They always demonstrate an *anterograde amnesia* (an inability to retain new information) and they may also demonstrate *retrograde amnesia* (an inability to recall information from prior to their injury). In terms of the retrograde impairments, *remote memory* (e.g., a memory of events from several years ago) typically remains more intact than does *recent memory* (e.g., a memory of events from a few days or even a few hours before the injury).

Patients with amnestic disorder often demonstrate **confabulation**—that is, they fill in memory gaps or inconsistencies with recollections of events that never occurred. (In some cases, a collateral informant is required to discern whether the patient is confabulating.) Confabulation occurs without any intent to deceive the examiner.

Of note, contrary to Hollywood portrayals, retrograde amnesia can extend from a few seconds prior to the brain injury to a few years prior to the injury, but it doesn't include amnesia for personal identity or all of the patient's previous life. Patients with such a presentation likely don't have a true amnesia. They either are feigning illness (as in **malingering** or **factitious disorder**), or have **conversion disorder**, or have a **dissociative disorder**. (These diagnoses are discussed in Chapters 13 and 14).

The presence of an amnestic disorder indicates that there is a lesion affecting some element of the *medial temporal lobe circuit*. This neural network consists of the hippocampus, fornix, mammillary bodies of the hypothalamus, and medial thalamic nuclei. The most common causes of amnestic syndrome are listed in Table 6–2.

The most common cause of amnesia is **head**

Table 6–2. Most Common Causes of Amnestic Difficulties

Head trauma
Wernicke-Korsakoff syndrome
Stroke (posterior cerebral artery)
Subarachnoid hemorrhage (anterior cerebral artery rupture)
Anoxic brain injury (anoxia, hypoperfusion, carbon monoxide poisoning)
Herpes simplex encephalitis
Alzheimer's disease
Brain tumors or metastasis
Temporal lobectomy
Transient global amnesia
Electroconvulsive therapy
Benzodiazepines

trauma. When the skull receives a severe impact, acceleration (coup) and deceleration (contracoup) cause the brain to slam against adjacent skull, which can cause intracranial hemorrhage, brain swelling, or both. The frontal lobes and anterior poles of the temporal lobes are most susceptible to this type of injury, regardless of the site of initial impact, as they lie against areas of skull with bony prominences. Rotational and horizontal movement of the brain also produces shearing of axons that travel along central white matter pathways, along with shearing of their associated penetrating blood vessels. This shearing also contributes to the establishment of diffuse deficits in cognitive and emotional regulation, again unrelated to the site of initial impact. (Of note, some of these injuries will not be apparent on routine neuroimaging studies.)

Following more severe impact, individuals typically experience some change in their level of consciousness. This can range from a transient lapse in consciousness or a confused or "dazed" state (either of which would be considered a *concussion*) to longer-term loss of consciousness (i.e., *postconcussive delirium or coma*). Following resolution of this acute change in mental status, individuals may be left with a combination of anterograde memory deficits and retrograde memory deficits. The latter can extend as far back as several years prior to the injury. As the anterograde deficits begin to improve (i.e., as the patient regains the ability to retain new information), the period covered by the retrograde amnesia also begins to shorten, often down to a period of time lasting for as little as seconds or minutes prior to the head injury.

However, some patients experience more extensive, irreversible cognitive and emotional deficits. Such patients demonstrate what has been termed *postconcussive syndrome*. This syndrome includes not only amnestic difficulties but also personality changes and behavioral disturbances, likely reflecting injury to not only the hippocampus but also the frontal lobes and associated limbic structures. The most common symptoms reported by these individuals besides memory difficulties are *apathy, irritability, emotional lability*, and difficulty with *executive function* (i.e., in their ability to plan ahead or to shift from one thought process or task to another).

Lesions involving the **orbitofrontal area** are more often associated with disinhibition and irritability, while lesions involving the **dorsolateral frontal area** are more often associated with apathy and social withdrawal. In clinical practice, though, many patients with frontal lobe injury display a combination of both features. Depending upon the severity of injury, some patients will experience a full-fledged dementia.

These patients traditionally have been labeled as having a "frontal lobe syndrome." However, this term is overly restrictive, since it is now understood that the frontal lobes constitute but one part of a larger system that includes the frontal, parietal, and temporal lobes as well as the limbic cortex and subcortical structures. This network contains the areas of cortex that are the most evolutionarily advanced, and they are critical to the regulation and integration of attention, emotional tone, memory, perceptions of external reality, attitudes, future plans, and motivated behaviors.

It is worth noting at this point that "frontal-type deficits" have been described in association with several major psychiatric disorders, including major depressive disorder, schizophrenia, and obsessive-compulsive disorder. Further, the results of structural and functional neuroimaging studies, while sometimes inconsistent with each other (likely due to varying patient populations and methodologies), have consistently revealed evidence that points along this circuit are involved in these disorders.

Amnesia also can result from **stroke**, particularly strokes that involve elements of the medial hemispheric limbic circuit, such as the hippocampus and the thalamus, along with the anterior fornix (which runs between them). The hippocampus is supplied by branches of the posterior cerebral artery (PCA). Each cerebral hemisphere's posterior cerebral artery arises out of a single basilar artery, which runs along the brain stem. Most hippocampal infarctions are caused by emboli from the basilar artery to the PCAs; therefore, patients tend to present with bilateral hippocampal lesions. The PCAs also supply the optic radiations, and patients therefore also may present with homonymous hemianopsia, a clue to a vascular etiology for the amnesia. Also note that the anterior fornix is located right at the posterior end of the medial frontal lobe, such that a ruptured anterior communicating artery or ruptured arteriovenous malformation in the area of the fornix can lead to both amnesia and frontal lobe symptoms similar to those encountered in patients with closed head injury.

In one particular presentation of amnestic disorder, called **transient global amnesia**, patients acutely develop both anterograde and retrograde amnesia such that they abruptly begin to ask the same questions repeatedly. This state then resolves fully within a few hours. Most cases likely reflect transient ischemic attacks involving the thalamus or another area along the medial limbic circuit, but the syndrome also has been described in association with migraine, epilepsy, brain tumor, small cerebral hemorrhages, and drug ingestion.

Amnesia can also result from **anoxia**—for example, following a cardiac arrest with associated hypoperfusion injury. Amnesia in the absence of other cognitive sequelae occurs because the hippocampus is more sensitive than other brain regions to anoxia. Similarly, an isolated but dense amnesia can occur following herpes simplex encephalitis, since the herpes simplex type I virus has an unusual predilection for attacking the temporal and frontal lobes. Such patients typically present in an acute delirious state that includes fever, agitation, focal neurologic deficits, and seizures. An MRI may reveal temporal and frontal lobe injury. Treatment must be initiated as soon as possible with an antiviral agent such as acyclovir or vidarabine, since 40%–70% of untreated patients die. Even when treated appropriately, the majority of patients are left with amnestic disorder, as well as with aphasia or dementia in more severe cases.

Temporal lobectomy is performed for seizures that are refractory to anticonvulsant medications. The neurosurgeons who introduced this procedure originally resected both temporal lobes, and their patients were found postoperatively to be left with an amnestic disorder. The most famous of these cases was "H.M.," who became the subject of several classic neuropsychological studies.

One major finding that emerged from this research was that H.M. had retained his *procedural memory* but had lost his *declarative memory*. For example, one could teach H.M. to perform a complex puzzle or to read words backward in a mirror, and his performance would improve over consecutive testing sessions. All of this was similar to what would be found for a person without any memory problems. However, whenever H.M. was asked to *repeat* these tasks, he expressed no conscious recall of ever having performed such a task before, despite his improved performance. These findings indicated that the memory of *how* to perform a task (procedural memory) is related to a different brain region than is the memory of having performed it (declarative memory).

Another important research finding was that H.M.'s *distant* retrograde memory of events from the years before his temporal lobectomy remained intact, despite his inability to consolidate *new* information (anterograde amnesia). It was as if he had been "frozen in time." Again, this suggests the existence of separate anterograde and retrograde systems, and that distant memories are not stored in the temporal lobes.

Currently, neurosurgeons only perform unilateral temporal resections. Preoperatively, they perform a "Wada test," in which they infuse a short-acting barbiturate, amobarbital, through the carotid artery that serves the hemisphere of interest. The amobarbital temporarily inhibits that hemisphere's function. If the patient immediately develops amnesia following the infusion, the surgeon has the option of either aborting the surgery or performing a more limited, hippocampal-sparing resection.

Another important cause of amnestic disorder is the **Wernicke-Korsakoff syndrome**, caused by thiamine deficiency. Malnutrition is one cause of the deficiency, but far more common is chronic alcoholism, and *DSM-IV* labels this condition **alcohol-induced persisting amnestic disorder**. The condition is associated with bilateral lesions of the *mammillary bodies and dorsomedial thalamus*.

Classically, the initial phase of this syndrome is an acute delirious state that is accompanied by ataxia and opthalmoplegia (**Wernicke's encephalopathy**). Following resolution of the delirium, patients are left with a chronic amnestic disorder (in this case called **Korsakoff's syndrome**). The treatment of both conditions involves giving thiamine supplementation. However, many alcoholic patients don't present with the classic accompanying neurologic signs. For example, in one retrospective patient series, only about 25% of patients with Korsakoff's syndrome had previously been diagnosed with Wernicke's encephalopathy. Sometimes the onset of the amnesia is more insidious, and all that is noted clinically are vague cognitive difficulties (which clinicians sometimes call "wet brain"). Korsakoff's syndrome may show some improvement if the patient receives thiamine and can remain abstinent from alcohol for at least several months. Given this, *treat all alcohol-dependent patients with thiamine*. Alcohol-induced persisting amnestic syndrome should also be distinguished from a more global syndrome, **alcohol-induced persisting dementia**. The latter syndrome includes amnesia as one feature, along with more extensive deficits.

One final cause of amnesia worth noting is amnesia due to treatment with **benzodiazepines**. These medications are prescribed for many indications, especially for their sedative, hypnotic, and anxiolytic effects. However, they can also cause memory problems distinct from their therapeutic effects. Amnesia occurs more commonly in association with the use of *shorter half-life agents*, such as midazolam (Versed) and triazolam (Halcion), when benzodiazepines are given in *higher doses*, and when they are *intravenously administered*.

Anesthesiologists often use benzodiazepines' amnestic effects to advantage by giving intravenous short-acting agents as part of an anesthesia induction. However, in the outpatient medical setting, while these drugs have an excellent margin of safety, some patients are particularly vulnerable to their cognitive side effects, particularly patients who take the medication along with alcohol and elderly patients who take them on a chronic basis. In the latter case, the benzodiazepine may accumulate over time, causing an insidious onset of memory difficulties despite the prescribed dosage remaining the same. The amnesia is most often anterograde, covering the period immediately after the patient has taken the medication. Longer-term consolidation of recently learned material may also be affected.

PATHOLOGY AND ETIOLOGY

About 50%–60% of dementia is due to Alzheimer's disease, 10%–20% is due to vascular disease, and 10%–20% is due to a combination of these two disorders. The remaining 10%–15% is due to a variety of other causes, as listed in Table 5–1.

Some researchers have proposed distinguishing between those dementias that are predominantly *cortical* (such as Alzheimer's disease, Pick's disease, and cortical strokes) and those that are predominantly *subcortical* (such as Huntington's disease, Parkinson's disease, multiple sclerosis, small-vessel vascular disease, and dementia due to the HIV virus). Differences between these two presentations are summarized in Table 6–3.

In both cortical and subcortical dementia, impairments of attention and concentration are noted early on. However, in cortical dementia, where the primary pathology involves specific cortical areas, *aphasia* is an early finding, recognition memory and recall memory are equally impaired, and the patient appears to have a normal speed of both thought process and motor movement.

In contrast, the pathologic processes leading to *subcortical dementia* involve the basal ganglia, which is part of both the extrapyramidal motor system and the frontal lobe system. Given this, patients present early on with a movement disorder (for example, choreiform movements, tics, dystonia, or tremor). Cognitive and motor slowing typically are present. Patients may appear apathetic but they may also be irritable (as noted in the above discussion of "frontal lobe syndromes"). While they may be *dysarthric*, they usually aren't *aphasic* (at least until late in the course of illness, when aphasia and other cortical signs do ultimately appear). Their recall

Table 6–3. Distinction of Cortical from Subcortical Dementia Syndromes

Cortical Dementia	Subcortical Dementia
Examples: Alzheimer's disease, Pick's disease, cortical strokes	Examples: Parkinson's, Huntington's, basal ganglia strokes, HIV, depression, alcohol
Decreased attention–concentration early	Decreased attention–concentration early
Aphasia early in course	Dysarthria early in course, but not aphasia
Recognition and recall memory both impaired	Recall memory more impaired than recognition memory
Normal speed of thought	Slowing of thought
Impaired executive functioning in proportion to other deficits	Impaired executive functioning out of proportion to other deficits
Normal motor exam early in course	Movement disorder common early in course

memory tends to be more impaired than their recognition memory: in other words, while memories are "laid down," they have difficulty *accessing* this information.

How might early cortical and subcortical deficits appear during screening with the Mini-Mental State Examination (MMSE)? In early *cortical* dementia, the patient might have difficulties performing serial 7s (attention) and recalling three objects (recall). Unfortunately there is no test of recognition on the MMSE, although when patients fail to recall an item, the examiner can offer several choices as a test of recognition memory. (The results would not be scored.) The patient also may also have difficulty copying pentagons accurately and naming items. In contrast, the MMSE contains mostly tests of cortical functioning and therefore is less sensitive to early subcortical dementia. In such cases, the patient may display difficulties with serial 7s, due to impaired attention. The patient also might have some difficulty with delayed recall. Often, such patients complain of being "unable" to recall the three objects but can in fact recall them after encouragement. What follows is an example of a patient with a subcortical dementia:

Psychiatric consultation is requested for a patient with late-stage AIDS. He demonstrates profound psychomotor slowing, with little spontaneous movement and a very blunted affect. He exhibits a paucity of spontaneous speech and offers only brief responses to direct questions, but demonstrates no evidence of aphasia. He denies feeling "depressed," or "sad," and he also denies feelings of guilt or low self-esteem. He appears more apathetic than sad. His MMSE score is 26, due to his missing one out of three objects and spelling WORLD backward as "DL . . . ," and then trailing off.

In contrast to the patient's relatively high score on the MMSE, his family reports that he is completely unable to function at home. While cooking, he gets distracted and then forgets to turn off the stove. He also drops cigarettes on the sofa or carpet without concern about the risk of starting a fire. He can't seem to do two things at once: for example, he is unable to drive a car and have a conversation at the same time. His personality also is changed. Whereas he previously had always been attentive to personal hygiene, he now is disheveled and doesn't even bother to zip his fly. He is apathetic and mostly sits on the sofa smoking cigarettes. He also is more irritable and becomes particularly explosive when faced with changes to his daily routine. When the examiner asks the patient to alternate between counting and reciting the alphabet—for example, "A 1 B 2 C 3 . . . "—he makes several perseverative errors: "A 1 B 2 C 3 . . . um, 4 5 6 . . . wait, C 4 C 5 C 6. . . . "

This patient's MMSE score reflects relatively intact cortical functioning. Given this, one might miss the dementia and assume that all of his problems are due to some other psychiatric disorder, such as major depressive disorder. However, his history is consistent with a profound, progressive dementia. He has psychomotor slowing, impaired motivation, and personality change. He also has impaired executive function—that is, an impaired ability to think abstractly, to plan ahead, to monitor his behavior, and to shift from one cognitive set to another and back again. Such abilities are a necessity in our daily lives. For example, people typically prepare different parts of a meal simultaneously or talk to associates while simultaneously performing other tasks.

Neuropsychological tests have been devised to assess for impairments in different aspects of executive function. One such test is the Wisconsin

Card Sorting Test. The examiner holds up cards containing different geometric figures of different colors. The examiner then asks that the patient to tell him which card pile to place each card in. The patient has to "figure out the rule" in order to do so. However, as the test progresses, the examiner "changes the rule." The test measures the patient's ability to generate alternative strategies in response to feedback without perseverating on earlier strategies.

Another test of executive functioning is the Trail Making Test. Here, the patient is timed while she attempts to "connect the dots" on a piece of paper where numbers and letters from the alphabet are scattered. This task measures the ability to integrate attention, working memory, and sequencing and also measures processing speed. A simple bedside version of this task asks patients to alternate between the alphabet and counting—that is, "A 1 B 2 C 3"—can be helpful in eliciting these difficulties.

The validity of the distinction between cortical and subcortical dementia has been debated. For example, many cortical dementias (including Alzheimer's disease), also do affect subcortical structures. Further, some diseases associated with subcortical dementia also affect the cerebral cortex, particularly the frontal lobe region, and this area and subcortical limbic structures are closely interconnected. Despite these limitations, the phenomenologic distinction remains clinically useful, particularly early in the course of a patient's illness.

Alzheimer's disease (AD) is the most common cause of dementia. Despite this, the diagnosis currently remains one of exclusion, made only after other, potentially reversible, causes of dementia have been excluded. The typical workup for dementia includes the following elements:

A history and neurological examination, mental status examination, and careful review of the patient's medical status and medications are performed to assess for medical or psychiatric illnesses (especially major depressive disorder) that might account for the patients cognitive difficulties. Special attention should be paid to medications that carry the potential for anticholinergic or sedative effects. Blood levels of suspect medications should be checked when available.

Basic ancillary screening tests are performed, again to screen for other medical illnesses that might be mistaken for AD. The most important tests are a vitamin B_{12} level and thyroid function tests, since B_{12} deficiency and hypothyroidism both are common in the elderly and constitute potentially treatable causes of dementia. Other routine screening tests that might be ordered at this point include chemistry and electrolyte panels, a complete blood count, an erythrocyte sedimentation rate (to screen for collagen vascular disease), a urinalysis, and a chest X-ray.

Screening tests for syphilis, such as the venereal disease research laboratory (VDRL), rapid plasma regain (RPR), and fluorescent treponemal antibody (FTA) tests, also tend to be included in diagnostic workups. However, positive results are rare and most likely will be be "false positives" since these tests are nonspecific and since syphilis has a very low prevalence in the United States outside of a few geographical regions (located primarily in southern and midwestern states). Within the past 20 years, there have been no reported cases of tertiary syphilis in any of the incidence or prevalence studies conducted in North America. One should consider screening for syphilis for patients who reside in higher-prevalence regions or who have a history of specific risk factors or of prior syphilitic infection.

Most clinicians also will obtain a *structural neuroimaging study*, either a noncontrast CT scan or MRI scan. Neuroimaging can help rule out other causes of dementia such as brain tumor, stroke, subdural hematoma, or normal-pressure hydrocephalus. The most common radiological finding in AD is cortical atrophy, but this is a nonspecific finding. The MRI scan gives a more detailed picture than the CT scan, especially in assessing for small-blood-vessel disease, but it is more expensive, takes longer to obtain (a problem for agitated or claustrophobic patients), and in most cases doesn't alter the final diagnosis or treatment plan.

Other testing might be obtained, depending upon the results of the history, physical exam, and initial screening tests. If the clinician suspects the presence of a CNS infection or multiple sclerosis, a *lumbar puncture* would be performed. An *EEG* can help distinguish dementia from delirium (although slowing similar to that seen in delirium can be seen in late-stage AD). In AD, most of these tests will be normal. Other potential tests include serum and urine studies for porphyria, antinuclear antibody studies, HIV testing, and a serum copper level (to assess for Wilson's disease).

Functional neuroimaging might demonstrate findings typical of AD even at early stages, thereby helping differentiate dementia due to Alzheimer's disease from dementia due to vascular disease or depression. *Positron emission tomography (PET)* scans use radiolabeled glucose to measure regional brain metabolic activity. They usually reveal hypometabolism in the temporal and parietal lobes early on in the course of AD, as well as hypometabolism in the frontal lobes in later AD. *Single photon emission tomography (SPECT)* scans, which measure regional cerebral blood flow (which in turn parallels regional cerebral metabolic activity), provide similar findings.

Given issues of expense and availability, these studies are not routinely performed outside of academic research centers. Further, since the *DSM-IV* clinical criteria already are very sensitive and specific in diagnosing Alzheimer's disease (in some studies, the clinical criteria alone are more sensitive than the functional neuroimaging results) these neuroimaging studies provide little additional diagnostic benefit.

"Activation" PET and "functional" MRI imaging are even newer techniques, again currently used as research tools. Here, images are obtained first at rest and then while the patient is performing a verbal memory task. Interestingly, when these studies are performed on individuals who are currently asymptomatic but are at *greater risk* for developing AD (in this case, individuals expressing the apolipoprotein E4 phenotype, as described below), scans performed during activation demonstrate *increased* activity in the hippocampal and parahippocampal areas compared to scans obtained in a control group. (This finding stands in contrast to findings among patients with AD, who demonstrate decreased activity in these regions.)

At-risk individuals who demonstrate this finding are more likely to show evidence of a functional decline when their cognition is retested 2 years later. This finding suggests that *presymp-* *tomatic* individuals need to marshal *more* brain resources than do control subjects in order to perform the same tasks. However, once these compensatory mechanisms begin to fail and the individual develops overt AD, a pattern of *hypoperfusion* comes to predominate.

Alzheimer's disease can only be definitively diagnosed when a microscopic examination of the patient's brain has revealed the characteristic histopathologic changes of AD. (While a diagnosis of definite Alzheimer's disease most often is assigned postmortem following an autopsy, on rare occasions patients receive the diagnosis following a diagnostic brain biopsy.) More commonly, a diagnosis is made of "probable Alzheimer's disease" or, to use *DSM-IV* terminology, *dementia of the Alzheimer's type*. The *DSM-IV* criteria for dementia of the Alzheimer's type are presented in Table 6–4. Following these criteria allows the clinician to diagnose AD with a diagnostic accuracy exceeding 85% according to several studies where neuropathologists later confirmed or disconfirmed the AD diagnosis at autopsy.

Sometimes the workup reveals more than one potential cause of dementia. For example, the patient's MRI might reveal evidence of cerebrovascular disease despite the patient's slow, progressive course of decline being most consistent with the diagnosis of Alzheimer's disease. Another example would be when the workup reveals hypothyroidism, but despite this having been addressed the patient continues to demonstrate cognitive deterioration. In such cases, both types of dementia would be diagnosed.

The discovery of biomarkers that might allow one to confirm the diagnosis of AD is the holy grail of AD research, and research toward this end has proceeded at a rapid pace over the past decade. The ideal biomarker would have such high sensitivity and specificity that it would allow the clinician to screen for and diagnosis AD while it still asymptomatic, thereby allowing one to initiate prophylactic therapy. Unfortunately, neither the biomarker nor the therapy has been discovered at this point. Genetic tests (particularly Apo E4 genotyping) and CSF markers (including β-amyloid, tau, and AD7C protein) are available, but—like functional neuroimaging study—are neither sensi-

Table 6–4. *DSM-IV-TR* Criteria for Dementia of the Alzheimer's Type

A. The development of multiple cognitive deficits manifested by both:
  1. Memory impairment (impaired ability to learn new information or to recall previously learned information)
  2. One (or more) of the following cognitive disturbances:
    a. Aphasia (language disturbance)
    b. Apraxia (impaired ability to carry out motor activities despite intact motor function)
    c. Agnosia (failure to recognize or identify objects despite intact sensory function)
    d. Disturbance in executive functioning (i.e., planning, organizing, sequencing, abstracting)
B. The cognitive deficits in criteria A1 and A2 each cause significant impairment in social or occupational functioning and represent a significant decline from a previous level of functioning
C. The course is characterized by gradual onset and continuing cognitive decline
D. The cognitive deficits in Criteria A1 and A2 are not due to any of the following:
  1. Other central nervous system conditions that cause progressive deficits in memory and cognition (e.g., cerebrovascular disease, Parkinson's disease, Huntington's disease, subdural hematoma, normal-pressure hydrocephalus, brain tumor)
  2. Systemic conditions that are known to cause dementia (e.g., hypothyroidism, vitamin B or folic acid deficiency, niacin deficiency, hypercalcemia, neurosyphilis, HIV infection)
  3. Substance-induced conditions
E. The deficits do not occur exclusively during the course of a delirium
F. The disturbance is not better accounted for by another Axis I disorder (e.g., major depressive disorder, schizophrenia)

Source: Reprinted with permission from the *Diagnostic and Statistical Manual of Mental Disorders, Fourth Edition, Text Revision.* Copyright 2000 American Psychiatric Association.

tive nor specific enough to significantly increase diagnostic yield over the use of a careful history and mental status examination utilizing *DSM-IV* criteria.

ALZHEIMER'S DISEASE: THE MOST COMMON PATHOLOGY

Phenomenology

While a specific age of onset is not part of the diagnostic criteria for AD, cases where the onset is before age 65 are classified as being of "early onset," while cases after age 65 are classified as being of "late onset." When the psychiatrist Alois Alzheimer first described "presenile dementia" in 1907, his patient was a 51-year-old woman. For the next several decades the diagnosis of AD was restricted to patients with onset before age 65. Later-onset cases were considered to be due to "hardening of the arteries" (it was also Alzheimer who first described vascular dementia and distinguished it from presenile dementia on histopathologic grounds). However, the pathologic changes in early onset and late-onset cases of Alzheimer's disease have been found to be the same, and in fact the incidence of new cases increases with age.

Most commonly, AD begins at some point after age 55 (most commonly in the patient's 60s,

70s, or 80s). The course is one of a gradual, steady decline in cognitive functioning, with patients typically losing about 2–4 points from their MMSE score each year. Survival rates are quite variable, with death occurring from about 1 to 14 years from the time of diagnosis, the mean time of death being after 10 years.

The most common initial symptom of AD is *impaired short-term memory*. Early on, long-term memory remains intact; for example, patients usually are able to provide a detailed life history. Unlike patients with subcortical dementia (including "dementia of depression"), these patients don't demonstrate improved performance when given cues or multiple-choice options as memory aids. Patients might also show impaired visual–spatial performance from early on. For example, they may have difficulty drawing the interlocking pentagons on the MMSE or drawing a clock face with the hands set at a specified time. These bedside findings correspond to the typical complaint by these patients that they find themselves getting lost even in previously familiar areas. Patients also may demonstrate mild aphasic difficulties—for example, word-finding difficulties. (These deficits may be too subtle to be noted on the MMSE, where patients only have to be able to name a "pen" and a "watch.")

At first, the "social graces" tend to be preserved. This, along with the patient's intact long-term memory, likely accounts for the inability of most care physicians to detect AD early on in the absence of a formal cognitive examination. Not uncommonly, the clinician is quite taken aback when the MMSE reveals that a patient who appeared cognitively intact during casual conversation is not oriented to the year and can't recall any of three objects after a very brief delay.

As the disease progresses, these cognitive deficits become more obvious and more severe. In addition, other psychiatric symptoms appear. Early in the course of the disease, patients may become *demoralized* as they attempt to cope with having an irreversible dementing process. This feeling of helplessness is compounded by the loss of autonomy, especially when patients have to give up driving. Keep in mind, though, that true *major depressive disorder* also occurs frequently in AD, and if a patient meets the diagnostic criteria for major depression it is important to initiate appropriate treatment, as this can be a treatable condition. Paranoid delusions occur in up to half of AD patients, initially perhaps due to con-

fabulation after being unable to find personal belongings (e.g., "my family is stealing my money; I left it on the dresser but now it's gone"), but sometimes more systematized and requiring treatment with antipsychotic drugs. The patient may come to believe that family members have been replaced by impostors who closely resemble them (**Capgras syndrome**).

Other psychiatric symptoms typically include *wandering, agitation, severe anxiety,* and *sleep disturbance.* Their behavior may become especially more agitated and erratic at night ("sundowning"). Patients may rapidly escalate or explode into **catastrophic reactions** when cognitively challenged or forced to do something they don't want to do—for example, bathe or stay in the house. In later AD, the patient becomes unable to walk, speak, or remain continent. See Table 6–5 for a summary of the typical findings in early, middle, and late AD.

Pathology

The pathology of AD was described in Alzheimer's original report. Grossly, the brain is

Table 6–5. Clinical Stages of Alzheimer's Disease

	Stage 1	*Stage 2*	*Stage 3*
Duration of illness	1–3 years	2–10 years	8–12 years
Memory	Impaired short-term	Impaired short- and long-term	Severe impairment
Visuospatial skills	Poor complex constructions and geographic orientation	Poor simple constructions and spatial orientation	Severe impairment
Language	Anomia; poor verbal fluency	Fluent aphasia	Severe impairment
Other		Acalculia, ideomotor apraxia	Urinary and fecal incontinence
Personality changes	Indifference, irritability	Indifference, irritability	Severe impairment
Psychiatric symptoms	Possible delusions	Possible delusions	Severe impairment
Neurologic exam	Normal	Aberrant motor behavior (pacing, restlessness)	Limb rigidity; flexion posture
EEG	Normal	Background slowing	Diffuse slowing
CT/MRI	Normal	Normal or mild atrophy/ ventricular enlargement	Ventricular dilatation and sulcal enlargement
PET/SPECT	Bilateral posterior parietal–temporal hypometabolism/ hypoperfusion	Biparietal and frontal hypometabolism/ hypoperfusion	Biparietal and frontal hypometabolism/ hypoperfusion

Source: Adapted from Cummings JL, Benson DF: *Dementia: A Clinical Approach,* second edition. Boston, Butterworths, 1992.

atrophied, although the degree of atrophy is variable and doesn't correlate with the degree of cognitive decline. Histologically, the two major findings are *neuritic plaques* and *neurofibrillary tangles*. The neuritic plaques are extracellular, with a core of *β-amyloid* surrounded by dystrophic neuritic processes. The neurofibrillary tangles are intracellular, made up of abnormally phosphorylated microtubules. Other common histologic findings include neuronal loss with granulovacuolar degeneration, Hirano bodies, and microvascular amyloid angiopathy, especially in the cerebral cortex and hippocampus.

Several risk factors for developing AD have been elucidated. As noted above, increasing *age* is a major risk factor. There also appear to be *genetic risk factors*. About 40% of AD cases are *familial*, and the rest are *sporadic* (i.e., without a clear familial pattern). The age of disease onset tends to be consistent within a given family. Some early onset cases have been linked to chromosomes 1 and 14 (which code for *presenilin 2* and *presenilin 1*, respectively, although the role of these proteins in causing AD is unclear), as well as chromosome 21 (which codes for *amyloid precursor protein, APP*). Chromosome 21 has long been suspected to play a role in AD, since patients with Down's syndrome (trisomy 21) inevitably develop typical classic Alzheimer's symptoms and neuropathology at a young age. In theory, if their gene on chromosome 21 for APP is defective, the resultant APP protein may also be defective, making it more prone to aggregate into *β*-amyloid plaques.

Some late-onset and sporadic cases have been linked to chromosome 19. This chromosome contains the gene for *ApoE4*, one of the most promising aspects of recent AD research. *ApoE* is one of the apolipoproteins that helps to clear lipids from the bloodstream. It also is found in the brain. ApoE recently has been recognized as playing a possible role in the pathogenesis of AD. There are three primary alleles for the ApoE gene: ApoE2, ApoE3, and ApoE4. Each of us has two ApoE alleles, one from each parent. Inheritance of each copy of ApoE4 tends to increase the risk and decrease the age of onset of AD, while the opposite appears to be the case for inheritance of each copy of ApoE2. For example, people who inherit *one copy* of the ApoE4 allele develop AD three times more frequently

than do people with no E4 allele, while people who inherit *two copies* of the ApoE4 allele develop AD eight times more frequently.

Histopathologically, ApoE4 has been found to bind avidly to β-amyloid and to be present in plaques, tangles, and amyloid angiopathy. While the presence of the ApoE4 allele therefore is one risk factor for developing AD, it still remains unclear how ApoE4 interacts with β-amyloid. One theory is that ApoE4 increases the risk of developing AD by promoting amyloid deposition. Another theory is that ApoE2 binds to amyloid and facilitates its removal while ApoE4 is less effective at doing so, thereby allowing amyloid to build up.

Should all patients, even asymptomatic ones, receive early genetic screening for AD through ApoE testing? At this point, consensus opinion recommends against this. Early clinical interventions might help reduce the social morbidity of AD, but ApoE genotyping doesn't really provide clinically useful information in an asymptomatic population since the ApoE4 genotype is neither necessary nor sufficient to cause AD. In other words, patients without the ApoE4 genotype may be falsely reassured, while patients with the ApoE4 genotype may be falsely alarmed. Similarly, while testing might be a useful confirmatory measure in cases of "probable AD," the sensitivity of the diagnosis of AD on clinical grounds alone is already so high that the incremental gain resulting from the addition of this testing is relatively small. A better case could be made for using such testing (along with functional neuroimaging) in atypical cases or cases where other possible causes of dementia exist but AD is believed to be a likely contributor.

The fact that at least three different chromosomes have been implicated in AD indicates that the disease likely has a heterogeneous or multifactorial etiology. In fact, there is only a 40% concordance rate in monozygotic twins, a rate identical to that for dizygotic twins. Since monozygotic twins share identical genetic material and the concordance isn't 100%, environmental factors also must play a contributory role.

Head trauma may be one such environmental factor. There appears to be a higher rate of head injury in family members of AD patients who also have developed AD. (Of note, repeated blows to boxers' heads can lead to them developing a form of dementia called **dementia pugilistica**; on autopsy these individuals' brains also contain typical Alzheimer-like neurofibrillary tangles, but no plaques.)

After it was reported that *aluminum* is found in higher concentration in AD plaques and tangles, people discarded all of their aluminum cookware and antiperspirants and worried about trace aluminum contained in public water supplies. However, it isn't clear that increased exposure to aluminum *causes* AD lesions; rather, the lesions may simply *concentrate* the aluminum that already is present in the body. (For example, **dialysis dementia** in renal failure patients is noted to be associated with elevated brain aluminum levels but not with the presence of plaques or tangles).

Some dementias (e.g., **Creutzfeldt-Jakob disease**) have been found to be associated with atypical infectious etiologies, leading investigators to search for similar infections in patients with AD. (There are plaques in Creutzfeldt-Jakob disease, but their core is a prion rather than β-amyloid.) However, no such infections have been identified for AD patients to date.

Etiology

How can we explain these myriad pathologic findings? Several theories address the myriad potential etiologic factors in AD. We shall return to each of these theories in turn at the end of the chapter in discussing possible treatment strategies.

The Amyloid Hypothesis

Amyloid accumulation in the brain may be analogous to cholesterol accumulation in blood vessels: too much of it, whether due to excessive production or inadequate removal, may be dangerous. One theory is that defective DNA on chromosome 21 codes for defective amyloid precursor protein. Instead of being removed from the cell, it causes amyloid deposits. These in turn lead to plaques and tangles, which themselves ultimately cause cell death.

The ApoE Hypothesis

As noted above, perhaps the role of ApoE in the brain is analogous to the role of cholesterol-binding lipoproteins in the bloodstream. "Good ApoE" (ApoE2) may bind to and clear amyloid, while "bad ApoE" (ApoE4) might do so less

well, thereby allowing for a buildup of amyloid precursor protein, with the same end results as in the amyloid hypothesis.

The Acetylcholine Hypothesis

Degeneration of a neurotransmitter system leading to neurotransmitter depletion, analogous to the loss of dopaminergic neurons in the substantia nigra and a subsequent dopamine deficiency state in Parkinson's disease, may play a role in AD. In this case, the neurons originate in the *substantia innominata* (also called the *nucleus basalis of Meynert*) and its axons project throughout the brain. The neurotransmitter is *acetylcholine (ACh)*. While AD is associated with depletion of several other neurotransmitters, the ACh depletion is the most severe; possibly amyloid accumulates in the substantia innominata prior to causing more widespread damage. ACh plays an essential role in memory function, and patients taking drugs with anticholinergic effects may experience memory impairments.

The Glutamate/Excitotoxicity Hypothesis

Glutamate is an amino acid that also acts as an excitatory neurotransmitter. The NMDA receptor for glutamate is a *ligand-gated ion channel for calcium*. When glutamate binds to it, the channel opens, allowing calcium to flow into the neuron. Excessive calcium influx may "excite the cell to death," since excessive calcium activates enzymes that in turn produce free radicals which are toxic to the membranes of the neuron and its organelles.

OTHER PATHOLOGIES ASSOCIATED WITH DEMENTIA

Vascular Dementia

Vascular dementia refers to dementia caused by one or more strokes. In contrast to AD, where the onset of the cognitive disturbance is insidious, in vascular dementia the patient typically experiences an abrupt onset of cognitive disturbance followed by a "stepwise" decline accompanying successive episodes of vascular insult. The strokes are documented by history, focal neurological signs and symptoms, and/or imaging studies. The pattern of cognitive deficits is often "patchy," depending on which regions of the brain have been injured. Associated focal neurological signs and symptoms may include an extensor plantar response, pseudobulbar palsy, gait abnormalities, exaggeration of deep tendon reflexes, and extremity weakness. Structural imaging studies usually indicate multiple vascular lesions involving the cerebral cortex and subcortical structures.

The onset of vascular dementia may occur at any time during late life but after age 75 its incidence declines while the incidence of AD continues to rise. Comorbidity between AD and vascular dementia is common, although generally only one diagnosis is recognized during a person's lifetime. Their relationship is complex in that small strokes may lead to a more rapid decline in the patient with preexisting, mild AD. The disease course may be improved through early intervention aimed at treating hypertension and peripheral vascular disease.

It should be noted that the vascular changes noted on neuroimaging scans in themselves are not diagnostic of vascular dementia. Many nondemented elderly people also demonstrate cortical atrophy, enlarged ventricles, and ischemic changes in the deeper white matter and basal ganglia.

Dementia Due to Parkinson's Disease

Dementia occurs in from 20% to 60% of patients with Parkinson's disease, particularly later in the illness. The syndrome has an insidious onset with predominantly subcortical features. Some of these patients are found at autopsy to have findings consistent with comorbid Alzheimer's disease or Lewy body disease. Treatment of patients with dementia due to Parkinson's disease can be complicated and difficult, for several reasons: they are especially sensitive to the deliriogenic effects of psychotropic drugs; antiparkinsonian drugs are either anticholinergic (which can cause worsened dementia and/or delirium) or dopaminergic (which also can cause delirium or psychosis); antipsychotic drugs prescribed to treat delusions or agitation can lead to worsening of the patient's parkinsonian stiffness, tremor, bradykinesia, and postural instability; Parkinson's disease predisposes to major depressive disorder, which in itself can impair cognitive function.

Dementia Due to Lewy Body Disease

Lewy body disease resembles AD clinically but it tends to progress more rapidly and to be associated with parkinsonism and prominent visual hallucinations. It may account for up to 25% of cases of dementia. On autopsy, in addition to features of AD, *Lewy inclusion bodies* in the cerebral cortex are noted. As in the case of patients with Parkinson's disease, these patients may be particularly difficult to treat given both their more prominent psychotic symptoms and their increased sensitivity to the extrapyramidal side effects of antipsychotic medications due to preexisting parkinsonism.

Pick's Disease

Pick's disease also is often mistaken for AD, but it preferentially affects the frontal and temporal lobes. In contrast to AD, the initial signs are more "hypofrontal" changes in personality and cognition (such as apathy, behavioral disinhibition, and prominent language abnormalities). In contrast to AD, memory problems and apraxia tend to develop later in the course of illness. Neuroimaging typically reveals prominent frontal and/or temporal atrophy, with relative sparing of the parietal and occipital lobes. The diagnosis of Pick's disease can only be confirmed by the autopsy finding of characteristic *Pick inclusion bodies*. (Pick's disease is one of a family of socalled "frontotemporal dementias," the others of which don't demonstrate Pick bodies. At the bedside, it often can't be distinguished with certainty from an atypical form of AD. Pick's disease typically has its onset between ages 50 and 60, although it sometimes occurs in older individuals. Treatment is essentially the same as for AD, although treatment may be required earlier in the course of illness for psychiatric and behavioral disturbances.

Huntington's Disease

Huntington's disease is an autosomal dominant condition (i.e., with a 50% likelihood of inheritance, regardless of sex, should one have an affected parent) that usually has its age of onset in the late 30s or early 40s. It presents with an insidious onset of subcortical dementia, with the earliest symptoms typically being nonspecific emotional ones (depression, anxiety, irritability), followed by personality changes (apathy, irritability), executive dysfunction, and memory impairment, along with a progressive choreiform movement disorder.

Early in the disease, structural neuroimaging typically is unremarkable, although PET scans reveal hypometabolism in the caudate and putamen. As the disease progresses, the caudate atrophies, leading to characteristic enlarged and squared off lateral ventricles on structural brain imaging.

The clinical diagnosis has always been based on the patient having characteristic symptoms in the context of a positive family history. However, the single genetic mutation on chromosome 4 responsible for Huntington's disease was identified in 1993 and a genetic test is now available. The genetic aberration is not a point mutation but a string—the same 3 base-pair (bp) sequence (CAG), which is repeated over and over. Individuals with Huntington's disease have far too many of these trinucleotide repeat sequences, leading to instability of the gene's protein product (called *huntingtin*). The mutation is not only passed down to subsequent generations but may also be further amplified by the addition of yet more repeat sequences, accounting for the clinical phenomenon of *anticipation*, whereby successive generations demonstrate earlier onset of disease and increased disease severity.

How the huntingtin protein causes or contributes to neurotoxicity is still unclear. As with other neurodegenerative disorders, it may somehow trigger excessive excitotoxicity or apoptosis in the basal ganglia and ultimately the cortex. The disease is inevitably fatal within 10–15 years of the diagnosis having been made. As in AD, the primary treatment strategy is to manage the dyskinesia with dopamine receptor antagonists and to address secondary psychiatric syndromes through pharmacotherapy, counseling, and behavioral interventions.

Creutzfeldt-Jakob Disease

Creutzfeldt-Jakob disease (CJD) is one of a family of diseases called **subacute spongiform encephalopathies (SSEs)**. SSEs all appear to be caused by prions, which are normal proteins that fold into abnormal shapes and become infectious. Unlike traditional infectious agents, prions contain no genetic material. They accumulate in the brain, where they cause a distinctive microscopic neuropathology in the cortical and subcortical gray matter characterized by neuronal vacuolation, neuronal loss, and glial cell proliferation. Macroscopically, this vacuolation causes the cortex to assume the texture of a sponge. About 10% of CJD brains also contain amyloid plaques in the cortex and cerebellum. These differ from the plaques seen in Alzheimer disease amyloid because immunohistochemical techniques reveal their core to be made up of prion protein rather than of β-amyloid.

Patients present initially with nonspecific or flu-like symptoms such as lethargy, depression, and fatigue. Within weeks, they rapidly deteriorate, demonstrating progressive cortical pattern dementia, myoclonus, pyramidal and extrapyramidal signs, and psychiatric symptoms including mood swings, psychotic symptoms, and marked personality changes. The disease typically progresses to akinetic mutism, coma, and death over a period of months. Beyond symptomatic management, there is no effective treatment.

MRI scans are initially normal, although late in the illness they may show hyperintensities in the striatum and cortex on T2-weighted images. Blood and CSF studies are unremarkable. PET scans demonstrate marked decreases in regional brain metabolism throughout the brain. The EEG may demonstrate a characteristic pattern of diffuse, periodic sharp, often triphasic and synchronous discharges at a rate of 0.5–2 Hz at some point during the disease course, but it may also be normal. A definitive diagnosis of CJD can only be made at autopsy.

Creutzfeldt-Jakob disease usually occurs in the sixth or seventh decade of life. However, it is believed that prion diseases can incubate for up to several decades before declaring themselves in this fulminant manner. Prions appear to be transmitted through the direct inoculation of contaminated body matter. For example, one form of SSE, **kuru**, reached epidemic proportions in women and children in New Guinea who engaged in a cannibalistic mourning ritual in which they ingested the brain tissue of dead relatives. The disease disappeared following the cessation of this practice.

CJD also has been transmitted iatrogenically to humans through cornea transplants and contaminated human growth hormone (prior to the development of a synthetic supply). Up to 15% of cases demonstrate a familial component, suggesting the possibility of vertical transmission of prion in such cases (as opposed to inoculation with the abnormal protein in sporadically occurring cases).

One SSE, **bovine spongiform encephalopathy** (BSE, or "mad cow disease") appears to be etiologically related to a new variant of CJD and has prompted worldwide concern about the safety of the meat supply. BSE was first identified in Great Britain in 1986. It appears to have been introduced into the British cattle supply through the use of animal feed containing rendered animal parts, which included sheep's brains and other sheep byproducts that were infected with **scrapie** (yet another form of SSE known for the past two centuries to affect sheep). Later, the feed also included brain tissue taken from other cows, which themselves were infected with BSE. In 1988, the British government began a program of compulsory destruction of suspect animals and banned the use of rendered animal feeds. This led to sharp declines in cattle infection rates.

In the mid-1990s, a new variant of CJD was identified in humans in Britain, France, and Ireland. This disease differed from classical CJD in that the victims were younger (all below age 42) and the histopathology varied. It appears that these individuals may have had contact with BSE-infected cattle. It now has been confirmed that BSE can be transmitted to humans and can cause variant CJD. For example, brain tissue from BSE-infected cows and brain tissue from variant CJD-infected humans, injected into monkeys or mice, both cause identical neurodegenerative changes, which in turn differ from the degeneration caused by the injection of brain tissue from victims of classical CJD.

Concerns about BSE and CJD have forced countries throughout the world to pay scrupulous attention to how animal byproducts are used. For example, they make their way not only into animal feed but also into pharmaceuticals and cosmetics. To date, no cases of BSE or variant CJD have been reported in the United States. The Department of Agriculture has banned the import from Europe of any animal products, has banned the use of rendered animal products in cattle and sheep feed, and has increased the surveillance of

U.S. cattle for BSE (destroying any cattle with signs of CNS disease and conducting postmortem brain examinations).

Most references quote an annual incidence of CJD of one case per million each year. The actual incidence may be higher, however, given that CJD is only diagnosed after an autopsy and that active surveillance does not take place. In other words, the statistic is based only on the average number of times that CJD appears on death certificates each year (only about 250 times). Given the greatly increased worldwide attention to CJD and fears about the potential for epidemic spread, the reported incidence of CJD may climb due to increased recognition.

TREATMENT

Behavioral and Emotional Treatment

Treatment of dementia can be divided into two components: attempts to *treat the behavioral and emotional symptoms* and attempts to *prevent, slow, or reverse disease progression*. It is a mistake for the clinician to diagnose AD and then simply assume that there is "nothing more than can be done" beyond tracking the course of deterioration and recommending nursing home placement when the family is no longer able to cope.

The initial step in treatment is for the physician to *establish an alliance with the family and other caregivers*. They often are the key informants, particularly when the patient has become an unreliable historian. They also may require a great deal of education, support, and even treatment for their psychiatric symptoms that may develop as a result of the stress of being a caregiver for a severely demented patient. They can also benefit from instructions about how to redirect the patient and avoid getting into confrontations over cognitive problems. Children of the patient may request genetic counseling to better understand their own risk of developing the dementing illness in question. They may also need advice or referral about legal matters as the patient becomes less capable of making financial and medical decisions for himself. They may benefit from advice about available community supports, such as hospitals, churches, community support groups, private day care programs, or the local chapter of the Alzheimer's Association.

The physician also should *follow the patient's psychiatric status with serial evaluations.* This is important because most dementing illnesses are progressive and because demented patients are prone to develop both superimposed delirium and other superimposed psychiatric syndromes. Serial mental status exams, including the MMSE, are key. Depression tends to occur early in dementia, while delusions, hallucinations, "sundowning," sleep disturbance, and agitation typically occur in middle to late dementia.

The physician needs to *monitor for patient safety,* including inquiring into falls, wandering, or impairments in driving, and should help the family to intervene when necessary. Physicians also should be aware of the risk of *elder abuse or neglect* from caregivers. Nursing, occupational therapy, and/or physical therapy outreach services can be useful in providing an assessment of the patient's safety in the home setting.

In managing psychiatric symptoms with medications, the best strategy is to "start low and go slow," since these medications may prove to be toxic at typical doses, especially after they accumulate in the patient's system over a period of several days. Despite this, some patients require the full adult dosage.

Depression is treated with antidepressant medication, although psychotherapy can be helpful early in the course of illness before memory problems interfere with its effectiveness. Low doses of antipsychotic medications can be helpful for psychotic symptoms and agitation, although for agitation that occurs in the absence of psychotic symptoms, many clinicians will attempt to make use of nonantipsychotic medications. Atypical antipsychotic drugs may be better tolerated than traditional antipsychotic agents (as discussed in Chapter 8). Similarly, benzodiazepines to treat sleep disturbance or agitation carry the risk of cognitive side effects and confusion, and also withdrawal effects, although they may be tolerated in low doses by some patients.

The clinician should be aware that some behavior problems might be amenable to behavioral interventions. For example, sleep disturbance may respond to preventing the patient from napping during the day. Or, if there is adequate

supervision (as in a nursing home) the patient simply might be allowed to remain awake at night. Scheduled toileting and prompted voiding can be used to reduce urinary incontinence. Some nursing home units have reported decreased behavioral problems during meals and bathing by utilizing low lighting levels, music, simulated nature sounds, walking, and light exercises, particularly during meals and bathing.

A summary of some treatment options for various psychiatric symptoms is presented in Table 6–6 Target symptoms need to be clearly defined with the family in advance if the physician is to track whether symptoms are improving while the patient is being prescribed a given agent. One should attempt to avoid the "rollercoaster of polypharmacy," whereby more and more agents are added to the pharmacologic mix to the point where it becomes difficult to tell whether symptoms are due to the dementia or to the medications.

Cognitive Enhancers and Primary Prevention

For Alzheimer's disease in particular, attempts have been made to identify medications that might prevent or delay progression of the disorder. These will be discussed based on their associated theory of disease etiology:

Acetylcholine Hypothesis

Acetylcholine (Ach) is formed in cholinergic neurons from two precursors: choline (obtained from dietary and intraneuronal sources) and acetyl coenzyme A (synthesized in the neuron's mitochondria from glucose), in a reaction that requires the enzyme *choline acetyltransferase (CAT).* Once resleased ACh binds to two different types of neuroreceptors, nicotinic and muscarinic. Ultimately, ACh is broken down by another enzyme, *acetylcholinesterase (AChE).*

Initially, researchers tried administering choline to AD patients. The goal was to boost ACh synthesis, thus compensating for the underlyling ACh deficiency state. This strategy parallels that of giving dopamine precursors to remedy an underlying dopamine deficiency state in Parkinson's disease. Unfortunately, this strategy hasn't proven to be effective. Perhaps the doses of choline haven't been high enough (although higher doses wouldn't have been practical). Perhaps—since so many ACh neurons have been de-

Table 6–6. Pharmacologic Agents Useful in Treating Psychiatric Symptoms in Dementia

Symptom	Medication	Special Considerations
Depression	Tricyclic antidepressants	Anticholinergic side effects (impaired memory, confusion, constipation), orthostatic hypotension (increased fall risk), arrhythmia, and oversedation are risks. Titrate upward very slowly and monitor serum level and ECG. Desipramine and nortriptyline are the safest
	SSRIs	Increased anxiety, tremor, sleep disturbance are risks
	Mirtazapine	Appetite stimulant effects may be useful for cachectic patients; oversedation and orthostatic hypotension are risks
Anxiety	Benzodiazepines	Lorazepam and oxazepam don't have active metabolites. Confusion, over sedation, ataxia, memory disturbance, behavioral disinhibition are risks
	Buspirone	Dizziness, nervousness, headache, nausea are risks
Insomnia	Trazodone	Oversedation, priapism (low risk in older men) are risks
	Benzodiazepines	See above
Psychosis	Typical antipsychotics	Increased risk of tardive dyskinesia in elderly, parkinsonism (fall risk), akathisia (may contribute to increased anxiety/agitation), and oversedation are risks. Low doses (e.g., 0.5 mg/day) of higher-potency agents (e.g., haloperidol) preferred, despite greater risk of extrapyramidal symptoms, given their lower anticholinergic toxicity
	Atypical antipsychotics	Lower risk of tardive dyskinesia, less likely to require concomitant administration of anticholinergic medication. Sedation and extrapyramidal symptoms still risks
Aggression	Antipsychotics	See above. Also treat comorbid psychosis. Atypical agents may also treat aggressive, depressive, or manic symptoms. Because of greater neurologic risks, typical antipsychotic agents generally should be avoided if aggression is sole presenting symptom (i.e., in absence of psychosis). Periodic tapers should be attempted if patient stable
	Buspirone	See above. Delayed onset of effect (weeks). Less sedating than other options, but therefore may require use of second agent at night for sleep or "sundowning." Treats comorbid anxiety
	SSRIs	See above. Delayed onset of effect (weeks). Treats comorbid depression and anxiety
	Trazodone	See above. Treats comorbid sleep disturbance
	Anticonvulsants (carbamazepine/valproate)	Confusion, ataxia, bone marrow suppression, hepatoxicity are risks
	Lithium carbonate	Confusion and toxicity are risks, especially in patients with renal insufficiency or on drugs that raise levels (e.g. diuretics, ACE inhibitors). Monitor lithium levels, renal function, thyroid function
	Benzodiazepines	See above. Treats comorbid anxiety
	β-blockers (propranolol and others)	Best studied in patients with head injury. Slow onset of effects, and need for gradual upward titration. Exclude patients with asthma or COPD, diabetes, congestive heart failure, significant peripheral vascular disease, hyper thyroidism

stroyed, the remaining neurons can't synthesize enough ACh despite the increased amount of choline.

Another approach has involved administering direct muscarinic or nicotinic receptor agonists. In other words, this strategy attempts to perform an end run around the underlying ACh deficiency. Several potential agents are currently un-

der investigation, but none is currently available. One rationale for this approach is epidemiologic evidence that smokers have a lower incidence of developing AD.

More recently, agents are available to patients that boost ACh levels by inhibiting its *breakdown* by AChE. These *cholinesterase inhibitors* have the potential to modestly improve cognition and slow the course of cognitive decline, thereby improving the quality of life for both the patient and caregivers and delaying the need for nursing home placement. However, they don't slow underlying disease progression (just as providing dopamine doesn't slow the progression of Parkinson's disease). Three agents have been approved at this point, and these also are the only agents currently approved by the FDA specifically for the treatment of AD.

The first of these agents to be approved was **tetrahydroamino acridine or tacrine (Cognex)**. In clinical trials lasting for 6 months, 30%–40% of patients who completed the trial showed modest improvements in cognition and daily functioning, as opposed to 10% of patients taking placebo. However, while the patients most likely to respond were those taking higher dosages, only about 60% of patients were able to tolerate even modest doses of the drug. Just as anticholinergic drugs *slow* bowel motility, cholinergic drugs cause the opposite effects, *nausea and vomiting*. Other side effects caused by tacrine include increased gastric acid secretion (a problem for patients who already have peptic ulcer disease or who are taking nonsteroidal antiinflammatory medications) and bradycardia (a problem for patients with preexisting cardiac conduction problems).

Another significant problem with tacrine therapy is medication-induced hepatocellular injury. Approximately 30% of patients develop significant (three times the upper limit of normal) but reversible elevations in liver enzyme levels, and 5%–10% of patients have to stop taking tacrine due to even more marked elevations (10 times the upper limit of normal). However, perhaps 80% of patients who initially develop elevations in liver enzyme levels can be successfully rechallenged with more gradual increases in dose. Hepatotoxicity is more common in women and tends to occur about 6–8 weeks into treatment. Patients must take Cognex four times per day with the dose gradually titrated to the maximal tolerated dose. Since the hepatotoxicity is typically asymptomatic, patients taking tacrine must have liver enzyme studies checked every 2 weeks.

As can be imagined, tacrine has not been readily accepted by patients, their families, or clinicians. However, two newer cholinesterase inhibitors are now available and in widespread use, **donepezil (Aricept)** and **rivastigmine (Exelon)**. In contrast to tacrine's frequent dosing requirement, donepezil can be administered once daily (at doses of 5 mg/day increased to 10 mg/day after 4–6 weeks), rivastigmine twice daily. (The initial dose is 1.5 mg twice daily, and this can be increased to 3 mg twice daily, then 4.5 mg twice daily, and then 6 mg twice with a minimum of 2 weeks between dosage increases.) Another agent, **galantamine (Reminyl)**, is both a cholinesterase inhibitor and a nicotinic receptor modulator. It also has demonstrated efficacy in clinical trials and has been approved by the FDA in doses of 16 mg/day and 24 mg/day.

While these newer agents also commonly cause nausea, vomiting, diarrhea, or muscle cramps when therapy is initiated, side effects tend to decline during the first few weeks of treatment and can be further mitigated by starting with a lower dosage gradually titrating upward on the dosage. None of these three newer agents has been associated with hepatotoxicity.

As these agents don't prevent disease progression, patients who stop taking them may rapidly decline in their functioning—that is, down to the level that would have been expected in the absence of pharmacologic intervention. Also, cholinesterase inhibitors are generally believed to be less effective later in the course of disease due to significant declines in the number of ACh neurons at that point. This being said, a recent 6-month trial demonstrated that donepezil administered to moderate- and later-stage AD patients (whose average baseline MMSE score was 12) offered significantly more benefit in addressing cognitive disturbances and psychiatric symptoms than did placebo.

Amyloid Hypothesis

Research is currently underway to find some way of inhibiting the activity of the various secretases involved in amyloid precursor protein synthesis. The goal is to prevent the formation of the plaques and tangles assumed to lead to cell death.

Another novel strategy involves administering a vaccine to β-amyloid such that the immune system clears it. In one study, mice who previously had been implanted with a mutated human gene that triggers the overproduction of amyloid were immunized with a synthetic form of β-amyloid peptide that had been linked to an immune system stimulus. The vaccine prompted the mice's immune systems to attack the amyloid plaques. When this vaccine was injected into young mice, they grew up without ever developing plaques; when it was injected into diseased mice, the treatment eradicated the plaques, improved the condition of damaged neurons, and reduced inflammation in surrounding tissues.

It is not certain whether such a vaccine would prove to be of benefit to humans with AD. First, only the minority of AD patients who have the early onset, familial form of the disease have this mutation. Second, it is currently unknown whether the vaccine would affect the development of neurofibrillary tangles, since the latter are not present in the mouse model. Third, one can't accurately assess whether a mouse who has improved "neuropathologically" also has improved "clinically," since one can't accurately assess cognition in a mouse. Finally, as of 2002, the first human research trial involving this vaccine has had to be aborted following the development of encephalitis in several research subjects.

ApoE Hypothesis

Research is also underway looking into the possibility of either preventing the synthesis of ApoE4 or increasing the synthesis of ApoE2. This strategy would be similar to that undertaken to decrease cardiac morbidity and mortality by either boosting "good cholesterol" or lowering "bad cholesterol." No such remedies are currently available, however.

Glutamate/Excitotoxicity Hypothesis

The glutamate receptor is a calcium channel. The channel is allosterically modified when glutamate binds to it such that more calcium can flow into the cell. The calcium then triggers a chain reaction that ultimately leads to the production of free radicals. This receptor also contains binding sites for other substances, including glycine, zinc, and polyamine. These substances cause similar allosteric modifications and also increase calcium influx. In contrast, magnesium and phencyclidine (PCP) have binding sites that cause changes to the channel that inhibit calcium influx. Therefore, at least in theory, drugs might be designed that decrease calcium influx, thereby acting as *neuroprotective agents*. They could do so either by blocking the glutamate, glycine, polyamine, or zinc receptors or by stimulating the magnesium or PCP receptors. (These drugs aren't feasible, though, as they likely would cause deep sedation and psychosis). At this point, all of these remain only theoretical options.

However, one potential neuroprotective agent that has received a degree of empirical support from clinical trials is **vitamin E**. Vitamin E acts as a free radical scavenger and it therefore may be helpful in blocking the detrimental effects of the calcium influx. Another agent is **L-deprenyl (selegiline)**, an irreversible inhibitor of the B form of monoamine oxidase (MAO) that also has antioxidant properties.

A single double-blind, placebo-controlled study has compared the effect of the administration over a 2 year period of vitamin E alone, selegiline alone, both drugs combined, and placebo on patients with moderate AD. Both agents were associated with about a 7-month delay in measures of *functional* decline (e.g., how soon patients required institutionalization or died). (Oddly, the benefit of receiving both drugs together was a bit less than the benefit of taking either drug given alone.) Unfortunately, neither drug demonstrated any benefit in slowing patients' *cognitive* decline.

Vitamin E and selegiline have not been studied in combination with cholinesterase inhibitors. However, since vitamin E performed as well as selegiline, is inexpensive, and has few side effects, it appears to be reasonable to empirically prescribe this along with a cholinesterase inhibitor. It often is prescribed at 2,000 units per day, since this is the maximum dosage not associated with the development of gastrointestinal side effects, and since it was the dosage employed in the above-cited study. However, other experts have recommended lower dosages (60–1,000 units per day) to minimize the risk of developing a coagulopathy.

Other Strategies

Other medications have been proposed for the treatment of cognitive decline, including vasodilators, melatonin, botanical agents (e.g., ginkgo biloba), and chelating agents for aluminum. None at this point has been shown to be effective in controlled clinical trials.

Some epidemiologic studies have suggested that **nonsteroidal anti-inflammatory drugs** may be useful. Patient's taking these drugs on a daily basis for rheumatologic disease appear to be have a 30%–70% lower risk of developing AD than patients who do not do so. However, daily use of these agents can cause gastrointestinal bleeding, liver toxicity, and renal toxicity. Daily use of nonsteroidal agents also may interfere with the cardiovascular benefit associated with taking daily aspirin. All of these latter risks may outweigh these drugs' benefits in terms of AD prophylaxis, so daily use is not recommended solely for AD prophylaxis. As of this writing, prospective studies are underway. It was hoped that newer, more selective nonsteroidal agents, the COX-2 inhibitors, would be effective in treating AD while carrying a lower burden of toxicity. However, to date, placebo-controlled trials of the COX-2 inhibitors have revealed no benefits compared to placebo.

Similarly, epidemiologic research has suggested that **estrogen replacement therapy** decreases the risk of women developing AD by 30%–70%. However, recent prospective clinical trials have revealed the administration of conjugated estrogen to be of no benefit compared to placebo. Estrogen replacement therapy also increases a woman's risk of developing endometrial cancer, deep venous thrombosis, and pulmonary embolus. Given this, estrogen also is not currently recommended for routine use in all women (although the risk/benefit ratio should be considered in individual cases, especially in individuals for whom estrogen replacement therapies might be implemented for other reasons) It also remains possible that estrogen therapy may be of benefit when given in conjunction with

cholinesterase inhibitors. Research into this possibility is currently underway.

SUMMARY

Dementia, like delirium, offers an excellent example of a psychiatric disorder best viewed from the disease perspective. Again we find that the same clinical syndrome can be caused by multiple pathologies. Our evolving understanding of the etiologies of each of the pathologies associated with dementia—originally only at the gross and microscopic levels, but more recently at the biochemical and genetic levels—has stimulated an alliance between basic scientists and clinicians. The goal is to work from research hypotheses as to the causes of dementia in designing more specific treatments that are designed to remediate putative etiologic factors.

Currently, however, the most effective treatment for dementia is to treat its associated psychiatric symptoms and behaviors. This is one reason why psychiatrists frequently play an important role in managing demented patients.

In doing so, other perspectives besides the disease perspective also must be brought into play. The dimensional and life-story perspectives are particularly important early in the course of dementia, since at this stage psychotherapeutic interventions can help the patient and family come to grips with a severe illness that has disrupted all of their lives. At later stages of illness, the behavioral perspective usually plays the most important role, as it is the patient's problematic behaviors that are most important factor in the decision to move the patient into a nursing home. While targeting these behaviors through a combination of environmental, behavioral, and pharmacologic strategies doesn't alter the underlying progression of the disease, it may greatly improve the quality of life for patients with dementia and their families.

Chapter 7

Mood Disorders

Mood disorders are common. For example, each year in the United States, 1.2 million people are diagnosed with major depressive disorder, an incidence of 5%–10%. Major depressive disorder affects at least 20% of women and 12% of men at some point in their lives. Mood disorders also are costly. For example, major depressive disorder not only is more *prevalent* than arthritis, diabetes, or heart disease; it also causes more emotional and physical *impairment*. Further, it affects patients' health indirectly, by increasing the morbidity and mortality associated with coexisting medical conditions. A recent study of premature mortality and disability ranked major depressive disorder as the fourth leading cause of worldwide disease burden. Finally, mood disorders can be lethal; up to 15% of such patients die by suicide. Despite all of this (and despite the availability of effective treatments), mood disorders remain underrecognized and undertreated.

Mood disorders resist reductionistic explanatory theories. Substantial evidence suggests that mood disorders are diseases. However, they are diseases that become intertwined with patients' individual life stories and personalities. Adverse life events trigger or exacerbate mood disorders, and the illness may then become the major adverse event in a patient's life. Furthermore, up to 85% of depressed patients experience multiple

episodes of illness, such that it becomes increasing difficult to distinguish the "illness" from the "person."

Complicating matters further, while the *DSM-IV* diagnostic criteria for depressive episodes, manic episodes, mixed episodes, and hypomanic episodes are clear (see Tables 7–1 through 7.4, respectively), many patients "haven't read the textbook," presenting instead with symptoms that may be subtle or "subsyndromal." Some patients with clinical "depression" do not even present with the complaint of feeling "sad."

For example, at least 50% of patients who present for treatment in the primary care setting are found to have no diagnosable medical illness. Many of these patients leave the physician's office dissatisfied, which may lead them to seek one or more further evaluations in search of answers. When researchers examined a group of these "service overutilizers," using a structured psychiatric interview, they found that 86% of these patients had lifetime histories of a psychiatric disorder. As can be seen in Table 7–5, the most common diagnosis was major depressive disorder.

This chapter reviews the clinical phenomenology of mood disorders and then discussed the major etiologic theories. Historically, competing theories have emphasized either form (viewing

Table 7–1. *DSM-IV-TR* Criteria for Depressive Episode

A. Five (or more) of the following symptoms have been present during the same 2-week period and represent a change from previous functioning; at least one of the symptoms is either (1) depressed mood or (2) loss of interest or pleasure Note: Do not include symptoms that are clearly due to a general medical condition, or mood-incongruent delusions or hallucinations
1. Depressed mood most of the day, nearly every day, as indicated by either subjective report (e.g., feels sad or empty) or observation made by others (e.g., appears tearful). Note: In children and adolescents, can be irritable mood
2. Markedly diminished interest or pleasure in all, or almost all, activities most of the day, nearly every day (as indicated by either subjective account or observation made by others)
3. Significant weight loss when not dieting or weight gain (e.g., a change of more than 5% of body weight in a month), or decrease or increase in appetite nearly every day Note In children, consider failure to make expected weight gains
4. Insomnia or hypersomnia nearly every day
5. Psychomotor agitation or retardation nearly every day (observable by others, not merely subjective feelings of restlessness or being slowed down)
6. Fatigue or loss of energy nearly every day
7. Feelings of worthlessness or excessive or inappropriate guilt (which may be delusional) nearly every day (not merely self-reproach or guilt about being sick)
8. Diminished ability to think or concentrate, or indecisiveness, nearly every day (either by subjective account or as observed by others)
9. Recurrent thoughts of death (not just fear of dying), recurrent suicidal ideation without a specific plan, or a suicide attempt or a specific plan for committing suicide
B. The symptoms do not meet criteria for a mixed episode
C. The symptoms cause clinically significant distress or impairment in social, occupational, or other important areas of functioning
D. The symptoms are not due to the direct physiological effects of a substance (e.g., a drug of abuse, a medication) or a general medical condition (e.g., hypothyroidism)
E. The symptoms are not better accounted for by bereavement (i.e., after the loss of a loved one, the symptoms persist for longer than 2 months or are characterized by marked functional impairment, morbid preoccupation with worthlessness, suicidal ideation, psychotic symptoms, or psychomotor retardation)

Source: Reprinted with permission from the *Diagnostic and Statistical Manual of Mental Disorders, Fourth Edition, Text Revision.* Copyright 2000 American Psychiatric Association.

Table 7–2. *DSM-IV-TR* Criteria for Manic Episode

A. A distinct period of abnormally and persistently elevated expansive, or irritable mood, lasting at least 1 week (or any duration if hospitalization is necessary)
B. During the period of mood disturbance, three (or more) of the following symptoms have persisted (four if the mood is only irritable) and have been present to a significant degree:
1. Inflated self-esteem or grandiosity
2. Decreased need for sleep (e.g., feels rested after only 3 hours of sleep)
3. More talkative than usual or pressure to keep talking
4. Flight of ideas or subjective experience that thoughts are racing
5. Distractibility (i.e., attention too easily drawn to unimportant or irrelevant external stimuli)
6. Increase in goal-directed activity (either socially, at work or school, or sexually) or psychomotor agitation
7. Excessive involvement in pleasurable activities that have a high potential for painful consequences (e.g., engaging in unrestrained buying sprees, sexual indiscretions, or foolish business investments)
C. The symptoms do not meet criteria for a mixed episode
D. The mood disturbance is sufficiently severe to cause marked impairment in occupational functioning or in usual social activities or relationships with others, or to necessitate hospitalization to prevent harm to self or others, or there are psychotic features
E. The symptoms are not due to the direct physiological effects of a substance (e.g., a drug of abuse, a medication, or other treatment) or a general medical condition (e.g., hyperthyroidism)

Source: Reprinted with permission from the *Diagnostic and Statistical Manual of Mental Disorders, Fourth Edition, Text Revision.* Copyright 2000 American Psychiatric Association.

Table 7–3. *DSM-IV-TR* Criteria for Mixed Episode

A. The criteria are met both for a manic episode and for a major depressive episode (except for duration) nearly every day during at least a 1-week period
B. The mood disturbance is sufficiently severe to cause marked impairment in occupational functioning or in usual social activities or relationships with others, or to necessitate hospitalization to prevent harm to self or others, or there are psychotic features
C. The symptoms are not due to the direct physiological effects of a substance (e.g., a drug of abuse, a medication, or other treatment) or a general medical condition (e.g., hyperthyroidism)

Source: Reprinted with permission from the *Diagnostic and Statistical Manual of Mental Disorders, Fourth Edition, Text Revision.* Copyright 2000 American Psychiatric Association.

depression as a pathological biological state to be "explained") or function (viewing depression as a subjective state to be empathically "understood," with depressive symptoms even being seen as adaptive psychological defenses.).

Is an understanding of these latter theories relevant for the busy physician who has no intention of being a "psychotherapist"? Absolutely. All physicians, even primary care physicians and surgical specialists, should enter the exam room equipped with at least a rudimentary understanding of the most common ways that psychosocial interactions affect mental and physical functioning and vice versa. Given this, in addition to reviewing neurochemical and neurophysiologic models of mood disorder, this chapter in-

troduces psychodynamic and cognitive models. With these biological and psychological theories providing our conceptual framework, we then will discuss different treatment strategies.

THE CLINICAL SYNDROME

Phenomenology

Historical Classification Schemes

The phenomenology of mood disorder hasn't changed over the centuries, despite the evolution of classification schemes. Hypocrites described "mania" and "melancholia" in about 400 BC. He postulated that the state of melancholia was more

Table 7–4. *DSM-IV-TR* Criteria for Hypomanic Episode*

A. A distinct period of persistently elevated, expansive, or irritable *mood*, lasting throughout at least 4 days, that is clearly different from the usual nondepressed mood. (i.e., not simply feeling good because has come out of a depression)
B. During the period of mood disturbance, three (or more) of the following symptoms have persisted (four if the mood is only irritable) and have been present to a significant degree:
   1. Inflated self-esteem or grandiosity
   2. Decreased need for sleep (e.g., feels rested after only 3 hours of sleep)
   3. More talkative than usual or pressure to keep talking
   4. Flight of ideas or subjective experience that thoughts are racing
   5. Distractibility (i.e., attention too easily drawn to unimportant or irrelevant external stimuli)
   6. Increase in goal-directed activity (either socially, at work or school, or sexually) or psychomotor agitation
   7. Excessive involvement in pleasurable activities that have a high potential for painful consequences (e.g., the person engages in unrestrained buying sprees, sexual indiscretions, or foolish business investments)
C. The episode is associated with an unequivocal change in functioning that is uncharacteristic of the person when not symptomatic
D. The disturbance in mood and the change in functioning are observable by others
E. The episode is not severe enough to cause marked impairment in social or occupational functioning, or to necessitate hospitalization, and there are no psychotic features (i.e., not full-blown mania)
F. The symptoms are not due to the direct physiological effects of a substance (e.g., a drug of abuse, a medication, or other treatment) or a general medical condition (e.g., hyperthyroidism)

*Note: Hypomanic-like episodes that are clearly caused by somatic antidepressant treatment (e.g., medication, electroconvulsive therapy, light therapy) should not count toward a diagnosis of bipolar II disorder.
Source: Reprinted with permission from the Diagnostic and Statistical Manual of Mental Disorders, Fourth Edition, Text Revision. Copyright 2000 American Psychiatric Association.

Table 7–5. Lifetime Prevalence of Mental Disorders in 119 Distressed High Medical Utilizers

Mental Disorder	Percent
Major depressive disorder	68
Dysthymic disorder	32
Panic disorder	22
Generalized anxiety disorder	40
Somatization disorder	20
Alcohol abuse/dependence	24
Any lifetime disorder	86

Source: Adapted from Katon W, Von Korff M, Lin E, et al: "Distressed High Utilizers of Medical Care: *DSM-III-R* Diagnoses and Treatment Needs." *Gen Hosp Psychiatry* 12:355–362, 1990. Copyright 1990, with permission from Elsevier Science.

than something to be "understood" empathically. It was an illness, a reflection of an underlying biochemical abnormality, in this case the excessive production of black bile. This represents one of the earliest applications of the disease perspective to a mental condition.

Aretaeus of Capadocia, writing in about AD 150, recognized that manic and depressive states may be aspects of a single illness, noting: "The melancholic cases tend towards depression and anxiety only. . . . If, however, respite from this condition of anxiety occurs, gaiety and hilarity in the majority of cases follows, and this finally ends in mania." He also recognized that manic patients were not always "happy." In some cases, patients who initially presented with euphoria escalated into dysphoric, irritable, even homicidally violent states. Despite this, he concluded, "there are infinite forms of mania, but the disease is one."

Robert Burton wrote the first English-language text on depression, *Anatomy of Melancholy*, in 1621. Reviewing 2,000 years of descriptive literature, he linked mood disorders to chronic personality temperaments, particularly the "melancholic" temperament and the "sanguine" (hot-blooded) temperament. These constructs overlap with our current *DSM-IV* constructs of dysthymic disorder and cyclothymic disorder, respectively. Burton also described the high frequency of comorbidity between mood disorder and alcohol abuse that remains readily apparent today.

Until the 1850s, two major forms of "insanity" were recognized: "mania" described those people who were insane and agitated, while "melancholia" described those people who were insane and psychomotor retarded. However, in 1854 two Frenchmen independently concluded that these two illnesses actually were two aspects of the same syndrome. Falret described "circular insanity" (*la folie circulaire*), where individuals "live out lives in a perpetual circle of depression and manic excitement interrupted by a period of lucidity, which is typically brief but occasionally long lasting." Baillarger described "double insanity" (*la folie à double form*) in similar terms. In 1882 the German psychiatrist Karl Kahlbaum, describing a condition he called "cyclothymia," described alternating episodes of mania and depression.

However, it remained for Emil Kraepelin (1856–1926) to theorize in 1899 that the construct of "insanity" was even more complex, subsuming two separate conditions: *manic-depressive psychosis* (our current bipolar disorder) and *dementia praecox* (our current schizophrenia). In describing the former condition, Kraepelin opined that—while some patients only became depressed, others only became manic, and still others cycled between these two states— these likely constituted varying presentations of a single illness. Beyond these cross-sectional symptoms, however, Kraeplin focused on longitudinal course of illness. In this regard, most of these patients achieved interepisode *recovery*. However, Kraepelin went on to describe what appeared to be another group of patients who did not exhibit such recovery. Rather, they experienced exacerbations of illness superimposed on a longer-term course of progressive *deterioration* (hence his label of dementia praecox, or "premature dementia").

Why did Kraepelin "see" this distinction when his peers did not? Kraepelin emphasized disease reasoning grounded in clinical phenomenology. (This method was facilitated by his having lived within the same psychiatric facilities where he worked, giving him the opportunity to observe his patients constantly over periods of months to years.) Kraepelin's lectures always began with a detailed phenomenologic description of a patient, followed by a description of the patient's course of illness and ultimate prognosis. His goal was to link psychiatric syndromes to studies of inheritance, neuropathology, and pharmacology. In fact, the like-minded psychiatrists that Kraepelin recruited as colleagues included Alzheimer, Nissl, and Brodmann, all of whom are now best remembered for their contributions to neuropathology.

Many of Kraepelin's contemporaries—especially followers of Sigmund Freud—criticized him for stating that manic-depressive psychosis and dementia praecox were *diseases*, no different from general paresis of the insane (neurosyphilis) or Alzheimer's disease (the latter being a label, incidentally, coined by Kraepelin). They argued that no signs of neuropathology had ever been delineated in these two forms of insanity, consistent with their being psychological in origin. However, time has proven to be more kind to Kraepelin than to his detractors. Following a period of relative neglect by American psychiatry, Kraepelin's descriptions of the mood disorders and schizophrenia reemerged a half-century later, echoed in the current *DSM* diagnostic criteria. Further, his approach has become the model for modern psychiatric research.

Current Classification Scheme

No classification scheme attempting to categorize disorders involving pathological mood states has completely succeeded. However, there is general agreement as to what elements should be included in any such scheme. These include the *severity* of the change in mood, the *acuity or chronicity* of abnormal mood states, and the *relationship* of the mood states to external life events.

For example, if a patient's low mood appears to be more mild, more chronic, and more closely tied to external events, clinicians might postulate that the patient's state of depression might best be explained from either the dimensional perspective or the life-story perspective. From the *dimensional perspective* the patient might be formulated as having a dour or pessimistic temperament, a "depressive personality." From the *life-story perspective*, the depression might be seen as an understandable reaction to an internal conflict or to external life events.

However, personality traits, biological states, and reactions to life events usually are not so readily segregated from each other. What about the patient who has been "mildly depressed" for his entire life despite years of psychotherapy who then shows a dramatic response to treatment with an antidepressant medication? Are we to believe that the medication "changed his personality" (i.e., altered his *traits*)? Or should we postulate that at least some patients who present with life-long "depressive traits" in reality have a chronic, "subclinical" form of a disease (i.e., are in a chronic, abnormal biological *state*)?

We appear to have a natural tendency to break difficult phenomena into dichotomies ("guilty" versus "innocent," "liberal" versus "conservative," etc.). Not surprisingly, most classification schemes for mood disorders rely on such dichotomies. The most common schemes have been variants of the following:

> *"Endogenous" depression versus "reactive" depression.* The former is diagnosed when there has been no recent stressor and when "vegetative symptoms" such as disturbances in sleep and appetite are prominent; the latter is diagnosed when there are recent stressors, especially a significant loss, and when there are fewer vegetative features.
>
> *"Psychotic" depression versus "neurotic" depression.* The former is diagnosed when the patient demonstrates severe (even psychotic) symptoms, which represent an acute change from baseline functioning; the latter is diagnosed when the patient's symptoms are milder, more chronic, and appear to be more "characterologic" in nature.
>
> *"Primary" depression versus "secondary" depression.* The former is "idiopathic" or "functional"; the latter is etiologically related to some antecedent medical or "organic" condition, such as hypothyroidism or stroke.

Unfortunately, none of these schemes can adequately account for all features of depressive illness. To an extent, we still rely on the "endogenous versus reactive" dichotomy when we differentiate between a depressive episode (Table 7–1) and an "adjustment disorder with depressed mood" (Table 7–6). However, recall our example in Chapter 1 of the elderly woman who became depressed after a stroke. Her family preferred to think of her illness as being "reactive," given her stressful life circumstances, while the psychiatrist approached her case primarily as being "endogenous" as well as possibly being "secondary" (i.e., etiologically related) to her stroke. The patient ultimately did respond to treatment

Table 7–6. *DSM-IV-TR* Criteria for Adjustment Disorder*

A. The development of emotional or behavioral symptoms in response to an identifiable stressor(s) occurring within 3 months of the onset of the stressor(s)

B. These symptoms or behaviors are clinically significant as evidenced by either of the following:
1. Marked distress that is in excess of what would be expected from exposure to the stressor
2. Significant impairment in social or occupational (academic) functioning

C. The stress-related disturbance does not meet the criteria for another specific Axis I disorder and is not merely an exacerbation of a preexisting Axis I or Axis II disorder

D. The symptoms do not represent bereavement

E. Once the stressor (or its consequences) has terminated, the symptoms do not persist for more than an additional 6 months.

Qualifiers: One can have adjustment disorder with either: (1) depressed mood, (2) anxiety, (3) mixed anxiety and depressed mood, (4) disturbance of conduct, or (5) mixed disturbance of emotions and conduct.
Source: Reprinted with permission from the *Diagnostic and Statistical Manual of Mental Disorders, Fourth Edition, Text Revision.* Copyright 2000 American Psychiatric Association.

with antidepressant medication, although this is not to say that her current life predicament was not one etiologic factor.

If we diagnosed "endogenous" or "biological" depression *only* in those cases where we can identify *no* situational stressors, we likely would miss most cases. In other words, the presence of stressors in the patient's life doesn't "prove" that the patient doesn't have a disease. By analogy, would we say that the man who experiences a heart attack 2 months after his wife's death only had a "reactive" heart attack that wasn't biological in nature, one that could be readily "explained" by the fact that he was grieving his wife's death? Similarly, would we say that the medical student who developed a viral illness immediately after taking three final exams in a row had a "reactive" viral syndrome, triggered by life stress?

In fact, retrospective studies of patients presenting with "endogenous" depression reveal that about 70% of them were able to cite a recent stressor that preceded their depressive episode. Similarly, prospective studies of patients initially diagnosed with "neurotic" depression reveal that a significant proportion of them go on to later develop "endogenous" depression, or even to develop manic episodes or episodes that include psychotic symptoms. Overall, most patients with major depressive disorder or Bipolar Disorder have *both* endogenous and reactive components to their presentation, the relative contributions of which vary from case to case. Where one "draws the lines" remains a source of diagnostic uncertainty.

Similarly, we still rely on the "psychotic versus neurotic" dichotomy when we distinguish between *major depressive disorder* and *dysthymic disorder.* The latter condition is a milder but more chronic form of depression that is more closely associated with temperament. Again, longitudinal and family studies show that a pure, dichotomous differentiation is overly simplistic. Family studies, prospective and retrospective longitudinal studies, and studies of biological markers suggest that "psychotic" depression may simply be a more *acute* form of illness, while "neurotic" depression may simply be a more *chronic* form. For example, some patients with dysthymic disorder go on to develop a superimposed acute major depressive disorder at some point, while some patients with major depressive disorder never fully recover and are left with chronic, residual "dysthymia-level" symptoms. Dysthymic disorder and major depressive disorder also tend to aggregate within families, further suggesting that the two disorders are related.

We also continue to rely on the "primary versus secondary" scheme when making the distinction between *major depressive disorder* and *mood disorder due to a general medical condition.* However, to lump all "idiopathic" presentations of mood disorder into the "primary" depression category isn't particularly enlightening. Further, the depressive symptoms that occur in the context of medical illnesses such as hypothyroidism, stroke, pancreatic cancer, or Parkinson's disease may reflect pathological changes along the same "final common pathways" that are affected by "primary" mood disorders such as major depressive disorder or bipolar disorder.

The disease perspective forces us to place different clinical phenomena into distinct categories, and this engenders debate between the "lumpers" and the "splitters," even after 2000 years. One still hears clinicians who describe patients as having "reactive depression" or "neurotic depression," despite the fact that these terms are not found in the current, official psychiatric nosology.

The *DSM-IV* categorical distinctions are not fully validated because we still don't completely understand how the body regulates mood. However, we continue to strive toward greater validity through clinical, epidemiologic, family, and biological studies. For example, based on family studies, researchers have determined that those patients who *only become manic* (i.e., who might be called "unipolar mania") likely have the same underlying disorder as those patients who become manic and also become depressed. Hence, the current nosology makes no distinction between these two groups; both are labeled as having bipolar disorder. In contrast, patients who only become depressed ("unipolar depression") *do* appear have a different condition than patients who become both depressed ("unipolar depression") and manic. Thus, *DSM-IV* distinguishes the former (labeled major depressive disorder) from the latter (bipolar disorder).

DSM-IV Classification Scheme

The DSM-IV categories for the various mood disorders are listed in Table 7–7. In terms of unipolar depressive disorders, *DSM-IV* distinguishes between *depressive (unipolar) disorders* and *bipolar disorders*. There are two primary depressive disorders, *major depressive disorder* and *dysthymic disorder*.

Major depressive disorder is characterized by the presence of one or more *major depressive episodes*—that is, by at least 2 *weeks* of depressed mood or anhedonia plus at least four associated depressive symptoms. (For a useful mnemonic in recalling these associated symptoms, see Chapter 2, Table 2–4). **Dysthymic disorder** presents with the insidious onset (usually during childhood, adolescence, or young adulthood) of more chronic symptoms—that is, at least 2 *years* of depressed mood for more days

Table 7–7. *DSM-IV-TR* Classification of Mood Disorders (in *DSM-IV-TR*, Adjustment Disorder Constitutes a Separate Category)

DEPRESSIVE (UNIPOLAR) DISORDERS

Major Depressive Disorder

One or more major depressive episodes (i.e., at least 2 weeks of depressed mood or anhedonia and at least four other depressive symptoms)

Dysthymic Disorder

At least 2 years of depressed mood along with associated symptoms, but without meeting the full criteria for major depressive episode (two rather than four additional symptoms)

DEPRESSIVE DISORDER NOT OTHERWISE SPECIFIED (NOS)

BIPOLAR DISORDERS

Bipolar I Disorder

One or more manic or mixed episodes (usually, but not invariably, accompanied by major depressive episodes)

Bipolar II Disorder

One or more major depressive episodes accompanied by at least one hypomanic episode

Cyclothymic Disorder

At least 2 years of hypomanic and dysthymic symptoms

Bipolar Disorder Not Otherwise Specified (NOS)

MOOD DISORDER DUE TO A GENERAL MEDICAL CONDITION

SUBSTANCE-INDUCED MOOD DISORDER

ADJUSTMENT DISORDER WITH DEPRESSED MOOD OR WITH MIXED ANXIETY AND DEPRESSED MOOD

than not plus at least *two* additional depressive symptoms (i.e., not enough symptoms to fulfill the diagnostic criteria for having a chronic major depressive episode).

Patients with dysthymic disorder can experience superimposed major depressive episodes (what has been termed "**double depression**"). Often, when the superimposed episodes resolve, patients return to their "baseline" dysthymia-level depression. In these cases, patients are assigned *both* diagnoses. Such patients should have experienced at least 2 years of dysthymic-level symptoms *before* having entered the major depressive episode. Note that in cases where the patient *initially* experienced a full major depressive disorder that never completely resolved, such that the patient is now left with dysthymia-level symptoms, the appropriate diagnosis would be *major depressive disorder, in partial remission* rather than double depression. However, if the patient initially experienced a major depressive episode and the symptoms haven't even *partially* improved over time, the appropriate diagnosis would be *major depressive disorder, chronic.*

In attempting to characterize a patient's depression, one helpful technique is to *chart the longitudinal course of illness*, as in Figure 7–1. Case A displays the course of recurrent major depressive disorder with no antecedent dysthymic disorder and full remission between episodes. This pattern is associated with the best future prognosis. Case B displays the course of recurrent major depressive disorder with no antecedent dysthymic disorder but with the persistence of symptoms between the two most recent episodes. In other words, the patient was only able to achieve partial rather than full remission in between episodes. Case C shows the more rare pattern (present in fewer than 3% of persons with major depressive disorder) of recurrent major depressive disorder with antecedent dysthymic disorder but with full interepisode recovery between the two most recent episodes. Case D shows the course of recurrent major depressive disorder with an antecedent dysthymic disorder and with no period of full remission between the two most recent episodes. This pattern occurs in about 20%–25% of persons with major depressive disorder.

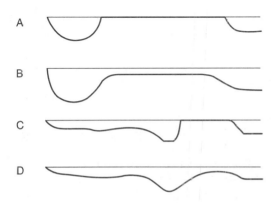

Figure 7–1. Longitudinal courses associated with depression. Reprinted with permission from the *Diagnostic and Statistical Manual of Mental Disorders, Fourth Edition. Text Revision.* Copyright 2000 American Psychiatric Association.

Depressive disorder not otherwise specified (NOS) is a residual category used to describe depressed patients who don't meet either of the above two diagnostic criteria but don't appear to have an adjustment disorder. These conditions, listed in Table 7–8, are included in the *DSM-IV* as diagnoses for which there was insufficient information to warrant acceptance into the official nomenclature but that are deserving of further study.

In terms of the bipolar disorders, the *DSM-IV* distinguishes between bipolar I disorder, bipolar II disorder, and cyclothymic disorder. In **bipolar I disorder**, the presence of one or more *manic or mixed episodes* is all that is necessary to make the diagnosis, although patients often will have a history of also having experienced major depressive episodes. In **bipolar II disorder**, the patient has had one or more major depressive episodes accompanied by at least one *hypomanic episode* but no "full-blown" manic or mixed episodes. In **cyclothymic disorder**, the patient has experienced numerous periods of hypomanic symptoms and of dysthymia-level depressive symptoms over at least a 2 year period but no full-blown depressive or manic episodes.

The course of a patient's symptoms over time reflects not only the impact of the underlying illness but also that of life events, psychotherapy interventions, and medication trials. Most clinicians don't construct formal timelines, but in more complex cases this strategy can help to clarify these interrelationships. Figure 7–2 presents an example of such a "life chart" for a patient with bipolar disorder.

The diagnostic criteria for depressive, manic, and hypomanic episodes all include "exclusionary criteria" indicating that the patient's depressive or manic symptoms should not be due to the direct physiological effects of a substance or of a general medical condition. In the latter cases, the more appropriate diagnoses would be **substance-induced mood disorder** or **mood disorder due to a general medical condition**, respectively.

"Substance use" can include the use of an illicit drug, of appropriately prescribed medication, or even of over-the-counter medications. Prominent mood changes can occur in association with **substance intoxication**, be it with alcohol, amphetamines, cocaine, hallucinogens, in-

Table 7–8. Types of Depressive Disorder Not Otherwise Specified in *DSM-IV-TR*

PREMENSTRUAL DYSPHORIC DISORDER

During most menstrual cycles over the past year, symptoms regularly occur during the last week of the luteal phase and remit completely within a few days of the onset of menses. Symptoms include markedly depressed mood and anhedonia, along with associated emotional symptoms (anxiety, anger, affective lability, anhedonia, rejection sensitivity, anhedonia and avoidance of social activities, increased interpersonal conflicts) and physical symptoms (lethargy, difficulty concentrating, overeating or food cravings, insomnia or hypersomnia, breast tenderness or swelling, headaches, weight gain). These symptoms must be severe enough to markedly interfere with work, school, or usual activities. The severity of the symptoms and the associated impairment distinguish this condition (which occurs in up to 5% of menstruating women) from the more prevalent "premenstrual syndrome" (which, variably defined, occurs in up to 50% of menstruating women). The presence of symptoms *only* prior to menses with complete remission following onset of menses distinguishes this condition from a premenstrual *exacerbation* of another mental disorder.

MINOR DEPRESSIVE DISORDER

One or more periods of depressive symptoms identical to major depressive episodes in duration (i.e., at least 2 weeks), but with fewer symptoms and less impairment (more than two but less than five additional symptoms). During the episode, these symptoms cause clinically significant distress or impairment in social, occupational, or other important areas of functioning. This is considered to be a residual diagnosis and therefore the diagnosis should not be made if the patient has ever had a major depressive, manic, mixed, or hypomanic episode or has had dysthymic or cyclothymic disorder

RECURRENT BRIEF DEPRESSIVE DISORDER

Depressive episodes with symptoms equal in number and severity to those seen in a major depressive episode but with a shorter episode duration (only 2 days to 2 weeks), most commonly 2 to 4 days. The episodes must occur at least once a month for 12 months and must cause clinically significant distress or impairment in social, occupational, or other important areas of functioning. They should not be associated exclusively with the menstrual cycle

POSTPSYCHOTIC DEPRESSIVE DISORDER OF SCHIZOPHRENIA

A major depressive episode occurs superimposed on the residual phase of schizophrenia (a phase which follows in the wake of an active phase of schizophrenia, characterized by the persistence of negative symptoms or of active-phase symptoms in more attenuated form). This diagnosis shouldn't be assigned if it appears that the mood symptoms are due to the direct physiological effects of a medication, a general medical condition, or a drug of abuse

MAJOR DEPRESSIVE EPISODE SUPERIMPOSED ON DELUSIONAL DISORDER, PSYCHOTIC DISORDER NOS, OR THE ACTIVE PHASE OF SCHIZOPHRENIA

A depressive disorder is present but the clinician is unable to determine whether it is primary, due to a general medical condition, or substance induced.

Source: Reprinted with permission from the *Diagnostic and Statistical Manual of Mental Disorders, Fourth Edition, Text Revision.* Copyright 2000 American Psychiatric Association.

halants, opioids, phencyclidine and related substances, or sedative/anxiolytic agents. Mood changes also can occur in association with **substance withdrawal** from these substances. Sometimes *psychological* withdrawal symptoms (such as depression, anhedonia, or irritability) continue for a prolonged period (even weeks to months) despite resolution of more acute *physical* withdrawal symptoms. These psychological symptoms not only cause subjective distress but also can heighten a patient's risk of resuming substance use.

Commonly prescribed medications that sometimes evoke mood symptoms include anesthetics, analgesics, anticholinergics, anticonvulsants, antihypertensives, antiparkinsonian medications, antiulcer medications (H$_2$-blockers), cardiac

medications (especially β-adrenergic antagonists), isotretinoin (Accutane), oral contraceptives, muscle relaxants, steroids, and sulfonamides. Medications that are especially likely to produce depressive symptoms include high doses of reserpine, corticosteroids, and anabolic steroids. Heavy metals and toxins (e.g., volatile substances such as gasoline and paint, organophosphate insecticides, nerve gases, carbon monoxide, and carbon dioxide) also can cause mood symptoms. This list is not exhaustive and patients' medication lists always should be examined in search of temporal associations between newly prescribed agents and the onset or exacerbation of mood complaints.

A variety of medical conditions are associated with pathologic changes in mood. These include

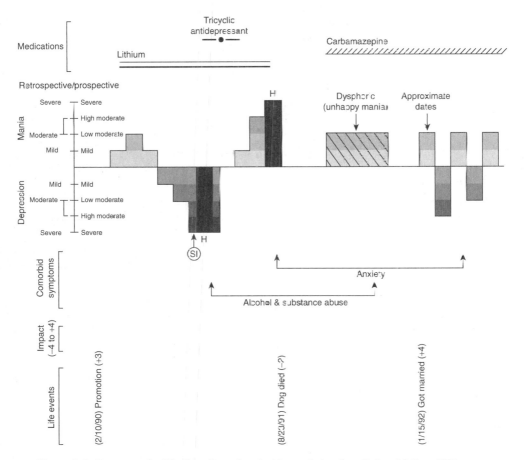

Figure 7–2. Prototype of a life chart. Reproduced with permission from Robert M. Post. "SI" connotes a suicide attempt; "H" connotes a hospitalization.

degenerative neurological conditions (such as Parkinson's disease and Huntington's disease), *cerebrovascular disease, metabolic conditions* (such as vitamin B_{12} deficiency), *endocrine conditions* (including hyper- and hypothyroidism, hyper- and hypoparathyroidism, hyper- and hypoadrenocorticism), *autoimmune conditions* (such as systemic lupus erythematosus), *viral or other infections* (such as hepatitis, mononucleosis, HIV), and *certain cancers* (e.g., carcinoma of the pancreas). Some of these illnesses affect the brain via *discrete localizable lesions* (e.g., stroke), while others do so via *scattered lesions* (e.g., Alzheimer's disease) or via a *pathology* that affects specific brain systems or regions (e.g., Parkinson's disease, Huntington's disease)

"Secondary" depressive (or more rarely, manic) symptoms in patients with these medical conditions can be as disabling as or more disabling than physical symptoms associated with the condition. While this in itself justifies re-

search into exactly how these mood changes arise and how best to treat them, another justification for this research is that—through inference and extrapolation—it will help us to gain a better understanding of the pathology underlying mood changes that occur in "primary" mood disorders.

One example of a mood disorder due to a general medical condition is **poststroke depression**. Among patients hospitalized for acute stroke, 22% meet the diagnostic criteria for major depressive disorder and an additional 17% meet the criteria for having dysthymic disorder if one excludes the 2-year duration criterion normally required to make this latter diagnosis. (For stroke patients examined in community settings at about the same time following their stroke as these hospitalized patients, the prevalence is a bit lower, at 13% and 10%, respectively.) The morbidity and mortality associated with poststroke depression are considerable. When all factors influencing physical recovery (such as lesion size and hours of physical therapy) are taken into account, depression has an independent effect inhibiting functional recovery over the first 2 years following stroke. Further, at both 15-month and 10-year follow-up, patients with poststroke major or minor depression are between four and eight times more likely to die than are nondepressed stroke patients, even taking into account other factors such as associated illnesses and previous strokes. Since poststroke depression is often responsive to therapy with antidepressant medications, it is important that clinicians keep this diagnosis in mind when examining stroke patients.

While strokes in all brain regions have been associated with the occurrence of depressive symptoms, when these symptoms occur during the first 1–2 months following a stroke, the most commonly associated lesion locations are *the left frontal lobe and the left basal ganglia*. In contrast, when the onset of such symptoms is later than this, the patient is just as likely to have a right hemisphere lesion (particularly a lesion in the right frontal lobe or right parietal lobe) as a left hemisphere lesion.

It is likely that strokes both cause *diffuse changes in brain monoamine levels* (either via direct injury to midbrain catecholamine neurons or via disruption of these neurons' cortical projections) and *disrupt established neurophysiologic pathways*. Supporting the former idea is the finding that brain lesions in animals cause decreases in norepinephrine, dopamine, and serotonin concentrations. While monoamine levels can't be directly measured in humans who have suffered strokes, CSF catecholamine *metabolites* can be measured and turn out to be lower in poststroke patients, and more severe decreases are associated with more severe depressive symptoms.

Supporting the latter notion is the finding that disruptions of two neurophysiological tracts are most likely to cause depression to develop: *(1)* pathways linking *the orbital and inferior frontal lobes to the basal ganglia* and *(2)* pathways connecting *the basal temporal areas to the basal ganglia*. These tracts, discussed in more detail in Chapter 4, are interconnected such that strokes in one location affect the metabolism of distant but related regions. For example, patients who become depressed following a basal ganglia stroke have been found on functional neuroimaging to have decreased metabolism in their bilateral frontal and temporal lobes. It is noteworthy that a similar pattern of decreased frontal and temporal metabolism has been noted in patients who have a "primary" major depressive disorder.

Stroke location isn't the whole story, however. Those poststroke patients who become depressed also are more likely to have more general risk factors for becoming depressed. These include having a past history of depression, a family history of depression, fewer social supports, a greater degree of impairment in activities of daily living, more life stressors preceding the stroke, and personality traits that render them more vulnerable to anxiety and depression in general (particularly having higher scores on psychological testing in the area of "neuroticism," an aspect of personality discussed in Chapter 10). These risk factors may be cumulative, such that the more "hits" one experiences, the more likely one is to become depressed.

Another example of a mood disorder due to a general medical condition is depression due to **Parkinson's disease**. This occurs in up to 50% of patients with the latter diagnosis. A loss of brain-stem monoaminergic neurons, along with degeneration of their mesocortical and mesolimbic projections, likely plays a contributory role here similar to that in poststroke patients. (While Parkinson's Disease is characterized by a dopamine deficiency, autopsy studies also reveal decreased stores of norepinephrine and serotonin.) Depression also occurs in up to 40% of patients with **Huntington's disease**, and the onset of depressive symptoms in these patients often precedes the onset of their motor and cognitive symptoms. As in the case of stroke and Parkinson's disease, limbic and prefrontal degeneration probably plays an important etiologic role.

Other Forms of Depression

Psychotic depression or mania also can present with **catatonic features**. While catatonia historically has been considered a subtype of schizophrenia, it actually occurs more commonly in patients with mood disorder.

Any of the forms of mood disorder (major depressive disorder, bipolar depression, or dysthymic disorder) also can present with **atypical**

features, and *DSM-IV* therefore considers this more of a "qualifying specifier" rather than a discrete diagnosis (e.g., "Bipolar disorder, depressive episode, with atypical features"). Atypical depression has several distinguishing features:

Preserved mood reactivity: Despite having a pervasive, sad mood more days than not, the patient retains the capacity to feel more happy or sad in response to positive or negative life events.

Reversed neurovegetative features: The patient sleeps more rather than less, eats more (especially carbohydrates and "junk food," often due to cravings for these foods) and gains weight.

Leaden paralysis: A heavy feeling especially noted in the arms and legs.

Heightened rejection sensitivity: The patient is overly sensitive to feeling rejected in interpersonal relationships. It must be significant enough to result in functional impairment. For example, the patient may be unable to sustain a long-term relationship, or may have to leave work early or use substances excessively after perceived criticism, or may avoid relationships in general.

DSM-IV specifies that the patient should have at least two of these four features during the period that the patient has been depressed. This presentation is two to three times more common in women than in men. It tends to demonstrate a younger age of onset (typically during high school) and also a more chronic, less episodic course, with only partial interepisode recovery. It may respond better to **monoamine oxidase inhibitors** than to tricyclic antidepressants. It also appears to respond to **selective serotonin reuptake inhibitors**, and most clinicians would initiate treatment with these agents first, given their greater margin of safety. Because of the overlap in phenomenology between atypical depression and depressive episodes experienced in bipolar disorder I and II disorders, one should also always inquire into a family or personal history of hypomanic or manic symptoms.

An overlap exists between atypical depression and **seasonal affective disorder (SAD)**, which the *DSM* again considers to be "specifier" rather than a separate disorder (e.g., "major depressive disorder, recurrent, moderate, with seasonal pattern"). Most mood disorders display seasonal variations. Unipolar depressive episodes most commonly occur in the spring; bipolar depression is more likely to recur in the fall, and manic episodes most commonly occur in the summer. Depressive episodes that occur in the spring tend to have typical features. However, in seasonal affective disorder ("winter depression") depressive episodes occur in the fall and winter months and remit in the spring. In this case, the symptoms are similar to those seen in atypical depression, although rejection sensitivity is less common. Again, there is a younger age of onset, a greater prevalence in women (four times more common than in men. The prevalence of SAD is also greater in higher-latitude areas, perhaps because these areas receive less light and have shorter days in the winter.

Seasonal affective disorder can be treated with either antidepressant medication or with bright light therapy. The latter therapy consists of sitting in front of a bright light (usually 10,000 lux) for about a half-hour early each morning. Lower intensities—for example, 2,500 lux—can be effective but require up to 2 hours in front of the lamp. Morning light appears to be more effective than evening light, although some patients do respond to the latter. Symptoms often improve within a few days, but without continued therapy throughout the winter symptoms typically recur. The most common side effects are transient headache and irritability. Again, one should explore for the possibility of bipolarity when patients with seasonal affective disorder are encountered, especially because light therapy—like all antidepressants—can increase the risk of "switching" from a depressive episode into a hypomanic or manic episode.

Depression and Personality Disorder

Many clinicians have had the experience of treating depression in a "difficult" patient labeled by the hospital staff as having a severe personality disorder only to find that the personality difficulties resolved (or at least substantially improved) once the depression had been addressed. In one study, half of patients who had received diagnoses of concurrent depression and personality disorder no longer met criteria for having a personality disorder once their depression had been treated. One way to distinguish between an Axis I mood disorder from an Axis II personality disorder is by taking a detailed social history and questioning the patient and collateral informants about the patient's traits and behaviors prior to the onset of depression.

However, and equally important, in some cases an isolated Axis II personality disorder may be the primary disturbance. Patients in these cases lack vegetative depressive symptoms but complain of chronic loneliness, emptiness, boredom, anger, and of having emotional needs that the people around them are failing to meet. These patients sometimes receive multiple unsuccessful trials of antidepressant medication with little benefit. But not all patients who are unhappy are clinically depressed, and not all aspects of the human condition respond to antidepressant medication, despite the desire on the part of many physicians and many patients to reach for quick fixes. Failure—by clinicians who feel more comfortable with medication management than psychotherapy—to recognize and address the underlying personality disorder while continuing to pursue one medical trial after another also does the patient a disservice: not only does it expose the patient to the risks of these medications, but it also reinforces the sick role and underemphasizes the importance of the patient taking responsibility for addressing maladaptive attitudes and behaviors.

Perhaps the most common scenario encountered in clinical practice, however, is one where the patient has *both* a mood disorder and a concurrent personality disorder. Between 30% and 70% of depressed patients fall into this category. Why such a high rate? Having a personality disorder may contribute to the development of depression, especially if the personality disorder is characterized by excessive perfectionism and self-criticism, as in obsessive-compulsive personality disorder, or if it is characterized by intense needs for emotional support from others that people can't fully meet, as in dependent, histrionic, and borderline personality disorders. Depressed patients with comorbid personality disorders also appear to have a poorer prognosis and to be more refractory to treatment (regardless of whether the treatment consists primarily of psychotherapy or medication).

Diagnostic boundaries may be the murkiest in cases where the mood disorder is chronic and complicates what appears to be a comorbid, lifelong personality disorder:

> A 22-year-old patient is diagnosed as having previously untreated dysthymic disorder, recurrent superimposed major depressive episodes, substance–induced mood disorder, and borderline personality disorder. (The last condition is characterized by chronic instability of moods, relationships, and self-image, as well as by impulsiveness.)
>
> The patient describes having been a "colicky" baby and a "difficult" child. Her mother also experienced depression throughout the patient's childhood. This led to her mother feeling overwhelmed by the patient's childhood behaviors, to the point where she became emotionally unavailable and verbally abused the patient throughout her childhood. The patient also reports a history of sexual abuse by a cousin that further contributed to her low self-image and impaired interpersonal functioning.
>
> She first became clinically depressed during late childhood and depressive symptoms continued into adolescence. Typical for depression presenting in adolescence, she not only experienced sadness but also increased irritability and conduct problems. She had difficulty making friends, began using alcohol and drugs at age 14, and became sexually precocious at that time as well. She described this behavior as having constituted attempts to "to feel better, or just to feel something." However, her behavior also reinforced her low self-esteem. While her substance use has been associated with increased depressive symptoms, she also describes having been sad throughout periods of abstinence lasting up to 9 months.

This clinical scenario is a common one. By the time that this patient is finally diagnosed with a mood disorder in her 20s and antidepressant medication therapy is initiated, her view of the world and of herself already has become entrenched to the point where she also has a *personality disorder*. Medications *alone* are not going to "cure" her of her lifelong personality vulnerabilities. However, the clinician shouldn't overlook the presence of a mood disorder simply because her personality disorder is so "out there" that he can't see past it.

Depression and Bereavement

It also is important to distinguish major depressive disorder from **bereavement**, since depressive symptoms constitute one part of the normal grief response that occurs following the death of a loved one. For example, 10%–20% of people suffer from severe, unremitting depression during the year following the death of a spouse. Given this, how can we distinguish "normal" grieving from a major depression triggered by this severe life stressor? Here are some guidelines.

First, while patients with bereavement may have enough symptoms to fulfill the diagnostic criteria for a major depressive episode, they generally don't display a pathological change in *self-attitude*. While they may demonstrate "survivor guilt" about actions they never took prior to the loved one's death, or wishes to have been the one who died rather than the loved one, or wishes that they had died along with the deceased, they typically don't voice attitudes that they are bad people in general or are worthless.

Second, bereaved patients who display *severe psychomotor retardation or functional impairment* likely are experiencing a superimposed major depressive episode. Similarly, while bereaved patients may report having very transiently "heard" or "seen" the deceased at some point, *hallucinations or delusions* beyond these limited ones are beyond the scope of the normal grief reaction and suggest the presence of a psychotic depression.

Third, sadness occurring in the setting of grief tends to be *circumscribed*, centering on thoughts about the deceased and arising unbidden when the survivor is confronted with reminders of the deceased. In major depressive disorder, sadness tends to be more *pervasive and autonomous*.

Fourth, sadness in grief tends to be more *self-limited*, often *improving* over a period of several months. (Given this, *DSM-IV* specifies that a new diagnosis of major depressive disorder shouldn't be made during the first 2 months after a loss.) When grief becomes prolonged, one should be alert to the possibility of a superimposed major depressive episode.

Finally, patients who develop major depressive disorder following a loss often have a *family history or past personal history* of major depression.

These distinctions having been made, clinicians should be aware that major depressive disorder commonly complicates bereavement and that in these cases *both* diagnoses should be assigned. For example, in a 2-year longitudinal study of 350 bereaved spouses conducted by Zisook and colleagues (1994), depressive symptoms were found to be very common. Table 7–9 shows the typical symptoms that these individuals experienced. Many of these individuals felt lonely or "blue" and voiced nonspecific somatic complaints even 2 years later.

At 2 months, 21% of bereaved individuals met the diagnostic criteria for having a major depressive disorder; 12% remained depressed at 13

Table 7–9. Depressive Symptoms in Widows and Widowers Versus a Married Comparison Group*

	PERCENTAGE			
	2 Months (n = 350)	13 Months (n = 286)	25 Months (n = 274)	Married Comparison Group (n = 126)
Trouble sleeping	57	29	26	14
Feeling blue	40	25	17	2
Trouble concentrating	20	13	9	2
Poor appetite	19	8	6	0
Anhedonia	18	15	8	2
Thoughts of death/dying	15	11	10	1
Feelings of guilt	12	8	5	0
Feelings of worthlessness	8	6	6	0
Thoughts of ending life	2	3	1	0

*The widows and widowers have significantly higher percentages of each depressive symptom at each point in time than the comparison group.
Source: Adapted from Zisook S, Shuchter SR, Sledge PA, et al: "The Spectrum of Depressive Phenomena after Spousal Bereavement." *J Clin Psychiatry* 55 (suppl 4), 29–36, 1994. Copyright 1994, Physicians Postgraduate Press. Adapted by permission.

months and 7% remained depressed at 2 years. In contrast, only 1% of members of a control group of still-married subjects were diagnosed with major depressive disorder during this time frame.

When depressive symptoms complicate bereavement, they carry a high social and emotional burden. Depressed widows and widowers, compared to widows and widowers not suffering from depression, show much greater functional impairment: they have poorer social functioning; they are less likely to become involved in a new relationship by 2 years after the spouse's death; they experience less satisfying relationships with friends and children; they are more likely to require counseling; they are not doing as well at work; they are more likely to begin drinking alcohol more heavily than they did previously; and they have worse medical health and visit the doctor more.

One might imagine that perhaps the circumstances surrounding the spouse's death or the "quality" of the marriage might play significant roles in whether or not the surviving partner experienced a greater or lesser degree of depression. However, at 2 months, among the factors that *weren't* predictive of significant depressive symptoms were: number of years married, sex of the survivor, whether the spouse's death was sudden or unanticipated, the extent of social support, the survivor's degree of belief in religion, and how the survivor rated the "quality of the relationship" with the deceased. In contrast, factors that *were* predictive of depression at 2 months were as follows: age of the survivor, a previous personal or family history of depression, and physical health problems. Notably, these all are risk factors for developing major depressive disorder even in the absence of bereavement.

Some bereaved survivors experience pervasive but less severe depressive symptoms that constitute a "*subsyndromal*" *depression*. Their severity of depression would fulfill the diagnostic criteria for dysthymic disorder except for the 2 year duration requirement. It is important to identify such individuals since this condition is as common as major depressive disorder (27% at 2 months, 19% at 13 months, and 12% at 25 months), is associated with similar, if slightly less morebidity (falling between the degree of

impairment seen in widowers with no depression and that seen in those with major depressive disorder), and can persist if treatment is not provided. (While 63% of individuals with subsyndromal depression at 2 months were no longer depressed when reexamined at 13 months, 28% of them remained at this same level of depression while 9% had progressed to a full major depressive disorder.)

Depression associated with bereavement constitutes a significant public health problem. About 7% of the U.S. population consists of widows and widowers, and 800,000 people become widows or widowers yearly. By age 65, over 50% of women and 14% of men are widowed. Two years after the partner's death, 14% continue to have major depressive disorder and 12% have subsyndromal depression. Depression can interfere with cognitive and emotional processing, thereby preventing the patient from successfully negotiating the grieving process, and it is associated with functional morbidity.

Equally concerning is how commonly this condition goes untreated. In Chapter 1, the point was made that physicians are less likely to diagnosis major depressive disorder when the patient's depression appears "understandable." The San Diego study reinforces this point. Most cases of depression diagnosed in the course of the study went unrecognized and untreated over the entire 2 years. Fewer than 40% of depressed subjects received any counseling during the 2 years, and fewer than 25% of subjects with major depressive disorder received any antidepressant medication despite more frequent doctors' visits than nondepressed widowers. When they were prescribed, antidepressants tended to be given in ineffective doses and little follow-up was provided to assess for clinical response. When primary care doctors did prescribe medication, they most often prescribed benzodiazepines (45% of depressed subjects were prescribed these shortly after the spouse's death). However, while benzodiazepines are useful in treating anxiety, they don't effectively treat major depressive disorder.

In *DSM-III-R*, sadness after a death that didn't fulfill the full diagnostic criteria for major depressive disorder was called "uncomplicated bereavement"—that is, grief not considered "complicated" by the development of a clinical depression. However, research demonstrating that even patients with subsyndromal depression remain impaired over the next 2 years led the *DSM-IV* committee to eliminate the category of "uncomplicated bereavement." Using *DSM-IV*, one now simply diagnoses "bereavement."

This classification scheme still tends to minimize the significance of depressive symptoms that occur in the setting of grief. There is no other diagnosis, psychiatric or medical, that is "negated" on the basis of a recent life event. For example, bereaved men die of cardiovascular disease at a higher rate than nonbereaved men, but no internist would postulate that the patient who experiences a myocardial infarction 1 month after his wife's death had "bereavement" and didn't also have cardiac disease. Should depression be treated differently? Similarly, clinical depression that occurs in the wake of a divorce or having received a diagnosis of cancer is still called major depressive disorder. Should depression that occurs in the setting of bereavement be treated differently? Recent research trials bolster the notion that depression occurring in the setting of grief does respond to treatment with antidepressant medications, while more specific grief-related symptoms persist.

Depression and the Elderly

The rate of depression increases with age during younger adulthood and middle age but doesn't continue to increase linearly throughout the life span. Contrary to popular belief, community surveys using standardized instruments reveal a rate of major depressive disorder in elderly individuals that is *lower* than that seen in the general population—about 1%–2% (with an additional 2% meeting the diagnostic criteria for dysthymic disorder).

Given this lower rate of depression in the elderly, one should avoid the temptation to "explain away" an older patient's depression as being "due to" factors associated with aging. Most people in later life are relatively happy. While they experience sadness over the loss of friends and relations, they usually expect such losses and respond better to them than younger people do.

When clinical depression occurs in older patients, it may present somewhat differently than it does in younger patients. Presenting symptoms are more likely to emphasize new somatic complaints, including weight loss, fatigue, anhedonia, and anxiety. Complaints of sadness and decreased self-esteem may be less prominent. Complicating matters further, some older patients won't admit to depressive symptoms, feeling it improper to complain. Given these two factors, many depressed older patients won't fulfill the *DSM-IV* diagnostic criteria for major depressive disorder. However, their depression, while subsyndromal, is associated with significant morbidity.

While major depressive disorder is less common among elderly individuals who reside in the *general community setting*, its prevalence is much higher in the *hospital and nursing home settings*. These settings are not included in community surveys. In these latter settings, the prevalence of major depressive disorder is about 12%, and an additional 25%–30% of patients have subsyndromal (dysthymia-level) depression.

Further, despite the lower overall prevalence of major depressive disorder among the elderly, the *impact* of their depression may be greater in older patients than in younger patients, both in terms of morbidity (conferring a poorer prognosis to comorbid medical problems) and higher mortality (from completed suicide). The severity of illness is often greater as well, and psychotic symptoms occur more commonly in older depressed patients. In such cases, combined antidepressant–antipsychotic therapy or electroconvulsive therapy (ECT) is typically required.

Many older patients have comorbid medical conditions and take multiple medications. These should be scrutinized to assess for the possibility that the patient actually has a mood disorder due to a general medical condition or a substance-induced mood disorder. This should especially be the case when the patient does not have a past history of depression.

Of note, older individuals with major depressive disorder are more likely to demonstrate cerebral atrophy and subcortical leukoencephalopathy on MRI scans than are age-matched, nondepressed individuals. This suggests that some cases of late-onset depression may occur secondary to subclinical cerebrovascular disease. Many of these depressed subjects do not demonstrate significant cognitive deficits, although depression can also be an early presenting symptom of dementia.

Course of Illness

Bipolar disorder typically is first *diagnosed* when patients are in their early 20s. However, some symptoms may have been present by the patient's early adolescence. Studies stratifying the age of onset of symptoms into 5 year periods reveal a peak between ages 15 and 19, followed closely by ages 20 to 24. On average, a 5–10 year lag occurs between the age at onset of symptoms and the age of first treatment or hospitalization. Why this long delay?

First, in childhood and adolescence, patients later diagnosed with bipolar disorder may demonstrate irritability, conduct problems, or rapid mood swings, and they often are diagnosed with *attention-deficit hyperactivity disorder* or *conduct disorder*. Bipolar disorder may not be diagnosed until the patient has experienced an acute manic episode.

Second, the patient may have experienced several major depressive episodes before ultimately having had a manic episode, leading to an initial diagnosis of major depressive disorder having been assigned. About 5%–10% of patients initially diagnosed with major depressive disorder ultimately have their diagnosis revised to one of bipolar disorder following a manic episode. Generally, this occurs 6–10 years after the first depressive episode has occurred, and during this interval two to four additional depressive episodes have taken place. In such cases, bipolar disorder isn't diagnosed until the patient has reached age 32, on average.

Given this, the clinician always should keep in mind the possibility of bipolar disorder when treating younger depressed patients, particularly since antidepressant medications can trigger a "switch" from depression into mania and can increase the frequency and severity of "cyling." (Notice in Fig. 7–2 how this patient's second episode of mania closely followed the initiation of treatment with a tricyclic antidepressant.)

In such cases, the patient may have an underlying bipolar *genotype*, despite having a clinical *phenotype* that to date has consisted only of depressive episodes. (Genetics researchers have labeled this latter phenomenon **pseudounipolar depression**.) Clinicians hoping to distinguish between unipolar depression and possible bipolar depression do so based on several historical and phenomenologic clues.

One such clue is *age of onset*. The age of onset for major depressive disorder tends to be later than that for bipolar disorder. In major depressive disorder, the mean age of onset is the late 20s, and 50% of cases first appear after age 40. While bipolar disorder also can have its onset in later life, it occurs less commonly. When a first episode of mania occurs after age 40, it should trigger a search for some underlying medical condition, most commonly cerebrovascular disease or a medication reaction.

A second clue is a *family history* of either major depressive disorder or bipolar disorder since these two illnesses tend to "breed true." Third, one should explore for a history of *previous hypomanic episodes*. The symptoms might be relatively subtle and therefore may have been paid little heed. Should these have occurred, the diagnosis would be modified to one of bipolar disorder, type II.

A fourth clue is the *phenomenology* of the depressive episode. Bipolar depressive episodes are more likely to present with "atypical" symptoms such as hypersomnia and psychomotor retardation. The episodes also usually are briefer than those that occur in major depressive disorder, lasting from several weeks to several months. In bipolar disorder, depressive episodes tend to end more abruptly. In 50%–60% of cases, they immediately precede or immediately follow a manic or hypomanic episode, with no intervening period of euthymia.

Frequently, the first episode of either major depressive disorder or bipolar disorder is temporally associated with some *stressful life event*, especially a loss. For example, the patient in Figure 7–2 experienced the onset of illness following a job promotion.

However, as the mood disorder progresses, it becomes increasingly *independent of life events*. For example, in untreated bipolar disorder, an average of 5 years intervenes between the first and second episodes of illness. A life stressor often precedes this second episode. Over time, the duration of episodes increases while the duration of the interval between them decreases. By the third or fourth episode, one might occur spontaneously, unpredictably, in the absence of a life stressor. By about the fifth episode, the interepisode interval has decreased to 6–9 months.

While most patients return to a normal mood state (called **euthymia**) about 20%–30% of patients never fully return to their premorbid level of functioning. Some remain chronically ill, others **rapidly cycle** (defined operationally in the *DSM-IV* as having four or more episodes of depressive or manic episodes within a single year).

While rapid cycling is associated with a poorer prognosis, even patients who return to a euthymic state suffer ongoing morbidity, as they now are faced with having to "pick up the pieces" of their lives. For example, they may have spent themselves into debt, lost their jobs, or become pregnant. They may be unable to return to work if job stress triggers episodes of illness, and may accept less challenging (and less satisfying) jobs. They may have difficulty determining whether their good or bad moods are appropriate feelings or are signs of impending relapse. All of these factors impair the patient's quality of life.

Bipolar disorder is associated with a less favorable prognosis than major depressive disorder. Following their first manic or depressive episode, 90% of bipolar patients go on to experience subsequent episodes. The mean number of lifetime episodes is nine, but 40% of patients experience more than 10 episodes. Only 15% of patients ultimately achieve a stable euthymic state. In contrast, 45% of patients experience euthymia punctuated by multiple relapses, 30% achieve a state of "partial remission," and 10% remain chronically ill.

Many patients with chronic bipolar illness experience a more chronic state that isn't quite "manic" or "depressed." Rather, it is a labile state that includes admixed symptoms of depression, mania, anxiety, and irritability and is called a **mixed state**. Given this, it would be overly simplistic to conceptualize bipolar disorder as an illness where the person resides only at one extreme pole or its opposite pole at a given time. Based on such considerations, Goodwin and Jamison (1990) have suggested that we return to Kraepelin's original label, "manic-depressive illness."

Major depressive disorder also is characterized by a vulnerability to recurrent or chronic illness. In the absence of treatment, 50% of patients who have experienced one major depressive episode will have a recurrence later in life. After two episodes, the recurrence rate is 70%, and after three episodes, recurrence is nearly inevitable, with a rate of 90%. As was the case with bipolar disorder, after several recurrences, episodes begin to recur more frequently and to last longer. Over a 20-year period, the average patient experiences five to six episodes.

Morbidity and Mortality

Major depressive disorder is associated with significant social and physical morbidity. In a survey of patients over 40,000 doctor visits, depression was associated with a greater degree of social and physical disability than were diabetes, chronic lung disease, hypertension, and arthritis across six different variables of functioning (as can be seen in Fig. 7–3). While coronary artery disease did surpass depression in its level of associated physical morbidity, it still was associated with a lesser degree of social impairment than depression.

Major depressive disorder also conveys a high risk of mortality, largely due to suicide. Suicide has been described as accounting for up to 15% of all deaths that occur in persons with mood disorder. This figure likely is an overestimate, as it is based on how often suicide occurs among former *inpatients* (many of whom were admitted specifically because they had suicidal ideation or had made a suicide attempt) who met older criteria for depression that were stricter than current criteria and that emphasized the presence of multiple melancholic symptoms.

Regardless, the risk of suicide clearly is higher among depressed individuals than among the general population. Viewed retrospectively, about 60% of all suicides are found to have been associated with the presence of a mood disorder. Viewed prospectively, the risk of suicide among patients with mood disorders varies depending on the setting. The lifetime prevalence of suicide for a mixed inpatient–outpatient population is 2%. For depressed patients who have been psychiatrically hospitalized for any reason, the lifetime risk of suicide is about 4%, while among patients who have been hospitalized specifically due to suicidality, the lifetime prevalence is 9%. (In contrast, the rate for nonaffectively ill population is less than 0.5%.)

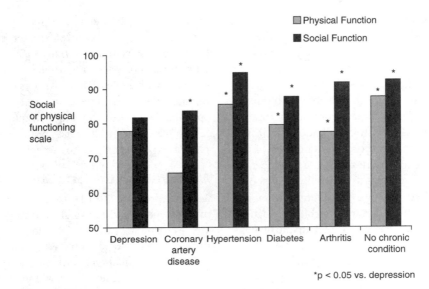

Figure 7–3. Physical and social functioning in depression and other chronic medical conditions. Adapted with permission from Wells KB, Stewart A, Hays RD, et al: "The Functioning and Well-Being of Depressed Patients: Results From the Medical Outcomes Study." *JAMA* 262:914–919, 1989.

The suicide risk is similar for major depressive disorder and bipolar disorder. In the latter case, suicide almost always is associated with depressive episodes rather than hypomanic or manic episodes, although agitated or mixed affective states also convey an increased risk. Suicide risk also is increased in depressed patients who have comorbid psychiatric conditions, particularly alcohol and substance abuse and/or a personality disorder.

Depression is also associated with greater morbidity and mortality from co-occurring medical illnesses. Individuals over age 55 who have major depressive disorder have a fourfold greater risk of dying from any cause than do age-matched individuals without depression. Patients admitted to medical and surgical inpatient units who are found on admission to meet the diagnostic criteria for major depressive disorder are more likely to die during that hospital stay than are nondepressed patients. Similarly, nursing homes residents who are depressed at the time of admission have an increased likelihood of dying during their first year at the nursing home compared to nondepressed nursing home residents.

The link between depression and cardiovascular disease is impressive. Otherwise-healthy individuals with depression, followed prospectively over time, experience ischemic heart dis-

ease at a much higher rate than do nondepressed individuals. One potential confounding variable in this regard is cigarette smoking, since a mere history of major depression (even in the absence of current illness) increases the likelihood that a person will smoke and increases the likelihood that attempts at quitting will fail. However, even when one controls for smoking history and for a myriad of other biological and social risk factors, the association between depression and excessive cardiac mortality persists.

When one examines all patients who have just had a myocardial infarction, one finds that 15%–20% of them describe symptoms fulfilling the diagnostic criteria for having a major depressive disorder. Members of this subgroup have a 10% greater mortality rate at 3 months than do nondepressed postinfarction patients; at 6 months they have a 15% greater mortality rate. As can be seen in Figure 7–4, at 6 months, 17% of the depressed patients have died, versus 3% of the nondepressed patients.

The reasons for this increased cardiac mortality in depressed individuals are not fully understood. Perhaps depression acts indirectly (e.g., perhaps depressed patients are less compliant in taking medications or following an exercise regimen), but this can't fully account for the above findings. For example, the excess mortality

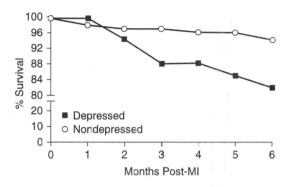

Figure 7–4. Mortality after myocardial infarction with and without comorbid depression. Reproduced with permission from Frasure-Smith N, Lesperance F, Talajic M: "Depression Following Myocardial Infarction: Impact on Six-Month Survival." *JAMA* 270:1819–1825, 1993. Copyrighted 1993, American Medical Association.

among depressed postmyocardial-infarction patients is due almost exclusively to sudden death, which itself usually is due to ventricular arrhythmia. Since major depressive disorder can be associated with changes in autonomic tone, depression may more directly increase the risk fatal arrhythmia after a myocardial infarction.

Autonomic changes can't explain why younger, depressed, but otherwise healthy individuals have a greater risk of developing ischemic heart disease later in life. Given this, researchers have directed their attention to platelet functioning. Platelet aggregation plays a key role in the development of occlusive vascular disease, and the platelets of depressed patients appear to have a greater propensity to aggregate. In addition, platelets contain serotonin, and antidepressants appear to decrease platelet aggregation. Depression also is associated with unfavorable alterations in lipid metabolism, and this may also increase a patient's risk of vascular disease. It remains to be determined whether treating depression, whether earlier in life or postinfarction, influences the course of the patient's cardiovascular disease.

Another explanation for the link between cardiovascular disease and depression is that some of these patients have subclinical cerebrovascular disease, since the latter is known to be a cause of depression. In other words, the relationship between atherosclerotic disease and clinical depression appears to be a two-way street: depression may increase one's risk both of developing

atherosclerotic disease and of having a less favorable prognosis, while atherosclerotic disease (at least cerebrovascular disease) potentially increases one's risk of becoming depressed.

It isn't clear at this point that depressed but otherwise healthy younger patients have an increased risk of having a stroke later in life, but individuals who have a stroke do appear to be predisposed to develop major depression. As was the case for depression in the post–myocardial-infarction patient, depression in post-stroke patients is associated both with impaired functional recovery and with increased mortality. (For example, at 15 month and at 10 year follow-up, depressed post-stroke patients are from 3.5 to eight times more likely to die than are nondepressed patients, even when one takes into account other factors such as associated medical illnesses and prior stroke.)

In fact, individuals who experience an onset of depressive symptoms only later in life are less likely to have a family history of depression and they are more likely to have hypertension, diabetes, and/or evidence of subclinical white matter hyperintensities on their brain MRI scans. This finding suggests that *subclinical* cerebrovascular disease plays a role in causing late-life depression.

Epidemiology

Major depressive disorder is common, with an overall lifetime prevalence of about 15%. The prevalence in women is about twice as high (25%) as in men (12%). (Of note, the Epidemiologic Catchment Area study [Weissman et al., 1991] found a lower prevalence, at 7% and 2.5%, respectively, perhaps related to the use of non-clinician interviewers and a structured interview). The greater prevalence of major depressive disorder in women has been noted almost universally in cross-cultural studies and doesn't appear to be due to gender bias in assigning diagnoses. Factors that might play a role include hormonal differences between women and men and different psychosocial stressors placed on women. In contrast, bipolar disorder has a lifetime prevalence of 1% and is equally distributed among men and women.

We have discussed *increasing age* as a risk factor for developing a mood disorder. The prevalence of mood disorder doesn't appear to vary among people of different *racial backgrounds*, although clinicians do tend to underdiagnose mood disorder in patients from minority groups while overdiagnosing schizophrenia, probably because of limited recognition of cultural variations in the clinical presentation.

Marital status appears to place some individuals at greater risk for major depressive disorder: separated and divorced people have higher rates of depression. Of note, while married men have a lower rate of depression than never-married men, married women have a higher rate than never-married women. Mood disorder hasn't been related to *socioeconomic status*. (While bipolar disorder may be more prevalent in individuals from higher social classes, this may reflect diagnostic bias.)

As noted above, *acute life stressors* appear to play a role both in triggering first episodes of illness and in relapses. The most common contributory stressors are the absence of close interpersonal relationships; marital discord or separation; not being employed outside of the home; having more than three children under age 14 living at home; and a recent death or illness in the family. *Early life stressors*, especially loss, have also been described. Perhaps early loss "sensitizes" the individual, increasing the propensity for depression later in life. In particular, the death or loss of the patient's mother prior to age 11 has been noted to be more common in depressed patients in several studies.

Women are at increased risk of becoming depressed during the *postpartum period*. Many women experience mild **"baby blues"** (crying, irritability, mood swings, with onset about 3–10 days postpartum and usually resolving in about a week). This syndrome may reflect the interaction of hormonal changes following delivery, stress, and sleep deprivation. However, true **postpartum depression** meeting the full diagnostic criteria for a major depressive episode also can occur, and this syndrome appears to be etiologically related to major depressive disorder.

Postpartum depression occurs in from 10% to 15% of new mothers. While the period of greatest risk is the first 2 weeks postpartum, women are at higher risk for becoming depressed for up to several months postpartum. Approximately 20%–30% of women who have had a prior depressive episode will experience postpartum depression. Conversely, 30% of women diagnosed with postpartum depression report having had a prior depressive episode. Once a woman has experienced a postpartum depression, she is at greater risk for a subsequent postpartum depression (between 30% and 50%).

Pathology, Etiology, and Treatment

We have discussed how mood disorders present in the clinical setting. When seeing a patient, one makes the diagnosis through the use of operational criteria. But how does one know if the patient "really" has major depressive disorder? By definition, the patient has major depressive disorder if he or she reports symptoms that fulfill the *DSM-IV* diagnostic criteria for major depressive disorder. While this appears tautological ("The criteria are based on the symptoms of the disease, and you have the disease if you meet the criteria"), using these criteria at least ensures greater diagnostic reliability.

But what about diagnostic validity? What lies *behind* the clinical presentation of mood disorder? While the *DSM-IV* criteria allow us to reliably delineate a particular group of patients, they are of little explanatory value. In discussing delirium and dementia, our primary point of view was that of "form" rather than "function." In other words, if a patient either becomes acutely confused or displays a progressive decline in cognition, it is more productive to initiate a medical workup to determine what disease is *causing* the patient's difficulties than to attempt to empathically understand the patient's "motivations" for "behaving in such a way."

While the patient's life history and personality affect the *content* of his or her symptoms, we couldn't say that they *explain* the presence of the pathological mental experiences. For example, a woman with dementia due to Alzheimer's disease who continues to grieve the loss of her deceased husband might believe that he is still alive, or a man with delirium due to sepsis who is going through a divorce might experience hallucinations of his estranged wife in his hospital room, tampering with his intravenous medications in an attempt to kill him.

In contrast, mood disorder is a syndrome that can be viewed from either form *or* function. The ancients viewed mood disorder from the perspective of form, describing it as an abnormal state resulting from an imbalance of bodily humors. Similarly, modern theories tend to view it as an abnormal state resulting from an imbalance of brain chemistry. However, theories in the early part of this century emphasized depression as the understandable reflection of a vulnerable individual's attempts to cope with adversity, whether consciously or unconsciously. Given that major depressive disorder and bipolar disorder become so entangled with patient's lives, any theory of etiology must attend to both aspects of mental life.

The most significant theories involving *function* (typically referred to as "psychological" theories) are the **psychodynamic** and **cognitive–behavioral** models. The most significant theories involving *form* (typically "biological" theories) are the **biogenic amine model** and the **neurophysiologic model**. As we discuss each model, we will discuss related treatment implications.

The Psychodynamic Model

Psychodynamic theory postulates that depressive symptoms reflect an *internal, unconscious conflict*. We will discuss two variants of this theory: the **classical psychoanalytic theory** and the more recent **object relations (ego psychology) theory**. (Psychotherapy in general is discussed in more detail in Chapter 17.)

Classical Psychoanalytic Theory

The classical psychoanalytic view posits that depression results from the *loss of an ambivalently loved object* and from *anger turned inward*. Sigmund Freud (1856–1939) first outlined this theory in his seminal 1917 paper, "Mourning and Melancholia." Freud, having trained as a neurologist, had initially—like Kraepelin—hoped to uncover the neuroanatomical basis of mental life and of psychiatric symptoms. However, he ultimately abandoned this project and turned to a *metaphorical* model of mind. The latter reflected the influence of the physics of the Industrial Revolution, emphasizing hydraulics. For example, Freud's initial papers on anxiety proposed that sexual ("libidinal") energy that is repressed from conscious awareness can begin to "build up." In the absence of an appropriate outlet, this energy ultimately is "discharged" in the form of anxiety.

While some subsequent psychoanalysts have treated Freud's theories as *scientific explanations*, on closer inspection one readily appreciates that his theories are actually *meaningful interpretations*. Using facts presented by the patient, they help the therapist to construct a "story" that "makes sense" of the facts. They help the listener appreciate *why* a patient might create such symptoms. In contrast to the disease model, here the patient is seen as playing an active role (although sometimes this role is unconscious), not in the pathogenesis of the disorder, but in its treatment.

In other words, Freud proposed that we view psychiatric symptoms not as reflections of some underlying "thing," or "disease," that the patient "has"; rather, they are seen as reflections of what a patient is "doing" as a defense against anxiety-laden thoughts or emotions. Unfortunately, sometimes what the patient is doing isn't working particularly well. It might even be causing other, bigger problems. Given this, psychoanalytic treatment involves first attempting to uncover why the patient has adopted these defenses and then trying to teach the patient more effective ways of dealing with his or her problems.

Freud struggled to understand *why* a patient might become depressed. He began by noting that—phenomenologically—depression resembles grief. However, while grief occurs in response to some clear *external loss*, many of Freud's depressed patients hadn't suffered any such loss. Therefore, perhaps clinical depression arises in response to an *unconscious or symbolic loss*. Freud further noted that in depression, patients tend to demonstrate *decreased self-attitude and guilt* and that these aren't typically seen in patients with grief. Finally, Freud noted that many depressed patients, despite readily expressing anger toward themselves, have difficulty expressing anger toward other people.

Putting all of this together, Freud suggested that the depressed patient has suffered from the loss (whether real or symbolic) of a significant figure in her life during early childhood, often the patient's mother. The patient has had difficulty dealing with the grief associated with this loss and so has identified with and even internalized (introjected) the image of this lost person into herself.

However, the loss is an ambivalent one. While the patient *loved* the lost person, she also remains *angry* with the person for having abandoned her. The anger can't be expressed, both because the lost person isn't there and because the patient has difficulty expressing anger in general. However, since the patient has introjected the image of the lost person into herself, she *turns this anger inward* at the internal representation of that person—that is, *onto herself.* (Again, note the analogy to hydraulics, where energy must "go" somewhere.) Later in life, a more recent loss, even a relatively mild one, brings this *latent* conflict back to the fore, such that the ensuing "depressive reaction" appears to be much more severe than would have been expected, given the circumstances.

There are some problems with this model, not the least of which is that many depressed patients do readily express anger toward others (and sometimes these individuals even become *less* angry following effective treatment of their depression). Also, many patients don't report any history of a childhood loss. While the therapist always can attributed significance to some relatively common childhood event described by the patient following an extensive interview, is the therapist then just the person who has a hammer who sees everything described by the patient as being a nail? Another problem with this theory is that it doesn't explain mania very well; Freud viewed mania as a defense against depression, and subsequent psychoanalytic theories have added little to our understanding of mania.

Object Relations Theory

Psychoanalytic theory has evolved in the years since Freud, however. The object relations school of psychoanalysis placed less emphasis on the sexual or aggressive urges of the unconscious *id* and focused more on the *self (ego)* and its relationships with significant other people from the outside world. (In this model, these other people are called "objects.") This model doesn't focus on the patient's *actual* mother, or girlfriend, or boss, but rather on the patient's *internalized representations* of these significant figures. We all have such internal representations, but clearly they are not exact replicas of the actual person; they are distorted, to greater or lesser degrees, depending on the person and on the particular "object." In psychiatric disorders, the internal representations tend to be more

distorted, usually due to early interpersonal difficulties. In this way, impaired early relationships pave the way for impaired future relationships. Given this, exploring past conflicts between "self" and "object" offers a way of understanding the patient's present symptoms.

While the object relations model of depression places little or no emphasis on "anger turned inward," it resembles the classical model in its emphasis on *disturbed interpersonal relations in early life* (usually involving a *loss or disappointment*) that impair subsequent interpersonal relations, thereby causing the patient to become depressed. Note that this model, unlike Freud's, doesn't view the childhood loss as being *directly responsible* for the current state of depression. Rather, the early loss contributes to the development of *character pathology*, which in turn renders the patient more *vulnerable* to later interpersonal difficulties and to even further losses, all of which ultimately result in the patient experiencing depressive symptoms.

Psychoanalytic treatment treats the patient's depression as a symptom of another problem rather than as the problem itself. Traditional psychoanalytic therapy sets a broader goal than symptomatic relief from depression; it seeks to help the patient develop more effective, more appropriate ways of seeing and reacting to the outside world *in general.*

One analyst who laid the theoretical foundations for the object relations school was John Bowlby (1907–1990), who wrote about childhood *attachment and loss.* Bowlby worked during World War II with displaced children and later worked with adolescents who presented with behavior problems. Bowlby also had an interest in *ethology*—the study of animal behavior in the natural environment. Bowlby noted that human infants, like other primate infants, have an innate predisposition to form a strong attachment to some primary figure, usually the infant's biological mother (although the child also forms other attachments, including to the father, siblings, or other caregivers).

These attachments begin to form at birth and are facilitated by factors such as skin-to-skin contact and frequent proximity. Infants and children display "preprogrammed" behaviors that encourage adults around them to reciprocate, including eye contact, clinging, smiling, laughing, vocalizing, and following. When an infant becomes anxious (for example, when startled or hungry), the mother soothes and provides for the infant: this leads to the infant developing a sense of *security* (the opposite of anxiety), and this feeling in turn becomes associated with the mother's presence. The formation of such attachments assures the safety of infants, especially in species such as mammals and birds where infants are faced with a prolonged period of physical dependence.

By around age 7–10 months, the child has formed an internal representation of the mother or other primary attachment figure but still lacks a sense of confidence that, were this person to leave, he or she would ever return. This leads to **separation anxiety**. While separation anxiety is normal, primate children can develop **pathological anxiety** in the setting of longer separations from their primary attachment figure. Bowlby described a characteristic sequence of emotional reactions: *protest*, followed by *despair*, followed by *detachment*. If the attachment figure returns after this, the child may react with indifference, even hostility.

Children subjected to maternal deprivation, whether because their mothers are physically unavailable (due to death, incarceration, or abandonment) or emotionally unavailable (due to postpartum depression poor parenting skills), frequently display these characteristic depressive symptoms. In contrast, when a parent remains present but demonstrates behavior toward the child that is abusive, rejecting, or fear-inducing, the child's attachment behaviors toward that parent may actually *increase*.

Psychoanalytic theory postulates that the quality of one's early attachments exerts great influence on the quality of one's later attachments, especially later attachments to significant figures (such as teachers, employers, lovers, or children). Adolescents and adults also tend to *recreate their earlier relationships*, even when the earlier attachment figures were abusive or rejecting. Having formed only *insecure attachments* earlier in life, the individual in later life risks experiencing feelings of low self-esteem, anxiety, and depression in the context of their later relationships. Their interpersonal style usually is characterized by excessive dependency, lack of trust, and fears of being rejected or abandoned.

However, opportunities may remain to redress such deficits. If the individual, later in life, *is* able to achieve such a sense of security with a stable attachment figure, this might provide—in the words of analyst Franz Alexander—a "corrective emotional experience." Thus, the child initially brought up in an abusive home environment, who is removed from this home and placed into a caring foster home and who also receives support from schoolteachers, may demonstrate improvement in his emotional and social functioning.

Similarly, one goal of psychoanalytic psychotherapy is to allow the patient to form a secure emotional attachment to the therapist while *refusing* to allow the patient to sabotage the relationship by recreating earlier pathological attachments. In doing so, the therapy aims to provide a corrective emotional experience. It also provides an opportunity for the patient to examine misperceptions about the outside world, especially as they become more apparent in this relationship. Ultimately, the patient may both achieve both a greater sense of security and may be able to modify dysfunctional attitudes.

How does the analytic therapist avoid being sucked into an inappropriate and potentially damaging relationship? One way is by striving to maintain a *neutral stance*. "Therapeutic neutrality" does not require that the therapist be cold or indifferent (although this is the popular misconception); rather, it requires that the therapist be caring while avoiding "taking sides." When the patient attempts to recreate a dysfunctional relationship by behaving in seductive, angry, or manipulative ways, the therapist attempts to point this out to the patient through the appropriate (i.e., noninjurious) use of *interpretation* while abstaining from responding in kind. For example, the therapist might point out that the patient appears to be *displacing* feelings held toward earlier attachment figures onto the therapist, a process called **transference**.

The therapist in turn attempts to avoid the trap of responding in kind to the patient's provocative behavior, a process called **countertransference**. For example, the patient may "test the limits" of the therapist's support. He might engage in immature or insulting behavior or might refuse to take medication, to abstain from alcohol, or to abstain from self-injurious behavior. The patient is goading the therapist, and if the therapist responds by becoming angry and rejecting, that will simply confirm the patient's worldview. The therapist will have been proven to be "just like everybody else." Surprisingly, the patient often demonstrates little or no recognition that he has *provoked* this situation.

The object relations model of depression is conceptually stronger than the traditional Freudian one. We have already noted that several studies have shown that people who lose their mother during childhood are at greater risk for becoming depressed later in life, and we have also noted the association between depression and the more recent loss of a significant attachment figure (i.e., in the setting of grief). A particular strength of this model is its usefulness when working with patients with comorbid depression and personality disorder who who experience chronic, more "characterologic" depressive symptoms in the setting of ongoing interpersonal difficulties.

However, such data don't "prove" that depression is psychological in origin. For example, early loss and bereavement might neurophysiologically "prime" the brain to experience similar responses later in life. Or, since depression runs in families, children who have a depressed parent may also be more likely to experience psychological or physical abandonment (through neglect or even through the suicide of the parent).

Time-Limited Psychodynamic Therapies

Traditional psychoanalytic psychotherapy is intensive and sets broad, ambitious goals. It requires frequent patient-therapist interaction (up to several times per week) over an extended period of time (sometimes years). It attempts to tap into the patient's unconscious thoughts by discouraging the censoring of unacceptable or embarrassing material, a technique called **free association**. This high degree of intensity and intimacy encourages the patient to develop strong transference feelings, both **negative transference** (irrational or excessive anger toward the therapist) and **positive transference** (irrational idealization of the therapist, who might come to be seen as infallible or all-caring).

The therapist attempts to remain neutral while assisting the patient to analyze these feelings. Note that some of the patient's complaints about

the therapist might be appropriate and reality based. (For example, the patient might be justifiably annoyed if the therapist habitually starts appointments late or appears distracted during sessions.) The therapist therefore must also attempt to distinguish transferential feelings from reasonable criticisms, which requires respect for the patient and honest introspection.

Many patients simply aren't able to tolerate such an intensive form of therapy, particularly patients with more severe psychopathology. Others don't wish to commit that much time and money. Further, many insurance companies aren't willing to invest in longer-term, more intensive psychotherapy. Given this, various psychoanalytically based (also called psychodynamic) **short-term therapies** have been devised. They share several features.

First, they all involve a *greater degree of participation by the therapist* than is the case in classical psychoanalysis. The therapist actively collaborates with the patient and—in the case of depression—provides education about depression. Second, the *scope of therapy is deliberately more limited*. Early on, one or two particular occupational or relationship problems are delineated and selected to be the primary focus of the therapy.

Third, *free association is discouraged*, since it can contribute to patients becoming more regressed. In traditional therapy, regression and the "acting out" of childhood problems within the therapy sessions are seen as necessary challenges that the patient must "work through" if she hopes to achieve longer-term therapeutic progress. In short-term therapy, they are viewed as impasses. Fourth, while the therapy still emphasizes the analysis of the patient's attitudes toward significant attachment figures—particularly as they play out in the patient's "transference" toward the therapist—*transference is more explicitly addressed almost from the outset of the therapy*.

Short-term therapies may be *close-ended*. In other words, the therapist may prescribe a fixed number of sessions, usually around 12 sessions, sometimes as many as 24 sessions. This stands in contrast to traditional therapy, which is open-ended and indeterminate in duration. When patients know that therapy is scheduled to terminate at a specific date, it "concentrates" the entire process (the forming of a therapeutic alliance, the working through of problems, and the need to deal with feelings of abandonment and resent-ment in the face of the impending termination of therapy). It also discourages the patient from re-gressing or from becoming excessively depend-ent on the therapist.

The short-term psychodynamic psychotherapy that has received the most empirical study is **interpersonal psychotherapy (IPT)**. First de-scribed in 1984 by Gerald Klerman and Myrna Weissman, this approach attempts to merge Bowlby's concepts with current psychobiologi-cal theories of depression. IPT views depression as a medical illness, but as one with both bio-logical and psychological roots. Given this, it encourages the physician to tell the depressed pa-tient that he has an illness and to prescribe med-ication in more severe cases, but it also encour-ages the physician to link the patient's depression to his interpersonal situation and to offer psy-chotherapy aimed at addressing dysfunctional at-titudes. It doesn't view these two approaches as coming into conflict. For example, it doesn't view medication as a "Band-Aid" fix that re-lieves the patient of the incentive to address un-derlying psychological issues.

IPT, like other psychodynamic therapies, em-phasizes how the depressed person relates to the significant figures around her, and postulates that one's current ability to form meaningful inter-personal attachments has been shaped by early childhood relationships and reinforced by all subsequent significant relationships. IPT pro-poses that the patient's ability to engage in sat-isfying relationships became even more dis-rupted at some point shortly before the onset of depressive symptoms by a recent life event. The four most common disruptive events are unre-solved grief, interpersonal role disputes, role transitions, and interpersonal deficits.

In *unresolved grief*, depression occurs follow-ing a significant loss and persists despite the pas-sage of time beyond what would be expected for acute bereavement. Depression also can arise in the setting of *interpersonal role disputes*—that is, arguments that occur within a relationship where each person has a different view of what each party's role should be. Examples include marital disputes, parent–child disputes, em-ployer–employee or coworker disputes, or dis-putes within the extended family or within a net-work of friends.

For some patients, depression begins in the setting of a *role transition*. High school or col-lege graduation, leaving home, entering the mil-itary, entering the labor force, being promoted or demoted, losing a job, marrying, divorcing, hav-ing a child, moving to a new state, and retiring all require an individual to relinquish an old role and make the transition to a new one. Some pa-tients find this particularly difficult.

Finally, some patients have significant *inter-personal deficits*. They lack the skills for initiat-ing meaningful relationships because they lack a repertoire of interpersonal skills. They tend to be shy, isolated, and lonely. Some of them have the skills to initiate attachments but cannot sustain them, particularly close ones when the attach-ments require commitment, intimacy, and ex-pectations of fidelity and loyalty.

In IPT, the first goal is to appropriately diag-nose the patient's depression through a detailed history and mental status examination. Second, the clinician provides the patient with education about depression, emphasizing that it has both biological and psychological underpinnings. In more severe cases, pharmacotherapy is offered early in the course of treatment. However, the clinician also offers an interpersonal formulation to the patient and explores the four areas outlined above with the patient. In contrast to traditional psychodynamic therapies, the assessment em-phasizes *current* relationships, especially re-cently disrupted ones. The clinician and the pa-tient agree on a preliminary formulation and an explicit treatment plan. This latter includes which specific target symptoms of depression will be fol-lowed, which specific area of interpersonal func-tioning will be addressed in psychotherapy, and how medications will be utilized.

A 53-year-old college professor presents for treat-ment of recurrent depression. The patient describes his premorbid personality as perfectionistic and self-critical but he is also cognizant of his above-average intelligence and his occupational success. He tends to become more anxious and irritable when under stress. The patient reports a history of previous depressive episodes at ages 25 and 31. These episodes, as well as the current episode, all have been characterized by sadness, anxiety and rumination, anhedonia, decreased energy, poor ap-petite with mild weight loss, passive death wishes, and sleep disturbance (middle insomnia with early morning awakening at about 4:30 or 5:00 AM). The patient notes that, despite his symptoms, he has continued to be able to work (although less efficiently), and casual acquaintances might not know that he is depressed, as he has remained able to maintain normal social behavior.

His first episode of depression occurred in the setting of his feeling stressed while completing his doctoral dissertation while also having "relationship difficulties." He recovered spontaneously after several months without clinical intervention. The second episode occurred in the setting of occupational stress (having to teach several classes while also trying to finish a book.) He was treated with psychotherapy with only partial relief of symptoms, followed by treatment with the tricyclic antidepressant imipramine over several months, with some further improvement in his symptoms. He did well after this for several years without any further need for clinical intervention.

The patient's wife died of ovarian cancer 3 years ago, and after this he experienced moderate symptoms of grief as well as some difficulties adjusting to living without her. However, he distinguishes these feelings from symptoms experienced during his depressive episodes, both in quality and intensity. He felt that he was coping well overall until several months ago, in the context of dating a woman in her late 30s. He describes this as having been an intense relationship that was satisfying sexually but that left him feeling "more anxious than content" because of his guilt over their age difference and different frames of reference, and also because this woman was a much more emotional person than himself, which led her to accuse him of being detached and to him feeling that she was overly "dramatic." After 10 months, after she pressed for them to move in together, he broke off the relationship. Following this, he found himself beginning to experience his typical depressive symptoms. He has continued to date intermittently but has continued to dwell on the recent breakup. He also has just finished a book that required several years of research and is not sure that he has anything left to say in his field of study. He could continue to "repackage" previous lectures, but he knows that this would not be intellectually satisfying.

The patient's primary care physician initially prescribed the antidepressant fluoxetine, which provided partial relief of his depressive symptoms but also was associated with worsening of his insomnia and complaints of erectile dysfunction. The patient encountered similar difficulties during a trial of another antidepressant, venlafaxine. At this point, the patient was referred for psychiatric consultation.

The psychiatrist discusses the diagnosis of major depressive disorder. She and the patient agree to a trial of the antidepressant bupropion since this agent is less likely to cause sexual dysfunction than serotonin reuptake inhibitors such as fluoxetine and venlafaxine. The psychiatrist also prescribes a short-term course of a benzodiazepine hypnotic agent to address the patient's insomnia.

The patient also agrees to a course of psychotherapy aimed at elucidating and addressing life circumstances that might be associated with his depressive episodes, particularly role transitions. Over the next several weeks, the patient is encouraged to recognize and accept painful emotions associated with the losses of both his wife and of his girlfriend. He examines his ambivalence toward his ex-girlfriend and is encouraged to explore what for him would constitute a "successful" romantic relationship. He becomes more accepting of his ex-girlfriend's personality, but also feels more comfortable that his decision to end their relationship had been the correct one. He also explores the role that academic success has played throughout his adult life and his fears that if he can't sustain his previous degree of success his life will no longer have "purpose." After several weeks, he reports both an improved mood and an increased sense of mastery in his attitudes toward interpersonal and professional issues.

Like other short-term dynamic therapies, IPT is time-limited and sets limited goals. It doesn't attempt to modify the patient's underlying personality structure and instead emphasizes symptomatic relief through education and medication. Further distinguishing IPT from psychoanalysis is its focus on current rather than past relationships and on interpersonal rather than intrapsychic phenomena. While the therapist may notice that the patient engages in characteristic unconscious defenses (such as denial, projection, or repression), she doesn't allow exploration of these defenses to become the *focus* of the therapy. Rather, the therapist tries to keep the discussion centered on specific "here and now" interpersonal conflicts and stressors and on the use of appropriate coping skills.

In further contrast to traditional analytic therapy, the goals of interpersonal therapy and the steps that will be taken to achieve them are very explicit. In fact, "how to" manuals have been written. These in turn have allowed IPT to be studied through objective research protocols, which have documented the efficacy of IPT in a variety of patient populations, in a variety of settings, and in head-to-head comparisons with medication therapy, cognitive psychotherapy, and no therapy.

Some of these studies have demonstrated that, regardless of whether they are treated with talk therapy or medication therapy, depressed patients are at greater risk of relapsing if therapy is discontinued. In the case of interpersonal psychotherapy, therapeutic gains are more likely to be maintained if, following an initial "index" course of the psychotherapy, the patient returns for "maintenance" or "booster" sessions (typically one session every few weeks).

IPT was first studied as a short-term individual psychotherapy for patients with major depressive disorder. Since then, however, its effectiveness has been demonstrated in other settings and with other patient populations. For example, it has been used for patients receiving group psychotherapy for bulimia nervosa, for patients receiving long-term psychotherapy for chronic dysthymic disorder, and for patients in the primary care setting with depression complicating a chronic medical illness.

The Cognitive–Behavioral Model

Like Klerman and Weissman, Aaron Beck was trained as a psychoanalyst. In the early 1960s, he became frustrated with the limited results he obtained using analytic methods to treat his depressed patients. He saw little evidence in these patients of "anger turned inward." However, he did notice that depressed patients tended to express similar types of thoughts. These thoughts weren't really "unconscious." They were more unnoticed, or unappreciated. He therefore called these *automatic thoughts*.

> A 36-year-old secretary presents for treatment of depression. She discusses how ineffective she is at getting through the day at work, and how she feels that she is disappointing everybody around her. The clinician asks her to describe in detail a period of time while at work when she felt especially sad:

PATIENT: I gave the typed dictation to my boss, and he pointed out where I had spelled some words wrong.
CLINICIAN: How did you feel when he did this?
PATIENT: Oh, just awful.
CLINICIAN: What thoughts were going through your head right at that moment?
PATIENT: I just felt like a total failure, like, "I just can't do anything right. I'm letting him down."

CLINICIAN: Did your boss actually say that you were letting him down?
PATIENT: Well . . . he never said it, but he seemed sort of annoyed when he pointed them out.
CLINICIAN: Are you the only one to whom he acts that way?
PATIENT: Not really. I mean he's kind of curt in general. But that's just the way he is.
CLINICIAN: Are there any times that he's ever done the opposite? Complimented you on your work?
PATIENT: Sometimes he says I've done a good job.
CLINICIAN: You feel sad when he criticizes you. Do you feel happy when he praises you?
PATIENT: (Laughs.) Not really.
CLINICIAN: What thoughts are going through your head when he praises you?
PATIENT: I guess I'm thinking, "He's just taking pity on me. He's just trying to be nice."
CLINICIAN: So, let me get this right. When he criticizes you he really means it, but when he praises you he doesn't really mean it?
PATIENT: (Hesitates.) I guess so. I guess that's kind of stupid on my part to think that way.
CLINICIAN: No, not stupid at all. But it is something worth questioning together. Why don't we examine the *evidence* to try to get a better sense of whether this really is the objective reality of the situation? But, before we do this, let me ask you something else. We've been discussing your perceptions of what your boss is thinking about you when you make a mistake. How about yourself? What are your thoughts about yourself when you make a mistake?
PATIENT: Oh, God. I feel like, "I'm just a total screwup. I'm going to get fired."
CLINICIAN: Do you feel that's being fair to yourself? Let's assume that *everybody* makes *some* mistakes—is that a fair assumption?
PATIENT: Sure.
CLINICIAN: Okay, so in your case, how many mistakes would you say is a reasonable number, an acceptable number, of mistakes to make *before* you allow yourself to get upset with yourself?
PATIENT: I'm not sure I've ever thought about it that way.

This dialogue demonstrates several features of cognitive therapy (CT). First, like interpersonal therapy, its focus is on the patient's "here and now" functioning rather than on distant childhood causes of the current problems or on the biochemical changes caused by depression. (Again, it's not that these factors aren't important; they simply aren't the focus of the therapy.) However, unlike IPT, CT doesn't emphasize the patient's current interpersonal role dispute with her employer. Rather, it focuses on how the patient experiences certain characteristic, negative, *automatic thoughts* when she is faced with certain types of situations.

The negative automatic thoughts most commonly encountered in depressed patients are listed in Table 7–10. Each of these thoughts can be recognized in the above dialogue. In cognitive therapy, the depressed mood is viewed as being secondary to negative thoughts, rather than the other way around. When the patient sees that her mood rapidly improves after having challenged negative thoughts, it gives her immediate, positive feedback.

A second feature of CT that makes it similar to IPT is that here, too, the therapist takes an active role in educating the patient about depression and in challenging maladaptive attitudes. In both forms of therapy, the therapist emphasizes that it isn't *external life events* that "cause" the patient's to feel sad; rather, the patient feels sad because of how she *perceives* and *interprets* these life events. While the patient may have come to believe that she has no say over her attitudes, over the course of therapy this belief is called into question. CT calls this questioning

Table 7–10. Typical Automatic Thoughts with Depression

Automatic Thought	Definition
Selective abstraction ("mental filter")	Drawing a conclusion based on only a small portion of the data
Arbitrary inference	Drawing a conclusion based on inadequate data or ignoring contradictory data
Absolutist ("all or none") thinking	Rigid dichotomies; patient is all good or all bad, perfect or completely flawed, a success or a total failure, etc.
Magnification and minimization	Overvaluing flaws, negative life events, or future bad outcomes, while undervaluing strengths, positive events, or potential good outcomes
Personalization	Taking blame or self-criticizing for events that are outside of one's control
Catastrophic thinking	Predicting the worst possible outcome while ignoring more likely events

Table 7–11. Recognizing Automatic Thoughts

Situation	Automatic Thoughts
Call from boss to submit a report	I can't do this. I don't know what to do. It won't be acceptable
My wife asks me to help more around the house	Nothing I do is ever enough. She thinks I don't try.
Car won't start	I was stupid to buy this car. Nothing works right anymore. This is the last straw.

Source: Reproduced with permission from Wright JH, Beck AT: "Cognitive Therapy." *American Psychiatric Press Textbook of Psychiatry*, 3rd edition. Edited by Hales, RE, Yudofsky SC, Talbott JA. Washington, DC, American Psychiatric Press, 1999.

process *collaborative empiricism*. The therapist and patient work as partners to examine the patient's automatic thoughts to see if they do in fact "hold water." The thoughts are treated as hypotheses that the patient—after having examined them objectively—might choose to retain without change, to modify, or to reject.

CT attempts to help patients learn to recognize these cognitive errors not only during therapy sessions but in the course of their daily lives. Patients often are asked to perform written "homework" assignments. First, patients are educated about automatic thoughts and about how they are closely associated with mood swings. Then, patients may be instructed to carry a pad around and to write down negative thoughts as soon as they are noticed. An example is given in Table 7–11. Next, patients are asked to try to challenge these thoughts and to note how doing so affects their moods. Table 7–12 presents one such patient's worksheet.

Finally, the therapist teachers the patient to recognize underlying maladaptive *cognitive schemas*. Schemas are deeper cognitive structures that contain a person's basic rules for screening, filtering, and coding information from the environment. They are formed in the course of early childhood experiences and modified as a result of subsequent formative influences. While schemas can be highly adaptive, most patients with psychiatric disorders demonstrate clusters of maladaptive schemas that perpetuate their dysphoric moods and their ineffective or

Table 7-12. Example of Daily Record of Dysfunctional Thoughts

Situation	Automatic Thought(s)	Emotion(s)	Rational Response	Outcome
Describe: a. Actual event leading to unpleasant emotion, *or* b. Stream of thoughts, daydream, or recollection, leading to unpleasant emotion, *or* c. Unpleasant physiologic sensations	a. Write automatic thought(s) that preceded emotion(s); rate belief in automatic thought(s), 0%–100%	a. Specify sad, anxious, angry, etc. b. Rate degree of emotion, 1%–100%	a. Identify cognitive errors b. Write rational response to automatic thought(s) c. Rate belief in rational response, 0%–100%	a. Once again, rate belief in automatic thought(s), 0%–100% b. Specify and rate subsequent emotion(s), 0–100%
Date: 4/15/93 I wake up and I'm immediately troubled, I start to worry about work	1. I can't face another day (90%) 2. The big project is due in 2 weeks; I'll never get it done (100%) 3. Everybody knows I'm ready to fall apart (90%) 4. It's hopeless (85%)	Sad (90%) Anxious (80%)	1. Magnification. Even though it has been rough, I have been able to get to work every day. Get a shower and make breakfast that will get things started (80%) 2. Catastrophizing, all or nothing thinking. About half of the work is done. Don't panic. Break it down into pieces. Taking one step at a time helps (95%) 3. Overgeneralization, magnification. Some people know I've been in trouble, but they haven't gotten down on me. I'm the one who puts me down. (95%) 4. Magnification. I know my job well and have a good track record. If I stick with this, I can probably make it. (90%)	Sad (30%) Anxious (40%)

Source: Adapted with permission from Wright JH, Beck AT: "Cognitive Therapy." *American Psychiatric Press Textbook of Psychiatry*, 3rd edition. Edited by Hales, RE, Yudofsky SC, Talbott JA. Washington, DC, American Psychiatric Press, 1999.

Table 7–13. Adaptive and Maladaptive Schemas

Adaptive Schemas	Maladaptive Schemas
No matter what happens, I can manage somehow	I must be perfect to be accepted
If I can work at something, I can master it	If I choose to do something, I must succeed
I'm a survivor	I'm a fake
Others can trust me	Without a woman, I'm nothing
I'm lovable	I'm stupid
People respect me	No matter what I do, I won't succeed
I can figure things out	Others can't be trusted
If I prepare in advance, I usually do better	I never can be comfortable around others
I like to be challenged	If I make a mistake, I'll lose everything
There's not much that can scare me	The world is too frightening for me

Source: Reproduced with permission from Wright JH, Beck AT: "Cognitive Therapy." *American Psychiatric Press Textbook of Psychiatry*, 3rd Edition. Edited by Hales, RE, Yudofsky SC, Talbott JA. Washington, DC, American Psychiatric

self-defeating behaviors. Examples of common adaptive and maladaptive schemas are listed in Table 7–13.

Maladaptive schemas can lie dormant until they are triggered by stressful life events, at which point they influence more "superficial" cognitive processing such that automatic thoughts occur that are consistent with the rules of the underlying schema. This theory applies primarily to episodic disorders such as depression and anxiety disorders. In chronic conditions such as personality disorder, schemas that pertain to the self are more consistently apparent and may prove to be more resistant to change.

CT, like IPT, lends itself to greater standardization and to empirical research. To date, it is the most extensively studied psychotherapy. For example, in the National Institute of Mental Health (NIMH) Treatment of Depression Collaborative Research Program, 250 outpatients with major depressive disorder were randomly assigned to one of four groups for 16 weeks of treatment: IPT, CT, imipramine plus routine clinical management, and placebo plus routine clinical management. While all four treatment conditions were associated with significant improvement in depressive symptoms, subjects assigned to the two psychotherapy groups and to the imipramine group all improved to a significantly greater extent than did those assigned to the placebo group. For *severely depressed patients*, while both IPT and CT performed significantly better than placebo, subjects in the imipramine group had the best outcome, and also experienced more rapid improvement. However,

subjects in the CT group demonstrated the most *sustained* improvement when followed up 18 months after the study was completed. (Their relapse rate was 36%, as opposed to 50% for patients in the imipramine group.)

CT, like IPT, has also been shown to be helpful in preventing recurrence of depressive episodes through the use of "maintenance visits" after completion of the acute course of psychotherapy. However, in more severe cases of depression the relapse rate for patients receiving maintenance CT remains higher than for patients maintained chronically on antidepressant medication.

In conclusion, research suggests that both IPT and CT are as effective as antidepressants for milder cases of major depressive disorder, while in more severe cases an antidepressant should be used. There is also some evidence to suggest that the *combination* of psychotherapy and medication has a synergistic effect, and this therefore is the practice of many clinicians, particularly in cases that have proven to be refractory to either treatment modality used alone.

The Biogenic Amine Model

Depression as a Disease

The above discussion has centered on theories emphasizing psychological factors that *contribute* to the development and perpetuation of mood disorders. However, these theories cannot fully account for the *existence* of mood disorders. Clinical depression is not the same as ordinary sadness, and several lines of evidence argue that mood disorders are best approached from the disease perspective. This evidence includes genetic studies, findings of associated abnormalities of biogenic amine and neuroendocrine systems, and findings suggesting diffuse and regional pathophysiologic changes.

Both major depressive disorder and bipolar disorder demonstrate a strong *genetic* component, as evidenced by family, twin, and adoption studies and by genetic linkage studies.

Family studies reveal that first-degree relatives of patients with bipolar disorder, compared to relatives of non-ill control subjects, are 4 to 18 times more likely to have bipolar disorder and 2 to 10 times more likely to have major depressive disorder. Similarly, first-degree relatives of patients with major depressive disorder have a 2 to 3 times greater risk of having major depressive disorder than do relatives of control subjects. (There may be an increased risk of having bipolar disorder but this isn't clear from available studies.) The finding that major depressive disorder is more common even in the relatives of bipolar disorder patients suggests a genetic link between these two illnesses. About half of all patients with bipolar disorder have one parent who also has a mood disorder, usually major depressive disorder. Conversely, if one parent has bipolar I disorder, his or her child has a 25% chance of developing a mood disorder (about half of these will have bipolar I or II disorder, while the other half will have a unipolar depression), and if both parents have bipolar I disorder, the child has a 50%–75% chance of developing a mood disorder.

The problem with family studies is that the increased prevalence of an illness within a family also might be explained by other, nongenetic factors, such as a shared home environment, shared stressors, or learned behavior patterns. *Twin studies* attempt to control for this by comparing monozygotic (identical) and dizygotic (nonidentical) twins. The latter are raised as twins but do not share an identical genetic profile. Studies of both major depressive disorder and bipolar disorder show an average concordance rate for monozygotic twins of 60% as compared to an average concordance rate of only 12% for dizygotic twins. This finding suggests that genetic factors play a role in the familial aggregation of the illness. However, the finding that the concordance rate for monozygotic twins isn't 100%

suggests that genetic factors alone are not enough to account for a person developing the illness, and that environmental or psychological factors likely play a contributory role.

Adoption studies attempt to further control for the contributory role of such environmental variables by comparing patients with mood disorder who were adopted with those who weren't adopted. These studies reveal that the rate of mood disorder is the same in the biological parents of either adopted or nonadopted mood disorder patients. Further, the rate of mood disorder in the adoptive parents of adopted mood disorder patients is the same rate as is seen in the general population. Both of these findings argue for mood disorder having a strong genetic component.

Linkage studies, which examine restriction fragment length polymorphisms (RFLPs) in families with mood disorders, have presented conflicting results consistent with the hypothesis that mood disorders likely are a heterogeneous *group* of conditions that likely are polygenic in origin, with variable phenotypic penetrance. Different genes may play a contributory role in different families, or several affected sets of genes may interact with each other in complex ways, leading to the development of the illness. These studies, which have involved different populations, have identified genetic markers for mood disorder on chromosomes 5, 11, and X.

Chapter 4 reviewed several neurobiological theories of depression. These included: *(1) monoamine theories*, which related mood disorders to dysregulation of serotonin, norepinephrine, dopamine, and their respective neuroreceptors; *(2) non-monoamine theories*, which related mood disorders to dysregulation of other stress-regulatory systems including the glucocorticoid, neurotrophic, excitatory amino acid, and endocrine systems; *(3) global neurophysiologic theories*, which related mood disorders to dysregulation of dysregulation of neuronal electrolyte balance and circadian rhythms; and *(4) neurophysiologic theories*, which related mood disorders to abnormal activity in specific brain regions responsible for the regulation of emotion, particularly the dorsolateral and ventral prefrontal cortex, the cingulate gyrus, the basal ganglia, and the temporal lobes.

Chapter 4 then presented a *stress diathesis model* of mood disorder, represented in Figure

4–4. This model proposes that genetically predisposed individuals' first depressive or manic episode is triggered by provocative life circumstances, but that once the illness has been "kindled," neurophysiologic changes occur that perpetuate the illness. Episodes beget further episodes. The episodes then begin to occur closer together, become more independent of life events, and become more refractory to psychotherapeutic and pharmacologic interventions. The discussion of antidepressant and mood-stabilizing medications that follows is based upon the above conceptualization.

Antidepressant Medications and Monoamines

All antidepressants discovered to date affect the activity of one or more of three primary monoamine neurotransmitters: serotonin (5HT), norepinephrine, and dopamine. Monoamine oxidase inhibitors (MAOIs) increase levels of all three of these monoamines by inhibiting their metabolism, while all of the other antidepressants affect their neurotransmission either by blocking their reuptake proteins or having agonist or antagonist effects at their respective receptors.

Newer antidepressant medications are more *selective* for one or more of these neurotransmitter systems than are the tricyclic antidepressants (TCAs) and the MAOIs. As a result, they tend to be associated with fewer adverse side effects and with greater patient acceptance. However, none of the newer agents has demonstrated itself to be more *efficacious* than the older agents.

During the following discussion, it should be kept in mind that psychopharmacology is a rapidly evolving field and that this presentation is an oversimplification. The goal is simply to convey some basic principles, thereby allowing the reader to choose one pharmacologic agent over another (or to combine different agents in more refractory cases) with a more clear rationale.

Basic Principles of Antidepressant Pharmacology

None of the antidepressants takes effect rapidly, despite all of them exerting immediate effects either on one or more neurotransmitters or on their receptors. While most of these medications raise the intrasynaptic concentration of a neurotransmitter within a single dose, there is generally a lag of from 2 to 3 weeks before the onset of clinical effects, with a 6–8 week lag before the full antidepressant response is reached.

As discussed in Chapter 4, this delay in clinical action likely correlates with the time required for postsynaptic neurons to "adapt" to these medication-induced alterations in monoamine homeostasis. These adaptations likely include downregulation of postsynaptic β-noradrenergic receptors, downregulation of postsynaptic serotonin receptors (particularly 5-HT$_{2A}$ receptors), and postreceptor, intracecellular mechanisms such the increased expression of genes coding for critical proteins such as neurotrophins.

Not all patients respond to antidepressant medications, and many other patients are only "partial responders." While it would be tempting to hypothesize that "nonresponders" do not have a "biological" depression, one can't generalize about whether or not a patient has an illness based solely on whether his condition responds to currently available treatments. In some cases, past medication trials involved inadequate dosages of medication. In other cases, medication trials have been too brief or have been limited by side effects. Finally, it is likely that some patients simply have a more refractory form of depression. Many clinicians have found that treatment-refractory patients require serial trials of different classes of agents, combinations of different medications, or treatment with electroconvulsive therapy.

All antidepressants provide similar response rates. In the average controlled clinical antidepressant trial, about two out of three patients respond to antidepressant treatment. The remaining one-third of patients are considered to have been "nonresponders." In contrast, about one out of three patients respond to treatment with a placebo ("placebo responders"), while the other two-thirds are considered to be "placebo nonresponders."). Note that some of the "actual drug" response may also include superimposed placebo effects.

While one-third of patients on average are "nonresponders" across clinical trials, this is not to say that that this would be the *same* one-third of patients across trials involving different medications. Given this, when a patient either doesn't respond to a medication or only demonstrates a partial response, they might still achieve a clinical response by *switching* to an alternative medication (perhaps one from a different chemical class) or by *augmenting* the first drug with a second, additional medication.

The U.S. Food and Drug Administration defines **response** in randomized clinical trials as a greater than 50% reduction in symptom severity on a standardized rating instrument such as the Hamilton Rating Scale for Depression. However, keep in mind that response is not the same as **remission**. The latter refers to *full recovery* from depression. Obviously, this is the goal in real-world settings. For example, a patient who presents with a very high depression score might experience a 50% reduction in symptoms (and thus be considered a "responder") but her score might remain so high that the next day she would still be ill enough to qualify for another clinical trial. While two-thirds of patients enrolled in the average antidepresssant trial are responders, only about two-thirds of these respondors achieve a state of remission.

Patients in the real-world setting of clinical practice are looking for more than 50% reductions in their symptoms. They want to be well again. Research backs up the validity of their desire. Responders who have not achieved remission continue to experience significant impairment in their occupational and social functioning. Further, patients who achieve response without remission also have a much higher rate of relapse into another depressive episode than do patients who achieve remission.

Given this, current antidepressant therapy leaves something to be desired. About 10% of patients in clinical trials are unable to tolerate the side effects of the medication and drop out of the trial. One-third of the remaining patients don't achieve a clinical response. One-third of the remaining group show a greater than 50% reduction in their symptoms but continue to suffer with depressive symptoms. True, some patients are diagnosed with depression by their primary care physician and achieve a prompt and gratifying response to their very first medication trial. However, many depressed patients treated in the primary care setting—and virtually *all* of the patients referred to a psychiatrist for more specialized care—are "treatment refractory." In these cases, serial medication trials, medication combinations, and medication–psychotherapy combinations are the norm.

Table 7–14 lists the primary agents used to

Table 7–14. Antidepressants Grouped by Presumed Mechanism of Action

MAO INHIBITORS

Irreversible Inhibitors of MAO-A and -B

    Phenelzine (Nardil)
    Tranylcypromine (Parnate)

Reversible Inhibitors of MAO-A (RIMAs)

    Moclobemide

TRICYCLIC ANTIDEPRESSANTS

Tertiary Amine Tricyclics

    Imipramine (Tofranil)
    Amitriptyline (Elavil)
    Doxepin (Sinequan)
    Trimipramine (Surmontil)
    Clomipramine (Anafranil)

Secondary Amine Tricyclics

    Desipramine (Norpramin)
    Nortriptyline (Pamelor)
    Protriptyline (Vivactil)
    Maprotiline (Ludiomil)

SELECTIVE SEROTONIN REUPTAKE INHIBITORS (SSRIS):

    Fluoxetine (Prozac)
    Sertraline (Zoloft)
    Paroxetine (Paxil)
    Fluvoxamine (Luvox)
    Citalopram (Celexa)
    Escitalopram (Lexapro)

SELECTIVE NOREPINEPHRINE REUPTAKE INHIBITOR (NRI)

    Reboxetine (Vestra)

DOPAMINE–NOREPINEPHRINE REUPTAKE INHIBITOR (DNRI)

    Bupropion (Wellbutrin)

SEROTONIN–NOREPINEPHRINE REUPTAKE INHIBITOR (SNRI)

    Venlafaxine (Effexor)
    Duloxetine (Cymbalta)

SEROTONIN (5-HT$_2$) ANTAGONIST/REUPTAKE INHIBITORS

    Trazodone (Desyrel)
    Nefazodone (Serzone)

SEROTONIN (5-HT$_2$ AND 5-HT$_3$) ANTAGONIST AND ALPHA-2 ANTAGONIST

    Mirtazepine (Remeron)

SEROTONIN (5HT$_{1A}$) PARTIAL AGONIST

    Buspirone (BuSpar)

MONOAMINE RELEASING AGENTS ("STIMULANTS")

    Dextroamphetamine (Dexedrine)
    Methylphenidate (Ritalin, Concerta, Metadate)
    Pemoline (Cylert)
    Amphetamine Mixture (Adderall)

Table 7–15. Comparison of Mechanism of Action of Different Antidepressants

Mechanism	Tertiary TCA	Secondary TCA	SSRI	Bupropion	Venlafaxine	Nefazodone	Mirtazapine
5HT uptake inhibition	*Yes*	No (slight)	*Yes*	No	*Yes*	*Yes*	No
5HT$_2$ blockade	No (slight)	No	No	No	No	*Yes*	*Yes*
5HT$_3$ blockade	No	No	No	No	No	No	*Yes*
NE uptake inhibition	*Yes*	*Yes*	No	*Yes*	*Yes*	No	No
Alpha-1 NE blockade	No (slight)	No	No	No	No	*Yes*	No
Alpha-2 NE blockade	No	No	No	No	No	No	*Yes*
Histamine-1 blockade	*Yes*	No	No	No	No	No	*Yes*
Acetylcholine blockade	*Yes*	Yes (mild)	No	No	No	No	No

Italics indicate clinically significant differences.

treat mood disorders, grouped by presumed mechanism of action. Table 7–15 presents a summary of relevant receptor effects. Finally, some prescribing guidelines are offered in Table 7–16.

The older antidepressants (the TCAs and MAOIs) are "dirtier"—that is, they act not only at the desired site of action but also at various other receptors, including the histamine, muscarinic, and α-1 and α-2 adrenergic receptors. This additional receptor activity accounts for many of their side effects (Table 7–17). More recently introduced, more "selective" antidepressants, while "cleaner," come with their own side effects. For example, the TCAs and MAOI are sedating and constipating due to their antihistaminergic and anticholinergic effects, but these effects *balanced* the tendency of increased norepinephrine and serotonin to cause nervousness, insomnia, diarrhea, nausea, and headache. Thus, newer drugs such as the SSRIs and venlafaxine more often cause these latter side effects. (Fortunately, these side effects most often are relatively mild and also are more likely to be transient than the antihistaminergic and anticholinergic side effects associated with the older agents.)

Monoamine Oxidase Inhibitors

The two MAOIs currently available in the United States, **phenelzine (Nardil) and tranylcypromine (Parnate)** bind *irreversibly* to the enzyme monoamine oxidase in the presynaptic neuron, thereby "poisoning" it and preventing it from metabolizing norepinephrine, dopamine, serotonin, leading to an increase in synaptic levels of these transmitters. MAOIs do not directly affect monoamine receptors or reuptake. While these medications are the oldest agents, they are

powerful antidepressants. Psychiatrists rarely prescribe them these days, though, for several reasons.

First, MAOIs are associated with virtually all of the side effects listed in Table 7–17. While free of anticholinergic side effects, they commonly cause a frustrating combination of insomnia and daytime somnolence, clinically significant hypotension (including orthostatic hypotension), anorgasmia, weight gain, myoclonus, and pedal edema. However, the major factor that relegates the MAOIs to "last resort" drug status in the minds of most clinicians is their potential to cause both the **tyramine ("cheese") reaction** and the **serotonin syndrome**.

There are two forms of monoamine oxidase, MAO-A and MAO-B. *MAO-A* metabolizes serotonin, norepinephrine, dopamine, and tyramine. *MAO-B* doesn't affect serotonin or norepinephrine and is thought to convert some amine substrates (protoxins) into toxins that can damage neurons. Traditional MAOIs irreversibly inhibit both MAO-A and -B. It takes 2 weeks following MAOI discontinuation for new MAO to be synthesized and put into effect.

Shortly after psychiatrists began prescribing these medications in the early 1960s, reports began to appear of some patients suffering from severe hypertensive reactions, in some cases leading to cerebral hemorrhage. It turned out that these patients had ingested foods high in *tyramine*. Tyramine is a precursor of norepinephrine, which in turn is a pressor. Normally, MAO destroys any excess norepinephrine but since this activity is irreversibly inhibited by the MAOI, patients can experience severe hypertension when exposed to certain foods. To help prevent

Table 7–16. Clinical Characteristics of Antidepressants

Class	Medication	Usual Adult Daily Dosage (mg/day)	Side Effects	Comments
TCA	Imipramine	100–300	Dry eyes/mouth, constipation, urinary retention, somnolence, orthostatic hypotension, sexual dysfunction, arrhythmia (tertiary tricyclics are more serotonergic, more antihistaminergic, anticholinergic, and antiadrenergic and so have more side effects than secondary tricyclics)	Also effective for chronic pain (usually amitriptyline or nortriptyline) and clomipramine is approved for OCD (maximum dose of 250 mg with clomipramine due to increased risk of seizures); titration to final dose required; QHS dosing minimizes daytime sedation; All TCAs can be fatal in overdose (>2000 mg, which is less than a 2 week supply), can slow cardiac conduction and lower seizure threshold; serotonin syndrome can occur when combined with MAOIs (2 week washout recommended when switching between TCAs and MAOIs); monitoring plasma level useful (with amitriptyline or imipramine, aim for "amitriptyline + nortriptyline" or "imipramine + desipramine" levels of 150–250; with nortriptyline or desipramine alone, aim for levels of 50–150, with this being a "therapeutic window" for nortriptyline)
	Amitriptyline	75–300		
	Doxepin	75–300		
	Trimipramine	75–300		
	Clomipramine	75–250		
	Desipramine	75–300		
	Nortriptyline	50–150		
	Protriptyline	20–60		
	Maprotiline	100–225		
MAOI	Phenelzine	30–90	Restlessness, dizziness, blurred vision, diarrhea, sedation, insomnia, weakness, arrhythmia, headache, sexual dysfunction	Also effective in panic disorder and phobic disorders; twice daily dosing; strict dietary cautions required; avoid in patients with cardiac or cerebrovascular disease; avoid amphetamines, asthma inhalers (except pure steroid inhalers), cold and sinus medications, narcotics (except codeine), sympathomimetics dopaminergic medications, antihistamines; avoid combinations with other antidepressants (stop MAOI at least 2 weeks before starting others; stop others at least 2 weeks before starting MAOI, 5 weeks for Prozac)
	Tranylcypramine	20–60		
SSRI	Fluoxetine	10–80	Nausea, diarrhea, anxiety, restlessness, dizziness, insomnia, headache, low libido, orgasmic delay/ anorgasmia	Also effective in panic disorder, generalized anxiety disorder, OCD, eating disorder, social phobia, post-traumatic stress disorder, premenstrual dysphoric disorder; low doses may be effective for many patients, higher doses in bulimia nervosa, OCD, and impulse control problems; many patients can start at final dose, but initial side effects can be minimized by giving half-doses for several days; fluoxetine's long half-life minimizes SSRI withdrawal and can improve long-term compliance, but washout takes longer; citalopram and sertraline have least potential for cytochrome-related drug interactions paroxetine's shorter half-life increases risk of SSRI withdrawal); citalopram and fluvoxamine are the least highly protein-bound
	Sertraline	50–200		
	Paroxetine	20–60		
	Fluvoxamine	100–300		
	Citalopram	20–60		
	Escitalopram	10–20		

(*continued*)

Table 7–16. Clinical Characteristics of Antidepressants (*Continued*)

Class	Medication	Usual Adult Daily Dosage (mg/day)	Side Effects	Comments
	Bupropion BupropionSR	150–450 200–400	Anxiety, restlessness, insomnia	Also effective for smoking cessation, but not effective for panic disorder, generalized anxiety disorder, or OCD; activating effects are potentially useful in patients with psychomotor retardation and involve no significant risk of weight gain or sexual dysfunction; greater seizure risk at higher doses and peak blood levels (give regular form as 75–150 mg TID or SR form as 100–200 mg BID) and in vulnerable populations (avoid in patients with seizure disorder, brain injury, alcohol or drug withdrawal, and bulimia nervosa)
	Venlafaxine VenlafaxineXR	75–375 75–375	Similar to SSRIs; increased blood pressure at higher doses (clinical significance uncertain)	Also effective for panic disorder and generalized anxiety disorder (lower doses often as effective as higher doses in the latter); may allow for a higher remission rate in depression than SSRIs; primarily serotonergic at lower doses (75 mg), gaining noradrenergic effects at higher doses (150–225 mg) and then dopaminergic at highest doses (>300 mg), so increasing dose may enhance efficacy in refractory depression); BID–TID dosing for regular form, daily dosing for XR form
	Mirtazapine	15–60	Somnolence, fatigue, increased appetite, weight gain, dizziness, diarrhea, dry mouth	Lower risk of sexual dysfunction than SSRIs; appetite stimulation and weight gain may be useful for cachectic patients but unacceptable to other patients; has antiemetic effects; sedation may be greater at lower doses, mitigated by continued use and sometimes by increased dosage; may offer more rapid onset of response than SSRIs (perhaps due to early sedative/anxiolytic effects); QHS dosing
	Trazodone	150–600	Somnolence, dizziness, postural hypotension, headache, nausea, insomnia	Too sedating for many patients, but effective as a hypnotic (in range of 50–200 mg QHS) and for treatment of agitation in brain injury as alternative to antipsychotics; low (1:1000–1:10,000) risk of priapism
	Nefazodone	300–600	Same as trazodone, but less sedating	Less sedating than trazodone (and no reports of priapism), but often more than SSRIs, which minimizes need for concomitant hypnotic; gradual dose titration required to minimize side effects; BID dosing, but can also try shifting most or all of daily dose to bedtime if daytime sedation occurs lower risk of sexual dysfunction than SSRIs; avoid concomitant drugs metabolized by CYP3A4, since nefazodone increases their serum and have linear pharmacokinetics; levels and risk of cardiac arrhythmia; low risk of hepatotoxicity

Table 7–17. Side Effects of Various Antidepressants, by Receptor Activity

Receptor	Side Effects
Histamine (H-1)	Sedation, weight gain, hypotension, delirium
Ach muscarinic	Dry mouth/eyes, blurred vision, urinary retention, constipation, memory impairment, delirium, resting tachycardia
Alpha-1	Orthostatic hypotension, reflex tachycardia, potentiation of antihypertensive effect of prazosin
Alpha-2	Block antihypertensive effect of clonidine, methyldopa, guanfacine
5HT$_2$	Anxiety, insomnia, ejaculatory dysfunction, hypotension
5HT$_3$	Nausea, cramps, diarrhea

this, patients taking MAOIs must be given a list of which foods to avoid. Many clinicians also give the patient a supply of rapidly acting antihypertensive medication to carry with them, such as nifedipine, to help ensure rapid intervention if the patient experiences any symptoms that might indicate that a tyramine reaction is starting. More recently, foods on the classic food-restriction list have been analyzed for tyramine content and the restrictions have been relaxed a bit, as described in Table 7–18. (Of note, one item on the list, fava beans, actually is high not in tyramine but in L-dopa, the precursor to dopamine. The latter also acts as a pressor when it accumulates due to the absence of MAO activity.)

Another problem with MAOIs is that they can be dangerous when combined with other drugs that increase serotonin through serotonin reuptake inhibition, including the tricyclic antidepressants and the selective serotonin reuptake inhibitors. *Serotonin syndrome* likely is caused by overstimulation of the central serotonin receptors that regulate autonomic activity. This leads to a variety of effects, potentially including abdominal pain, diarrhea, sweats, fever, tachycardia, hypertension, myoclonus, irritability, hostility, mood changes, and delirium. Severe manifestations of the syndrome include hyperpyrexia, cardiovascular shock, and death.

To avoid precipitating a serotonin syndrome, clinicians should discontinue MAOIs 2 weeks before prescribing an SSRI (long enough to allow for synthesis of fresh monoamine oxidase). They should discontinue SSRIs five half-lives

Table 7–18. Sunnybrook Health Science Center MAOI Diet

Food Group	Food to Avoid	Food Allowed
Cheese	All matured or aged cheese all casseroles made with these cheeses (pizza, lasagna, etc.); all cheeses are considered matured or aged except those listed opposite	Fresh cottage cheese, cream cheese, ricotta cheese, processed cheese slices, fresh milk products (sour cream, yogurt, ice cream)
Meat fish, poultry	Fermented/dry sausage (pepperoni, salami, mortadella, summer sausage, etc.); improperly stored meat, fish, or poultry; improperly stored pickled herring	All fresh packaged or processed meat (e.g. chicken loaf, hot dogs), fish, or poultry; store in fridge immediately, eat ASAP
Fruits, vegetables	Fava or broad bean pods (not beans); banana peels	Banana pulp; all others except those listed opposite
Alcoholic beverages	All tap beers	No more than two domestic bottled or canned beers or two 4 oz glasses of wine (red or white) per day; also applies to nonalcoholic beer. (Note: red wine can produce a headache unrelated to increased BP)
Miscellaneous	Marmite concentrated yeast extract; sauerkraut; soy sauce and other soybean condiments	Other yeast extracts (e.g., brewer's yeast) Soy milk

Source: Adapted, with permission, from Gardner DM, Shulman KI, Walker SE, et al: "The Making of a User Friendly MAOI Diet." *J Clin Psychiatry* 57:99–104, 1996. Copyright 1996, Physicians Postgraduate Press.

(about 10–14 days) before initiating treatment with an MAOI. (The exception to this rule is fluoxetine, whose active metabolite norfluoxetine has a half-life of about 1 week, necessitating at least a 5 week washout of fluoxetine before initiation of an MAOI.)

The other drug interaction with MAOIs that one should be familiar with occurs when MAOIs are administered along with **meperidine (Demerol)**. This combination causes a similar syndrome. (Less severe reactions also have been described as a result of the combination of MAOIs and other opiate agonists, such as morphine, and partial agonists such as buprenorphine, butorphanol, and pentazocine). Patients taking MAOIs also should be wary of taking amphetamines or sympathomimetic-containing decongestants or "diet pills."

Given these difficulties, why do clinicians still prescribe MAOIs? For some subtypes of mood disorder, MAOIs still may be the most efficacious agents. These subtypes include dysthymic disorder, "atypical" depression, seasonal affective disorder, and possibly depressive episodes occurring in the setting of bipolar disorder. Even in these subtypes, however, most clinicians initiate treatment with an SSRI, bupropion, or venlafaxine given their greater margin of safety. While clinical research suggests that these alternative agents also are useful in these forms of depressive illness, MAOIs remain the gold standard and should be considered in the treatment of refractory cases.

Clinicians have attempted to use **selegiline (Deprenyl)**, a selective inhibitor of MAO-B used in the treatment of Parkinson's disease. Unfortunately, at the doses necessary to obtain an *antidepressant* effect, selegiline loses its MAO-B selectivity (and therefore its advantage over the other MAOIs). In contrast, **moclobemide** is a *reversible* inhibitors of MAO-A. It binds to MAO-A, but not permanently, such that if dietary tyramine ingestion causes norepinephrine levels to rise, the norepinephrine *competes* with moclobemide, displacing it off of MAO-A and allowing the MAO to again metabolize the norepinephrine. Moclobemide is available in Canada and Europe but not in the United States.

Tricyclic Antidepressants

All of the tricyclic antidepressants represent modifications to the first tricyclic agent, imipramine. Most of the original clinical studies of the pharmacologic treatment of depression used imipramine and even today it remains the gold standard comparison treatment in clinical trials of new antidepressant agents. The oldest TCAs (**imipramine**, **amitriptyline**, and **doxepin**) have *tertiary amine side chains*. This side chain makes them more prone to cross reactions with a variety of other types of receptors, thereby causing more side effects. The latter include *antihistamine* effects (sedation and weight gain), *anticholinergic* effects (dry mouth, dry eyes, constipation, memory problems, or even frank delirium), and *antiadrenergic effects* (orthostatic hypotension, a significant problem in elderly patients since they are more sensitive to this side effect, are more prone to falls due to gait instability, and have a higher risk of suffering fractures following a fall due to preexisting osteoporosis).

The *tertiary amine TCAs act predominantly on serotonin receptors rather than on norepinephrine receptors*. However, these TCAs have active metabolites. These metabolites, which also are tricyclic antidepressants, have *secondary amine side chains*. For example, the metabolite of imipramine is **desipramine**, while the metabolite of amitriptyline is **nortriptyline**. These *secondary amine TCAs primarily block norepinephrine reuptake rather than serotonin reuptake*.

Later, the secondary amine TCAs were synthesized and marketed as antidepressant agents in their own right. Their advantage over the tertiary amine agents is that their side effect profile, while the same as that of the tertiary amine agents, is generally less severe. In cases of depression refractory to one TCA, switching to another one isn't typically an effective strategy. All of these agents have weaker serotonin reuptake effects than do the SSRIs with the notable exception of **clomipramine**, a tertiary amine agent most commonly used in the treatment of obsessive-compulsive disorder.

TCAs can have significant effects on cardiac conduction. They are class I antiarrhythmic agents. Like quinidine, disopyramide, and procainamide, they depress fast sodium channels and prolong cardiac repolarization. Patients with ventricular arrhythmia who are already taking another class I antiarrhythmic agent but require tricyclic drug therapy should receive careful medical supervision given the potential for additive cardiac effects. As with quinidine, TCAs can provoke bradyarrhythmia in patients with preexisting but subclinical sinus node dysfunction. TCAs also can lengthen the QT interval, even in the presence of "therapeutic" serum drug levels. Among patients with preexisting asymptomatic conduction defects (such as interventricular conduction delay and bundle-branch block) tricyclic treatment can induce symptomatic conduction defects. Clinicians also should be aware that such cardiotoxicity has occurred even in patients with normal pretreatment ECGs. Some patients have developed an atrioventricular block that reverted to normal following drug discontinuation. Some individuals with prolonged QT intervals (whether preexisting or due to coadministration of other agents) have developed ventricular tachycardia during in the setting of TCA treatment.

As newer antidepressants tend to have no effects on cardiac conduction, they have become first-line drugs for most depressed patients with cardiac disease. This being said, however, TCAs have been used for decades in patients with cardiac disease. Patient should be carefully monitored and the ECG should be followed, particularly following dosage increases. Older patients should receive an ECG before treatment with a TCA is initiated.

Clearly, the most serious problem with TCA therapy is that *overdoses of TCAs can be lethal*. Even a 10 day supply can cause cardiac arrhythmia, seizures, and death. Therefore, in significantly depressed patients, clinicians should only provide a small supply. (Note that even when one takes such precautions, patients still can *hoard* pills in preparation for an overdose.) Also, clinical lore suggests that some patients may enter a period of higher risk for suicide shortly *after* the initiation of antidepressant therapy, even when the patient appears to be showing early signs of improvement. Perhaps such patients remain sad, self-deprecating, and hopeless but regain enough energy, motivation, and concentration to follow through on suicidal thoughts or plans. Patients who are "improving" after 1–2 weeks of antidepressant treatment still are not "out of the woods," and clinicians should continue to monitor patients closely at this stage.

Given the variety of potential adverse effects associated with TCAs, it is impressive how many primary care physicians continue to prescribe them in lower doses primarily for their hypnotic effects without taking into consideration their significant potential for morbidity (particularly in elderly and postoperative patients). It also is noteworthy that patients usually are not given extensive disclosures about these side effects.

We still use TCAs because they are very effective in treating depression. They may be more effective in cases that are refractory to SSRIs and they are also useful in the treatment of patients with chronic pain syndromes (treating both the pain itself and the depression that often accompanies chronic pain). The least likely TCA to cause orthostasis is nortriptyline, and both this and desipramine, two secondary amine agents, are usually the best-tolerated TCAs. In general, there is rarely a reason to prescribe a tertiary amine agent rather than a secondary amine agent, with the exception of *clomipramine*, which is used as an alternative to SSRI therapy in the treatment of obsessive-compulsive disorder.

TCAs should be started at a low dose and then titrated gradually upward as tolerated over a period of several days to weeks. Patients with anxiety disorders and elderly patients should be started at even lower doses. Half-lives of TCAs are long enough to allow for once daily dosing, usually at night (to help with sleep and to minimize daytime sedation, since their antihistaminergic effects tend to be greatest at peak blood levels).

One advantage of the TCAs over other agents is that serum levels are readily obtainable and can be clinically useful. Most TCAs show a sigmoidal dose-response curve (Fig. 7–5), with the onset of clinical effects occurring at serum levels of between 150 and 200 ng/ml and "diminishing returns" above this level (particularly relative to increasing side effects). The exception to this rule is nortriptyline, which appears to have a "therapeutic window" of between 50 and 150 ng/ml (Fig. 7–6), with lesser clinical responses being obtained at serum levels both below and above the "window."

Clinicians don't obtain serum TCA levels in every case, but they are quite useful in specific situations. Patients who aren't responding to therapy who are found to have blood levels just below the therapeutic level can demonstrate a

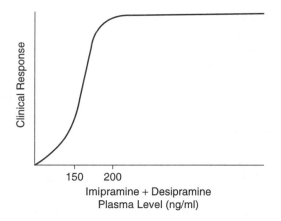

Figure 7–5. Sigmoidal curve for imipramine. Reproduced with permission from Schatzberg AF, Cole JO, DeBattista C: *Manual of Clinical Psychopharmacology*, 3rd edition. Washington, DC, American Psychiatric Press, 1997.

dramatic response to just a slight upward dosage titration. Alternatively, patients who have responded to treatment but are experiencing side effects who are found to have serum TCA levels significantly above the therapeutic zone may have "room" for a dosage reduction without greatly increasing the risk of relapse. Finally, when a patient fails to respond to TCA therapy, the determination that the patient has been maintained at a therapeutic serum level for an adequate period of time assists the clinician in determining that the patient is unlikely to demonstrate a further response to the TCA and

that it is time to move on to other treatment strategies.

Blood levels also can be helpful since patients vary significantly in their ability to metabolize drugs. TCAs are metabolized by the *cytochrome P450 system*, mostly by the enzyme *CYP2D6*. About 10% of patients are "poor metabolizers" and develop significantly higher blood levels (up to eightfold higher). The presence of side effects isn't a reliable indicator of the serum level, since side effects occur even at low levels. Also, some drugs saturate the CYP2D6 enzyme. When given along with a TCA, the TCA level can increase to two- to threefold-higher levels than might otherwise be expected. Some SSRIs do this, especially **fluoxetine** and **paroxetine**. Some clinicians, not aware of this potentially lethal interaction, have added one of these SSRIs to the regimen of a patient already receiving amitriptyline for sleep or vice versa.

One "near-TCA" that is worth mentioning but that is rarely used is **amoxapine**. This agent is a heterocyclic antidepressant that also blocks dopamine receptors. It is more effective than TCA monotherapy in cases of psychotic depression, where an antidepressant–antipsychotic combination strategy is otherwise typically required to achieve efficacy. However, amoxapine can cause all of the side effects associated with traditional antipsychotic agents, including tardive dyskinesia (discussed further in the next chapter). Further, with a combination drug strategy, the antipsychotic agent can be titrated independently of the antidepressant medication, offering greater flexibility than one can achieve with amoxapine.

Serotonin Reuptake Inhibitors

Selective serotonin reuptake inhibitors (SSRIs) block the presynaptic neuron's serotonin transporter protein, thereby inhibiting serotonin reuptake while having little effect on other neurotransmitters or receptors. Their selectivity allows for a greatly improved side-effect profile. These agents have not been demonstrated to be have greater *efficacy* than MAOIs or TCAs in randomized controlled clinical trials. However, they are much more likely to be prescribed in therapeutic dosages (due to their ability to be prescribed at full doses from the outset of treatment and for an adequate length of time (due to lower

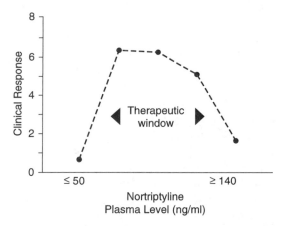

Figure 7–6. Curvilinear curve for nortriptyline. Reproduced with permission from Schatzberg AF, Cole JO, DeBattista C: *Manual of Clinical Psychopharmacology*, 3rd edition. Washington, DC, American Psychiatric Press, 1997.

rates of premature medication discontinuation). Therefore, the SSRIs appear to be more *effective* than the older agents in real-world treatment settings. Further—and especially important given how many patients experience chronic depression and require lifelong treatment—SSRIs carry a lower burden of "tolerable, but still unpleasant" chronic side effects.

The greater serotonergic activity associated with these agents likely accounts for their usefulness in treating other psychiatric conditions including most of the anxiety disorders (including panic disorder, post-traumatic stress disorder, generalized anxiety disorder, social phobia, and obsessive-compulsive disorder), as well as in impulse control disorders such as bulimia nervosa and pathological gambling or shopping. They also are useful in the treatment of the irritability, dysphoria, impulsiveness, and self-injurious behaviors that can be associated with "cluster B" personality disorders such as borderline personality disorder. Many of these conditions commonly co-occur with major depressive disorder or dysthymic disorder, and prescribing an SSRI in such cases potentially allows the clinician to "kill two birds with one stone."

SSRIs allow for once daily dosing and in many cases don't require dosage titration. Given this, and given their favorable side-effect profile, patients typically can start on and remain on a therapeutic dosage throughout the entire course of treatment. One caveat, however, is that while *most* patients can initiate treatment at the full dose, side effects associated with initial medication exposure still can be minimized by having the patient take a half-dose (even a quarter-dose) for at least the first few days. This is particularly the case for patients presenting with either an "anxious depression" or a comorbid anxiety disorder, since these patients tend to be more sensitive to medication side effects.

Two other major advantages of the SSRIs over the TCAs and MAOIs are that they carry little risk of cardiotoxicity and that they are much safer in the event of an overdose.

Unlike the TCAs, the chemical structure of each SSRI differs substantially from those of the other SSRIs. Therefore, it is possible that a patient who doesn't respond to trial of one SSRI might benefit from switching to another SSRI. However, given the variety of currently available agents, a more reasonable clinical strategy when faced with a patient who hasn't responded to an agent from one chemical class might be to switch to an agent from a different class. For example, one might switch a primarily *serotonergic* agent to a primarily *noradrenergic* agent (such as bupropion, reboxetine, or desipramine). Alternatively, one might try adding the noradrenergic agent to the SSRI to allow for synergistic effects or might switch to a *mixed* noradrenergic–serotonergic agent such as venlafaxine or mirtazapine.

The major considerations influencing clinicians' choice of one SSRI over another are *drug life span*, the potential for *drug–drug interactions*, and *marketing factors* (such as out-of-pocket expense to the patient). The longer half-life of fluoxetine allows it to have the lowest likelihood of causing discontinuation symptoms. Research in actual treatment settings reveals that 30%–60% of patients don't take medication as prescribed and that 15%–25% of patients wait 2 weeks or more to refill their antidepressant prescriptions after their supply runs out. Given this, fluoxetine may be particularly useful for patients in whom sporadic compliance might be expected. (Fluoxetine even is available in a 80 mg dosage form, allowing for once weekly dosing.) However, fluoxetine's long half-life may prove to be problematic for patients who develop side effects or for patients whose depression occurs in the setting of bipolar disorder. In the latter case, if the patient enters a manic state, the long half-life of fluoxetine frustrates the usual goal of immediately discontinuing any antidepressant medications. Further, as noted above, one needs to allow for a 5 week washout of fluoxetine prior to initiating MAOI therapy as opposed to a 2 week washout for other SSRIs.

The most common *side effects* associated with SSRI therapy are anxiety, nervousness, restlessness (even to the point where it could be considered akathisia), insomnia (broken sleep, associated with decreases in the amount of time spent in REM sleep), fatigue or sedation (even when there is co-occurring insomnia), headache, weight loss, dizziness or lightheadedness, sexual dysfunction, and gastrointestinal upset. These side effects likely reflect increased serotonin activity, particularly at the level of the **5-HT$_2$ receptor** in most cases, or of the **5-HT$_3$ receptor** (in the case of gastrointestinal symptoms). Some of these symptoms can be mitigated by initially prescribing a low dose followed by gradual dosage escalation.

Many patients find that most of these symptoms resolve spontaneously after several days of therapy. However, some side effects (particularly sleep disturbance and sexual dysfunction) are more likely to persist for the duration of therapy. Many clinicians treat insomnia with a low dose of trazodone (which blocks the $5HT_2$ receptor and also has antihistaminergic properties) or with a short-acting benzodiazepine. Weight loss is usually only a few pounds and requires no specific intervention. A minority of patients have complained of weight gain, which typically only occurs following several months of therapy, ranging from about 1 to 3 kg. Rates may be a bit higher for paroxetine than for the other SSRIs, perhaps because this SSRI has a small amount of anticholinergic effect. In some cases, weight gain might reflect patients having regained weight previously lost during the episode of depression.

Sexual side effects also are prevalent with SSRIs. They include decreased libido, delayed orgasm or anorgasmia, and impotence. The original controlled clinical trials with the first of these agents, fluoxetine, estimated that sexual dysfunction occurred only in about 2% of treated patients. Trials of the next three agents to reach the market (sertraline, paroxetine, and fluvoxamine) revealed rates of about 15%. However, all of these studies are of limited value because they only involved patient's *spontaneous reports* of side effects. Clinical drug trials follow this practice to avoid introducing bias through direct inquiry into particular side effects. In the case of sexual side effects, however, which are so embarrassing to many patients that they may not spontaneously report them, this practice likely led to gross underestimations of the prevalence of this problem.

More recent studies, using formal questionnaires, have estimated that sexual side effects actually occur in 30%–50% of patients treated with SSRIs. Similar rates of sexual dysfunction occur with other serotonergic antidepressants, including the MAOIs, the TCAs, and venlafaxine. Since patients may not mention these side effects, clinicians should discuss them with patients both at the in initiation of therapy and throughout the course of treatment.

Many patients experience low libido as part of their depression, and—as with apathy—one way to distinguish a medication side effect from recurrence of depression is to examine whether all of the other symptoms of depression have improved *with the exception* of sexual dysfunction. When this is the case, it is more likely that the sexual dysfunction reflects a medication side effect than a symptom of depression. Prior to the initiation of treatment, some patients will say that they don't mind risking sexual dysfunction since "sex is the least of my concerns right now." However, patients' willingness to tolerate sexual side effects may change considerably after their depression has lifted, particularly since these side effects can persist for months or even years.

The sexual dysfunction that occurs in a major depressive episode may be caused by decreased dopaminergic activity along the mesolimbic "pleasure circuit" described in Chapter 4. This circuit mediates a wide variety of motivated behaviors including sexual activity, substance use, and compulsive behavior. Sexual side effects from SSRIs occur shortly after the initiation of treatment (even after a single dose of medication), suggesting that they are caused by increased serotonin levels rather than receptor or postreceptor changes. The serotonin receptor that has received the most attention in this regard is the $5HT_2$ receptor. Stimulation of $5HT_2$ receptors on dopamine neurons results in the inhibition of dopamine release. In other words, in this case serotonin and dopamine have a reciprocal relationship. Given this, increased serotonin levels may cause even further decreases in mesolimbic dopamine, resulting in worsening of sexual dysfunction. However, increased serotonin also may exert independent effects on sexual functioning, via descending serotonergic pathways from the brain stem to spinal neurons influencing excitement and orgasm.

Patients who experience SSRI-induced sexual dysfunction who otherwise are benefiting from the medication might respond to the prescription of an "antidote" shortly before intercourse, such as the α-2 blocker **yohimbine** or the serotonin antagonist **cyproheptadine**, or the antiviral medication **amantadine**. (The mechanism of action of amantadine is unknown, but it is believed to have dopaminergic properties given its beneficial effects in early Parkinson's disease.) Another strategy has been to add a standing dose of nefazodone or mirtazapine (antidepressants with $5HT_2$ receptor antagonist activity) or bupropion (an antidepressant with noradrenergic and dopaminergic effects). While each of these strategies helps in some cases, none is universally beneficial.

Another strategy for patients in remission from depression has involved having the patient take a "drug holiday" on Friday and Saturday and having intercourse only on weekends. This not only reduces the spontaneity of sexual activity but also increases the risk of the patient experiencing serotonin discontinuation syndrome or discontinuing the medication outright The strategy is ineffective for patients taking fluoxetine given this drug's long half-life.

A final strategy is to switch the patient to an alternative agent not associated with sexual dysfunction or simply to not use an SSRI as one's initial medication choice (particularly in those cases where the patient isn't suffering from a comorbid condition that preferentially responds to serotonergic therapy such as obsessive-compulsive disorder). The noradrenergic antidepressants *bupropion* and *reboxetine* are not associated with sexual dysfunction, while *nefazodone* and *mirtazapine* have lower rates of sexual dysfunction than the SSRIs, likely due to their 5-HT2 antagonist effects.

While SSRIs have useful anxiolytic effects, some patients taking them complain that they not only feel less anxiety but also feel "less of anything." As discussed in Chapter 4, such SSRI-induced *apathy* also may reflect decreased mesolimbic or frontal dopamine activity due to serotonin–dopamine antagonism. Alternatively it may reflect a drug-induced alteration in the normal balance between serotonin and the catecholamines. Catecholamines play a important role as mediators of "drive" and "novelty-seeking," while serotonin helps to keep such drives in check by encouraging emotional and behavioral inhibition. Therefore, the benefits and the side effects of enhanced serotonergic activity may be two sides of the same coin.

When such apathy appears, it tends to arise only after a few weeks into the course of treatment, often shortly after patients had just begun to report improvement in their moods. Given this, distinguishing apathy from a recurrence of depression along with worsening depressive *anhedonia* can be difficult. Some clinicians incorrectly conclude that the SSRI has "stopped working," which prompts them to *increase* the SSRI dosage, sometimes leading to an even further worsening of apathy. It is important for clinicians to elicit and document a detailed history of the patient's complete symptom profile prior to the initiation of antidepressant therapy and to then track these symptoms during the course of treatment. Relapses of depression associated with anhedonia are likely to be accompanied by other symptoms that existed prior to the initiation of therapy, while anhedonia due to SSRI therapy may be a new complaint that occurs in isolation or may occur in conjunction with other SSRI side effects such as sexual dysfunction or sleep disturbance.

Fluoxetine has received some bad press due to concerns that it might cause depressed but previously nonsuicidal patients to become suicidal. Some patients refuse to take fluoxetine as a result. The initial report that raised these concerns described only six patients; a later reanalysis of over 1000 cases revealed no evidence that fluoxetine induces suicidal thinking. In contrast, untreated depression clearly is associated with an increased risk of suicide. This being said, clinical wisdom (not borne out in research studies at this point) suggests that all antidepressant drugs can potentially exacerbate suicidal ideation in depressed patients, particularly early on in therapy, and that suicidal ideation must be carefully monitored in all depressed patients *regardless* of which antidepressant agent the patient is taking. Some commentators have speculated that perhaps uncomfortable, drug-induced *akathisia or anxiety* accounts for the development of suicidal thoughts in patients taking SSRIs who have experienced this problem.

Some SSRIs are potent inhibitors of enzymes in the **cytochrome P450 system.** This system is made up of heme-containing proteins—located mostly in the smooth endoplasmic reticulum of cells in the liver, intestine, kidney, lung, and brain—that catalyze oxidative reactions, including drug metabolism. While over 500 such enzymes have been identified to date, many of these are very similar and only a few are responsible for drug metabolism in humans. The two most important enzymes in terms of drug metabolism are **cytochrome 2D6** and **cytochrome 3A4**, which together account for the metabolism of over 80% of marketed medications.

Genetic polymorphism plays a role in the extent to which an individual expresses these various enzymes. For example, cytochrome 2D6 is inactive in 10% of Caucasians and 2% of Asians, while cytochrome 3C19 is inactive in 5% of Caucasians and 20% of Asians. Therefore, depending on the medication in question and its degredative pathway, some individuals will be "poor metabolizers" while others will be "extensive metabolizers."

Complicating matters, though, some medications *induce* the expression of these enzymes, typically over a period of days to weeks. Examples include *carbamazepine, alcohol,* and *tobacco smoke.* In other words, carbamazepine induces the production of cytochrome 3A4. This in turn increases the metabolism of carbamazepine, leading to a lowering of its own serum levels and a need to subsequently increase the daily dosage if one wishes to maintain clinical efficacy. Obviously, the induction of 3A4 by carbamazepine also will increase the metabolism of any *other medications* oxidized by 3A4.

In contrast, other medications, including some of the SSRIs, *inhibit* the activity of different P450 enzymes, thereby *raising* these medications' own serum levels and the levels of any coadministered medications that also happen to be metabolized by that particular enzyme. Table 7–19 describes some common interactions. For example, in the case of enzyme 2D6 (which is inhibited by both paroxetine and fluoxetine), one can see increases not only in SSRI levels but also in the levels of coadministered *tricyclic antidepres-*

sants. Further, 2D6 metabolizes *codeine* to its active form (morphine), so these two SSRIs can potentially prevent codeine from exerting any analgesic effect. In the case of enzyme 3A4 (inhibited by nefazodone and to a lesser extent by fluoxetine and fluvoxamine) there is a risk of raising the levels of anticonvulsant medications and benzodiazepines, leading to sedation or confusion in vulnerable patients. More concerning, there is the risk of raising the levels of some medications that cause QT prolongation and potentially fatal torsades de pointes. Three such medications, terfenadine (Seldane), astemizole (Hismanal), and cisapride (Propulsid), have been removed from the market in the United States due to this risk.

The SSRIs that are least likely to affect any of the various cytochrome P450 enzymes to a significant extent are **citalopram** and **escitalopram** (which therefore aren't listed in Table 7–17). (Other agents also not associated with significant P450 interactions are venlafaxine, bupropion, and mirtazapine.)

Because SSRIs can inhibit their own metabolism, patients might not complain of signs of SSRI toxicity until *several weeks* after the initiation of treatment due to the accumulation of both the therapeutic agent and active metabolites. These later-appearing side effects (including apathy, fatigue, weight gain, and sexual dysfunction) are distinguished from early appearing side effects such as anxiety and gastrointestinal discomfort in that they often do not improve over time. Such patients might benefit from SSRI dosage reduction at this point.

SSRIs originally appeared to carry the advantage of not causing "discontinuation" or "withdrawal" symptoms such as were seen with the

Table 7–19. SSRIs and the Cytochrome P450 System

Isoenzyme	Inducers	Inhibitors	Main Drug Interactions
1A2	Tobacco, charbroiled foods	Fluvoxamine, grapefruit juice, favinoids, ciprofloxacin, norfloxacin	Theophylline, clozapine, haloperidol, olanzapine, propranolol, caffeine
2D6		Fluoxetine, paroxetine	Tricyclics, codeine
2C		Fluoxetine, fluvoxamine	Phenytoin, diazepam
3A4	Carbamazepine, phenobarbital	Nefazodone, fluoxetine, fluvoxamine, ketoconazole, cimetidine, erythromycin	Terfenadine, astemizole, cisapride, ziprasidone, carbamazepine, alprazolam, triazolam

MAOIs and TCAs upon abrupt discontinuation. However, it now is recognized that such *discontinuation symptoms* commonly occur. Symptoms range from mild, transient anxiety and insomnia to severe dizziness, fatigue, weakness, nausea, headache, myalgias, and paresthesias or "electric sensations."

Discontinuation symptoms often resolve after several days, but in a minority of patients they last for weeks and are disabling. The syndrome can occur with all of the SSRIs, even after only a few weeks of treatment. However, it is more likely to occur with agents that have a *shorter half-life* (it most commonly occurs with paroxetine and least often occurs with fluoxetine) following the prescription of *higher doses* and after *more extended treatment* (months to years).

A rapid onset of symptoms followed by an equally rapid cessation of symptoms following resumption of SSRI use suggests serotonin withdrawal is responsible. Patients should be educated about the nature of these symptoms, the importance of consistent therapy, and the need to, if necessary, formulate a discontinuation schedule with their physician. When discontinuing SSRIs, a gradual taper is recommended. In some cases, this may require several weeks. Benzodiazepines may mitigate withdrawal symptoms in more severe cases. Some patients who wait several days before refilling their SSRI prescription experience discontinuation symptoms but mistake them for symptoms of relapse of their underlying mood or anxiety disorder.

SSRI discontinuation symptoms also sometimes are mistaken for side effects of the new antidepressant medication being prescribed in the wake of the SSRI. When switching from an SSRI to a new antidepressant, a "cross-titration" may be better tolerated than a "washout" of the first agent, both because this minimizes the risk of SSRI withdrawal and because it decreases the risk of the patient experiencing a depressive relapse during the washout. (The exception to this suggestion is the combination of an SSRI and an MAOI; they should not be overlapped due to the risk of causing serotonin syndrome.)

Bupropion

Bupropion (Wellbutrin) doesn't interact with any of the receptors associated with causing side effects in the setting of TCA or MAOI treatment, a major advantage. While its mechanism of action remains uncertain, it appears to have weak norepinephrine and dopaminergic reuptake inhibitor effects. It also has been used to treat attention-deficit hyperactivity disorder (as an alternative to the psychostimulants, which have more potent dopaminergic effects) and to treat nicotine dependence (under the trade name Zyban). Some data suggest that bupropion is less likely to induce mania or rapid cycling than the TCAs when used to treat depressive episodes occurring in the setting of bipolar disorder. Its mild stimulant effects may be useful in the treatment of anergic, anhedonic patients. Another advantage of bupropion over the SSRIs is that treatment is not associated with sexual side effects. The flip side of this lack of serotonergic activity, however, is that does not have the anxiolytic properties of the SSRIs and is not useful in treating comorbid anxiety disorders (such as panic disorder, obsessive-compulsive disorder, or generalized anxiety disorder).

As might be expected given its catecholaminergic profile, the most commonly reported side effects of bupropion are anxiety, agitation, and insomnia. Rarely, patients have experienced psychotic symptoms. Bupropion also has a higher risk of causing seizures than do other antidepressants, although the risk must be placed in perspective. At typical doses (150–300 mg/day), in typical patients, the effect is negligible (0.4%, versus 0.1% for the SSRIs). However, at doses between 450 and 600 mg/day, the risk increases 10-fold, to 4%. Patients at higher risk for experiencing seizures include those with a history of a preexisting seizure disorder or of a head trauma, a brain tumor, or an eating disorder (this last because starvation and purging can cause electrolyte imbalances). The risk of seizures is greatest at peak serum levels.

For the regular-release formulation, the average dose is 100 mg three times daily, with a maximum daily dose of 450 mg and no individual dose greater than 150 mg. (This necessitates three times daily dosing, even for the patients taking 300 mg per day.) A sustained-release preparation is available (WellbutrinSR), which allows for individual doses up to 200 mg, since delayed absorption leads to lower peak serum levels. This allows for once or twice daily dosing, with the average dose being 150 mg twice daily. Patients typically initiate therapy at 150 mg once per day, increasing the dosage to 150 mg twice daily after 3 days as tolerated. The maximum recommended daily dose is 400 mg (given as 200 mg twice daily). Despite the risk of seizures, bupropion is generally safe in overdose and is not cardiotoxic.

Venlafaxine and Duloxetine

The pharmacologic profile of **venlafaxine (Effexor)** resembles that of a TCA in that it inhibits the reuptake of both norepinephrine and serotonin. However, unlike the TCAs, venlafaxine is not associated with antihistamine, antiadrenergic, or anticholinergic side effects. In other words, it is a selective serontergic–noradrenergic reuptake inhibitor. At lower doses (75–150 mg/day) it appears to be primarily a serotonin reuptake inhibitor, while at higher doses (150–300 mg/day) it gains more noradrenergic effect. At even higher doses (300–450 mg/day) it appears to have dopaminergic effects as well. (Note that venlafaxine is only FDA-approved for dosages of up to 225 mg/day.) Venlafaxine formerly required twice daily dosing, but a sustained-release preparation (EffexorXR) allows for daily dosing and improved tolerability.

Venlafaxine's side effects are similar to those associated with SSRIs, including sexual dysfunction. More patients complain of initial gastrointestinal symptoms and anxiety with venlafaxine than with the SSRIs, but these symptoms usually subside within the first 1–2 weeks of treatment. Gradual upward dosage titration and use of the extended-release form also help to minimize these side effects. Like the SSRIs, drug cessation or dosage reductions of venlafaxine can cause serotonin discontinuation symptoms, necessitating gradual dosage reduction.

Venlafaxine also can cause elevations in diastolic blood pressures in about 10% of patients given higher dosages higher than 300 mg/day. Perhaps this is caused by the drug's increased dopaminergic effects at such dosages. Not all patients require these doses, and for those who do the increase in diastolic blood pressure only averages about 8 mm of mercury. Whether this is clinically relevant is uncertain, but blood pressure should periodically be monitored at higher dosages. Despite these concerns, venlafaxine is not associated with cardiac side effects and gen-

erally has been found to be safe in overdose. It should not be combined with MAOIs.

The wide dosage range and the need for dosage titration are potential disadvantages of venlafaxine when compared to the SSRIs. However, an advantage of venlafaxine is that it may be moderately more efficacious than the SSRIs: there is some evidence that although rates of *response* are similar for venlafaxine and the SSRIs, more patients taking venlafaxine successfully achieve a full *remission* from their depressive symptoms than do patients taking SSRIs. One meta-analysis of eight double-blind randomized clinical trials comparing venlafaxine to fluoxetine, paroxetine, fluvoxamine, or placebo found final remission rates of 45% for venlafaxine, 35% for the SSRIs, and 25% for placebo. Although the protocols of the studies differed, the favorable ranking of venlafaxine relative to an SSRI was consistent across the studies.

This apparent clinical advantage may relate to venlafaxine's dual mechanism of action involving both serotonin and norepinephrine. Given that relatively higher doses of venlafaxine might be necessary to achieve significant noradrenergic effects, patients who fail to respond to lower doses should be titrated to higher doses.

Another agent with a dual mechanism of action is **duloxetine (Cymbalta)**. Early studies suggest it may offer the advantage of having significant noradrenergic inhibitory effects even at the initiation dose of 60 mg. As of this writing, duloxetine has been approved by the FDA but has not yet been released to the market.

Trazodone and Nefazodone

Trazodone (Desyrel) is only a weak serotonin reuptake inhibitor, and its main effect is as a direct *5-HT$_2$ receptor antagonist*. (Its main metabolite is a 5-HT$_2$ *agonist*, but it is likely that the antagonist effects of the parent compound outweigh this effect.) An advantage of trazodone is that, by blocking this receptor, it avoids side effects such as sexual dysfunction, anxiety, and insomnia.

Trazodone also acts at the postsynaptic α-1 receptor and so can cause significant orthostatic hypotension and sedation. While the drug is an effective antidepressant, these side effects greatly limit its usefulness, and many patients simply are unable to tolerate an antidepressant dosage. However, in smaller doses, trazodone is commonly used as a hypnotic, particularly in conjunction with SSRIs.

This combination strategy is appropriate from the perspective of "rational polypharmacy," since the SSRI provides a potent reuptake inhibitory action that trazodone lacks, while trazodone provides a blockade of the receptor subtype that likely causes the side effects associated with SSRI therapy.

Trazodone also has proven to be useful in treating elderly patients with dementia who experience severe agitation or nocturnal combativeness. In such patients, one should start with low doses and monitor for the development of excessive sedation or hypotension.

One rare but significant side effect of trazodone in men is *priapism*. While only occurring in perhaps one in every 6,000 men, it is a urological emergency. It is treated in the emergency room by injecting α-adrenergic agents directly into the penis.

Trazodone does not have anticholinergic side effects and is generally safe in cardiac patients, although there are a few case reports of cardiac irritability. It is safe in overdoses. It should not be used in combination with MAOIs due to the risk of serotonin syndrome. (While in theory combining trazodone with an SSRI also carries the potential for serotonin syndrome, in practice this combination has been well tolerated by a large number of patients.)

Nefazodone (Serzone) was created by modifying trazodone's chemical structure in order to decrease its α-adrenergic antagonist activity. As a result, nefazodone is less sedating than trazodone and doesn't cause orthostatic hypotension or priapism. Unlike the SSRIs, nefazodone doesn't interfere with REM sleep and it is less likely to cause sexual dysfunction—again, probably because of its $5HT_2$ antagonist effects. It also is less likely to cause initial anxiety and restlessness than the SSRIs, perhaps for the same reason. It has little or no affinity for other receptors including cholinergic and dopamine receptors and other serotonin receptor subtypes.

Nefazodone's side effects include sedation, dizziness, weakness, headache, dry mouth, nausea, and constipation. It is not significantly associated with weight gain. While nefazodone's sedative effects are less severe than those associated with the tertiary TCAs and trazodone, they still can be troublesome for many patients, es-

pecially at higher dosages. While the package labeling suggests initiating therapy in healthy adults at 100 mg twice a day, 50 mg twice a day tends to be better tolerated by many patients. Then increase the dosage by 50–100 mg every 3 or 3 days up to 300 mg/day. The final dosage range is generally 300–600 mg.

There may be a "therapeutic window" for nefazodone dosing, similar to that previously discussed for nortriptyline. In clinical trials involving patients with major depressive disorder, the response rate has been about 70% for patients taking 300–500 mg/day but only 50% for those taking either 200–300 mg/day or taking the maximum recommended dosage of 600 mg/day. Therefore, one might observe the patient for 2 weeks on 300 mg per day, monitoring for side effects and therapeutic response before increasing the dosage to 500 or 600 mg if the response has been unsatisfactory and if the increased dose is tolerated. While pharmacokinetic considerations suggest twice daily dosing, patients who experience significant daytime sedation or fatigue may fare better taking the bulk of the daily dose at night.

Nefazodone isn't cardiotoxic and generally is safe in overdoses. However, it inhibits *cytochrome enzyme 3A4* in a manner similar to erythromycin and ketoconazole, and it therefore can raise the serum levels of *other* potentially cardiotoxic medications. As noted above, three such agents (terfenadine, astemizole, and cisapride) have been removed from the U.S. market given the availability of safer alternative medications. Nefazodone can be administered safely with other antihistamines, including loratidine (Claritin), fexofenadine (Allegra), and cetirizine (Zyrtec).

While these coadministered antihistamines appear to be safe in terms of their *pharmacokinetics*, one still should observe for synergistic sedative effects due to *pharmacodynamic* interactions. Similarly, two benzodiazepines— *alprazolam (Xanax)* and *triazolam (Halcion)*— are metabolized by enzyme 3A4 and the addition of nefazodone therefore significantly increases their serum levels, potentially leading to excessive sedation and impaired psychomotor performance. Again, sedative effects of *other* benzodiazepines also may be exacerbated due to nefazodone's own sedative effects, even when their serum levels are not significantly increased.

Occasionally, patients "paradoxically" complain of agitation, excessive stimulation, or insomnia at higher doses. This may be more likely when the patient is concomitantly taking a cytochrome 2D6 inhibitor, such as fluoxetine or paroxetine (or still has fluoxetine in the system following recent discontinuation). As noted above, the *parent* compound of nefazodone is metabolized primarily by enzyme 3A4, but a *metabolite* of nefazodone, called m-chloro-phenyl-piperidine (mCPP), is metabolized primarily by enzyme 2D6. This metabolite is a mixed serotonin agonist–antagonist (depending on the particular serotonin receptor) that has *anxiogenic* effects when administered in research protocols to either lab animals or humans subjects who have anxiety disorders.

There have been rare reports of liver failure with nefazodone. Initially, four patients were cited in two reports. After 14–28 weeks of treatment, patients developed jaundice, followed by encephalopathy 2–6 weeks later despite having discontinued nefazodone within a week after the onset of symptoms. Liver failure and death have been reported with other antidepressants, including the SSRIs, but no firm causal relationship has been demonstrated. The rate with nefazodone, while apparently higher than that associated with other antidepressants, is still relatively low (about one in every 250,000–300,000 patients). Given such a low frequency, routine monitoring of hepatic enzyme levels doesn't appear to be warranted, but patients should be educated about potential warning signs of hepatic disease.

Mirtazepine

Mirtazepine (Remeron) is similar to nefazodone in that it is a $5HT_2$ antagonist, but in addition it also is a *$5HT_3$ receptor antagonist*, which probably accounts for its being less likely to cause gastrointestinal side effects and nausea than are the SSRIs. (Another $5HT_3$ receptor antagonist, ondansetron, is used to treat nausea associated with chemotherapy and surgical anesthesia.) Another difference from nefazodone is that it not only raises levels of serotonin but also of norepinephrine. In other words, mirtazapine, like venlafaxine, has a dual mechanism of action, which may prove to be useful in treatment-refractory cases.

Unlike venlafaxine, however, mirtazapine

doesn't raise levels of norepinephrine or serotonin by inhibiting their reuptake. Rather, it blocks the *presynaptic α-2 norepinephrine autoreceptor*. This receptor, like a thermostat, monitors synaptic levels of norepinephrine and—when they are too high—inhibits the release of norepinephrine. Therefore, antagonizing this receptor "blocks the thermostat" and causes the neuron to increase norepinephrine output. Of note, blocking the norepinephrine autoreceptor also appears to cause the neuron to increase its serotonergic output.

Like nefazodone and the SSRIs, mirtazapine has a low affinity for muscarinic and α-1 adrenergic receptors, leading to an improved side-effect profile compared to the TCAs. It also poses little risk of cardiac toxicity and is safe in an overdose. However, it is similar to the TCAs in that it has significant antihistaminergic effects, which may account for mirtazapine causing *sedation and weight gain* in significant percentages of patients.

The sedation is decreased by giving the drug in a single bedtime dose. For depressed patients experiencing prominent insomnia and anxiety, these initial sedative effects may be advantageous and may eliminate the need for concurrent benzodiazepine therapy. Other patients can't tolerate the sedation, however. In placebo-controlled studies in the United States comparing mirtazapine to amitriptyline and to placebo, 54% of patients in the mirtazapine group complained of somnolence compared to 60% of patients in the amitriptyline group and 18% in the placebo group. Ten percent of patients in the mirtazapine group dropped out of the trial due to somnolence versus 2% in the placebo group.

However, like the TCAs and nefazodone, patients who remain on the drug typically find that the somnolence improves within a few days and usually is gone within the first few weeks. Also, it is noteworthy that in European studies only 15% of patients complained of significant somnolence. This may reflect the higher starting dosage used in the European studies (15–20 mg/day) compared to the U.S. studies (5–10 mg/day). It is likely that mirtazapine's antihistaminergic properties are so potent that sedation occurs even at very low doses; in contrast, countervailing noradrenergic activating effects only appear at higher doses (e.g., 15–60 mg/day).

Given this, clinicians vary as to whether they start patients at low doses (7.5 mg), medium doses (15 mg), higher doses (30 mg), or very high doses (45–60 mg), and in their titration schedules. Some patients experiencing excessive sedation might improve with a dosage increase (something that likely will bewilder them unless an explanation is provided), while other patients might benefit from the traditional strategy of dosage reduction.

Mirtazapine is more likely to cause increased appetite and weight gain than other antidepressants. In the U.S. trials, 17% of mirtazapine-treated patients complained of increased appetite, compared with 6% of patients in the amitriptyline group and 2% of patients in the placebo group. A weight gain of at least 7% of body weight was reported by 8% of patients in the mirtazapine group, by 6% in the amitriptyline group, and by none of the patients in the placebo group

Like the sedative effects, weight gain may prove to be advantageous for some patients (particularly older, cachectic patients presenting with an "agitated depression") but may be intolerable for other patients. When weight gain does occur, it usually appears early in the course of treatment; patients who have not gained weight during the first 6 weeks of treatment are unlikely to do so over the course of more prolonged therapy.

Buspirone

Buspirone (BuSpar) is marketed as a nonbenzodiazepine anxiolytic agent and is approved by the FDA only for treatment of generalized anxiety disorder. However, while it has primarily anxiolytic properties at lower doses (15–30 mg/day), premarketing studies found it to have antidepressant properties when prescribed at higher doses (40–60 mg/day or even higher).

While buspirone isn't used as monotherapy for depression, it sometimes is used as an augmenting agent for patients who exhibit only a partial response to an SSRI. However, the results have been variable. Initial case reports and open trials were encouraging, but a subsequent placebo-controlled trial revealed no benefit from buspirone over placebo. (This latter result remains inconclusive due to the high rate of placebo response, about 50%, observed in both the placebo and the buspirone groups.)

Unlike other serotonergic antidepressants, buspirone doesn't act on the serotonin reuptake protein. Rather, it directly interacts with presynaptic and postsynaptic serotonin $5HT_{1A}$ receptors, where it is a *partial agonist*. The differential effect of lower and higher doses may relate to these partial agonist properties, although its precise mechanism of action remains unclear.

Let us first consider the *postsynaptic* serotonin receptor. At *lower* doses, buspirone competes with serotonin for receptors, but—being only a *partial* agonist—it takes up receptors that serotonin otherwise would have occupied. Since it has less intrinsic activity, the net result is a weak serotonin antagonist effect, which may be particularly useful in treating anxiety. At *higher* doses (and perhaps in cases of serotonin depletion due to depression), there is so much more buspirone than serotonin that it reaches many more receptors, and the net result is a weak serotonin agonist effect, since a partial agonist is better than no receptor stimulation at all.

However, buspirone also acts on *presynaptic* neurons, which contain $5HT_{1A}$ *autoreceptors* that decrease serotonin release through feedback inhibition. One theory suggests that buspirone augments the effects of SSRIs by acting as an autoreceptor agonist, thereby slowing the neuronal firing. This might "quiet the neuron" in cases of anxiety or might allow for greater repletion of presynaptic serotonin stores in the case of depression. An alternative theory posits that chronic stimulation by buspirone desensitizes the autoreceptor, thereby "blocking the thermostat" and enhancing neuronal serotonin output. Yet another possibility is that, in cases of depression, buspirone's postsynaptic serotonin agonist effects outweigh its presynaptic agonist effects on the autoreceptor.

Buspirone has a relatively benign side-effect profile, although some patients do experience dizziness, nausea, headache, nervousness, lightheadedness, or excitement. Like trazodone, it can be useful in treating some patients with dementia who experience anxiety or agitation.

Monoamine Releasing Agents ("Stimulants")

The stimulant drugs (**dextroamphetamine, methylphenidate,** and **pemoline**) increase synaptic release of dopamine (and, to a lesser extent, norepinephrine and serotonin). This increase in dopamine likely contributes to their ability to increase attention, concentration, energy, and motivation. As opposed to all of the other agents discussed so far, their onset of therapeutic effect is rapid (within hours), but short-lived. The short half-life of dextroamphetamine and methylphenidate necessitates giving several doses per day to maintain the effect, and the clinical response therefore can be uneven. Some patients only achieve transient effects.

Stimulants have been used in medically ill patients with depression, since they are generally safe and since their rapid onset of clinical effect may offer significant benefit to medical, surgical, or cancer patients who aren't getting out of bed, aren't eating well, and aren't participating in physical therapy. They also have been used with SSRIs both to counteract the SSRI-induced apathy syndrome and to augment therapy in cases where there has only been a partial response. Stimulants also have been used to combat apathy and attention deficits in patients with closed head injury or subcortical dementia.

Side effects of the stimulants can include headache, nervousness, and insomnia. They also can have appetite-suppressive effects, although when used to treat depression, improvements in motivation may outweigh these effects such that the patient's oral intake may improve. They have minimal cardiac side effects. At higher doses, stimulants' dopaminergic effect can lead to psychosis, but this is quite rare. Dextroamphetamine and methylphenidate are controlled substances and could potentially lead to abuse. "Refills" and "phoned-in" prescriptions are prohibited by the Drug Enforcement Agency (DEA). However, the number of patients who are receiving these agents for treatment of depression who become addicted to them or use them in an abusive way appear to be small.

Reboxetine

While some of the TCAs, such as desipramine, have significant inhibitory effects on norepinephrine reuptake, **reboxetine** is even more potent in this regard and is a *selective* reuptake inhibitor. Like the SSRIs, it lacks the adverse effects associated with the TCAs. Despite its selectivity, European studies have demonstrated it to be as effective in treating severe melancholic depression as imipramine, desipramine, and flu-

oxetine. Given the possible role of norepinephrine as a mediator of depressive symptoms such as fatigue, anhedonia, inattention, and cognitive complaints, and given the persistence of some of these symptoms in patients treated with serotonergic agents, this agent may be useful for such patients either alone or in combination with an SSRI.

Reboxetine has minimal effects on cytochrome P450 enzymes, has no reported cardiotoxic effects, and appears to be safe in overdose. It is generally well tolerated: while some patients complain of dry mouth, constipation, headache, sweating, insomnia, nausea, and dizziness, the frequency of these reports was no higher than that observed in patients who received placebo. Most patients started on 4 mg twice daily do not require further titration, although occasional patients require an increase to 5 mg twice daily after several weeks.

Reboxetine is currently available in over 50 European countries. As of this writing, it remains under review with the U.S. Food and Drug Administration (FDA) pending review of a larger study of the drug's efficacy and safety.

Lithium

For over 150 years, **lithium** was a primary ingredient in various "home remedies," "mineral cures," and medicinal preparations advertised as being effective in treating a wide variety of ailments such as gout and rheumatism. In 1948 it was marketed in the United States as a salt substitute for cardiac patients on low-sodium diets, some of whom became lithium toxic and died, leading to lithium's being removed from the U.S. market in 1949. That same year, however, an Australian psychiatrist and hospital superintendent named John Cade experimented with injecting lithium into guinea pigs. He found that the guinea pigs appeared more lethargic, and he therefore concluded that lithium might effectively treat mania. He administered lithium to several manic patients, to great effect.

Not surprisingly, his findings were met with significant skepticism, particularly in the United States. This state of affairs persisted until the 1960s, when Mogens Schou, a Danish psychiatrist, treated a series of bipolar disorder patients with lithium and carefully documented both how their acute episodes of illness were shortened and how their overall longitudinal course of illness dramatically improved following the introduction of lithium to their treatment regimen.

Lithium, the third element on the periodic table, is a salt that is present in trace amounts in water, food, and all living tissue. Following ingestion, it is rapidly and completely absorbed. It is not protein bound and isn't metabolized, being eliminated almost entirely by the kidneys. It is distributed everywhere in the body because it is soluble in body water. It is more concentrated in some tissues, however, such as thyroid and kidney, which may account for its potential to cause hypothyroidism and renal disease. It penetrates the central nervous system but exits the CNS relatively slowly, perhaps explaining why symptoms of lithium intoxication can persist for several days beyond declines in serum lithium levels.

How lithium treats symptoms of both mania and depression and how it helps to stabilize the cycling of mood that occurs in bipolar disorder remain uncertain. There is no evidence that bipolar disorder is caused by a bodily deficiency of lithium (and in fact the serum concentrations of lithium created in the course of clinical treatment are 100 times greater than the normal physiologic level). Researchers have identified several putative sites of action. The major current theory is that lithium modifies second messenger signal transduction. It likely does so at multiple levels. These include alterations in the coupling of neuroreceptors to their respective G-proteins, alterations in the configuration of the G-proteins themselves, and interactions at several stages of the intracellular signaling chain (including the formation of cAMP, inositol triphosphate, and protein kinase C). Chronic lithium administration appears to provide additional benefits beyond acute administration, and these effects may reflect even longer-term alterations in the nuclear regulatory factors that mediate neuronal gene expression.

Lithium has myriad other effects, however. For example, lithium substitutes for sodium at the Na-K-ATPase pump, thereby slowing the influx of sodium and stabilizing neuronal membranes. It augments serotonin function throughout the central nervous system, acting at all stages of serotonin metabolism (precursor uptake, synthesis, storage, catabolism, release, re-

ceptor activity, and receptor-mediated effects). This may contribute to its antidepressant effects, its ability to augment the therapeutic activity of other antidepressants, and its ability to help quiet aggressiveness and impulsiveness. Lithium also may correct desynchronizations in circadian rhythms hypothesized to occur in bipolar disorder patients, perhaps by altering the activity of the brain's "circadian pacemaker" at the level of the suprachiasmatic nucleus of the hypothalamus.

Lithium monotherapy is effective for about 70%–80% of patients with bipolar disorder, and it is useful in treating both manic and depressive episodes. When used in *acute manic episodes*, there is a latency of 5–10 days before it takes effect. Given this, agitated or hyperactive patients typically also receive adjunctive antipsychotic or benzodiazepine medication followed by a gradual taper of these agents once the patient is more stable. (While benzodiazepines tend to have fewer acute side effects, antipsychotic agents may be more effective since they primary antimanic and antipsychotic effects.) Manic patients also tend to improve once their disturbed sleep–wake cycle has been addressed (suggesting an underlying phase-shift disturbance), and the bulk of adjunctive medication therefore is given at night.

In younger patients, lithium is usually initiated at 300 mg two to three times per day, using a slow-release preparation if dose-related side effects become problematic. The target blood level is between about 0.8 and 1.0 mEq/L, but some patients require higher levels if tolerated. Since older patients may develop neurotoxic side effects even at these same serum levels, and since their renal clearance of lithium is lower, clinicians should aim for smaller daily doses and lower serum levels.

Sometimes a patient demonstrates an increase in his plasma lithium level after his manic episode has subsided, necessitating decreased lithium dosing. It isn't clear whether this effect reflects increased uptake of lithium into excitable tissue during mania, or increased renal blood flow and glomerular filtration rate during mania, or both. Similarly, patients may experience more side effects at the same blood level following recovery from mania such that the typical *maintenance* blood levels are a bit lower. At serum levels of 0.4–0.6 mEq/L, side effects are milder but the relapse rate is higher than when levels are kept at 0.8–1.0 mEq/L. Many clinicians and their patients ultimately settle on a range of 0.6–0.8 mEq/L The relapse rate is still probably a bit greater at these serum levels than at higher levels, so that patient education about signs of worsening illness and how to manage problematic side effects is essential.

Some acute cases of mania don't respond as well to lithium. Predictors of poor response include a dysphoric or agitated manic state (as opposed to the more "classic" euphoric mood), a "mixed" state (with co-occurring manic and depressive symptoms), the presence of rapid cycling between depression and mania, and mania presenting with comorbid substance abuse. Such cases may respond better to treatment with anticonvulsants such as valproate and carbamazepine.

Lithium also is effective for about 80% of the depressive episodes that occur in bipolar disorder. As with antidepressants, the onset of clinical effect lags behind the initiation of treatment by about 6–8 weeks. Using lithium to treat bipolar depression is preferable to using a primary antidepressant (especially a TCA) because antidepressants can have a destabilizing effect, treating the acute depressive state but ultimately contributing to an increased number of manic and depressive episodes, to a greater likelihood of rapid cycling, and to the illness being more refractory to treatment with agents such as lithium. When antidepressant agents must be added to the regimen, one should start with low doses and discontinue them as quickly as possible. (This strategy stands in contrast to the strategy used to treat major depressive disorder, which emphasizes longer-term maintenance therapy at the same dosage of medication dose that led to remission.)

Lithium can be used by itself to treat depressive episodes that occur in major depressive disorder, but it doesn't appear to be as effective as the primary antidepressants. However, it is commonly added to other antidepressants as an *augmenting agent* in treatment-resistant cases. About 30% of patients achieve complete remission following the addition of lithium while another 25%–35% experience substantial improvement without achieving remission. Sometimes this clinical response occurs rapidly (within days) and only requires a low lithium dose. However,

other patients may require several weeks of treatment at full doses. Lithium augmentation has been most extensively studied with the TCAs, and only a few small studies have examined lithium augmentation of newer agents such as SSRIs, venlafaxine, or bupropion. It appears possible that the response rate may be lower, so patients who fail to respond to an SSRI may benefit more from a switch to an antidepressant with a broader spectrum of activity than to lithium augmentation. As of this writing, no large-scale, controlled study has addressed this question.

Lithium also has been used in *schizoaffective disorder* (described in Chapter 8). In general, it is more effective in cases where there is a significant "affective component." However, sometimes patients with *schizophrenia* (even those without a notable "affective component") respond to lithium augmentation treatment with antipsychotic medication. Lithium has also been used to treat *aggression and impaired impulse control* in a variety of conditions, including schizophrenia, mental retardation, dementia, and more severe cases of personality disorder.

Lithium is not the perfect treatment for bipolar disorder. First, while it has offered profound relief for many patients, it has not been a panacea. As noted above, it is less effective for the up to 40% of patients who present with dysphoric mania, mixed states, and rapid-cycling illness. In terms of its ability to prophylax against relapse, while lithium does reduce the frequency and severity of depressive and manic episodes, about a third of patients taking lithium continue to have relapses. Of course, this relapse rate still is clearly better than that which occurs in patients who are placed on placebo (80% of such patients relapse) or who stop taking their lithium (50% of such patients relapse within the next 6 months). The relapse rate also is higher among patients who discontinue lithium abruptly rather than slowly tapering it.

Second, lithium treatment can be associated with many side effects and carries a high potential for inadvertent toxicity. While many patients remain safely on this agent for years, 75% of them experience side effects. Lithium has a narrow therapeutic index and monitoring of lithium plasma levels can be essential.

Some side effects are dose-dependent, while others are idiosyncratic. *Idiosyncratic side effects* include: facial rash resembling acne, alopecia, and aggravation of psoriasis. *Dose-related side effects* include the following:

1. *Tremor.* This tends to be worse shortly after each dose, when serum levels are at their peak. It is a postural tremor, similar to that caused by caffeine, best observed when the patient's hands and fingers are outstretched. It can interfere with writing, which appears shaky (in contrast to a parkinsonian tremor, where the writing is often micrographic), and can interfere with routine activities such as drinking from a cup. It can become a significant source of embarrassment for the patient. If it doesn't improve with mild dosage-reduction, adding a β-blocker such as propranolol may be useful.

2. *Renal.* Lithium inhibits the effect of antidiuretic hormone (ADH) on the distal tubules (probably by inhibiting cAMP production). This causes polyuria with a secondary polydipsia in about 25% of patients. It can progress to frank diabetes insipidus (urine output greater than 3 L/day, "normal" being 1–2 liters/day), and in rare cases urine output can be as high as 8 L/day. When in doubt, a 24 hour urine sample should be collected. When patients experience polyuria, it is important to assess whether they can maintain their fluid balance through increased water intake, since they are at risk for becoming dehydrated and lithium toxic. Sometimes polyuria responds to dosage reduction or to giving all of the lithium in a single nighttime dose (if tolerated). The latter strategy leads to higher peak levels, but the polyuria probably reflects trough levels, which are lower with single daily dosing. Another strategy is to give the patient a thiazide diuretic. While coadministering thiazides and lithium is relatively contraindicated (since thiazides decrease lithium clearance by about 50%, thereby doubling lithium levels), the strategy still can be useful provided that the lithium dosage is halved and serum lithium levels are closely monitored. Rarely, lithium therapy has been associated with decreased renal function or even renal failure, apparently by contributing to minimal-change glomerulonephritis or interstitial nephritis.

3. *Gastrointestinal.* Lithium can cause nausea, vomiting, and diarrhea. The nausea is related both to local gastric irritation and to the rapidity of rise in serum lithium levels. Therefore, nausea tends to be worse at the initiation of therapy and can be minimized by giving the lithium along with food, by using smaller but more frequent dosing, or by using a sustained-release preparation. While diarrhea also can reflect a rapid rate of absorption, it also can be an osmotic effect. In the latter case, slow-release preparations can worsen diarrhea, and one option is to switch from lithium carbonate to lithium citrate, since the citrate form is absorbed more rapidly.

4. *Thyroid.* Lithium causes a benign goiter in about 5% of patients, perhaps due to physical accumulation of lithium in the thyroid. This generally doesn't require intervention. However, about 5% of patients (more often women) develop hypothyroidism during chronic lithium treatment. When it occurs shortly after the initiation of treatment, it tends to be a transient effect, but when it occurs during chronic treatment it is more likely to be a sustained effect. While this often resolves following discontinuation of lithium, if the patient is doing well the clinician might simply prescribe thyroxine. It is important to monitor for hypothyroidism with routine blood testing rather than simply waiting for "classic signs" to appear, since even subtle or subclinical hypothyroidism can contribute to treatment refractoriness or rapid cycling.

5. *Cardiac.* Lithium displaces intracellular potassium and therefore its effects on the ECG resemble hypokalemia—that is, T-wave flattening or inversion. This is usually benign, but lithium still should be prescribed with caution in patients with cardiac disease. A pretreatment ECG should be obtained. Lithium has very rarely been reported to depress sinus node function and lithium therefore is contraindicated in patients with sick sinus syndrome, where it can lead to dysrhythmia and syncope.

6. *Weight gain.* The mechanism for this isn't clear. Lithium may cause changes in carbohydrate metabolism, patients may develop

water retention or edema, and lithium may increase patients' appetites. Also, patients with polydipsia may be drinking high-caloric fluids such as soda or fruit juice rather than water, and should be cautioned against this.

7. *Cognitive problems*. Patients taking lithium may complain about impaired memory, cognitive slowing, apathy, or a loss of spontaneity and creativity. Clinicians may be tempted to ascribe these symptoms to depression or to the patient regretting the loss of chronic hypomanias or "natural highs" that they enjoyed prior to their having received treatment for their bipolar disorder. However, normal research subjects placed on lithium have described similar cognitive disturbances. These effects tend to be dose-related and therefore sometimes respond to dosage reduction or to a switch to once nightly dosing. When patients complain of cognitive problems, clinicians also shouldn't forget to assess for lithium-induced hypothyroidism, which also might be the cause.

8. *Hematologic*. Lithium can cause a leukocytosis, which is benign and doesn't require intervention.

9. *Birth defects*. Lithium exposure during the first trimester has been associated with cardiac malformations, especially Ebstein's anomaly of the tricuspid valve. The risk of cardiac defects was initially reported to be as high as 11%, but this figure represents overreporting of bad outcomes and also doesn't control for the effects of the illness itself, other medications, or the spontaneous rate of malformations. More recent controlled epidemiological studies have reported a much lower rate of Ebstein's anomaly, in the range of 0.1% to 0.7%. While low, this is still approximately 20–140 times greater than the rate in the general population. The risk of major congenital malformations with first-trimester lithium treatment is now thought to be in the range of 4% to 12%, versus 2%–4% in an untreated comparison group.

10. *Toxicity/overdose*. Since lithium in the body is basically a salt dissolved in water, toxicity arises either when the intake of the salt is increased (via intentional or unintentional overdose) or when there is a loss of body water. The latter occurs with increased sweating (e.g., with vigorous exercise during summer months or in the course of illnesses accompanied by fever), from diarrhea or vomiting (e.g., due to an illness or due to lithium toxicity itself), or from increased urination (due to lithium-induced diabetes insipidus).

Patients taking lithium therefore should be warned to maintain adequate hydration, especially in the summer or when ill. They also should be educated about the early signs of lithium toxicity and told that they should stop taking lithium and arrange for an immediate serum assay when such symptoms appear.

Other medications also can contribute to the development of lithium toxicity. Fluid loss is increased when patients take *loop diuretics* such as furosemide, while *thiazide diuretics* not only increase fluid loss but also directly interfere with lithium clearance. *Nonsteroidal anti-inflammatory drugs (NSAIDs)* all raise lithium levels with the exception of sulindac (Clinoril). (This is of even greater concern now that several NSAIDs are available over the counter.) Acetaminophen and aspirin are preferable alternatives, as they do not affect lithium levels. *ACE inhibitors* also raise lithium levels.

Symptoms of lithium toxicity become more severe as serum lithium levels increase. In *mild-to-moderate intoxication (1.5–2.0 mEq/L)*, patients experience tremor, dysarthria, and ataxia along with lethargy, weakness, and gastrointestinal symptoms. In *moderate-to-severe intoxication (2.0–2.5 mEq/L)*, the nausea and vomiting become persistent, syncope or seizures can occur, and the ataxia is now accompanied by muscle fasciculation and myoclonus. Patients can experience impaired consciousness that progresses from delirium to stupor and ultimately to coma. Finally, *severe intoxication (>2.5 mEq/L)* causes seizures, renal failure, and death.

In mild cases, patients should be instructed to stop the lithium and push oral fluids. In more severe cases, the patient's lithium level, electrolytes, renal function, and ECG should be quickly evaluated and intravenous fluids should be administered. In cases of lithium overdose, the clinician should force emesis and perform a gastric lavage, since lithium can form a clump in the stomach (bezoar) that slowly dissolves. Hemodialysis may be performed when patients have more severe symptoms or very high blood levels. This is the only reliable way to eliminate lithium from the body more rapidly. Patients may require serial lithium blood levels and repeated hemodialysis every 6–10 hours since lithium can redistribute from tissue stores to the periphery, causing "secondary peaks."

Note that some symptoms of toxicity (polyuria, vomiting, diarrhea) can further exacerbate dehydration and toxicity. Further, patients who develop delirium due to lithium toxicity might become further unable to keep up with fluid intake or might even take repeated doses of lithium accidentally, both of which can further compound lithium toxicity.

Some patients experience a persistent change in mental status following a lithium overdose despite lithium having declined to an acceptable level. The clinician might presume that the patient must now be displaying a new form of psychopathology, such as a manic episode. More likely, the patient is still delirious: lithium accumulates in the central nervous system, and delirium can persist for several days following restoration of lower serum levels.

Patients who are to be prescribed lithium should first receive an initial workup, both to determine the potential safety of treatment and to provide baseline values. The workup should include a general medical history and physical examination, BUN and creatinine levels, a pregnancy test, thyroid function testing, and an ECG with rhythm strip for patients over age 40. Some authorities also suggest obtaining a baseline complete blood count (CBC).

Serum lithium levels should be assayed before and after dosage increases; steady-state levels are likely to be reached approximately 5 days after a dosage adjustment, but levels might be checked sooner when rapid dosage increases are necessary (e.g., during the treatment of an acute manic episode) or when toxicity is suspected. As serum levels approach the upper limits of the therapeutic range (1.0 mEq/L), levels should be checked at more frequent intervals following dosage increases in order to decrease the risk of toxicity.

Thyroid tests, renal tests, and lithium levels should be obtained every 2–3 months during the first 6 months of maintenance therapy. Subsequently, they can be obtained every 6 months to 1 year if patients are stable. They also should be obtained when clinically indicated (e.g., when breakthrough affective symptoms occur or when new medical complaints arise).

Carbamazepine (Tegretol)

Carbamazepine (CBZ) structurally resembles imipramine, a TCA. However, it has a very different pharmacologic profile, especially when one considers that TCAs lower the seizure threshold and—in bipolar disorder—can induce mania or rapid cycling, while CBZ is an anticonvulsant that can treat both mania and rapid cycling. CBZ is effective in the treatment of simple partial, complex partial, and generalized tonic–clonic ("grand mal") seizures. It is ineffective against (and may even exacerbate) absence seizures. It also effectively treats neuropathic pain, such as trigeminal neuralgia. CBZ usually causes fewer cognitive side effects than do anticonvulsants such as phenytoin and phenobarbital.

CBZ demonstrates complex pharmacokinetics. It is metabolized by the cytochrome P450 system, primarily by enzyme 3A4. Its main metabolite, CBZ-10,11-epoxide, is as powerful an anticonvulsant as the parent compound. CBZ is 75% bound to plasma proteins. This is significant because only unbound (free) drug penetrates to the CSF. Further, the epoxide metabolite reaches concentrations in the plasma and the brain that are 50% that of the parent compound. However, typical plasma levels reflect only the amount of parent compound and reflect the *total* (i.e., bound plus free) CBZ level.

To complicate matters further, CBZ speeds up its own metabolism by inducing increased production of cytochrome enzyme 3A4. This usually occurs after about 2–4 weeks of therapy. Therefore, a patient who is initially improving on the drug may acutely deteriorate, with the blood level being discovered to have declined. (Another possibility in such cases is that the blood level of *other* medications that the patient was taking—for example, those of an antipsychotic or antidepressant drug—may have *also* declined due to enzyme induction.)

CBZ isn't FDA approved for the treatment of bipolar disorder, but it has been well studied over the past decade. Its efficacy in treating acute mania is comparable to lithium or antipsychotic monotherapy. The latency period prior to onset of its antimanic effects is about the same as that seen with lithium. CBZ may be more effective than lithium in treating dysphoric mania, rapid cycling, and mixed states. It also is modestly effective for treating major depressive disorder, with a response rate of about 30% (as opposed to up to 70% for primary antidepressant agents). Like lithium, it isn't a panacea. Fifty percent of patients maintained on CBZ for chronic prophylactic treatment still experience breakthrough symptoms.

Carbamazepine's mechanism of action in treating bipolar disorder remains unclear. Like lithium, it causes a multiplicity of effects, making it difficult to determine which one plays the primary role in controlling bipolar disorder. While it would be tempting to suggest that its mood-stabilizing effects are related to its anticonvulsant effects, there is no evidence that bipolar disorder is related to epilepsy. Further, the time of onset of carbamazepine's antimanic effects is much later than the time of onset of its anticonvulsant and analgesic effects.

Carbamazepine rapidly binds to and inactivates sodium channels, leading to decreased neuronal excitability. This may account for its anticonvulsant and antinociceptive properties. However, with longer-term administration, CBZ affects a variety of neurotransmitter systems, including adenosine, norepinephrine, dopamine, glutamate, GABA, substance P, and aspartate. It also exerts more direct inhibitory effects on both of the known second messenger systems.

Like lithium, CBZ can have both dose-related and idiosyncratic side effects. The typical dose range for use in epilepsy is 4–12 μg/ml, and clinicians use similar dosages in treating bipolar disorder. CBZ causes fewer cognitive side effects at therapeutic doses than does lithium. However, *dose-related side effects* occur in 30%–50% of patients, particularly at serum levels above about 9 μg/ml. They are most prevalent shortly after the initiation of treatment. They include gastrointestinal effects (nausea, vomiting, cramps, diarrhea) and CNS effects (confusion, drowsiness, ataxia, hyperreflexia/clonus, tremor).

Some populations, especially the elderly and those with brain injury, are more prone to developing such neurotoxicity. The goal is therefore to "start low and go slow," especially when longer-term treatment compliance is the goal. Of note, when CBZ is used *in combination with lithium and/or antipsychotic drugs*, there is a synergistic risk of neurotoxicity.

While CBZ can decrease cardiac conduction at the A-V node, this effect occurs less commonly than with TCAs, and the drug generally only poses problems for patients with preexisting conduction disease. An ECG therefore should be obtained prior to starting therapy with older patients. As with TCAs, CBZ can be fatal in overdose, with drowsiness progressing through stupor and coma, heart block, seizures, hypotension, and respiratory depression as its serum levels increase.

CBZ treatment is also associated with potential *idiosyncratic side effects*. While these are less common than the dose-related side effects, they are potentially lethal. They most commonly involve effects on bone marrow, skin, and liver. *Transient leukopenia* occurs commonly (in about 10% of patients) but doesn't predispose to infection and usually doesn't require intervention. *Mild thrombocytopenia* also occurs and often responds to dosage reduction or (in more severe cases) discontinuation of the medication. (Sometimes CBZ can then be successfully restarted at a lower dose.)

Aplastic anemia and agranulocytosis are unrelated to these milder side effects. They occur in somewhere between 1 in 10,000 to 1 in 100,000 patients. They don't appear to be dose-related. Most, but not all, cases arise in the first 3–6 months of treatment, and some clinicians advocate checking CBCs every 2 weeks for the first 2 months and then every 2 to 6 months after this. However, there is no evidence that long-term repeated testing is of benefit. The warning symptoms are fever, sore throat, rash, petechiae, bruising, and easy bleeding. Patients should receive education about these symptoms and should be instructed to seek immediate medical attention should they experience them.

Similarly, while about 10% of patients develop a pruritic rash in the first few weeks of treatment that is transient and benign, a small percentage of these patients can go on to develop life-threatening *exfoliative dermatitis, erythema multiforme, Stevens-Johnson syndrome,* or *toxic epidermal necrolysis.* One clinical strategy might be to educate patients to report any fever, bleeding, or exfoliative lesions but to continue treating with CBZ when the rash appears to be benign. However, given the severity of these syndromes, most clinicians opt to discontinue CBZ when any rash occurs. If the drug is essential, the CBZ might be reintroduced at a later time, often following pretreatment with corticosteroids in an attempt to prevent a recurrence of the rash.

About 10% of patients treated with CBZ develop either *elevation of liver enzymes* from chemical hepatitis or *elevation of bilirubin and alkaline phosphatase* due to cholestasis. These effects usually occur within the first few weeks of therapy. If the elevations are mild, they may respond to dosage reduction with close follow-up. There have been rare cases of fatal hepatic failure, though. Patients should be warned to call if they experience any symptoms of hepatitis (such as malaise, anorexia, nausea/vomiting, edema, or abdominal pain).

Two other noteworthy idiosyncratic side effects can occur with CBZ therapy. From 10% to 30% of patients treated with CBZ develop *hyponatremia and/or hypo-osmolality that reflects an ADH-like effect.* Finally, among the drugs whose metabolism is increased by CBZ (with a resultant lowering of their serum drug levels and loss of effectiveness) are the *oral contraceptives.*

Overall, however, most patients do tolerate CBZ, and its use in bipolar disorder has become more popular over the past decade. Typically, clinicians educate patients about the warning symptoms of neurotoxicity, hepatic injury, bone marrow suppression, and rash, and check blood levels, liver function tests, and a CBC every few weeks initially and then every few months.

Valproate (Depakote)

The molecular structure of **Valproate (VPA)** contains no rings, a rarity for a psychopharmacologic agent. It first was synthesized in the 1880s and for years it was used as a chemical solvent. Its anticonvulsant properties only were discovered in the 1960s, when every drug tested at a particular laboratory in France seemed to demonstrate anticonvulsant properties. Upon further investigation, it was determined that all of these drugs were being administered in a vehicle of valproic acid and that the vehicle was in reality the active drug.

Unlike carbamazepine, valproate is FDA-approved for the treatment of mania in bipolar disorder, in addition to being approved for the treatment of simple and complex partial seizures. VPA is available in two forms, generic valproic acid and divalproex sodium (Depakote), with "valproate" being a general term that connotes either form. The latter form consists of two valproic acid molecules joined by a sodium moiety that also has an enteric coating. This strategy allows for slower absorption and, consequently, fewer gastrointestinal side effects. Another advantage of the divalproex sodium formulation is that acutely manic patients can be administered a single "oral loading dose" of about 20 mg/kg followed by treatment at the final standing dose. This allows patients to achieve a more rapid onset of therapeutic effects (usually within a few days). The valproic acid form doesn't allow for this because it causes significant gastrointestinal side effects unless it is started at lower doses and gradually is titrated upward over several days.

VPA causes fewer cognitive side effects than does lithium or CBZ, and it isn't associated with the extrapyramidal side effects that can occur when antipsychotic drugs are used to treat acute mania. The therapeutic plasma level for treatment of seizure disorder is 50–100 μg/mL, but there is no upper dose level for bipolar disorder and some manic patients require levels of 120 μg/mL or higher. While obtaining blood levels can be important in monitoring the patient's status, it is most important to determine what appears to be the "clinically effective dose" and to weigh this against any dose-related side effects.

The efficacy of VPA appears to be similar to that of lithium in treating the euphoric form of mania, and it is comparable to CBZ in treating patients with dysphoric, mixed, or rapid-cycling states. Data so far suggest generally good efficacy for longer-term prophylaxis of bipolar disorder. While there is scant literature on VPA as a treatment for major depressive disorder, it may not be as effective as lithium.

Like lithium and CBZ, VPA has many effects on neuronal activity, making it difficult to establish its precise mechanism of action in either epilepsy or bipolar disorder. VPA enhances the effect of GABA by inhibiting its catabolism, increasing its release, decreasing its turnover, and increasing receptor density.

The most common *dose-related side effects* associated with VPA are *sedation, nausea, vomiting,* and *diarrhea*. As with lithium and CBZ, these side effects are more common at the time that treatment is initiated. They are less frequent with the sustained-release divalproex sodium preparation. Other side effects resemble those of lithium, including a *fine tremor* (even more of a problem if VPA and lithium are used together) and *weight gain*. Like CBZ, some patients develop elevated liver enzymes and bone marrow suppression (most commonly thrombocytopenia). Both of these may respond to dose reduction along with close monitoring.

VPA has been associated with rare, potentially fatal *idiosyncratic side effects* including *fatal hepatotoxicity, hemorrhagic pancreatitis,* and *agranulocytosis*. The major risk factors for fatal hepatic failure are being under 2 years of age (there have been no fatalities in patients over 10 years of age), coadministration with other anticonvulsants, and the presence of other medical problems in addition to epilepsy. With recognition of these risk factors, the fatality rate from hepatotoxicity has declined from 1 in 10,000 cases to 1 in 50,000 cases. As was the case with CBZ, periodic routine blood monitoring does not appear to decrease mortality, although many clinicians do monitor the CBC and liver enzymes every few months. Caution should be exercised with patients taking *aspirin or warfarin* due to their increased bleeding risk.

Like CBZ, VPA is highly protein-bound, and only the unbound (free) portion reaches the CNS. Also like CBZ, the typical serum level reflects the *total* (bound plus free) drug. Thus, in cases of hypoalbuminemia, or if VPA is given along with a drug such as CBZ, a complex picture will emerge. First, CBZ will compete for protein binding with VPA, thereby increasing free (and therefore CNS) levels of VPA. Second, VPA will increase the free (and therefore CNS) levels of both CBZ and of its active epoxide metabolite. Note that despite these two changes, the *total* serum levels of both CBZ and VPA will appear to both be in the "therapeutic" range, even after the patient suddenly appears toxic. Third, neurotoxicity from these two drugs can occur in synergistic fashion, leading to increased neurotoxicity even when *free* drug levels for each agent are below "toxic" levels. Fourth, and complicating matters even further, over time CBZ induces hepatic enzymes, thereby leading to increased metabolism of both CBZ and VPA. At this point, the serum levels of both drugs will decline. In fact, patients who are taking the full dose of CBZ may have difficulty reaching a therapeutic level of VPA even when they are prescribed high doses of the latter. Therefore, when using these agents in combination, the CBZ dose may need to be decreased and the VPA dose increased. When these agents are used in combination, it is recommended that clinicians obtain *free plasma levels* for both agents.

Gabapentin (Neurontin)

Gabapentin (Neurontin) was released in 1994 and at this point is only FDA-approved as an adjunct treatment for focal seizures with or without secondary generalization. It originally was synthesized to be an analogue of GABA (by integrating GABA into a lipophilic cyclohexane moiety to facilitate transport across the blood–brain barrier). The plan was for the compound to increase GABA receptor activity, thereby inhibiting seizures. While the compound did turn out to inhibit seizures, it was found (remarkably) not to be binding to the GABA receptor. Gabapentin's mechanism of action therefore remains uncertain. It is possible that it interacts with the GABA transporter, thereby indirectly increasing GABA levels.

In the original treatment studies involving epileptic patients, some patients were noted to experience an improvement in their mood and quality of life. Given the success of carbamazepine and valproate in treating a variety of psychiatric conditions, including chronic pain, alcohol withdrawal, aggression/impulsivity, and bipolar disorder, gabapentin also has been studied as a treatment for all of these conditions. Preliminary reports suggested that gabapentin was well tolerated and was potentially effective in treating mania, generalized anxiety disorder, panic disorder, social phobia, and chronic pain.

However, gabapentin's effectiveness as an antimanic agent, especially when used as monotherapy, remains uncertain. While several large case series in which gabapentin was used as an adjunctive treatment in mania suggested that it helped to improve mood, decrease irritability, and decrease frequency of cycling, two later controlled trials (one using gabapentin monotherapy and the other using it as an adjunctive agent) have not shown it to be superior to placebo. Limitations in the studies' designs may have contributed to this negative finding, however. Typically, treatment with gabapentin is initiated at 300 mg three times per day and it then is titrated upward to dosages as high as 2000 or even 3600 mg/day.

Gabapentin is an extremely "clean" drug. It is well absorbed, does not bind to plasma proteins, has few if any drug interactions (making it especially useful in combination with other mood stabilizers or antidepressants), and is not metabolized in humans (it is excreted unchanged by the kidneys). Patients tolerate gabapentin extremely well, even at very high dosages. The most frequent side effects are drowsiness, dizziness, and gastrointestinal upset, especially during the first week of treatment.

Gabapentin is rapidly absorbed (over 2–3 hours) and has a short serum half-life (6–7 hours). While its absorption is not affected by food, it is treated by the gut like an amino acid: it is absorbed through *active transport*. Given this, its absorption slows at higher doses as the transporter becomes more saturated. This, plus its serum half-life, necessitates dosing at three to four times daily, a significant disadvantage. *Pregabalin*, a structurally modified form of gabapentin, may have a longer half-life and greater potency. It is currently undergoing clinical trials.

Lamotrigine (Lamictal)

Lamotrigine (Lamictal) is FDA-approved only as an adjunctive treatment for partial epilepsy. As with other anticonvulsants, findings during initial trials with epileptic patients suggested that it also might be helpful as a mood stabilizer or antidepressant. Like phenytoin and carbamazepine, lamotrigine inhibits voltage-gated sodium channels, thereby reducing the presynaptic release of glutamate. However, it may also have other, as-yet-undetermined mechanisms of action, including serotonin reuptake.

Open-label studies with lamotrigine used both as an adjunctive treatment and as monotherapy as well as a recent large double-blind, placebo-controlled study suggest that it is effective in controlling rapid cycling and mixed bipolar states and that it also demonstrates efficacy in treating depressive episodes without unduly increasing the risk of "switching" into mania.

Most patients tolerate lamotrigine well. The most common side effects are sedation, dizziness, tremor, headache, and nausea. However, as was the case with carbamazepine, the most significant concern with this agent is the risk of developing a *rash*, which in rare cases can progress to life-threatening *Stevens-Johnson syndrome* or *toxic epidermal necrolysis*.

About 10% of patients treated in the clinical trials for epilepsy developed a rash. It occurred twice as often as this when the drug was used in combination with valproate, possibly because valproate inhibits lamotrigine's metabolism. (In contrast, lamotrigine itself does not affect the metabolism of other anticonvulsant agents.) This rash is most likely to occur during the first 6–8 weeks of treatment and occurs more frequently with a higher starting dose or a more rapid titration schedule. Life-threatening rashes also occur more commonly in children than in adults, with rates of 2% versus 0.1%, respectively.

While more severe rash is a rare complication, patients need to be educated about the warning signs, and a slow, fixed titration schedule is commonly employed even for patients who aren't experiencing side effects. For example, in a recent large study of patients with bipolar disorder, lamotrigine monotherapy was initiated at 25 mg/day for 2 weeks, followed by an increase to 50 mg/day for the next 2 weeks. The dosage then was increased in increments of 50 mg/week up to a maximum daily dose of 500 mg/day. For patients taking concomitant valproate, lamotrigine was initiated at 25 mg every other day, followed by 25 mg/day for 2 weeks, and then increased by 25 mg daily every 2 weeks up to a maximum daily dose of 200 mg. For patients taking carbamazepine (which induces the metabolism of lamotrigine), dosages and incremental increases were doubled over the dosages used with lamotrigine monotherapy, with a maximum dosage of 700 mg/day.

Topiramate (Topamax)

Topiramate (Topamax) is FDA-approved for the adjunctive treatment of partial-onset seizures.

While it has been studied in bipolar disorder, as of this writing such research has consisted only of open-label and retrospective studies. However, these suggest that it has efficacy both as a monotherapy and as an adjunctive treatment. Topiramate is a sulfamate-substituted monosaccharide that inhibits firing of the voltage-dependent sodium channel, enhances the effect of GABA at its receptor, and antagonizes the effects of kainate on the glutamate receptor.

As with the other anticonvulsants, the most commonly occurring side effects are somnolence, dizziness, ataxia, headache, and gastrointestinal upset. In addition, however, topiramate therapy is associated in up to 25% of cases with cognitive symptoms that include difficulty concentrating, psychomotor slowing, and word-finding difficulties. These symptoms often have insidious onset after 2–3 weeks of therapy and are the primary reason that patients stop taking the medication, although they sometimes respond to dosage reduction. Treatment with topiramate also is associated with a small but significant increased risk of developing kidney stones. (Its prevalence in patients of 1.5% is two to four times greater than the rate observed in similar, untreated populations.) Topiramate weakly inhibits carbonic anhydrase, thereby reducing urinary citrate excretion and increasing urinary pH, which likely increases the rate of kidney stone formation. Topiramate shouldn't be given concomitantly with other carbonic anhydrase inhibitors and patients should be encouraged to maintain adequate fluid intake in order to lower the urinary concentration of substances involved in renal stone formation.

On the positive side, in contrast to almost all of the previously discussed psychotropic agents, topiramate is more likely to cause *weight loss* than weight gain, a distinct advantage. Some clinicians have even prescribed topiramate as an "antidote" to weight gain induced by other psychotropic agents such as clozapine and olanzapine.

Topiramate does not affect liver enzymes and remains largely unbound to plasma proteins. It does not affect the plasma levels of carbamazepine or valproate but can increase phenytoin levels by as much as 20% in some patients. In the presence of a hepatic-enzyme-inducing agent such as carbamazepine, its dosage may need to be doubled in order to maintain the same serum level. Like carbamazepine, topiramate can interfere with the efficacy of oral contraceptives. The typical starting dose is 25–50 mg/day, with dosages increased by 50 mg/day at weekly intervals, using twice daily dosing. Final dosages have typically ranged from 200 to 400 mg/day.

Electroconvulsive Therapy (ECT)

The first reported use of induced grand mal seizures to treat mental illness was by the Swiss physician Paracelsus, who in the sixteenth century "gave camphor by mouth to produce convulsions and cure lunacy." The first published citation was by Leopold von Auenbrugger (originator of the "percussion method" of cardiac and lung examination), who in the eighteenth century treated "mania vivorum" with camphor every 2 hours to the point of convulsions. About 20 years later, Oliver (in England) and Weikardt (in Russia) also used camphor to treat mania, not knowing about Auenbrugger's earlier work or about each other's work.

Convulsive therapy disappeared for the next hundred years. In 1932, however, Ladislas von Meduna (again unaware of any of any previous work) used camphor to treat a catatonic schizophrenic who had stopped eating, was incontinent, and hadn't moved in 4 years. Over a course of six treatments, the patient reportedly achieved a complete recovery.

Why induce seizures to treat severe mental illness? Meduna postulated that a "biological antagonism" existed between epilepsy and psychosis. He noted that psychiatric illness and epilepsy seemed to co-occur less frequently than otherwise might be expected. (We now know that this is incorrect.) A colleague of Meduna's even had injected blood from schizophrenic patients into epileptics in the hope of discovering an endogenous anticonvulsant.

Meduna also observed that some schizophrenic and catatonic patients' symptoms seemed to improve after they had experienced a spontaneous seizure. This second observation proved to be more prescient. His camphor therapy (he later used pentylenetetrazol) was remarkably successful in spite of the fact that the clinician (and the unanesthetized patient) had to sit for over a half-hour following medication administration anxiously awaiting the seizure.

In 1938, Cerletti and Bini, in Italy, searching

for a safer and more reliable way to induce seizures, applied electricity to the scalp, and this quickly became the preferred means of eliciting a seizure. Electroconvulsive therapy spread throughout Europe in the 1940s. Chlorpromazine was not to be introduced as a treatment for psychosis until 1952, while the MAOIs and TCAs were not to be introduced as treatments for depression until the late 1950s. ECT therefore represented the first effective biological therapy for mental illness. Even now, despite the availability of all of the antidepressant and mood-stabilizing agents previously discussed, many patients either cannot tolerate the medications or have a medication-refractory illness. In the United States, about 100,000 individuals receive ECT annually.

ECT carries the undeserved reputation of being used as a punishment that causes permanent brain damage, a reputation perpetuated by films such as *One Flew Over the Cuckoo's Nest*. ECT, as currently practiced, is safe and efficacious. While it can potentially cause various side effects, this is the case with all medical therapies, including treatment with medications and psychotherapy. Further, psychiatric *illnesses*, especially untreated or partially treated mood disorders, carry significant competing risks. Patients need to be informed of the facts about ECT if they are to make informed decisions rather than having to rely upon misinformation and stigma.

ECT remains the most effective available treatment for mood disorder. In patients with *major depressive disorder* who are receiving ECT either as their first treatment intervention or who previously have received only inadequate courses of pharmacotherapy, its efficacy is 80%–90%. While its efficacy is lower in patients referred for ECT because they have not responded to one or more adequate antidepressant trials, 50%–60%, this response rate is still substantial. There is a delay between the initiation of therapy and the onset of therapeutic effect, but the full therapeutic response generally occurs earlier than it does with medication therapy— that is, after only about a 2–4 week delay in the case of ECT as opposed to a 4–8 week delay with medication.

The efficacy of ECT in *bipolar depression* is similarly high, and its efficacy in treating *mania* is about the same or better than treatment with lithium or antipsychotic medications. ECT may be the treatment of choice for *catatonia*, whether due to mood disorder or schizophrenia. ECT is less effective for treating dysthymic disorder unless one is using it to treat a superimposed major depressive episode.

The most common indications for ECT are medication-ratefractory illness, an inability to tolerate medication side effects, the need for a more rapid and certain response (as occurs in treating patients who are acutely suicidal or who aren't maintaining their basic physical needs such as eating and sleeping), recurrence of symptoms in patients who have previously demonstrated a good response to ECT, and patient preference. ECT also is used to treat schizophrenia that has proven to be refractory to treatment with antipsychotic medications. Less common indications for ECT include Parkinson's disease, neuroleptic malignant syndrome, and intractable epilepsy.

During the ECT procedure, patients receive a muscle relaxant (most commonly succinylcholine), which attenuates motor seizure activity and virtually eliminates the risk of spinal or extremity fractures or dislocations. A bite block also is used to prevent dental injury. Before receiving the muscle relaxant, patients are placed into a state of light anesthesia with a short-acting barbiturate (typically methohexital). Throughout the procedure, patients receive supplemental oxygen by mask, appropriate airway management, and monitoring of their pulse oximetry, blood pressure, cardiac rhythm, and EEG activity. Electrically induced seizures typically last between 30 and 90 seconds. A full course of treatment usually consists of between 4 and 12 sessions given two to three times per week.

Following a successful acute course of treatment, patients remain at high risk for relapse over the next several weeks to months. While most patients receive maintenance medication therapy following ECT, this is more likely to be effective for patients who have received an inadequate course of medication treatment prior to having received ECT than for those referred after they have already had one or more adequate medication trials. In the latter case, ECT responders should not simply be placed back on the same antidepressant medications that they were taking prior to having received ECT. More appropriately, one could try adding an "augmenting" agent (such as lithium or an atypical antipsychotic medication), switching to an alternative antidepressant (perhaps one with a different or broader spectrum of activity), or both.

An increasingly popular alternative strategy is to follow up the acute course of ECT with "maintenance treatments" spaced out over a more extended time frame. For example, a patient might receive one treatment every few weeks on an outpatient basis. This strategy is associated with significantly lower relapse and rehospitalization rates than is maintenance medication therapy.

The risks of ECT involve the cardiac, vascular, and cerebral systems. The electrical stimulus initially triggers a *parasympathetic* discharge that can lead to bradyarrythmias and even a few seconds of asystole. This almost never leads to complications, although some clinicians advocate routine pretreatment with a vagolytic agent such as atropine or glycopyrrolate. In contrast, during the seizure a *sympathetic* discharge occurs, leading to hypertension and tachycardia. This usually only lasts for the duration of the seizure.

While the risks associated with this sympathetic discharge aren't that different from asking patients to walk briskly up two or three flights of steps, many patients referred for ECT are elderly, frail, and even bed-bound. Some of them have already experienced previous heart attacks or strokes. The risks associated with the sympathetic response in these latter situations can be attenuated through the use of short-acting intravenous β-blockers or nitrates.

Prior to receiving ECT, patients should receive a detailed medical evaluation, with the emphasis on identifying specific conditions that might increase the patient's risk of complications. The most important conditions are: *(1)* unstable or severe cardiovascular conditions (a recent myocardial infarction, unstable angina, poorly compensated congestive heart failure, or severe valvular cardiac disease), *(2)* an aneurysm or vascular malformation that might be susceptible to rupture with increased blood pressure, *(3)* increased intracranial pressure (as may occur with some brain tumors or other space-occupying cerebral lesions), *(4)* a recent stroke, pulmonary conditions (such as severe chronic obstructive pulmonary disease, asthma, or pneumonia), or

(5) patients who are rated at level 4 or 5 on the American Society of Anesthesiology (ASA) physical status classification scheme (typically because of severe cardiopulmonary or other organ system disease).

The evaluation also may include an electrocardiogram, chest X-ray, and neuroimaging. Potentially deliriogenic medications also should be minimized or discontinued. There are no absolute contraindications to ECT. When significant medical conditions are discovered, they should be stabilized to the extent that this is possible, and the risks posed by ECT should be weighed against the gravity of the patient's psychiatric condition and also the risks of alternative treatments.

The rate of mortality associated with ECT is estimated to be approximately the same as that associated with minor surgery or childbirth, about 1 per 10,000 patients or 1 per 80,000 treatments. Despite the frequent use of ECT in patients who are elderly or who have significant medical problems, the mortality rate appears to have declined in recent years. The morbidity and mortality associated with ECT may be less than that those that are associated with some medications (particularly the TCAs). Further, some longitudinal follow-up studies have suggested that mortality rates following psychiatric hospitalization are lower among those depressed patients who received ECT than among those who received other treatment modalities or no treatment.

During all three trimesters of pregnancy, ECT may be a safer treatment for depression or mania than are many psychotropic drugs. Exposure during ECT to medications that cross the placenta only occurs for a few minutes, thereby minimizing the risk of teratogenic complications. In contrast, the administration of anticonvulsants during pregnancy has been associated with a low risk of a variety of fetal birth defects, including facial deformity and spina bifida. Similarly, the administration of lithium during the first trimester is associated with a low risk of fetal cardiac malformations.

Cognitive side effects related to ECT are the major complications limiting its use. More severely depressed patients who receive ECT often have difficulty attending to, processing, and recalling information prior to treatment, as a result of their illness. Therefore, shortly after completion of an ECT course, many of these patients report *improved* subjective cognitive functioning which is confirmed by improved scores on a variety of neuropsychological tests. Against this background, however, patients also may experience transient confusion or delirium as well as a characteristic pattern of anterograde and retrograde memory deficits.

Patients experience a *transient postictal confusional state* for 30–60 minutes following each treatment session. Some patients in the midst of a series of treatments also experience a mild, transient *delirium*. This clears upon completion of the treatment course. Elderly patients and patients with a preexisting neurologic disease or insult (such as a stroke, Parkinson's disease, or Alzheimer's disease) are at greater risk for becoming delirious. Patients with only "subclinical" evidence of neurologic disease (basal ganglia lesions or severe white matter hyperintensities on a pretreatment MRI scan) also are at greater risk, as are patients who receive anticholinergic medications during the treatment course. Monitoring patients' cognitive status during a course of ECT is essential, particularly when patients are receiving outpatient therapy. When the patient is safe to return to work, drive, live independently, and make important financial or personal decisions needs to be determined on a case-by-case basis, since the extent of cognitive side effects is quite variable. The presence of supportive family or friends can be of particular importance in the outpatient setting.

ECT also can be associated with the development of two kinds of amnesia. *Anterograde amnesia* refers to difficulty laying down new memories for events that occur shortly after the treatment session. Retrograde amnesia refers to a loss of memory for events that occurred prior to treatment that previously had been remembered. ECT produces retrograde deficits for both autobiographic and more impersonal memories (e.g., memories of public events), but loss of personal memories is likely to be less severe, perhaps reflecting these memories being more deeply encoded. Events closest in time to the administration of ECT seem to be most vulnerable, and personal events of less objective significance are more likely to be forgotten than events that are more important to patients, again perhaps reflecting deeper encoding of the latter type of memory. These losses improve substantially after completion of the ECT course, but residual difficulties do persist in some patients. The severity and persistence of retrograde memory loss is greater when a bitemporal stimulus electrode placement is utilized than when both electrodes are placed over the nondominant hemisphere. While some patients have complained of *permanent* loss of autobiographical memories dating back even years prior to having received ECT or have complained of *persisting memory problems* years after ECT, objective neuropsychological tests have not confirmed such deficits. The nature of this subjective amnesia therefore remains unclear. While psychological factors may play a role, it also is possible that some cognitive deficits are too subtle be detected by existing techniques. Of note, many of these patients are still depressed, and depression itself can contribute to memory impairment. Autopsy and MRI studies have found no evidence that ECT itself causes brain damage.

Confusion and memory loss can be decreased if the ECT stimulus is given at a dose just above the seizure threshold and/or if the stimulus electrodes are both placed in a unilateral position over the nondominant hemisphere, rather than placing one over each temporal area. However, lower stimulus energy and unilateral placement, while associated with lower rates of cognitive problems, can be associated with a lower response rate. The decreased efficacy associated with unilateral stimulation delivered at just suprathreshold energy levels occurs even when a typical motor seizure occurs. One therefore can't predict how effective a treatment session will be based solely on whether the patient experienced a seizure or whether the seizure lasted for a certain duration.

While the delivery of a *subconvulsive* electrical stimulus is clearly inadequate (the patient must seize to get well), inducing the motor seizure is necessary but not sufficient to guarantee treatment efficacy. Perhaps this is because the seizure must adequately *generalize* to involve deeper limbic structures in order to be effective. Adequate seizure generalization is more likely to occur using a bilateral lead placement or—in the case of a unilateral lead placement—when energy doses several orders of magnitude above the patient's seizure threshold are delivered.

As is the case with all antidepressant and mood-stabilizing treatments, the mechanism of action of ECT is uncertain. It does appear to affect monoamine neurotransmission, but in a different manner than currently available medications. Like most antidepressants, ECT is associated with downregulation of the norepinephrine β-receptor, but unlike most antidepressants, it is associated with *upregulation* (rather than downregulation) of serotonin $5HT_2$ receptors. Unlike the SSRIs, ECT is not effective in the treatment of obsessive–compulsive disorder.

Similarly, ECT is different from typical *antimanic drugs*. Like carbamazepine and valproate, ECT has anticonvulsant effects. During a course of therapy, a patient's seizure threshold (the amount of energy that must be delivered to induce a seizure) increases, while seizure duration decreases. However, unlike the anticonvulsants, ECT *decreases rather than increases GABA synthesis and release*. This has led to speculation that perhaps inducing seizures leads to the release of some other endogenous anticonvulsant that decreases "limbic kindling" through a mechanism that is distinct from increased GABA activity. Also, unlike the anticonvulsants, ECT offers profound antidepressant effects.

ECT is especially effective in treating psychotic depression. Despite this, while antipsychotic medications *block* dopamine receptors, ECT *increases* dopamine receptor sensitivity. ECT even has been utilized as an adjunctive therapy for patients with later-stage Parkinson's disease (a condition characterized by dopamine deficiency). ECT may be the treatment of choice for patients who have both Parkinson's disease and psychotic depression, since it allows clinicians to treat both the psychotic symptoms and the extrapyramidal symptoms simultaneously, rather than being forced to treat one symptom complex at the expense of exacerbating the other symptom complex.

Experimental Therapies

Two promising new therapies that are still in the empirical testing stage are transcranial magnetic stimulation (TMS) and vagal nerve stimulation. Both have the potential to offer antidepressant efficacy due to direct electrical brain stimulation while allowing lower dosages of energy to be ap-

plied. Therefore, they are not burdened with the cognitive side effects that can complicate treatment with ECT.

Transcranial magnetic stimulation is a noninvasive technique in which neurons are stimulated by repetitive, brief, electromagnetic pulses. In contrast with ECT, which triggers a generalized convulsion and requires higher amounts of current, TMS allows one to stimulate *targeted* brain regions by placing a large electromagnet over that particular region (the frontal region having received the most study). The procedure is performed in awake patients, without any need for anesthesia. The most common side effect is a muscle tension headache, which occurs in 10%–20% of patients. It tends to be mild and readily alleviated with over-the-counter analgesics. Current research is attempting to delineate the efficacy of the treatment, the optimal stimulation parameters, the duration of the clinical response, and the brain regions associated with greatest clinical efficacy when stimulated.

Vagal nerve stimulation entails the subcutaneous implantation (usually under the left axilla) of a small, lightweight, pacemaker-like pulse generator that extends two electrodes to the left vagus nerve. (The procedure is typically performed as an outpatient and takes about an hour. The device can operate for about 8–12 years.) One implanted, the device applies mild intermittent pulses to the vagus nerve. The vagus nerve in turn sends widespread direct and indirect connections throughout the brain, particularly to the limbic region.

Stimulating the vagus nerve appears to cause changes in brain neurophysiology such that this treatment has proven useful in suppressing seizure activity in epileptic patients who have not fully responded to antiepileptic medications. In some of these patients, improvements in mood have been noted that exceed what might have been expected solely due to improved seizure control. Given the efficacy of anticonvulsant medications as mood stabilizers and antidepressants, prospective trials now are underway to delineate the extent to which vagal nerve stimulation offers efficacy in treatment-refractory depression. Early results are promising, and the treatment already has been approved for the treatment of depression in Europe and Canada.

Stages of Treatment

Treatment of mood disorder should progress along three stages, the acute phase, the continuation phase, and the maintenance phase. These stages are depicted in Figure 7–7 and are defined by the patient's current degree of symptom severity. The "five R's" of clinical treatment are response, relapse, remission, recurrence, and recovery.

In the **acute phase** of treatment, the physician *makes the diagnosis* and *decides on a treatment strategy.* The choice of treatment often is made based on a guess as to whether the effects of a particular class of medication will work to the patient's benefit or detriment. The clinician might consider factors such as: *(1)* the patient's risk of becoming delirious, *(2)* the patient's risk of overdosing on medication, *(3)* whether the patient has responded (or failed to respond) in the past to particular types of medication or psychotherapy, *(4)* whether the patient appears to have a bipolar diathesis that places her at greater risk of becoming manic or of rapid cycling, *(5)* whether family members who have had similar symptoms have responded to particular forms of treatment, and *(6)* the presence of comorbid medical or psychiatric conditions.

For example, in atypical depression, a MAOI might be chosen for its greater efficacy, but such a choice would be contraindicated in a patient judged to be at high risk for an overdose attempt or believed to be unreliable in following through with strict dietary restrictions. An SSRI might be a better initial choice in such a case. In geriatric depression, a serotonergic agent, bupropion, or venlafaxine might be chosen due to their safer cardiac profile and lower risk for causing anticholinergic delirium, but a secondary TCA might still be chosen due to it potential for offering greater efficacy in more severe cases. A TCA might be chosen when there is a comorbid chronic pain condition. Wellbutrin might be chosen in bipolar depression that hasn't responded to mood stabilizers alone due to the possibility that it offers a lower risk of inducing mania. MAOIs may be more effective than other antidepressants in refractory cases of bipolar depression. SSRIs or clomipramine are usually chosen when depression accompanies obsessive–compulsive disorder, since drugs with strong serotonergic effects are required to effectively treat the latter condition. ECT or the combination of an antidepressant and an antipsychotic are usually chosen when depression is accompanied by psychotic features, given the low response rate of psychotic depression to antidepressant monotherapy.

When the patient has not responded to a single agent, the clinician has several available options: *(1)* she might *increase the dose* of the single med-

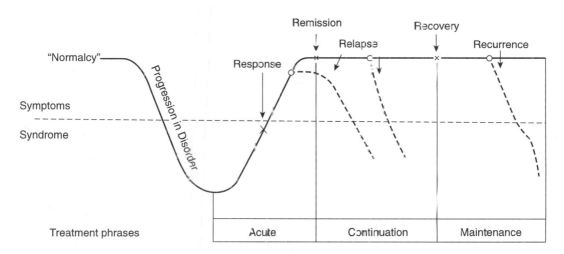

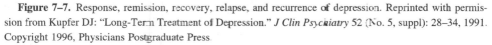

Figure 7–7. Response, remission, recovery, relapse, and recurrence of depression. Reprinted with permission from Kupfer DJ: "Long-Term Treatment of Depression." *J Clin Psychiatry* 52 (No. 5, suppl): 28–34, 1991. Copyright 1996, Physicians Postgraduate Press.

ication, *(2)* she might *switch* to a different medication, *(3)* she might *combine two classes of medication*, or *(4)* she might "augment" the first medication with a second medication.

The third strategy differs from the fourth strategy in that in the latter case, one isn't adding a
second primary treatment but is adding a medication that is known to have lesser efficacy when
used as monotherapy but may have particular
value in giving primary medications a needed
"boost." For example, in treating depression, the
most common augmenting techniques are to add
lithium, thyroid hormone, or an atypical antipsychotic medication. Some patients demonstrate a
rapid and gratifying response to such strategies.

Much of the "art" of psychopharmacology
consists of determining which of these routes to
take. Several considerations should be taken into
account. First, has the patient demonstrated at
least *some* response (i.e., a "partial" response) to
the first medication trial? If so, a dose increase
or augmentation might be appropriate. If not, a
switch or a combination strategy may offer
greater therapeutic yield. Is the patient willing to
take more than one antidepressant? If not, a dose
increase or a switch would be most appropriate.
Is the patient able to withstand potential adverse
drug reactions that might arise from these strategies? If the patient already is experiencing significant side effects on the first medication (e.g.,
sexual dysfunction) despite little therapeutic benefit, a switch might be most appropriate.

When employing combination strategies, the
potential for pharmacokinetic interactions should
be considered, especially the risk of toxicity due
either to one drug inhibiting the metabolism of
another (e.g., an SSRI inhibiting the metabolism
of a TCA due to inhibition of cytochrome enzyme 2D6) or to the risk of precipitating a serotonin syndrome (especially when serotonergic
agents are combined with an MAOI).

Also, pharmacodynamic interactions should
be considered. Theoretical considerations suggest that a "rational" combination of two drugs
with *different* mechanisms of action offers the
potential for greater synergistic effect, and therefore greater efficacy, than a combination of two
drugs with *similar* mechanisms of action.

For example, rather than combine two SSRIs,
"rational polypharmacy" suggests that it would
be preferable to combine an SSRI (which affects

serotonin) with bupropion (which affects norepinephrine and dopamine). The latter combination
might allow not only for synergistic treatment of
different dimensions of the *symptom complex*
(with the bupropion helping address symptoms
of anergia and the SSRI helping to address symptoms of anxiety and worry) but for synergistic
side effect profiles (with the bupropion helping
to counteract sexual dysfunction or apathy potentially induced by the SSRI). Or, one might
combine mirtazapine (which promotes greater
presynaptic *release* of all of the monoamines)
with venlafaxine (which inhibits the *reuptake* of
monoamines), thereby allowing for substantial
synergistic effect involving all of the
monoamines, as well as allowing for the possibility that mirtazapine's serotonin receptor antagonist effects might help to minimize gastrointestinal upset or sexual dysfunction induced
by venlafaxine. One must keep in mind that many
of these "rational" strategies—while theoretically gratifying—have not been subjected to controlled, empirical research.

One advantage of the combination antidepressant strategy over the augmenting strategy is that
some patients who respond to the two-drug combination might ultimately be transitioned to
monotherapy with the second agent. The first
agent might be gradually tapered while the clinician continues to assess the patient's symptoms
to assure that they do not worsen. When the latter occurs, it suggests that the patient does in fact
require both medications, and the dose of the first
medication should be titrated upward again.

For patients with bipolar disorder who are in
manic, mixed, or rapidly cycling states, the most
appropriate primary treatment is either a mood
stabilizer or ECT. For patients who become
manic while already taking a particular mood stabilizer, the clinician should ensure that the patient has been compliant with medication and—
if so—that the dosage has been maximized. One
should attempt to achieve a high enough serum
level in an attempt to maximize monotherapy and
decrease the risk of relapse (although, not uncommonly, compromises are necessary in order
to minimize dose-related side effects). Clinicians
should avoid or discontinue antidepressants if
possible. If treatment with a mood stabilizer has
been optimized but the patient remains manic, a
second (or even a third) mood stabilizer might

be added. Alternatively, one might add an adjunctive medication such as an antipsychotic or benzodiazepine. The patient's general medical condition should be checked to rule out the presence of potential contributory conditions (especially thyroid disease for patients taking lithium or prescribed or illicit substances with mood-elevating properties).

For patients with bipolar disorder who are currently depressed, the primary goal is to effectively treat the depression while avoiding precipitating mania or increasing "cycling." Ideally, one should maximize the use of mood stabilizers first rather than immediately adding an antidepressant. TCAs in particular should be avoided since these appear to be the most destabilizing class of antidepressants. Among the mood-stabilizing agents, lithium appears to be the most effective antidepressant (as well as being the only one demonstrated to reduce the risk of suicide in bipolar disorder). If lithium currently is not being employed, it could be added to the regimen, while if lithium already is in use, one should ensure that its serum levels are in the most effective range (0.8 mEq/L or higher). Lamotrigine also appears to be a mood stabilizer with notable antidepressant properties. An alternative to adding a second mood stabilizer, especially for the patient who is already taking lithium or who has already been found to have difficulty tolerating lithium, is to add either an antidepressant or an atypical antipsychotic agent while continuing treatment with the present mood stabilizer.

For the depressed bipolar patient with psychotic symptoms, the first additional agent would likely be an antipsychotic agent. Even for the nonpsychotic patient, the atypical antipsychotic agents appear to possess antidepressant properties distinct from their antipsychotic effects, possibly related to their serotonin receptor antagonism. Another advantage of the atypical agents is they are less likely to cause tardive dyskinesia, which bipolar patients appear especially vulnerable to developing when treated with the traditional antipsychotic agents. (For example, in one study, tardive dyskinesia was observed in one-third of patients with bipolar disorder who were receiving treatment with traditional antipsychotic medication; none of the patients in the group treated without antipsychotic medication showed signs of tardive dyskinesia.) An-

tipsychotic medications are described in greater detail in Chapter 8.

When an antidepressant is added to the regimen of a patient with bipolar disorder, the goal of treating depression while minimizing the risk of precipitating a manic or mixed state or rapid cycling necessitates different strategies than when it is used to treat major depressive disorder. Here, rather than attempting to maintain the patient over an extended period of time on the full antidepressant doses, attempts are made to start with lower doses, only escalating to full doses if necessary, followed by attempts to discontinue the antidepressant after a relatively brief course (weeks to months). The long-term strategy will be influenced by the patient's clinical characteristics. (For example, a previous history of rapid cycling or of antidepressant-induced mania or cycling would be cause for a more conservative strategy.) Bupropion may be less likely to induce mania than other antidepressants, although the SSRIs may be equally efficacious and also appear to carry a lower risk of inducing mania than the TCAs. Many clinicians avoid using fluoxetine in patients with bipolar disorder since its long half-life prevents it from being eliminated from the patient's system quickly following discontinuation in the event that the patient becomes manic. In less severe cases, adjunctive psychotherapy also is a valuable intervention.

Some patients with bipolar II disorder who present in a depressive episode might benefit from antidepressant monotherapy. These patients appear to be less prone to experience antidepressant-induced mood elevations; when this does occur it more often takes the form of a milder hypomanic state than a full-blown manic episode. Since these patients often aren't troubled by their hypomanic periods and may even be at their most productive during these periods, and since they might tolerate antidepressant monotherapy better than combined therapy with both an antidepressant and a mood stabilizer, antidepressant monotherapy might be attempted. At least, this *appears* to be the case based on a small number of short-term, uncontrolled studies involving small numbers of patients. Whether patients with bipolar II disorder who are maintained on antidepressant monotherapy are rendered more refractory to treatment or more prone to cycling over the longer term remains open questions. One might decide to avoid monotherapy when treating patients who have a higher risk profile, such as a history of more than a few past episodes of hypomania or who are rapid cycling (i.e., who demonstrate four or more mood swings per year), or who have experienced functional impairment during hypomanic phases.

One goal in the acute phase of depression therapy is to help the patient *adhere* to the treatment, be it medication, psychotherapy, or a combination strategy, despite the nihilistic attitudes and increased sensitivity to medication side effects that often accompany depression. Side effects must be closely monitored and addressed. The acute phase extends until there is a clinical response to treatment. **Response** refers to a decrease in clinically significant symptoms following the initiation of treatment. In uncomplicated cases, this phase lasts for 1–3 months. After this, the patient is considered to be in **remission**.

Remission indicates that the patient has entered the **continuation phase** of therapy, which typically lasts for at between 4 and 9 months (typically about 6 months). During this phase, the goal is to *monitor for completeness of response, for relapse, and for any late-appearing side effects*. The patient is still "convalescing" during this phase, and discontinuation of medication during or before this phase is associated with a *higher rate of relapse*. **Relapse** refers to the return of some symptoms during or upon cessation of treatment. Note that rapid discontinuation of medication rather than a slow taper may increase the chance of the patient experiencing a relapse.

If the patient doesn't experience a relapse and remains in a more extended state of clinical remission, he is considered to have *recovered* from the depressive episode and to have entered the **maintenance phase** of therapy. The goal during this phase is to prevent future episodes from occurring. During the continuation phase, a return of symptoms is considered to be a relapse of the original depressive episode; however, if the symptoms return during the maintenance phase, this is considered a **recurrence**—that is, a new depressive episode. The diagnosis would be relabeled at this point as "recurrent" depression.

During the continuation or the maintenance phases, clinicians should watch closely for signs of *"roughening"* of mood. This term refers to a recurrence of subsyndromal depressive or hypo-

manic symptoms despite the patient otherwise still meeting the criteria for having recovered. For example, the patient may complain of difficulties sleeping, mild fatigue, or increased procrastination. While these symptoms are nonspecific and might reflect the effects of stress or of a viral illness, they also might be harbingers of an impending depressive episode. Similarly, increased creativity and a decreased need for sleep might be harbingers of an impending manic episode. If particular subsyndromal symptoms always have tended to precede affective episodes for particular patients, these symptoms should routinely be inquired about, and patients and their families also should be educated about these "red flags." While these symptoms don't inevitably indicate that a recurrence of illness is imminent, clinicians who observe the presence of roughening should strongly consider raising the dose of the patient's prophylactic medication at that point rather than waiting to find out.

Traditionally, antidepressants are discontinued and psychotherapy is terminated during the maintenance phase, particularly if this has been the patient's first episode of major depressive disorder. In such cases, most clinicians attempt to taper medications during a period when the patient is likely to be under less stress. For example, summer vacation would be a better time for college students to attempt a medication taper rather than shortly before their final exams. If symptoms return during the taper, the dose should be increased. In the case of bipolar disorder, long-term maintenance medication therapy is appropriate even after only a single episode of mania.

For many patients, depression is a chronic disease. These patients can benefit from ongoing maintenance antidepressant therapy and/or "maintenance psychotherapy." They should be maintained on the same dosage of antidepressant that proved to be necessary to treat their symptoms during the acute phase, since lower doses tend to be associated with a greater risk of symptom recurrence.

Patients often ask, "Do I need to take these medications for the rest of my life?" Since answering this question involves applying statistics to an individual case, there is no single correct answer. However, the clinician and patient should take several factors into account. First, there is convincing evidence that patients with three or more major depressive episodes benefit from maintenance-phase treatment and that—even at 5 years—maintenance medication has prophylactic efficacy. When patients only have experienced two major depressive episodes, the choice is less clear. Factors associated with a greater risk of recurrence in such cases include poor interepisode recovery between these two episodes, the two episodes having occurred within the last 3 years, and the presence of a family history of major depressive disorder or bipolar disorder. Even when the patient and physician decide to discontinue medication, the patient still should be followed up for monitoring at regular intervals. Finally, since early intervention can shorten the duration of an episode, the "door should always be left open" for the patient to immediately return for a resumption of care should his or her symptoms recur.

More detailed recommendations about the treatment of mood disorders are offered in several consensus guidelines and algorithms that have been advanced. These include guidelines for the treatment of major depressive disorder and for bipolar disorder authored by the American Psychiatric Association, recommendations for the treatment of depression in primary care from the Depression Guideline Panel of the U.S. Public Health Service Agency for Health Care Policy and Research, and the Texas Medication Algorithm Project (Crimson et al., 1999).

SUMMARY

Major depressive disorder is among the most common disorders seen by the primary care physician; up to 10% of patients entering the outpatient clinic are in the midst of a current episode. Despite this, and despite the profound morbidity and mortality associated with depression, this disorder remains underdiagnosed and undertreated.

One goal of this chapter has been to instill an appreciation of the most common presentations of mood disorders. A second goal has been to introduce the relevant psychological and biological approaches to the treatment of mood disorders.

A final goal has been to demonstrate how disease reasoning can be applied to a psychiatric illness even when we don't yet have a full understanding of the condition's underlying pathology

and etiology. In the case of the mood disorders, genetic factors appear to predispose individuals to develop the illness, although environmental factors (particularly significant losses or blows to self-esteem) likely play an important role in triggering and perpetuating the illness.

Once established, the illness progresses over time. Episodes beget future episodes, and untreated (or undertreated) illness tends to become more severe and more treatment-refractory. This clinical picture likely reflects a host of progressive biological and psychological changes. In more severe and more chronic cases, neuroimaging reveals a loss of hippocampal and frontal lobe volume, likely caused by an exaggerated stress response which includes elevated cortisol levels, increased neurotoxicity, and decreased activity by neuroprotective proteins such as brain-derived neurotrophic factor. These brain changes also are associated with the development of progressive cognitive symptoms such as impaired learning, memory, and problem-solving. Patient's attitudes—even their personal identities—come to revolve around the depression, further perpetuating the illness.

Effective treatment intervenes at multiple points along this cascade. In milder cases, psychotherapy directed toward depressive attitudes and behaviors can both improve mood (as measured with various rating scales) and affect brain metabolism (as measured with serial functional neuroimaging studies). Antidepressant medications, mood-stabilizing medications, and electroconvulsive therapy act through other mechanisms which still haven't been fully elucidated. While they all acutely influence monoamine metabolism or neuronal excitability, they likely also exert even more profound neuromodulatory and neuroprotective activity following chronic administration over a period of weeks to months. Medication combinations offer the greatest potential for synergistic effects but also offer the greatest potential for toxicity. The choice of a particular treatment strategy should be tailored to the patient's particular case based on factors such as the current presentation, past treatment response, risk of side effects, and the presence of comorbid medical and psychiatric conditions. Combination treatment with medication and psychotherapy offers the greatest promise in more severe or refractory cases.

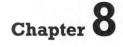

Schizophrenia and Other Psychotic Disorders

Schizophrenia is a prevalent condition and a significant source of morbidity and mortality. It affects 1% of the population worldwide. In the United States, it accounts for 25% of hospital days, 20% of Social Security benefit days, 10% of the disabled population, and 2% of the gross national product. Thirty percent of patients with schizophrenia attempt to kill themselves at some point; 10% of patients with schizophrenia die by suicide.

Schizophrenia can be difficult to treat. Twenty percent to 30% of patients respond poorly or not at all to currently available pharmacologic therapies. Relapse rates are very high: 20% of patients who take their medications appropriately experience relapses despite this, while 70% of patients who stop taking their medication relapse within 1 year. Noncompliance rates are also very high: 40% of patients are not taking their medications as prescribed by 6 months following an acute episode of illness.

For several reasons, all clinicians need to know about schizophrenia. First, schizophrenia is extremely common and therefore clinicians are certain to encounter it. Second, patients with schizophrenia have higher rates of medical morbidity and mortality than do people in the general population, and these associated medical illnesses often are unrecognized and untreated by physicians. Third, various medical conditions and medications can cause symptoms that re-

semble those occurring in schizophrenia, and therefore all clinicians needs to be able to recognize which symptoms are most typical of true schizophrenia. Fourth, the antipsychotic medications used to treat schizophrenia are associated with a variety of general medical complications that may require treatment.

Schizophrenia is characterized by the *presence* of characteristic psychotic symptoms (hallucinations, delusions, and/or thought disorder) in the *absence* of either a change in level of consciousness (which distinguishes it from delirium), a significant disturbance of cognition (which distinguishes it from dementia), or a primary change in mood (which distinguishes it from a depressive episode or manic episode). Before diagnosing schizophrenia, one also must attempt to rule out the possibility that the patient's psychotic symptoms reflect central nervous system manifestations of a general medical illness or of a medication, toxin, or substance of abuse.

Schizophrenia is distinguished from mood disorder associated with psychotic symptoms since the distinction carries important treatment implications. Schizophrenic patients likely will require chronic treatment with antipsychotic medications but not antidepressant or antimanic medications while the reverse is the case for patients with mood disorder. This distinction also has important prognostic implications since the prognosis typically is worse for schizophrenia than for mood disorder.

While schizophrenia typically is diagnosed "by exclusion" (i.e., only after all other psychiatric illnesses that present with psychotic symptoms have been considered and ruled out) some symptoms are more commonly associated with schizophrenia than with other illnesses. These include characteristic impairments in patients' abilities to organize their thinking, to relate with people around them, and to distinguish their internal mental processes from sensory perceptions of the external world. These particular syndromal features have been recognized since antiquity and in every culture.

DSM-IV includes several diagnostic entities under the rubric of "psychotic disorders." These are listed in Table 8–1. These disorders share various features of schizophrenia, tend to be more common in the relatives of individuals who have schizophrenia, and are treated with similar medications. All of this suggests the existence of a "schizophrenic spectrum" of conditions. Given this, our discussion will emphasize schizophrenia but then will touch on these related syndromes. As was the case for delirium, dementia, and the mood disorders, we first will examine the characteristic clinical syndrome of schizophrenia (phenomenology, course, and epidemiology), and follow this up with a discussion of

Table 8–1. *DSM-IV-TR* Classification of Psychotic Disorders

SCHIZOPHRENIA

Symptoms persist for at least 6 months, including at least 1 month of active-phase symptoms, including hallucinations, delusions, thought disorder, disorganized or catatonic behavior, or "negative" symptoms (more on the latter momentarily), along with evidence of a decline in social or occupational functioning

SCHIZOPHRENIFORM DISORDER

Same criteria as schizophrenia except for its duration (1 to 6 months) and (given its shorter time span) the absence of a requirement that there be evidence of a decline in functioning

BRIEF PSYCHOTIC DISORDER

A psychotic disturbance lasting more than 1 day but remitting by 1 month

SCHIZOAFFECTIVE DISORDER

The patient meets criteria for both schizophrenia and mood disorder. There are acute episodes in which the patient demonstrates evidence of both mood disorder and active-phase symptoms of schizophrenia, but these are preceded or followed by at least 2 weeks of delusions or hallucinations *without* prominent mood symptoms (which is what distinguishes this from major depressive disorder or bipolar disorder with psychotic symptoms)

DELUSIONAL DISORDER

Nonbizarre delusions in the absence of other active-phase symptoms of schizophrenia, lasting for at least 1 month

SHARED PSYCHOTIC DISORDER (*FOLIE A DEUX*)

The disturbance develops in an individual who is strongly influenced by someone else who has an established delusion with similar content

PSYCHOTIC DISORDER DUE TO A GENERAL MEDICAL CONDITION

The psychotic symptoms are judged to be a direct physiological consequence of a general medical condition

SUBSTANCE-INDUCED PSYCHOTIC DISORDER

The psychotic symptoms are judged to be a direct physiological consequence of a drug of abuse, a medication, or toxin exposure.

PSYCHOTIC DISORDER NOT OTHERWISE SPECIFIED

The patient demonstrates either a presentation with psychotic symptoms that don't meet the criteria for any of the specific psychotic disorders or there is currently inadequate or contradictory information preventing a more specific diagnosis from being made

Source: Adapted with permission from the *Diagnostic and Statistical Manual of Mental Disorders, Fourth Edition, Text Revision.* Copyright 2000 American Psychiatric Association.

presumed pathology and etiology. Lastly, we will discuss the currently available treatments in relation to these theories.

THE CLINICAL SYNDROME

Phenomenology

Historical Diagnostic Schemes: Categorical Versus Dimensional Criteria

Descriptions of the characteristic symptoms of schizophrenia can be found in writings dating back to the fifteenth century BC. However, psychotic illness has been lumped together under the label of "insanity" or "moral weakness." By the end of the nineteenth century, psychological theorists had made a large number of dubious distinctions between forms of psychosis, including "old maid's insanity," "monomania," "moon madness," "masturbatory insanity," and "wedding night psychosis."

One hundred years ago, *Emil Kraepelin* made the greatest contribution to our current psychiatric nosology by distinguishing between manic-depressive psychosis (our current bipolar disorder) and dementia praecox (our current schizophrenia). Kraepelin noted that the former illness was characterized by the presence of significant mood symptoms (either depression or mania) and a cyclical course while the latter was characterized by an absence of pervasive mood symptoms and a more deteriorative course. This simple conceptual scheme revolutionized psychiatric thinking, and earlier classification schemes fell by the wayside.

Kraepelin's analysis emphasized both *cross-sectional description* and *course of illness*. This reflected his research methods. After examining each newly admitted patient, he and his residents would write down the patient's presenting symptoms and presumed diagnosis on an index card. At the time of discharge, the card was updated: the current symptoms again were written down, along with the discharge diagnosis.

Kraepelin kept these cards in a "diagnosis box" and frequently flipped through them (even taking them along with him when on vacations). Kraepelin was especially interested in which symptoms improved, worsened, or changed and

how these changes affected the patient's ultimate functional outcome. He recognized that a given patient's biography and culture influenced the *content* of his or her delusions and hallucinations, but he did not adhere to theories of "psychogenesis."

Thus, Kraepelin emphasized the *form* of the illness *across* patients rather than the unique details of any *particular* patient's life story. In doing so, he discovered that the mere presence or absence of prominent mood symptoms was a powerful predictor of the patient's prognosis. When prominent mood symptoms were present, the patient tended to improve or to have a cyclical illness; when they were absent, the prognosis was much poorer. This demarcation was simple but was far from obvious. Adolph Meyer, a leader in American psychiatry at the time, commented about Kraepelin's nosology: "The terms of a tradition of over 2000 years are overthrown."

Kraepelin's contributions to psychiatric nosology go even further. In addition to describing dementia praecox and its characteristic hallucinations and delusions (what we now refer to as the positive symptoms of schizophrenia), he described another syndrome, characterized by a *loss* of volition and by "emotional dullness" (what we now call negative, or deficit, symptoms). He believed these two symptom clusters represented distinct processes that tended to progress independently of each other.

Kraepelin also distinguished a separate group of patients who experienced circumscribed persecutory delusions in the absence of either hallucinations or of prominent mood symptoms. While they might be disabled by their symptoms, which persisted over time, they did not otherwise deteriorate over time. He labeled this condition "paranoia," and it corresponds to our current diagnosis of **delusional disorder**.

Another psychiatrist who attempted to delineate distinguishing features of schizophrenia was *Kurt Schneider*. He identified specific types of hallucinations and delusions, which he considered to be "**first-rank symptoms**." While these symptoms can occur in other psychotic conditions (including delirium, dementia and mood disorders), they do appear to occur more commonly in schizophrenia and therefore can help "tip the scales" in favor of diagnosing schizophrenia, particularly when *several* of these symptoms are present. It is useful for clinicians to specifically inquire about them because patients may not mention them spontaneously. These first-rank symptoms include the following:

1. *Thought echo:* The patient experiences auditory hallucinations that echo his own thoughts, either just as he is thinking them or almost immediately afterward, sometimes with a mocking tone.

2. *Voices commenting:* A voice (or voices) offers running commentary on the patient's behavior. For example, "Now he's walking across the room. Now he's sitting down. Maybe he should leave. Maybe he should kill himself." The voice most commonly addresses the patient in the *third person* ("he") rather than in the second person ("you").

3. *Voices arguing:* Here there is more than one voice, and they usually argue about the patient in the third person. Some voices tend to be disparaging while others rise to his defense. For example, "He should kill himself." "Oh, leave him alone. He should not kill himself, he's a good person."

4. *Thought insertion:* The patient believes that thoughts that are not his own literally are being inserted into his head. One must be careful when asking about this ("Do you ever feel that people are trying to put thoughts into your head?") to distinguish perceptions of thought insertion from perceptions that people are trying to exert undue *influence* over the patient. For example, if the patient replies, "I could tell from the way he talked to me that he was trying to put thoughts into my head to kill myself," this would not be an example of thought insertion. However, a patient's belief that his current thoughts are being beamed into his head via a small transmitter, surreptitiously implanted in his brain while he was sleeping, would be an example of thought insertion.

5. *Thought withdrawal:* The patient believes (again literally) that thoughts are being taken out of his head.

6. *Thought broadcasting:* The patient believes that his thoughts are being broadcast widely and that everybody knows about them.

7. *"Made" impulse, "made" affect, "made" volition, and somatic passivity:* Here, the patient believes that he is being controlled, almost like a puppet dangling from strings, such that his impulses, feelings, or desires aren't in fact his own; rather, his body and mind are being controlled by an outside force. In somatic passivity, the influences specifically are acting on the patient's body (e.g., alien beams are shooting into the patient's sternum) and these in turn are controlling his movements, thoughts, etc.

8. *Delusional perception:* An actual perception of some innocuous event in the environment triggers a full-blown delusion. The patient may already have been experiencing a vague, suspicious sense that "something isn't right" around him without specific delusions (so-called "delusional mood or "delusional atmosphere"), an experience associated with fear and perplexity. When the delusional perception finally occurs, it may be accompanied by a sense of relief and of finally having "figured out what's *really* going on," even when the themes involve persecution, as in the following example:

A 24-year-old medical student, on emergency room rotation, appears haggard and unshaven. The resident working with him at first makes little of this. However, the student appears perplexed as the resident interviews a patient lying on a stretcher and then discusses his formulation with the student. Finally, the student blurts out: "You know, you're not fooling anybody. I know that these aren't real patients." The resident asks the student what he is talking about, and the student states that over the past 2 weeks he has become increasingly concerned that something hasn't been "quite right" during his ER rotation. The ER staff has been subtly hostile or provocative toward him, for no clear reason. For example, they would say things to him such as, "Why don't you see the patient in room 3?" He interpreted these comments as "signs" that he was being "tested" and "observed." Tonight, while watching the resident interview the current patient, the student noticed that the patient's intravenous fluids weren't dripping. Suddenly, "it all came together." The student realized that the patient was in fact an actor, hired to *portray* a patient, simply to "test" the student.

The student's classmates who are on rotation with him can provide little information about him. They know that he initially had been in the class 1 year ahead of them but had "taken a year off for personal reasons." Since his return, he has engaged in minimal social interaction with his classmates.

The dean reports that the student in fact took the year off to stay with his parents due to "depression" as well as beliefs that he was being "treated unfairly" by the medical school faculty (who were making subtle references to him in their lectures). To date, the student has refused any psychiatric intervention. The dean consulted a psychiatrist from Student Health, who felt that the student couldn't be involuntarily treated as an outpatient and that civil commitment wasn't an option since the student hadn't shown evidence of being an acute danger to himself or others.

Eugene Bleuler, a contemporary of Kraepelin, emphasized the importance of negative symptoms in schizophrenia as opposed to psychotic symptoms or a deteriorating course of illness. He described four major *deficits* in his patients with schizophrenia, which have since come to be called Bleuler's "four A's": loss of **associations** between thoughts (i.e., formal thought disorder), an abnormal **affect**, **ambivalence** of thought, and **autistic** behavior and thinking (i.e., a fundamental deficit in one's ability to relate to other people).

In contrast to Kraepelin, Bleuler reported that not all of his patients demonstrated hallucinations and delusions; he therefore considered these symptoms to be *secondary* in importance to the deficit symptoms. Bleuler also believed that it was more appropriate to focus on patients' cross-sectional symptoms than on their course of illness, since—in some of *his* "dementia praecox" patients—deterioration was not inevitable (hence there was no "dementia") and the onset of illness wasn't always early (hence there was no "praecox").

Bleuler coined an alternative label, "schizophrenia," to emphasize what he saw as the key feature of the illness—not the progressive deteriorative course, but the "splitting of the mind" demonstrated by these patients. Patients with schizophrenia demonstrated rifts between *one thought and the next one*, or between *thoughts and emotions*, or between *thoughts and behaviors*. For example, a schizophrenic patient might laugh while discussing how sad he felt after his mother died. (Unfortunately, the term "schizophrenia" has been misused in popular language ever since. Most commonly, it is used to describe situations where a person demonstrates contradictory impulses, as in, "He led a schizophrenic existence, a loving father at home but a tyrant at work.")

Note that both Kraepelin and Bleuler distinguished **positive symptoms** (those symptoms *present* in schizophrenic patients but not in the general population) from **negative symptoms** (*deficits* that occur in schizophrenic patients but not in the general population). Positive symptoms include hallucinations and delusions while negative symptoms include lack of motivation (apathy), affective blunting, poverty of speech or thought content, social withdrawal, inability to relate to others, poor attention, poor grooming, and dishevelment.

Both men were prescient in making this distinction. While the positive symptoms of schizophrenia clearly are more dramatic, the negative symptoms account for the bulk of social and functional morbidity associated with schizophrenia. Negative symptoms typically persist after positive symptoms associated with an acute psychotic episode have diminished or resolved. Further, conventional antipsychotic medications are far more effective in treating positive symptoms than negative symptoms. (In fact, they can *exacerbate* negative symptoms given the overlap between negative symptoms and psychological manifestations of antipsychotic-induced parkinsonism, such as bradyphrenia.) The major, recent innovation in the treatment of schizophrenia has been the advent of newer, "atypical" antipsychotic medications which demonstrate greater efficacy in reducing patients' negative symptoms.

One model, proposed in 1980 by T.J. Crow, divided schizophrenia into two basic types based on the predominance of either positive or negative symptoms. **Type I schizophrenia**, characterized by predominantly positive symptoms, was associated with good premorbid functioning, an acute onset, a course characterized by remissions and exacerbations, a better response to traditional antipsychotic medications, relatively good cognition between episodes, and normal findings on routine neuroimaging. **Type II schizophrenia**, in contrast, was characterized by predominantly negative symptoms, poor (schizotypal) premorbid functioning, an insidious decline into illness rather than acute onset, a course characterized by chronic deterioration, a poorer response to traditional antipsychotics, prominent cognitive impairment, and cerebral atrophy and

Table 8–2. Distinctions between Type I and Type II Schizophrenia

Type I Schizophrenia	Type II Schizophrenia
Prominent positive symptoms	Positive symptoms less prominent
Good premorbid functioning	Poor (schizotypal) premorbid functioning
Acute onset	Insidious decline
Remissions and exacerbations	Chronic deterioration
Better response to traditional antipsychotics	Poor response to traditional antipsychotics
Good cognition between episodes	Prominent cognitive impairment
Normal findings on routine neuroimaging	Atrophy and enlarged ventricles on neuroimaging

enlarged ventricles on routine neuroimaging. These differences are summarized in Table 8–2.

While such a dichotomous model remains useful in identifying aspects of a patient's illness associated with a better or worse prognosis, as a classification scheme it is overly simplistic. For example, many patients' presentations *change* over time, with negative symptoms becoming more prominent and positive symptoms becoming less so. Other patients have *mixed* presentations, with prominent positive *and* negative symptoms. Given this, rather than dividing patients into two discrete *classes*, it makes more sense to identify *symptom clusters*. In the latter scheme, different patients are seen as demonstrating particular symptom clusters to greater or lesser extents.

Factor analysis of large groups of patients suggests the presence of *three*, rather than two, symptom clusters: *(1)* **psychoticism** (which includes hallucinations and delusions, i.e., the "positive" symptoms), *(2)* **negative or deficit symptoms**, and *(3)* **disorganization** (which includes both disorganized speech and behavior and also inappropriate affect). Some researchers have suggested that, in addition to disorganization, other symptom domains should be demarcated from the "negative symptom" cluster, particularly **depressive symptoms**, which occur in at least 25% of schizophrenic patients.

Note that for two primary reasons the Bleulerian criteria are much broader than the Kraepelinian criteria. First, Bleuler didn't require the presence of "positive" symptoms. (He even described a group of patients who had *only* negative symptoms, a condition he called "simple schizophrenia." These patients rarely were admitted to the hospital, since they lacked hallucinations or delusions but nonetheless demonstrated signs of psychopathology.) Second, while

Kraepelin emphasized *categorical* criteria (such as hallucinations or delusions, which clearly are pathological phenomena that are either "present" or "absent"), Bleuler emphasized *dimensional* criteria (apathy or social withdrawal, aspects of mental life which are present within the general population but which are evident to a much greater degree in individuals with schizophrenia).

In other words, under Kraepelin's scheme, one would never say that an individual is "a little schizophrenic" the way that one might say that a person is "a little shy." Either the patient has a psychotic mental illness or doesn't. In contrast, Bleuler's "four A's," being dimensional, allowed for the possibility of there being individuals who exhibit a "mild" loss of affect or "mild" autistic thinking. Bleuler therefore opened the door to psychiatrists considering a variety of patients to have milder, "subsyndromal variants" of schizophrenia.

There is some validity to the Bleulerian approach. For example, as discussed in Chapter 10, the "cluster A" personality disorders—schizoid personality disorder, schizotypal personality disorder, and paranoid personality disorder—are probably best considered as "schizophrenia spectrum" disorders. They are more prevalent in the relatives of patients with schizophrenia, they share similar findings on structural and functional neuroimaging, and detailed neurological and neuropsychological testing reveals a similar pattern of subtle deficits.

However, dimensional reasoning—when applied too broadly—obscures *any* distinctions between "normal" and "abnormal." For example, given that we *all* have experienced periods of moderate sadness, loss of enthusiasm, or sleep disturbance, do we all have "low-grade" mood disorders? In the case of schizophrenia, mid-twentieth-century psychoanalysts, relying heavily on dimensional criteria, viewed "psychotic" conditions such as schizophrenia as being more severe but otherwise fundamentally the same as "neurotic" conditions such as panic disorder, mood disorder, personality disorder, and eating disorder.

The psychoanalytic view was that—in all of the conditions—patients' symptoms reflected the use of various *defense mechanisms*. Patients used these defenses in order to protect themselves against or to retreat from painful conflicts or stressors. For example, in anorexia nervosa, self-starvation was seen as arising out of fears of being excessively controlled by one's parents or of one's own sexual or oral desires. By rejecting food, the patient symbolically expresses these fears while simultaneously defending against them, by asserting total control over her body.

Schizophrenic patients were seen as utilizing similar but more pathological defensive strategies. In this case, in the face of a painful stressor they might withdraw from the outside world completely (leading to negative symptoms). Or, they might disavow having unacceptable aggressive impulses by *projecting* them onto other people (leading to paranoid delusions and hallucinations). For example, the patient might be viewed as saying, "It's not *me* who wants to hurt other people. It's *they* who want to hurt *me*."

Psychiatric illness was seen as falling along a continuum. "Milder" conditions, such as less severe personality disorders or nonpsychotic depression or anxiety, were viewed as reflections of the use of less pathological, more "neurotic" defenses. Psychotic illness was seen as reflecting the use of more pathological defenses. At the "borderline" between these neurotic and psychotic conditions were the severe personality disorders such as borderline personality disorder (hence the name).

Bleuler's criteria were embraced by American psychoanalysts while Kraepelin's criteria were adopted throughout much of Europe. In the 1960s and 1970s, psychiatrists from different countries found themselves using similar *diagnostic labels* but very different *diagnostic criteria*. For example, the U.S.–U.K. Diagnostic Project, using standardized interviews, demonstrated that London psychiatrists diagnosed mood disorder in cases where New York psychiatrists diagnosed schizophrenia. This period also brought the advent of new pharmacologic treatments with

relatively selective benefit for either schizophrenia or mood disorder (the antipsychotic agents, the antidepressants, lithium carbonate, and electroconvulsive therapy). This further demonstrated the importance of establishing diagnostic criteria of sufficient reliability and validity.

Such categorical diagnostic distinctions cried out for at least *some* of the diagnostic criteria to be categorical in nature. Given this, the *DSM-III* established reliable, symptom-based diagnostic criteria for schizophrenia and for the mood disorders which have been retained with only minor changes for the past 20 years, up through the current edition of the diagnostic manual, the *DSM-IV*. These *DSM* criteria also have been adopted internationally in the 10th *Revision of International Statistical Classification of Diseases and Related Health Problems* (the *ICD-10*).

DSM-IV Criteria

The current *DSM-IV* criteria for schizophrenia, listed in Table 8–3, attempt to consolidate all of these earlier diagnostic schemes. Under *DSM-IV*, a patient must demonstrate at least two out of the following five symptoms: delusions, hallucinations, disorganized speech, grossly disorganized or catatonic behavior, and negative symptoms. Note that by requiring two symptoms rather than one symptom, schizophrenia is distinguished from more limited psychotic syndromes such as delusional disorder and visual or auditory hallucinosis.

Also, note how under the *DSM-IV* criteria, patients can present in a more "Bleulerian" way— that is, with predominantly disorganized and negative symptoms in the absence of hallucinations or delusions—and still qualify for the diagnosis of schizophrenia. The *DSM-IV* also gives Schneiderian first-rank symptoms "extra weight" since it makes an exception to the "two-symptom" rule if the patient expresses an isolated hallucination or delusion that is "bizarre." Finally, note that the criteria retain a "Kraepelinian" emphasis on the course of illness. The course must be *continuous* over at least 6 months and must be associated with *functional impairment*. (Earlier criteria, in *DSM-III*, required evidence of functional "deterioration," but this was modified in *DSM-IV* after longitudinal research revealed that some patients with schizophrenia don't experience a significant functional decline.)

Table 8–3. *DSM-IV-TR* Criteria for Schizophrenia

A. *Characteristic symptoms*: Two (or more) of the following, each present for a significant portion of time during a 1-month period (or less if successfully treated):
   1. Delusions
   2. Hallucinations
   3. Disorganized speech (e.g., frequent derailment or incoherence)
   4. Grossly disorganized or catatonic behavior
   5. Negative symptoms, i.e., affective flattening, alogia, or avolition
   Note: Only one criterion A symptom is required if delusions are bizarre or hallucinations consist of a voice keeping up a running commentary on the person's behavior or thoughts, or two or more voices conversing with each other

B. *Social/occupational dysfunction*: For a significant portion of the time since the onset of the disturbance, one or more major areas of functioning such as work, interpersonal relations, or self-care are markedly below the level achieved prior to the onset (or when the onset is in childhood or adolescence, failure to achieve expected level of interpersonal, academic, or occupational achievement)

C. *Duration*: Continuous signs of the disturbance persist for at least 6 months. This 6-month period must include at least 1 month of symptoms (or less if successfully treated) that meet criterion A (i.e., active-phase symptoms) and may include periods of prodromal or residual symptoms. During these prodromal or residual periods, the signs of the disturbance may be manifested by only negative symptoms or two or more symptoms listed in criterion A present in an attenuated form (e.g., odd beliefs, unusual perceptual experiences)

D. *Schizoaffective and mood disorder exclusion*: Schizoaffective disorder and mood disorder with psychotic features have been ruled out because either (1) no major depressive, manic, or mixed episodes have occurred concurrently with the active-phase symptoms; or (2) if mood episodes have occurred during active-phase symptoms, their total duration has been brief relative to the duration of the active and residual periods

E. *Substance/general medical condition exclusion*: The disturbance is not due to the direct physiological effects of a substance (e.g., a drug of abuse, a medication) or a general medical condition

F. *Relationship to a pervasive developmental disorder*: If there is a history of autistic disorder or another pervasive developmental disorder, the additional diagnosis of schizophrenia is made only if prominent delusions or hallucinations are also present for at least a month (or less if successfully treated)

Source: Reprinted with permission from the *Diagnostic and Statistical Manual of Mental Disorders, Fourth Edition, Text Revision.* Copyright 2000 American Psychiatric Association.

The *DSM-IV* doesn't include specifiers that indicate whether positive or negative symptoms are predominant in a given case, but it does require clinicians to designate a *subtype* of schizophrenia. These subtypes, listed in Table 8–4, include: *paranoid type* (primarily hallucinations and delusions), *disorganized type* (primarily disorganization), *undifferentiated type* (demonstrating both paranoid and disorganized features), *residual type* (demonstrating either an attenuated form of the initial presentation or isolated negative symptoms in the wake of an earlier episode of more active symptoms), and *catatonic type* (demonstrating catatonic features).

While the *DSM-IV* retains this traditional, categorical typology rather than embracing the three-dimension scheme described above, the reliability and validity of these subtypes are not well established. For example, family studies haven't found these subtypes to "breed true," and a given patient's presentation can even change over the time. (The *DSM* therefore requires clinicians to specify a subtype based upon only the

most recent episode.) While these subtypes do demonstrate some predictive validity, in that patients with the paranoid subtype (i.e., those with predominantly positive symptoms without prominent cognitive symptoms) tend to fare better than those with either the disorganized or the undifferentiated subtype, no significant differences have been found between the disorganized and undifferentiated subtypes. Essentially, the presence of significant disorganization or thought disorder is associated with a poorer prognosis.

Because of these limitations, *DSM-IV* includes an alternative three-dimension scheme (psychotic, disorganized, and negative) in its appendix under the heading of "Criteria Sets Provided for Further Study." The *psychotic factor* includes delusions and hallucinations; the *disorganized factor* includes disorganized speech, disorganized behavior, and inappropriate affect; and the *negative factor* includes all of the various negative symptoms.

Research suggests that such a three-factor model offers greater validity. For example, dif-

Table 8–4. *DSM-IV-TR* Criteria for Schizophrenia Diagnostic Subtypes

PARANOID TYPE

A type of schizophrenia in which the following criteria are met:
  A. Preoccupation with one or more delusions or frequent auditory hallucinations
  B. None of the following is prominent: disorganized speech, disorganized or catatonic behavior, or flat or inappropriate affect

DISORGANIZED TYPE

A type of schizophrenia in which the following criteria are met:
  A. All of the following are prominent:
    1. Disorganized speech
    2. Disorganized behavior
    3. Flat or inappropriate affect
  B. The criteria are not met for catatonic type

CATATONIC TYPE

A type of schizophrenia in which the clinical picture is dominated by at least two of the following:
  1. Motoric immobility as evidenced by catalepsy (including waxy flexibility) or stupor
  2. Excessive motor activity (that is apparently purposeless and not influenced by external stimuli)
  3. Extreme negativism (an apparently motiveless resistance to all instructions or maintenance of a rigid posture against attempts to be moved) or mutism
  4. Peculiarities of voluntary movement as evidenced by posturing (voluntary assumption of inappropriate or bizarre postures), stereotyped movements, prominent mannerisms, or prominent grimacing
  5. Echolalia or echopraxia

UNDIFFERENTIATED TYPE

A type of schizophrenia in which symptoms that meet criterion A are present, but the criteria are not met for the paranoid, disorganized, or catatonic type

RESIDUAL TYPE

A type of schizophrenia in which the following criteria are met:
  A. Absence of prominent delusions, hallucinations, disorganized speech, and grossly disorganized or catatonic behavior
  B. There is continuing evidence of the disturbance, as indicated by the presence of negative symptoms or two or more symptoms listed in criterion A for schizophrenia, present in an attenuated form (e.g., odd beliefs, unusual perceptual experiences)

Source: Reprinted with permission from the *Diagnostic and Statistical Manual of Mental Disorders, Fourth Edition, Text Revision.* Copyright 2000 American Psychiatric Association.

ferent symptoms within each dimension typically vary together in severity, both cross-sectionally and over time; this is less likely to be the case for symptoms from two different factors. In other words, delusions and hallucinations tend to co-vary in severity but are less related to the severity of negative or disorganized symptoms. The data do not suggest that each factor represents a completely different disorder, since it is relatively uncommon for symptoms from one dimension to be present in the complete absence of symptoms from either of the other dimensions. Under this scheme, a patient might be classified as follows: "Schizophrenia, continuous, with severe psychotic dimension, absent disorganized dimension, and moderate negative dimension."

Whether "schizophrenia" in fact constitutes a single disease process with varying presentations (like syphilis or cancer) or is really a constellation of different disease processes with similar presentations (like type 1 versus type 2 diabetes) remains unclear. Rather than close any doors prematurely, psychiatric researchers still categorize all of these presentations as schizophrenia while also attempting to isolate and validate subcategories through clinical, biochemical, and neuropathological correlations.

The above discussion draws attention to the limitations of a diagnostic system that is based on *clinical phenomenology* rather than on an underlying *mechanism of disease.* By analogy, were we to define cancer solely based upon its clinical presentation, we would face similar diagnostic dilemmas. Like schizophrenia, cancer presents with a great diversity of symptoms, disease severities, and clinical courses, depending upon the sites of cancer origin and where it tends to metastasize. Also like schizophrenia, cancer isn't caused by any single etiology: whether or not a patient develops cancer is influenced by the patient's exposure to a multitude of genetic and/or environmental "hits" (family history of cancer, exposure to viruses, exposure to carcinogens, exposure to radiation, suppressed immunity, etc.). However, *underlying* all cancers is a single disease mechanism: cell growth has become autonomous (i.e., is no longer regulated by external signals), and cells have gained the capacity to invade tissues and/or to metastasize to distant sites.

Presently, we don't have a full understanding of the disease mechanism that *underlies* schizophrenia. As a result, it isn't possible to tie together all of the strands of our current knowledge base, such as known risk factors, variations in symptoms between individuals, the typical course of illness, associated biochemical and neuroanatomical findings, and the known biochemical effects of various medications used to treat the illness. This being said, following our discussion of schizophrenia's clinical presentation, we will explore recent theoretical approaches along with associated treatment implications.

Course of Illness and Epidemiology

There are four phases of illness: the prodromal phase, the active phase, remission, and relapse. To this scheme, we might add a still-earlier phase, the premorbid phase.

The majority of affected individuals go through a **prodromal phase,** which is characterized by the gradual development of negative symptoms such as social withdrawal, loss of interest in school or work, deterioration in hygiene, unusual behavior, and angry outbursts. Family members typically find the patient's behavior difficult to comprehend. They may minimize or rationalize it.

Eventually, though, **active-phase symptoms** occur—hallucinations, delusions, gross disorganization, or catatonia. Sometimes these symptoms have insidious onset, but they may occur abruptly in the form of an "acute psychotic

break." (This is what occurred in the above example of the medical student on his emergency room rotation.) At this point, family and friends typically recognize that the affected individual has a mental illness and encourage him to seek treatment, often in the emergency room. The evaluator often recommends psychiatric hospitalization at this point, to better allow both for rapid evaluation and for the initiation of treatment in a monitored setting. This is particularly likely to be the recommendation when the patient is disorganized, acutely paranoid, potentially violent, unable to care for himself, or lacking in insight into the fact that he is ill.

Patients in the **residual phase** of illness, like those in the prodromal phase, may not display positive symptoms. However, treating clinicians should be aware of the nature of the active phase symptoms that the patient expressed earlier, since these symptoms often are in fact present in *attenuated form.* For example, hallucinations may appear as illusions and delusions as "odd" or "idiosyncratic" ideas held with a lesser degree of tenacity.

Depressive symptoms occur commonly in schizophrenia, either as part of the acute phase of illness or during the residual phase. In first episodes of schizophrenia, 75% patients present with prominent depressive symptoms while 50% meet the diagnostic criteria for major depressive disorder with psychotic features. The depressive symptoms usually improve along with the psychotic symptoms. About a quarter of patients with schizophrenia experience depressive symptoms during subsequent episodes, and depressive symptoms may appear as part of the prodromal syndrome heralding impending relapse.

After an acute psychotic episode has abated, patients can experience a *postpsychotic depression,* again resembling a major depressive episode. This syndrome often responds to treatment with antidepressant medications and doesn't simply represent demoralization over having had a relapse of symptoms. Many of the schizophrenic patients who ultimately commit suicide do so during these periods. Given this, close follow-up and psychosocial support *following* "successful" treatment of a psychotic episode are essential.

Two other postpsychotic syndromes resemble depression but should be distinguished since they require different interventions. *Negative symptoms of schizophrenia* include apathy, psychomotor retardation, and social withdrawal. However, patients with negative symptoms in the absence of depression generally don't report a prominent lowering self-attitude or "sadness." *Parkinsonism due to antipsychotic medication* can include psychomotor slowing and anergia (sometimes referred to as *secondary negative symptoms* or *akinetic depression*). Assessment therefore should include assessment for the presence of cogwheel rigidity, resting tremor, a blunted or masked facial expression, and gait disturbance. One way to assess for subtle parkinsonism is to have the patient walk across the room and to look for a decrease in the normal degree of arm swing.

Relapse from the residual phase into another episode of active-phase symptoms is often preceded by nonspecific prodromal symptoms. For example, patients may complain of worsening dysphoria, tension or nervousness, poor concentration, sleep disturbance, poor appetite, or depression. Ideas of reference may begin to emerge. Patients may demonstrate increasingly "bizarre" behavior.

It is important to warn patients and their family members in advance to be on the lookout for such "red flags." Sometimes patients in early relapse are diagnosed as being "depressed" and therefore are treated with antidepressant medication. However, a more appropriate intervention in many cases is to increase the dosage of *antipsychotic* medication, particularly when this medication previously was tapered downward in an attempt to minimize side effects or to decrease the risk of the patient developing tardive dyskinesia. Rapid intervention is essential in these cases since the "window" between the appearance of prodromal symptoms and full relapse may last only from a few days to a few weeks.

Schizophrenic symptoms tend to "plateau" after about 5 years. About 30% of patients ultimately have a "good" outcome (if good is defined as no further hospitalizations). Another 30% have a "bad" outcome (either continuous hospitalization or moderate-to-severe intellectual or social impairment necessitating intensive outpatient support and frequent hospital readmission). The remaining 40% have an "intermediate" outcome (occasional readmissions, some persistent symptoms, and chronic interpersonal difficulties).

However, schizophrenia can be a devastating illness even in "good-" or "intermediate-"outcome cases. About two-thirds of patients are unable to tolerate gainful employment, and 70% are unable to marry. Further, 10% of schizophrenic individuals ultimately commit suicide, often during episodes of depression that follow psychotic episodes. Ironically, higher-functioning patients, who have greater insight into having an illness and who retain greater cognitive organization, have a much higher risk of committing suicide than do lower-functioning patients, despite their better long-term prognosis.

The lifetime *prevalence* of schizophrenia, about 0.5%–1.5%, is the same in women and men. However, men have a lower mean age of onset between ages 15 and 25; in women onset is between ages 25 and 35. Men also are more likely to experience prominent negative symptoms, to demonstrate a more chronic, disabling course, and to never marry. The reasons for these differences are unclear. Perhaps they relate to estrogen having a protective effect in women, via attenuated dopamine-blocking effects. Also, since women on average marry at younger ages than do men, and since schizophrenia in women is associated with better premorbid functioning and a later onset, women with schizophrenia are more likely to have already developed significant interpersonal relationships before the illness intervenes.

The age of onset is variable, however, and schizophrenia can develop at nearly any age. It has been diagnosed in children as young as age 5, although childhood-onset cases are very rare. In children, delusions and hallucinations may be less elaborate and visual hallucinations may be more common. Before diagnosing schizophrenia in a child, one first should exclude other disorders that are more common in children. For example, communication disorders and pervasive developmental disorders can present with disorganized speech, while attention-deficit hyperactivity disorder is associated with disorganized behavior.

Individuals with an earlier age at onset likely have a stronger genetic component to their illness. They more often are male, demonstrate poorer premorbid functioning (likely representing an earlier onset of the prodromal phase of illness), have lower premorbid educational achievement, demonstrate more evidence of structural brain abnormalities on neuroimaging, have more prominent negative signs and symptoms, and have a greater degree of cognitive impairment when assessed through neuropsychological testing.

Less commonly, schizophrenia develops later in life, after age 45 or later. Later onset tends to be associated with a better prognosis As might be expected, more of these individuals are women, and they tend to have a history of having been married and having been successfully employed. Disorganized and negative symptoms occur less commonly than in younger-onset cases. While the course is usually chronic, these individuals may respond to low doses of antipsychotic medication. Patients with the *latest* age of onset (over age 60) are more likely to have conditions such as vision and hearing loss, suggesting that sensory deprivation plays a contributory role.

The *course* of illness also is variable. Some individuals experience exacerbations and remissions, while others remain chronically ill. *DSM-IV* offers several course specifiers, described in Table 8–5. While *DSM-IV* includes a specifier for "complete remission" (i.e., a return to full premorbid functioning), this outcome is uncommon over the longer term, occurring in only 5%–10% of cases. Of those individuals who remain ill, some have a relatively stable course,

Table 8–5. *DSM-IV-TR* Schizophrenia Longitudinal Course Specifiers*

1. Episodic, with interepisode residual symptoms
2. Episodic, with no interepisode residual symptoms
3. Continuous
4. Single episode, in partial remission
5. Single episode, in full remission
6. Other or unspecified pattern

*These should be applied only after at least 1 year has elapsed since the initial onset of active-phase symptoms. "Episodes" are identified by the reemergence of prominent psychotic symptoms. In the "continuous" course, prominent psychotic symptoms are present throughout the period of observation.
Source: Reprinted with permission from the *Diagnostic and Statistical Manual of Mental Disorders, Fourth Edition, Text Revision.* Copyright 2000 American Psychiatric Association.

Table 8–6. Factors Associated with a Better Prognosis in Schizophrenia

Female sex
Good premorbid adjustment
Acute onset of illness
Later age at onset
Good interepisode functioning
Minimal residual symptoms
Association of illness exacerbations with acute precipitating events
Presence of associated mood disturbances
Brief duration of active-phase symptoms
Absence of structural brain abnormalities on neuroimaging
Normal neurological functioning
Family history of mood disorder
Absence of family history of schizophrenia

while others experience a progressive decline into more severe disability. For many individuals, negative symptoms persist between acute exacerbations of positive symptoms, and these negative symptoms become more prominent over time. Factors associated with a *better prognosis* are listed in Table 8–6. However, one must use caution when attempting to extrapolate from epidemiologic data to individual patients. For example, a World Health Organization study involving nine different countries showed that 47 predictive variables combined predicted only 38% of the variance in patients' clinical courses.

The vulnerability to developing schizophrenia appears to begin early on, even at conception. A number of genes, somewhere between 5 and 30, have been implicated in conferring susceptibility to developing schizophrenia, with environmental factors then helping to convert vulnerability into active illness. Unfortunately, it has been difficult to identify both the risk-conferring genes and the nongenetic factors.

"Environmental" insults may include the simple element of *randomness* associated with the "wiring" of hundreds of trillions of brain synapses in utero. When one examines brain sulcal and gyral patterns, one finds that even identical twins don't have "identical brains" (although their brains do resemble each other more closely than do the brains of nonidentical twins). Epidemiologic studies suggest that superimposed in utero environmental insults may further increase the risk of an individual developing "faulty wiring." For example, schizophrenic individuals are more likely to have experienced perinatal complications than are nonaffected individuals. In northern latitudes, individuals with schizophrenia are more likely to have been born during the winter months, suggesting that a gestational viral insult plays a role in some cases. (No such virus has been identified, however.) Later in life, environmental factors such as family stress, academic setbacks, poverty, and substance abuse may add additional neurobiological "hits."

A very puzzling aspect of schizophrenia, though, is the fact that it doesn't manifest itself during early childhood. It's relatively late onset sharply contrasts with other genetic disorders that affect the brain, such as autistic disorder, Down's syndrome, and fragile X syndrome. While there are other conditions (most notably learning disorders such as dyslexia) that have strong genetic components but only are diagnosed after a delay, in these latter cases the delay relates to *recognition* of the disorder. In contrast, in schizophrenia there is a true period of *latency* lasting from 15 to 30 years. During this period, individuals who later develop schizophrenia are virtually indistinguishable from people around them who do not do so.

This is not to say that these individuals are completely normal prior to the onset of overt clinical symptoms. For example, the most commonly reported finding from neuroimaging studies comparing individuals with schizophrenia to nonaffected individuals is the presence of larger cerebral ventricles. Are these present from birth or do they only occur later? The former would suggest that schizophrenia is a developmental disorder while the latter would suggest a neurodegenerative disorder. One creative study looked at third-trimester three-dimensional prenatal ultrasounds obtained routinely during the course of pregnancy. Some of the expectant mothers had schizophrenia, and their ultrasounds were compared to those obtained on expectant mothers who did not have schizophrenia. The brains of the fetuses of the schizophrenic mothers demonstrated larger ventricles on average that did fetuses of nonschizophrenic mothers.

Another creative study examined Israeli Draft Board Register assessments, which are routinely performed on all 16-year-old and 17-year-old males in Israel. The researchers looked back at the testing results of those individuals who ultimately went on to develop schizophrenia in the subsequent decade. On average, this occurred 5 years from the time of testing. Compared to all other test subjects, the preschizophrenic subjects had lower I.Q. scores, lower social functioning, and lower autonomy. Again, this finding suggests that negative symptoms and cognitive symptoms are present during the latency period.

This premorbid at-risk state—characterized by a constellation of subtle findings that include negative symptoms, mild neuropsychological impairments (impairments in smooth-pursuit eye movement, poor coordination, poor perceptual–motor integration, abnormal speech, lower I.Q., and lower educational achievement), and characteristic structural brain on structural neuroimaging—has been termed **schizotaxia**. Not all individuals with schizotaxia go on to develop either schizophrenia or schizotypal personality disorder. Schizotaxic symptoms occur in 20%–50% of the first-degree relatives of patients with schizophrenia. In contrast, only about 10% of schizophrenic patients' relatives develop any psychotic illness, while under 10% of relatives develop schizotypal personality disorder. Further, some individuals who are functionally normal (i.e., who have no evidence of schizotaxia) later develop schizophrenia.

Still, these findings have important public health implications. Clinical research suggests that treatment interventions for schizophrenia (as with interventions for heart disease, stroke, diabetes, and cancer) are much more likely to be effective when they are initiated *early* in the course of illness, or even prophylactically if "high-risk" cases can be identified. Not only are the acute positive symptoms more likely to respond, but so are the negative and cognitive symptoms that later go on to become more "treatment refractory." For example, a large number of studies examining the outcome of first-episode treatment reveal that almost 90% of patients meet very stringent criteria for complete remission after the first episode. Even among treatment responders however, a longer duration of psychosis prior to intervention was associated with a longer period of treatment being necessary before they reached a state of remission.

At some point in the near future, individuals determined to be at higher risk for developing schizophrenia on the basis of historical factors such as a strong family history might receive a battery of tests including genetic screening, neuroimaging, and neuropsychological testing. This might allow either for prophylactic intervention during the prodromal stage or patient education and close monitoring, followed by rapid initiation of treatment at the first sign of psychosis.

It remains unclear at this point, however, whether early treatment slows or halts the progression of illness rather than merely mitigating its symptoms and decreasing associated morbidity. If prolonged psychosis in itself turns out to cause neurotoxicity, then antipsychotic medications may affect the underlying illness. Alternatively, antipsychotic medications might turn out to not only treat the disease's clinical manifestations but also its underlying pathology (by analogy to infectious diseases, if they turn out to treat the "infection" and not simply the "fever"). Currently, we don't have significant data to address these questions.

If these initial treatment interventions are so effective, how do patients ultimately end up becoming so disabled? Studies following first-episode treatment responders longitudinally reveal that by 1 year, about 20% of them have relapsed, by 2 years 50% of them have relapsed, and by 5 years 80% of them have relapsed. Subsequent episodes don't respond as well to treatment, and with each subsequent episode, symptoms improve progressively more slowly after initiation of treatment and patients are progressively less likely to achieve full symptom remission. This ultimately leads to an "end stage" of illness over the next 5 years, with the majority of patients ultimately exhibiting persistent symptoms even with treatment compliance. Deterioration is most pronounced in the early years of the illness (the first 5–10 years) and then usually reaches a plateau, although in more severe variants, patients continue to demonstrate functional decline over ensuing decades.

Clearly, the rate of relapse among patients who are compliant with medication is several orders of magnitude lower than among patients who discontinue their medication (although some patients who are compliant still do relapse). But it is a rare patient who, following recovery from a first episode of psychotic illness, continues to take antipsychotic medication indefinitely. Many patients stop taking the medication on their own, while others request a decreased dose or a trial off of medication, particularly if several months have gone by without any symptoms. Since making a diagnosis of schizophrenia with a high degree of certainty is difficult early in the disease's course, and since patients may be experiencing medication side effects (such as extrapyramidal symptoms, cognitive slowing, or weight gain), clinicians might end up agreeing to a trial of tapering or discontinuing the medication. Some practice guidelines suggest that this might be reasonable if patients have been symptom free for at least a year following a single episode of psychosis. However, the relapse rate for such patients off of medications turns out to be 96% over the following 2 years.

This is not to say that clinicians must adamantly insist on chronic maintenance therapy in all first-episode patients. Evidence from studies of large groups provides useful guidance but doesn't dictate clinical practice in individual cases. Many patients will only accept that ongoing medication therapy is worth the cost, the hassle, the stigma, and the side effects in the face of evidence that their symptoms return without it. Medication discontinuation, however, requires patient education and close monitoring, as well as an understanding that medications will be rapidly reinstated at the first signs of symptom recurrence. When this strategy is followed, the majority of patients can avoid rehospitalization.

Such a strategy theoretically could worsen patients' long-term prognosis due to the presumed neurotoxic effects of psychosis, but there is a difference between leaving full-blown psychosis untreated for months and quickly resuming antipsychotic drug therapy at the first appearance of subtle psychotic symptoms. There is no evidence for a worsened prognosis associated with this latter strategy. In any case, clinically supervised medication withdrawal is safer than covert patient noncompliance, and might contribute to better medication compliance in the long term and to the formation of a trusting relationship with the treatment provider.

PATHOLOGY, ETIOLOGY, AND TREATMENT IMPLICATIONS

A "stress diathesis" model of schizophrenia is proposed whereby environmental stressors act on a genetically vulnerable individual, and the disease ultimately becomes independent of these environmental stressors once it has taken hold. This model is similar to that previously discussed for mood disorders (Fig. 4–4). Current research has focused on the relative importance of each of the different risk factors, and on which of these factors are either *(1)* nonspecific predisposing risk factors, or *(2)* insults that are necessary but not sufficient in themselves to cause the illness, or *(3)* insults that are both necessary and sufficient in themselves to cause the illness (i.e., they are able to cause the illness with a "single hit").

As with mood disorder, explanatory concepts in schizophrenia historically have tended to focus on its symptoms from the point of view of either form or function. However, there is now ample evidence that schizophrenia is a disease. Especially as the definition of schizophrenia has narrowed to include only patients with psychotic symptoms, psychological theories of *causation* have become less relevant. While these theories still have some relevance in helping the clinician to understand the types of stressors that can lead to exacerbations of illness and also to appreciate patients' subjective experience, virtually no modern clinician would attempt to base a theory of schizophrenia solely on arguments from function. The primary treatment strategy is biological therapy, with psychosocial treatments playing an essential but supplemental role.

Genetic Factors

As was the case with mood disorder, the strongest evidence that schizophrenia is a disease comes from genetic studies, including family, twin, adoption, and linkage studies. Naturalistic studies of *family members* reveal rates of schizophrenia in family members that are much higher than those seen in the general population, and the risk increases dramatically the closer family members are genetically to the affected proband, as summarized in Table 8–7.

While family studies indicate that family factors play a role in schizophrenia, they don't distinguish between genetic factors and shared environmental factors. *Twin studies* attempt to isolate genetic factors to a greater degree by comparing monozygotic twins (who have identical genetic material) with dizygotic twins (who don't). In dizygotic twins, the concordance rate is what might be expected for siblings in general

Table 8–7. Risk of Developing Schizophrenia by Relationship to Schizophrenic Proband

Relationship to Proband	Risk of Schizophrenia
No relationship (general population)	1%
One parent	5–6%
One sibling	10%
One sibling and one parent	17%
Two parents	46%

(about 15%). However, in monozygotic twins, the concordance rate is much higher (somewhere between 30% and 80% depending on the ascertainment method; the average is about 50%). The elevated concordance rate in monozygotic versus dizygotic twins is consistent with an etiologic role for genetic factors. However, given that the concordance rate for monozygotic twins isn't 100%, nongenetic factors also must play a role. In other words, genetic factors appear to be either nonspecific predisposing risk factors or necessary but not sufficient insults.

Further evidence for the etiologic role of genetic factors comes from *adoption studies*. In one study, biological children of schizophrenic mothers were raised by nonschizophrenic adoptive parents. They were found to have a 16% risk of developing schizophrenia, which is about the same rate that would have been expected had they been raised by schizophrenic parents. (In a control group of adoptees from nonschizophrenic biologic mothers, none developed schizophrenia.) Similarly, a "cross-fostering" study examined children of healthy biologic parents raised either by a couple where one member had schizophrenia or where neither parent had schizophrenia. Children in both groups had the same (low) rate of developing schizophrenia.

How are these genetic factors transmitted? As was the case with the mood disorders, mathematical analyses of twin and adoption study data aren't consistent with single gene "Mendelian" inheritance. *Linkage studies* involving different families revealed several putative vulnerability genes, including regions on chromosomes 1, 6, 8, 10, 13, and 22.

Transmission likely is polygenic, with two or more defective genes interacting synergistically and with a greater number of "genetic hits" leading to a greater degree of vulnerability to ultimately developing schizophrenia. This might explain the findings from family studies indicating that an individual's risk of developing schizophrenia is greater when a larger number of family members also have the disorder. Transmission also appears to have incomplete phenotypic "penetrance." In other words, in the absence of a sufficient "environmental hit," a person with the schizophrenia genotype may not develop the disorder. This would explain why one monozygotic twin might have an affected sibling yet fail to develop the illness herself.

Incomplete penetrance also would help to explain the higher rate of "schizophrenia-spectrum disorders" (such as schizotypal personality disorder and schizotaxia) and biological "trait markers" (such as impaired smooth-pursuit eye movements) in the extended family members of schizophrenic probands than in the general population. For example, 40% of first-degree relatives of schizophrenic patients have impaired smooth pursuit eye movements compared to 10% of the general population.

Neurodevelopmental and Neuropathological Factors

Kraepelin was criticized for considering schizophrenia to be a biological illness in the absence of any detectable anatomic or histologic abnormalities. While the clinical *course* of schizophrenia suggested to Kraepelin that it was a neurodegenerative disorder like Huntington's disease and Alzheimer's disease, the most striking neuropathological finding has been the *absence* of gliosis (scarring). As a result, schizophrenia was called the "graveyard of neuropathology."

However, recent research with more sensitive techniques has revealed some characteristic findings. These findings are statistically significant when *groups* of schizophrenic patients are compared to *groups* of control subjects, although they also are nonspecific and may not be dramatic in individual cases. For example, an individual patient's MRI scan may appear to be "within normal limits."

The most consistent anatomic findings from structural neuroimaging and autopsy have been *decreased cortical volume* and *cerebral ventricular enlargement*. Many cases also demonstrate *sulcal dilatation* and *cerebellar atrophy*. These findings appear to reflect the underlying pathology in schizophrenia rather than chronic treatment with antipsychotic medications, since enlarged ventricles have been described in never-medicated first-onset patients and even in utero.

The presence of cerebral ventricular enlargement likely reflects atrophy of paraventricular brain regions. High-resolution MRI scans with volumetric measurements have revealed *temporal lobe atrophy*, particularly in the region of the *superior temporal gyrus*. This region contains the auditory association cortex, and it is noteworthy that a greater magnitude of atrophy correlates with the presence and severity of auditory hallucinations.

Early studies involving adult subjects previously diagnosed with schizophrenia examined prospectively through serial CAT scans found that cortical atrophy and ventricular enlargement remained stable over several years. This, along with absence of gliosis, suggested to investigators that the anatomic abnormalities may have been present since birth and may reflect a static neurodevelopmental abnormality. However, the other possibility would be that a progressive degenerative process caused these findings, but that it had run its course prior to the time of the first scan. The process would have to be different than that seen in other neurogenerative illnesses, though, in that it isn't associated with visible neuronal damage or gliosis. It now appears that both answers may be correct.

As noted above, ventricular enlargement has been discovered in at-risk individuals, in patients at the time of the first episode, and in relatives who have schizophrenia-spectrum conditions. This, along with the absence of gliosis, suggests that schizophrenia is a neurodevelopmental disorder. However, more recent prospective studies of children and adolescents with childhood-onset schizophrenia (a particularly severe and progressive form of the illness) as well as of first-break patients indicate that illness progression *is* associated with progression of neuroimaging findings and that the latter occurs even in the case of antipsychotic medications, and even when patients' symptoms are responding to treatment.

In addition, neuroimaging studies also reveal increases in *extracerebral* (sulcal) cerebrospinal fluid. This finding can only be explained by atrophy that occurs either in later childhood or in early adolescence since skull growth is caused by outward pressure on the skull by the brain, which more than triples in size between birth and age 5. The process continues until the skull sutures fuse, late in childhood. Given this, only a diffuse lesion that results in a *loss* of brain tissue—with its onset *following* this period of maximal brain volume expansion and skull suture fusion—could account for these increases in extracerebral cerebrospinal fluid. In other words, in the case of a nonprogressive developmental lesion, present since birth, any increase in extracerebral CSF would be "filled" in by subsequent outward brain growth.

Therefore, the presence of genetic factors, the presence of enlarged ventricles early in life, and the absence of gliosis suggest the presence of a neurodevelopmental diathesis rather than of a neurodegenerative disorder. However, the latency of illness onset and the progression of neuroanatomical findings over time both are consistent with an illness that is progressive rather than static. How, then, does the illness progress in the absence of obvious neurodegeneration?

One clue comes from a study of childhood-onset patients in which MRI scans were performed every 2 years. As already described, at the time of the first scan, subjects already had enlarged ventricles, which had progressed by the time of the second scan. However, by the time of the third scan (now 4 years after study entry) the changes had stabilized. Therefore, at least in this childhood-onset population, the process of brain atrophy appears to have had its onset prior to adolescence, with stabilization by about age 18 or 20. Further, on the initial MRI, these patients did not demonstrate significantly decreased cortical volume in the frontal or temporal lobes or in the hippocampal area (findings described in adult patients), but by the time of the second scan, the volume of these areas had diminished.

Of note, though, the *control* group in this study offered researchers their first opportunity to study changes in brain MRI scans that occur over time in *healthy* adolescents. The researchers discovered that members of the control group also experienced decreases in cortical volume in the frontal and parietal regions.

These decreases reflect the normal process of synaptic pruning that occurs at this age. As discussed in Chapter 4, during postnatal develop-

ment there is an overelaboration of axons and dendrites. A huge number of synaptic connections are formed, perhaps even at random. Subsequently, though, weaker connections are pruned away, and neurons are even lost through the process of apoptosis. Endogenous factors such as glutamate and neurotrophic factors likely play a significant role in this process, which also is influenced by life experience.

Ultimately, about 40% of synaptic connections are lost. In primary sensory areas, such as occipital cortex, the synaptic pruning process is largely complete by age 2. However, in prefrontal and association areas, the process begins at about age 5, becomes more robust in later childhood and adolescence, and declines to lower adult rates during the third decade. The changes are concentrated in the frontal and parietal lobes but not in the temporal and occipital cortical areas.

The volume loss experienced by control subjects in the frontal and parietal regions was relatively small (3%–4%). In contrast, adolescents in the schizophrenia group demonstrated significantly greater volume loss in these regions, 8%–11%. They also showed decreases of this same magnitude in the temporal lobe, an area that showed no volume loss in control subjects. This suggests that in this childhood-onset population, excessive synaptic pruning occurs during adolescence. Perhaps a similar process takes place in adult-onset cases, but here the most significant damage already has occurred prior to the time of the first scan.

However, it is not clear that this process is inevitable. Studies of monozygotic twins discordant for having developed schizophrenia reveal the affected twin to often have enlarged ventricles relative to the unaffected twin. Given their identical genetic makeup, environmental factors must play a role. Unfortunately, to determine when the twins' brain images began to diverge from each other would require serial radiologic examinations from a young age of a large number of twins who are only *at risk* for developing schizophrenia.

As discussed earlier, the presence of significant cortical atrophy and enlarged ventricles on neuroimaging correlates with the presence of more extensive negative and cognitive symptoms and with a poorer prognosis. This is not to say that there are two distinct groups (the "large-ventricle" group and the "small-ventricle" group). The extent of negative symptoms varies along a *dimensional gradient*, as do these neuroimaging findings. For example, in monozygotic twins, affected twins have bigger lateral ventricles than their siblings, but often the size still was "within the normal range," with the presence of ventricular enlargement being noted only when the affected twin's scan was compared to a perfectly genetically matched but unaffected control subject (i.e., his twin). This finding suggests that perhaps *all* schizophrenic patients have ventricles that are more dilated than they *would have been* in the absence of illness but that in many cases the changes are too subtle to be appreciated through a single neuroimaging study.

Consistent with this hypothesis, postmortem histopathologic studies reveal decreased size of some cortical limbic structures (including the amygdala, the hippocampus, and the parahippocampal gyrus), the prefrontal cortex, the thalamus, and the cerebellum. In the prefrontal cortex, despite the loss of cortical volume, neuronal density is *increased*. While the neurons themselves are retained, there is a loss of "neuropil"—the space *between* neurons, which represents axonal and dendritic arborization and synaptic connections.

Therefore, patients predisposed to develop schizophrenia appear to begin life with a lesser degree of synaptic density, likely due to a combination of genetic vulnerability and perinatal insult. The illness doesn't become apparent, however, until later in life, perhaps due to the density of synaptic connections finally falling below a critical level as a result of normal (and quite possibly excessive) synaptic pruning and/or apoptosis during childhood and adolescence. Mild dysfunctions associated with these deficits may begin to emerge during adolescence in the form of subtle social, behavioral, neurologic, and cognitive disturbances (schizotaxia). Ultimately, hallucinations and delusions occur. The latter may reflect either a deficit state—for example, the *loss* of the ability to dampen "background noise"—or a state of functional *excess* (due to a loss of normal frontal lobe inhibition of associated limbic centers).

Findings from *functional* neuroimaging studies also are consistent with this hypothesis. Both

PET and SPECT scans reveal evidence for *decreased frontal lobe metabolic activity and cerebral blood flow in schizophrenic subjects compared with controls*. These deficits are more evident when subjects are asked to engage in tests of *executive function* that require complex decision-making such as the Wisconsin Card Sort task. During such "cognitive challenges," frontal lobe activity does not increase in schizophrenic subjects to the extent seen in nonschizophrenic subjects. This discrepancy also occurs when one compares the scans of affected and unaffected monozygotic twins.

EEG studies also complement the anatomic studies, offering another window into brain activity. Up to 80% of patients with schizophrenia demonstrate EEG abnormalities, although most of these findings are nonspecific. The most reproducible finding is blunting and delay in the appearance of the *P300 wave*, which is a large evoked potential that occurs almost immediately (300 milliseconds—ms) following the delivery of an unexpected auditory or visual stimulus to the study subject. It is believed that this wave originates in the medial temporal lobe (perhaps in the hippocampus) and reflects an attempt by the brain to update its cognitive "image" of what to expect from the environment. The finding that this ability is dampened in schizophrenic subjects is consistent with theories suggesting they are impaired in their ability to filter out environmental input (so-called "sensory gating").

Psychological Factors

Life stress likely plays an important role in precipitating "first-break" episodes as well as later relapses. Helping patients learn to better manage stress and establish a predictable and structured environment are essential parts of treatment. The prevalence of illness appears to be greater in low-income urban areas. While it was hypothesized in the 1930s and 1940s that urban stress was the root cause of schizophrenia, more recent studies suggest that many schizophrenic individuals with higher-income backgrounds ultimately end up in the inner cities as a result of their illness (the *downward drift hypothesis*). Similarly, schizophrenia is somewhat more prevalent among immigrant populations, but lower-income groups (with a higher rate of mental illness) also are more likely to immigrate.

Family theories, especially popular in the 1950s, postulated that schizophrenia was the result of the patient "retreating from reality" due to having grown up in a dysfunctional family and as a result being unable to face the outside world. Particular emphasis was placed on the role of faulty mothering (the so-called "schizophrenogenic mother" theory), and mothers of schizophrenic patients were described as having been too invested, too aloof, or too hostile during patients' childhoods. These theories didn't take into account the effects on parenting style of living with a child displaying the early symptoms of mental illness. They also led to the parents of schizophrenic individuals being doubly victimized, first by having a child who developed a severe psychiatric illness, and second by the field of psychiatry placing the blame on them.

This having been said, research does suggest that a stressful home environment increasing the risk of relapse. Studies in the 1950s revealed that patients who returned from the hospital to families who were critical or overly involved (*high expressed emotion* or "high EE" families) had twice as high a rate of relapse. A recent review of 26 studies since then, involving more than 1300 patients in several countries, found this to be a robust finding. The median relapse rate for patients from high-EE families was 48% at 6–9 months after hospital discharge versus 21% for patients from low-EE families. While it is possible that more severely ill or noncompliant patients (who also have higher rate of relapse) lead their family members to become more critical, a higher relapse rate is seen even among *compliant* patients taking depot antipsychotic medication. Given this, family support and family education clearly are extremely important aspects of treatment. In fact, family education of high-EE families appears to decrease the degree of expressed emotion and also to decrease the relapse rate to the same rate that is seen in patients from low-EE families.

We have discussed in earlier chapters how each clinical perspective allows us to view patients from the point of view of both form and function. We have discussed schizophrenia from the disease perspective and have emphasized its form. In contrast, individuals with schizophrenia view their illness much differently. This "view from the inside" emphasizes the point of view of function. Patients in the midst of an episode of active illness don't tend to see themselves as having abnormal mental experiences, the content of which is shaped by their unique life experiences. Rather, they may see themselves as trying to live a normal existence despite having an illness that has caused repeated setbacks. They may fail to recognize that they have an illness, instead seeing themselves as being influenced by forces beyond their control. In some cases, delusional fears and feelings of loss of control have been reinforced by actual events. For example, many patients have been picked up by the police despite having committed no crime. They have been involuntarily locked in a hospital, perhaps as a result of testimony provided by a family member (about whom they already harbored persecutory delusions). They may even find themselves forced to take medications that they believe to be making them more ill.

Early psychological theories attempted to explain schizophrenia from the point of view of function, postulating that schizophrenia represented a "retreat from reality." While the above discussion has emphasized the disease perspective, psychotherapy continues to play an important role in the treatment of the disease and in supporting the affecting individual. *Intensive insight-oriented therapy*, aimed at helping the patient recognize unconscious motivations, is no longer a staple of treatment, and in fact this form of therapy is contraindicated in most patients since it is too stressful for them. In contrast, *supportive psychotherapy*, which places more emphasis on the development of a trusting therapeutic alliance, can enhance compliance with treatment while providing a model for appropriate interpersonal relationships.

Other types of therapy also play an important role in treatment. These include *social skills training* (teaching patients how to manage their finances, cook meals, and interact with peers), *vocational rehabilitation*, and *day treatment programs or clubhouses*. The goal of all of these programs is to help the patient to reintegrate into society while also attempting to avoid placing so much pressure on her in doing so that she experiences a relapse. Patients with schizophrenia may require not only a therapist but also a "case manager." The latter individual attempts to help them (and their families) negotiate the complex social service and public housing bureaucracy.

Neurochemical Factors and Antipsychotic Medications

The Dopamine Theory of Schizophrenia

The most important theory of schizophrenia to date has been the *dopamine theory*, which postulated that the symptoms of schizophrenia are somehow related to *overactivity in the dopamine system*. This theory originally was based on two observations. First, medications that increase brain levels of dopamine (such as amphetamine, cocaine, and L-dopa), especially when taken chronically, can cause a paranoid psychotic state resembling schizophrenia and also can exacerbate psychotic symptoms when they are taken by patients with preexisting schizophrenia. Second, not only do all known antipsychotic drugs block dopamine receptors, but their antipsychotic potency correlates with their binding affinities for the dopamine D_2 receptor, as indicated in Figure 8–1.

The dopamine system could be overactive for a variety of reasons, but research has failed to confirm any of them. One possibility is excessive dopamine production by dopaminergic neurons. Another possibility is that dopamine production is normal, but there is a deficiency of dopamine breakdown or reuptake, leading to a functional excess of synaptic dopamine. However, many studies examining cerebrospinal fluid and serum levels of the principal breakdown product of dopamine, homovanillic acid (HVA), have failed to demonstrate excessive levels of HVA in schizophrenic patients compared to normal control subjects. Some schizophrenic patients even had lower levels of HVA, which corresponded with the presence of more severe negative symptoms.

A third possibility is that in schizophrenia the dopamine receptor itself has either *increased in number* or has become overly *sensitive* to dopamine. Supporting this theory are postmortem studies and in vivo PET scan studies, both of which demonstrate an increase in D_2 receptor density. However, postmortem and PET receptor studies have been difficult to interpret due to the effects of chronic antipsychotic administration, which in itself causes dopamine receptor upregulation. (As we shall soon discuss, this may be a cause of tardive dyskinesia, a movement disorder that occurs in the setting of chronic antipsychotic usage.) One PET study, using never-medicated schizophrenic patients, failed to demonstrate an increase in dopamine receptor density over that seen in control subjects. Autopsy studies can be further confounded by

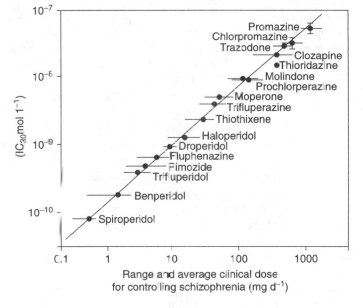

Figure 8–1. Potency and receptor affinity of typical antipsychotic medications. Reproduced with permission from Seeman P, Lee T: "Antipsychotic Drugs: Direct Correlation Between Clinical Potency and Presynaptic Action on Dopamine Neurons." *Science* 188:1217, 1975.

postmortem changes in the brain that might affect receptor density.

Another problem with the classic dopamine theory is that it fails to explain the negative symptoms of schizophrenia. Amphetamine and cocaine intoxication both can cause hallucinations and delusions resembling the positive symptoms of schizophrenia but they don't cause negative symptoms. Similarly, traditional D_2-antagonist drugs do provide some relief from negative symptoms but typically the response is modest at best. In many cases these agents *exacerbate* them, since drug-induced parkinsonism is associated with worsening of psychomotor slowing and apathy (so-called "secondary" negative symptoms).

More recent formulations have modified the classic dopamine hypothesis in an attempt to account for such clinical phenomena. One possibility is that there is hyperactivity in *one* dopamine pathway, leading to positive symptoms (which benefit from antipsychotic treatment), but underactivity along another dopamine pathway, leading to negative symptoms (which are exacerbated by traditional antipsychotic agents). Such a theory could also account for the variability in CSF levels of HVA, since one wouldn't expect to see either profound increases or decreases in the *overall* HVA level under this model. In addition, whether a patient presents with predominantly positive or negative symptoms might be explained by which dopamine pathway is most affected. Some recent preclinical and clinical studies lend support to this model, suggesting the presence of abnormalities in dopamine storage, release, reuptake, and metabolism in the mesolimbic system.

Other recent theories have suggested that *more than one neurotransmitter system* is out of balance in schizophrenia, not simply the dopamine system. The most significant findings have involved the serotonin and glutamate systems. These latter theories have been bolstered by the introduction of the newer class of "atypical" antipsychotics. These agents have only *weak* D_2-blocking effects but they appear to be at least as effective in treating positive symptoms as the conventional antipsychotic drugs and also probably demonstrate better (albeit mild) efficacy against negative and cognitive symptoms.

It remains possible, however, that dopamine is important in schizophrenia but that dopamine dysregulation is not the cause of the illness: First, antipsychotic medications block dopamine receptors, but while this effect is rapid, the onset of therapeutic effects can take up to several weeks. As we discussed in the previous chapter with regard to the relationship between the efficacy of monoaminergic antidepressant efficacy and the presumed etiology of major depressive disorder, it is possible in this case that it is not dopamine blockade per se that treats psychosis but rather the brain's "downstream" attempts to adapt to antipsychotic-induced alterations in homeostasis.

Second, dopamine is a neurotransmitter that plays a role in several complex circuits that involve multiple other neurotransmitters. The exact nature of these circuits remains poorly understood. Dopamine may simply be "the loudest voice in the chorus."

Third, we already have discussed in detail how the negative and cognitive symptoms of schizophrenia often appear earlier than do the positive symptoms and also respond more poorly to dopamine-blocking medications. Given this, the negative and cognitive features may be the "defining" features of schizophrenia, while the psychotic symptoms may be nonspecific aspects of severe mental disruption: the "fever" rather than the "infection." Evidence for this includes the fact that psychotic symptoms (even Schneiderian "first rank" symptoms) can occur in a wide variety of psychiatric, neurologic, and medical illnesses, including mood disorder, delirium and dementia (each of which can be caused by a long list of etiologies), and toxins. Genetic overlap also has been found between schizophrenia, schizoaffective disorder, and bipolar disorder. Antipsychotic medications have proven to be useful tools in managing all of these conditions, although they haven't been shown to reverse the underlying pathology in any of them. The limited response of the "core" features of schizophrenia to conventional antipsychotic medications suggests that schizophrenia may be no different.

To better understand these theories as well as the therapeutic and adverse effects of antipsychotic medications, we will first briefly review the dopamine system. Until recently, we only knew about two dopamine receptor subtypes, D_1

and D_2. The D_1 receptor is located in cerebral cortex and is linked to adenylate cyclase, while the D_2 receptor is located more subcortically and isn't linked to adenylate cyclase. More recently, D_3, D_4, and D_5 receptors have been identified. They are located primarily in limbic areas of the brain. Our current discussion, however, will focus on the D_2 system, which has been most strongly associated with the beneficial effects of antipsychotic medications.

There are four major D_2 pathways, as illustrated in Figure 8–2. Dopamine-containing cell bodies are located in a small area of brain stem. The substantia nigra sends fibers to the basal ganglia (**the nigrostriatal tract**) while the nearby **ventral tegmental area** sends fibers both to the nucleus accumbens (**the mesolimbic tract**) and to limbic cortical areas (**the mesocortical tract**). Dopamine is also contained in the arcuate nucleus of the hypothalamus, from which fibers project downward to the anterior pituitary gland (**the tuberoinfundibular tract**).

In each of these pathways, dopamine is but one neurotransmitter. It acts as one link in a network of cortical–subcortical *feedback loops* that are arranged in parallel, connecting discrete areas of cortex. For example, the occipital cortex is associated with the perception of vision and with visual memory, while the temporal cortex plays a similar role for the perception of sound. The frontal lobes are involved with attention, planning, and working memory. There are discrete loops for each type of function (thoughts, perceptions, emotions, motor behavior), and connections between neurons serve homologous functions in each brain region.

The subcortical basal ganglia and limbic areas appear to play a vital role in physical and mental well-being. While they don't receive direct afferent data from the eyes or ears, they help to integrate and modulate these data. For example, in patients with neurological disease affecting the basal ganglia, while the actual motor (or pyramidal) system remains intact, the ability to integrate and modulate movements is lost, leading either to excessive or deficient motor activity. It is possible that similar pathways modulate visual input, auditory input, thought associations, memory, planning, and attention to the outside world. Injury to these pathways could either lead to a decreased ability of the brain to "dampen" unwanted brain activity (perhaps leading to hallucinations, delusions, or thought disorder) or to a loss of "gain" in the system (perhaps leading to apathy, poverty of thought, social withdrawal, and attentional problems).

The nigrostriatal tract modifies motor activity via the extrapyramidal system. In Parkinson's disease, degeneration of this tract causes the characteristic symptoms of resting tremor, rigidity, bradykinesia, and postural instability. Antipsychotic-induced parkinsonism likely is caused by D_2 blockade within this pathway. In contrast, increased dopaminergic activity—for example, through excessive administration of L-dopa, leads to excessive (choreaform, dyskinetic, and/or dystonic) movements. The average person has an adequate reserve of dopamine in the substantia nigra such that 80% of striatal dopamine receptors must be occupied by antipsychotic medication before drug-induced parkinsonism becomes evident.

Increased dopaminergic activity in the mesolimbic tract may account for the positive symptoms of schizophrenia. The *nucleus accumbens* is thought to mediate the pleasurable sensations that act as internal reinforcers in motivated behaviors, including the euphoria that is associated with the use of addictive drugs. Excessive activity along this pathway might lead to

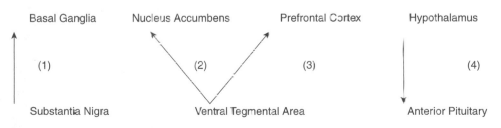

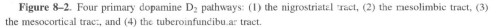

Figure 8–2. Four primary dopamine D_2 pathways: (1) the nigrostriatal tract, (2) the mesolimbic tract, (3) the mesocortical tract, and (4) the tuberoinfundibular tract.

hallucinations and delusions, while the thera-peutic effects of conventional antipsychotic agents may relate to their D_2-blocking effects in this pathway.

The mesocortical tract may mediate the effects of dopamine on attention and planning. In par-ticular, the frontal lobes, which have reciprocal connections with the basal ganglia, may play an important role in the genesis of negative symp-toms. The negative symptoms may reflect a rel-ative state of *dopamine deficiency* (rather than dopamine excess) along this pathway. For ex-ample, many of these negative symptoms re-semble the symptoms seen in patients who have suffered a frontal lobe injury. As discussed above, there also is evidence on functional neu-roimaging of decreased frontal lobe activity in schizophrenia, particularly when patients are asked to perform tasks that demand "executive function." Conventional antipsychotic medica-tions may cause "secondary" negative symptoms either by causing parkinsonian symptoms (via ni-grostriatal dopamine blockade) or by exacerbat-ing a preexisting dopamine deficiency state along the mesocortical tract.

Dopamine secreted via the tuberoinfundibular tract causes tonic inhibition of pituitary prolactin release. Thus, D_2 blockade by conventional an-tipsychotic agents results in an increase in serum prolactin, which in turn can cause gynecomastia, galactorrhea, amenorrhea, sexual dysfunction, and infertility and can contribute to the develop-ment of osteoporosis.

Conventional Antipsychotic Agents

There are several classes of conventional an-tipsychotic drugs, which are summarized in Table 8–8. No traditional antipsychotic has been shown to be superior to another. Therefore, drug selection is based on whether a patient has tol-erated and/or responded well to a particular agent in the past, as well as on consideration of po-tential side effects. A further consideration is that *haloperidol* and *fluphenazine* are the only agents available in "depot" form, suspended in oil, which allows for a single dose to be administered intramuscularly in the clinic or by a mental health outreach worker every few weeks. This strategy is associated with enhanced compliance and with a lower risk of relapse.

Like the older antidepressants, traditional an-

Table 8–8. Conventional Antipsychotic Classes and Agents

Class	Examples
Phenothiazines	Chlorpromazine (Thorazine)
	Fluphenazine (Prolixin)
	Trifluoperazine (Stelazine)
	Perphenazine (Trilafon)
	Thioridazine (Mellaril)
Butyrophenones	Haloperidol (Haldol)
Thioxanthenes	Thiothixene (Navane)
Dihydroindolones	Molindone (Moban)
Dibenzoxazepines	Loxapine (Loxitane)

tipsychotics are "dirty drugs," with antagonist activity at multiple receptors types, including the *H_1 histamine receptor* (causing sedation and weight gain), the *α-1 norepinephrine receptor* (causing hypotension), and the *M_1 muscarinic acetylcholine receptor* (causing blurred vision, dry mouth, and constipation, as well as mental slowing or confusion, sometimes incorrectly at-tributed to negative symptoms when in fact it is iatrogenic and a significant reason for medica-tion noncompliance).

All of these drugs, due to their dopamine-an-tagonist effects within the nigrostriatal system, can cause **parkinsonism** and other **extrapyra-midal symptoms (EPSs)**. Most often, these are treated with **anticholinergic medications** such as **benztropine (Cogentin)** and **trihexyphenidyl (Artane)**. Anticholinergic medications are ef-fective because acetylcholine has a reciprocal re-lationship with dopamine within the nigrostriatal pathway. Dopaminergic neurons from the sub-stantia nigra synapse on cholinergic neurons in the basal ganglia, thereby inhibiting acetyl-choline release. Given this, *blocking* dopamine receptors on these cholinergic neurons triggers *excessive* acetylcholine release, thereby trigger-ing excessive inhibition of motor behavior in the form of parkinsonism. Anticholinergic drugs combat this effect without affecting antipsy-chotic drugs' antidopaminergic effects along the mesolimbic pathway. Unfortunately, they also further exacerbate the burden of anticholinergic side-effects.

Table 8–9 lists the conventional antipsychotic agents by their relative potency in blocking the D_2 receptor, along with their sedative, anti-adrenergic, and extrapyramidal side-effect pro-

Table 8–9. Conventional Antipsychotic Drug Potency and Relationship to Side Effects

Drug	Equivalent Dose (mg)	Sedation	Autonomic	Extrapyramidal
Fluphenazine (Prolixin)	2	1+	1+	3+
Haloperidol (Haldol)	2	1+	1+	3+
Thiothixene (Navane)	4	1+	1+	3+
Trifluoperazine (Stelazine)	5	2+	1+	3+
Perphenazine (Trilafon)	10	2+	1+	2+/3+
Molindone (Moban)	10	2+	1+	1+
Loxapine (Loxitane)	15	2+	1+/2+	2+/3+
Mesoridazine (Serentil)	50	3−	2+	1+
Chlorpromazine (Thorazine)	100	3+	3+	1+/2+
Thioridazine (Mellaril)	100	3+	3+	1+

files. As can be seen, the least potent agents are the most likely to cause sedation and hypotension. However, a benefit of these lower-potency agents is that they also are the least likely to cause EPS, since they have a higher level of intrinsic anticholinergic activity. It is as if they have a "built in" anticholinergic medication. This combination of a greater degree of sedation and lesser EPS can be useful in the treatment of very agitated patients. However, the sedation also can become troublesome to some patients, especially since acute agitation subsides, but the patient may need to remain on a medication for years.

Similarly, the hypotension and anticholinergic effects associated with the lower-potency agents can become problematic. Elderly or brain-injured patients may become delirious while higher-functioning patients may find that they "just can't think as clearly." Weight gain can be associated with elevated blood glucose levels (even diabetes), elevated lipid levels, as well as with medication noncompliance.

The lower-potency drugs also are more likely to be associated with certain idiosyncratic side effects. They can cause photosensitivity reactions such as severe sunburn, rash, or blue–gray metallic skin discoloration. (Patients should be instructed to use sunscreens.) These reactions are particularly seen with **chlorpromazine**. Patients receiving long-term treatment with chlorpromazine also may develop granular deposits in the anterior lens and posterior cornea. These are only seen with slit-lamp examination and rarely affect vision. In contrast, high doses of **thioridazine** (greater than 1 g/day) can result in retinal pigmentation and lead to permanent decreased vi-

sion or even blindness. Given this, thioridazine shouldn't be prescribed at doses greater than 800 mg/day.

Many clinicians therefore opt to use a higher-potency agent (such as **haloperidol** or **fluphenazine**), typically in conjunction with an anticholinergic medication. Another option is to choose a medium-potency agent (such as **trifluoperazine** or **perphenazine**), which may be particularly useful when patients experience EPSs with higher-potency agents despite the addition of anticholinergic medication.

One extrapyramidal symptom that can be particularly troublesome, especially with the higher potency agents, is **akathisia**, a severe form of motor restlessness described in more detail in Chapter 2. It is important to recognize akathisia and to distinguish it from psychotic agitation because the treatment for these two conditions are diametric opposites, either cutting back the dose of medication (for akathisia) or increasing the dose of medication (for psychotic agitation).

Akathisia is very common and is likely the most frequently occurring type of EPS. In one study, following the administration of a single 5 mg dose of haloperidol (a relatively low dosage in schizophrenia treatment), 40% of patients experienced akathisia. After receiving 10 mg of haloperidol at bedtime for 1 week, 75% of patients were experiencing akathisia. This side effect tends to be less responsive to anticholinergic medication than is parkinsonism. Akathisia may respond to the addition of a β-adrenergic blocking medication (such as propranolol), to the addition of a benzodiazepine, or to a reduction in the dosage of antipsychotic medication. Another option is to switch from the conventional agent to an atypical antipsychotic medication.

Another form of EPS is **acute dystonia**. Characterized by sustained, involuntary muscle spasms, dystonia most often involves the muscles of the face, neck, and back (*opisthotonus*). The extraocular muscles may be involved, with the eyes locked in an upward gaze (an *oculogyric crisis*). When laryngeal spasm occurs, it can lead to difficulty breathing. Acute dystonia typically occurs very earlier in treatment, generally within the first week. It is more common in patients who have not been exposed previously to antipsychotic medications, and especially young males. It also is more likely to occur with the high potency antipsychotic medications.

Acute dystonia may be caused by abrupt nigrostriatal dopamine blockade or perhaps by an imbalance between postsynaptic dopamine blockade and dramatically increased dopamine release due to presynaptic blockade of the dopamine autoreceptor. Intravenous or intramuscular administration of anticholinergic medication (e.g., benztropine 2 mg) or antihistamine medication (e.g., diphenhydramine 50 mg) usually leads to rapid relief. Following this, standing doses of anticholinergic medications should be prescribed for at least a week. In some cases, the patient may benefit from a switch to a lower-potency agent, although the problem often doesn't recur. Rarely, though, patients contract a late-appearing, more chronic form of dystonia called **tardive dystonia**.

Imagine the effect an acute dystonic reaction can have on the state of mind of a young psychotic patient who lacks insight into being psychotic and who only has agreed (reluctantly) to a trial of medication based on the psychiatrist asking the patient to "trust her." Most commonly, given the circumstances, the patient hasn't been informed of this potential risk. Given the possibility that acute dystonia, akathisia, or parkinsonism can adversely influence long-term medication compliance—and by extension, the patient's entire course of illness—many clinicians advocate empirically prescribing a standing dose of anticholinergic medication along with initiation of antipsychotic treatment. Later, though, a taper of the anticholinergic medication always should be attempted.

The disadvantage of this strategy is that anticholinergic medications do carry side effects, including constipation, dry mouth, and confusion (even delirium) and might increase the risk of the patient subsequently developing tardive dyskinesia (see below). Still, in new-onset cases, especially those involving young males, empiric initiation of an anticholinergic medication is a prudent strategy.

Two other side effects also probably relate to nigrostriatal dopamine blockade, **tardive dyskinesia (TD)** and **neuroleptic malignant syndrome (NMS)**. These are the most serious potential complications of antipsychotic drug therapy. The risk of causing TD and NMS appears to be the same for all of the conventional antipsychotic medications.

Tardive dyskinesia consists of abnormal, involuntary twitching movements of the tongue and jaw (75%), limbs (50%), trunk (25%), or all of the above (10%). As its name suggests, it appears later than other forms of EPS. In many cases, it is very subtle (lip and tongue movements that might be confused with a nervous habit or a schizophrenic stereotypy). It often isn't detected by patients or their families (or even by clinicians who don't routinely inspect for TD at regular intervals in all of their patients who are taking maintenance antipsychotic medication). TD doesn't occur in all patients, and in many cases it isn't progressive. When detected early, it may still be reversible. However, in some cases TD is a socially disfiguring, progressive, irreversible complication. It is the major reason why conventional antipsychotic drugs are recommended only when reasonable alternatives aren't feasible.

The risk of developing TD is about 5% per year during the first several years of therapy, ultimately stabilizing after several years at about 20%–30%. However, the incidence of TD among elderly patients prescribed conventional antipsychotics is much higher: 25% after 1 year, 50% after 2 years, and 60% by 3 years. This is something one should consider when treating agitation in the setting of dementia. Antipsychotic agents sometimes are the drugs of choice, particularly when psychotic symptoms are present or when the patient is acutely delirious. Beyond this, particularly in cases of where the primary target symptom is "agitation," one should consider alternative agents, such as those listed in Chapter 6 in Table 6–6.

Risk factors for developing TD include *age, sex* (with equal prevalence among younger men and women, but in the elderly occurring more commonly in women), *coexisting neurologic conditions,* and *total lifetime cumulative exposure to antipsychotic medications.* Other potential risk factors include a greater number of lifetime drug-free *"drug holidays," diagnosis* (it occurs more commonly in mood disorder patients than in schizophrenia patients), the presence of *diabetes,* and a history of having experienced *acute dystonia.* Lifetime *exposure to anticholinergic medications* also may potentially increase the risk of developing TD.

The cause of TD is unclear. One theory is that chronic exposure to dopamine-receptor antagonists ultimately leads to upregulation and "supersensitivity" of the dopamine receptor. In other words, in acute parkinsonism, dopamine blockade causes a functional deficiency of dopamine, while in chronic dyskinesia, receptor upregulation causes a functional excess of dopamine. Consistent with this theory, the presence of TD might be "unmasked" when the dose of antipsychotic medication has been decreased. Similarly, TD can be "masked" by increasing the dose of antipsychotic medication. Note that transient "withdrawal dyskinesias" also commonly occur

with antipsychotic dosage decreases. These resolve after about a month and TD therefore shouldn't be diagnosed until a sufficient period of time has elapsed following a medication taper. Other theories involve noradrenergic hyperactivity or the production of free radicals that damage catecholamine and/or GABA receptors.

Not all that twitches is TD. Studies of unmedicated schizophrenic patients in the pre-antipsychotic era indicated that up to about a quarter of schizophrenic patients develop spontaneous dyskinesias. Patients with more prominent negative symptoms and cognitive dysfunction also are more likely to develop spontaneous dyskinesia. As previously discussed, these are the same patients who tend to have cortical atrophy and enlarged ventricles on structural neuroimaging. One possibility is that a mesocortical hypodopaminergic state ultimately causes a hyperdopaminergic state in both the mesolimbic and nigrostriatal tracts. The result of such a process would be a prodromal period of negative symptoms (mesocortical tract) followed by the development of positive symptoms (mesolimbic tract) and abnormal motor movements (nigrostriatal tract), as illustrated in Figure 8–3.

In addition to transient drug-withdrawal dyskinesia and spontaneous dyskinesia, other con-

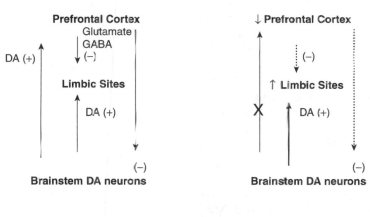

Normal State   **Schizophrenia**

Figure 8–3. Interactions between mesolimbic and mesocortical systems The "X" indicates injury to the mesocortical pathway, while dotted lines indicate the resultant loss of normal feedback inhibition of the limbic system both directly (via glutamate from the prefrontal cortex) and indirectly (via loss of feedback inhibition of brain-stem dopaminergic neurons in the ventral tegmental areas, thereby resulting in increased dopamine release by the ventral tegmental area along the mesolimbic pathway). The heavy line indicates increased mesolimbic activity. Not pictured are increased activity along the nigrostriatal pathway due to loss of feedback inhibition on dopaminergic neurons in the substantia nigra, which potentially causes spontaneous dyskinesias.

ditions that one should consider in the differential diagnosis of patients exhibiting dyskinesias include Huntington's disease, Wilson's disease, Sydenham's chorea, systemic lupus erythematosus, thyrotoxicosis, and heavy metal poisoning. One also should make sure to ask the patient to remove dentures if these are present before inspecting for buccolingual movements, since ill-fitting dentures can lead to mouth movements that resemble these.

The most effective treatment for TD is primary prevention. This includes attempting to treat patients at the lowest possible dose of antipsychotic medication that doesn't lead to exacerbations of illness, with consideration being given every few months to another gradual dosage taper if the patient is stable. Unfortunately, lower medication doses are associated with a higher risk of relapse, particularly during periods when the patient is under more stress. Gradual dosage reduction also should be attempted should signs of TD appear, although again this must be weighed with countervailing clinical considerations, especially when mild TD occurs in the setting of severe psychiatric illness that otherwise is responding to treatment.

Preliminary evidence suggests that vitamin E might help decrease the risk of developing TD or treat TD, lending credence to the theory that TD is caused by overexcitation and free radical formation. Finally, consider switching to an atypical antipsychotic medication. The primary benefit of these medications is their dramatically lower rate of extrapyramidal symptoms, including TD. Further, the risk of TD has been the primary reason that we do not simply maintain schizophrenic patients at the dosage of antipsychotic medication to which they initially responded, as we do with antidepressants in patients with major depressive disorder or mood stabilizers in patients with bipolar disorder. Given this, the atypical agents may allow patients to chronically take higher dosages of medications, thereby allowing for more effective prophylaxis against relapse.

Another potentially serious complication of antipsychotic treatment is NMS. This potentially fatal disorder occurs in up to 1% of inpatients treated with antipsychotics. Various criteria have been used in different research studies, but the essential features of NMS are *severe muscle rigidity and elevated body temperature*. The patient may have only a very mild temperature elevation (e.g., 99°F) but may experience severe hyperthermia (e.g.,106°F). This may be accompanied by *diaphoresis, dysphagia, tremor, incontinence, delirium* (which can progress to coma or death), *mutism, tachycardia, elevated or labile blood pressure, leukocytosis* (with WBC counts usually between 10,000 and 20,000) and *elevated creatinine phosphokinase (CPK).* (If the elevated CPK is mild, it may simply be an artifact of intramuscular injections or the use of restraints. However, these are unlikely to be the cause when CPK elevations are severe.) Severe CPK elevations also can cause *myoglobinuria* (with the urine dipstick reading positive for blood but with no red blood cells seen on microscopic exam) and ultimately *renal failure*.

Unfortunately, there is no way to predict who will develop NMS. In mild cases, the condition may be self-limited and might be mistaken for a benign viral syndrome. It usually develops within a month of first starting on antipsychotic medication, most often during the first week. However, some patients develop NMS after having been on a stable dose of medication for several months.

The risk of NMS appears to be higher among individuals who have experienced *previous episodes of NMS*. Other risk factors include *agitation* (perhaps with related motor activity and autonomic hyperactivity), *dehydration, high doses of neuroleptic medication, rapid increases in dosage, intramuscular antipsychotic injection*, and *use of high-potency agents. Mood disorder patients* may be more at risk, and *lithium carbonate* used in combination with antipsychotics may also increase the risk of developing NMS. Being in a warm or humid environment also may be a predisposing factor. Various *general medical illnesses* can place the individual at greater risk; conversely, NMS can cause complicating medical problems such as pneumonia, renal failure, cardiac or respiratory arrest, seizures, sepsis, pulmonary embolism, and disseminated intravascular coagulation (DIC).

A "classic case" of NMS might be a young, agitated manic patient who hasn't been eating or drinking (and who therefore is mildly dehydrated) in locked-door seclusion (with the seclusion room being warm and poorly ventilated) who has required high doses of antipsychotic medication (sometimes administered intramuscularly). He becomes increasingly agitated despite these interventions and ultimately becomes acutely febrile, stiff, and delirious. He is transferred to the intensive care unit in order to better manage his autonomic instability, but the combination of his ongoing mania and superimposed delirium cause significant behavioral problems (pulling of intravenous lines, assaultive behavior toward the staff, and a need for continuous physical restraint).

When symptoms of possible NMS are noted, this should trigger a workup for sepsis. One also should discontinue any antipsychotic medication, initiate treatment with antipyretic drugs, administer intravenous fluids, and provide cooling blankets. Following discontinuation of antipsychotic medication, NMS often resolves after about 2 weeks (or after about a month if "depot" antipsychotic medication has been prescribed). Dopamine agonists such as **bromocriptine** and peripheral muscle relaxants such as **dantrolene** may be useful adjuncts. **Electroconvulsive therapy** also can be very useful since it demonstrates efficacy in treating both NMS and acute psychotic illness.

Fatality rates associated NMS cited in the clinical literature range from 10% to 20%, but these may be artificially high due to reporting bias. With increasing recognition and treatment of NMS, fatality estimates have decreased somewhat. There also have been case reports of neurological sequelae that persist following recovery.

NMS may be caused by an acute hypodopaminergic state, especially in the nigrostriatal and hypothalamic pathways. As was the case with TD, similar symptoms rarely occur in patients with schizophrenia who are not taking antipsychotic medication. In this case, the spontaneously occurring form of NMS is **malignant catatonia**. Patients with malignant catatonia initially may present with symptoms of either a psychotic mood disorder or schizophrenia, but they then enter a catatonic state that is complicated by autonomic hyperactivity. The state is essentially indistinguishable from NMS except for the fact that the symptoms either occur in the absence of antipsychotic medication or precede the initiation of antipsychotic medication. One theory (among many) is that malignant catatonia reflects the body's attempts to compensate for a hyper-dopaminergic psychotic state through dopamine receptor downregulation. When this occurs too rapidly, it creates a dopamine imbalance and leads to an NMS-like state. Given this, one should be cautious when prescribing antipsychotic drugs (especially conventional agents) to catatonic patients.

Glutamate

While dopamine clearly plays a role in schizophrenia, other chemical transmitters also are implicated. The "modified" dopamine theory postulates that schizophrenia involves dysfunction of several interconnected transmitter systems. For example, it is possible that a deficiency of *glutamate* plays a role in the pathogenesis of the illness. We have already discussed how one argument supporting the dopamine hypothesis is that dopaminergic drugs such as amphetamines and cocaine can produce positive symptoms. Similarly, the effects of *phencyclidine (PCP)* argue for glutamate playing a role.

PCP binds to a site on the glutaminergic NMDA receptor, thereby causing an allosteric modification that inhibits the influx of calcium and antagonizes the effect of glutamate. In other words, PCP's effect on the NMDA receptor mimics what one might see in a *glutamate deficiency state*. Clinically, PCP intoxication can cause an acute psychotic state that resembles schizophrenia, including true hallucinations, thought disorder, negative symptoms, and cognitive deficits.

We have discussed the reciprocal relationship between dopamine and acetylcholine in the nigrostriatal system. Glutamate also has a reciprocal relationship with dopamine, such that a state of glutamate deficiency resembles a state of dopamine excess. *Glutamate fibers* from the cortex to subcortical limbic structures *stimulate* the activity of interneurons. These interneurons contain the inhibitory transmitter GABA, which allows them to play a modulatory role. Meanwhile, *dopamine fibers* to the striatum *inhibit* these interneurons. Therefore, it's possible that a similar final pathway involving decreased GABA could be produced either by *deficient corticolimbic glutamate activity* or by *excessive mesolimbic dopamine activity*. Since the frontal lobes are rich in glutamate receptors, it may turn out that in schizophrenia glutamate provides a crucial link between the negative–cognitive symptoms and the positive symptoms.

Figure 8–3 illustrates this model. Presumably, genetic and/or prenatal insults to the mesocortical pathway might lead to decreased cortical (particularly frontal) dopamine levels, contributing to the appearance of negative symptoms. At a later point, this in turn leads to a loss of normal inhibition of the mesolimbic system. This occurs both directly (through loss of corticolimbic glutaminergic transmission) and indirectly (through loss of feedback inhibition of the ventral tegmental area by the cortex, leading to increased dopamine transmission along the mesolimbic pathway).

Serotonin

Serotonin also may play an important role in schizophrenia. Again, a drug of abuse provides a relevant model. *Lysergic acid diethylamide (LSD)*, which produces a quasi-psychotic state, was noted in the 1950s to structurally resemble serotonin. Further, its main effect appears to be as a serotonin receptor agonist. A prevailing theory at the time was that schizophrenia would turn out to be due to serotonin dysregulation. However, phenomenologic studies revealed that—in contrast to what is seen in schizophrenia—LSD intoxication is associated more with visual *illusions* than with visual hallucinations, auditory hallucinations occur only rarely, insight is often preserved, and negative symptoms are absent. In the 1970s, as the role of dopamine became increasingly clear, attention turned away from serotonin.

However, serotonin, like glutamate, has a *reciprocal relationship with dopamine*. Serotonin fibers from the dorsal raphe area project to the substantia nigra, where they synapse on somatodendritic $5HT_2$ receptors located on the dopamine neurons that project to the striatum. Serotonin inhibits the firing of these neurons. Thus, serotonin has an *inhibitory effect* on the nigrostriatal dopamine system. Serotonin seems to exert similar effects in the mesocortical system.

In the last chapter, we discussed how SSRIs, which increase levels of serotonin in the frontal lobes, can cause *apathy symptoms* in some patients, especially when they are administered at higher doses. This syndrome resembles a state of

mesocortical dopamine deficiency. In fact, one strategy that has been used to treat SSRI-induced apathy is to add a stimulant agent such as **methylphenidate (Ritalin)**, which acts by increasing dopamine release. We have also discussed how in some individuals SSRIs can be associated with *akathisia*, which might be mediated by decreased nigrostriatal dopamine. Thus, serotonin appears to play a modulating role on dopamine transmission in the nigrostriatal system and possibly in the mesocortical system. It doesn't appear to play as important a role in the mesolimbic system. This distinction will have important implications as we move on to discuss the "atypical" antipsychotic drugs.

"Atypical" Antipsychotic Agents

The role of serotonin in schizophrenia likely still wouldn't be receiving much attention were it not for the drug **clozapine (Clozaril)**, the first—and prototypical—atypical antipsychotic agent. In the 1960s, researchers in Austria and Germany described clozapine as being particularly effective in treating schizophrenia. Many clinicians doubted that this could be the case, since clozapine violated the conventional wisdom, which stated that: *(1)* all antipsychotics require a significant amount of D_2-receptor blockade in order to be effective; *(2)* therefore, all antipsychotics cause EPS; and *(3)* one can estimate the most effective dosage of the antipsychotic agent by titrating the dosage upward until EPS first appears, since at this point 80% of striatal D_2 receptors are occupied.

In contrast, clozapine didn't cause EPS. In addition, it didn't cause tardive dyskinesia. Clozapine became quite popular in Europe in the 1970s. Unfortunately, after several years of use, it became evident that clozapine caused potentially fatal **agranulocytosis** in 1% of patients. Given this, clozapine wasn't approved for use in the United States until 1990, and then only with tight regulation.

The real twist in the clozapine story came as the drug was being tested in the United States. Investigators hoped to demonstrate to the Food and Drug Administration that clozapine, despite its risks, might be of utility for those patients unable to tolerate conventional antipsychotic drugs because of EPS. For ethical reasons, the drug was tested specifically in treatment-refractory patients (i.e., those who had remained severely ill despite trials of several different conventional agents). In this group of pateints, clozapine was found to offer *greater efficacy* in treating both positive and negative symptoms of schizophrenia than conventional agents.

In other words, clozapine more effectively treated *positive symptoms*, despite having weaker D_2 antagonist effects than typical agents have, suggesting that there can be more to treating psychosis than simply blocking dopamine. (Just what that "more" is remains an open question, though.) In addition, clozapine had a greater impact on *negative symptoms*. Some of this apparent benefit clearly related to improvement in "secondary" negative symptoms (i.e., subtle parkinsonism) in patients once they were switched from their previous, conventional agent to clozapine. However, this probably isn't the only explanation. Higher clozapine doses were more effective in treating negative symptoms than were lower doses; this wouldn't be consistent with the hypothesis that clozapine simply causes fewer cognitive side effects. Perhaps the drug, by blocking serotonin, *increases* dopamine in the *mesocortical system*, thereby decreasing negative symptoms.

How is it possible to treat psychosis without causing EPS? It turns out that clozapine has *weaker D_2 antagonist activity* than do conventional antipsychotic drugs (20%–60% receptor blockade versus 70%–90% blockade, respectively). However, clozapine also has powerful *$5HT_2$ receptor antagonist effects*. While traditional agents have little activity in this regard, clozapine causes up to a 90% $5HT_2$ blockade. Because of this, in the *mesolimbic system* (where serotonin doesn't playa a significant role), clozapine confers predominantly *D_2 antagonist effects* (leading to a lessening of positive symptoms) while in the *nigrostriatal system*, its serotonin antagonist effects counteract D_2-blocking effects, thereby allowing it to avoid causing EPS.

This, of course, is just one theory. Another theory is that since clozapine has a very high binding affinity for the D_4 receptor relative to its affinity for the D_2 receptor, the D_4 receptor might be a particularly important receptor in the positive symptoms of schizophrenia. However, it turns out that conventional antipsychotics also demonstrate high binding affinity for the D_4 receptor. (In fact, haloperidol's affinity for the D_4 receptor is higher than clozapine's.) In addition, experimental agents offering selective affinity for the D_4 receptor have been found to be devoid of antipsychotic benefit in clinical trials.

Yet another theory is that clozapine and other atypical antipsychotics cause less EPS than do conventional agents because they *more rapidly dissociate from the D_2 receptor*. The affinity of the antipsychotics for the D_2 receptor highly correlates with their rate of dissociation. In other words, drugs with a low binding affinity for the dopamine D_2 receptor, such as atypical agents, also dissociate from the receptor much more quickly. PET scan studies reveal that when D_2 binding in the striatum is high (as occurs with conventional antipsychotics), motor side effects still occur even when potent $5HT_2$ antagonists are added to the mix. (Perhaps this is why one can't simply add nefazodone, a $5HT_2$ antagonist, to haloperidol to alleviate EPS.) It may be that rapid dissociation allows the dopamine receptors to be free from antipsychotic antagonism for a brief period between medication doses. This brief exposure to natural dopamine may be just enough to prevent patients from developing EPS while still not being enough of a dopamine exposure for psychotic symptoms to return.

While it doesn't cause EPS and can be more effective than conventional agents, clozapine was used much less frequently than one might expect due to the fact that it can cause a wide variety of *other* side effects. It is a "dirty drug" that works on at least nine receptors, including the H_1 histamine receptor (leading to sedation) the M_1 muscarinic receptor (leading to anticholinergic side-effects), and the α-1 receptor (leading to significant orthostatic hypotension and tachycardia). It affects not only subcortical D_2 receptors but also cortical D_1 and D_4 receptors. It also blocks the $5HT_{2C}$ and $5HT_3$ receptors. Idiosyncratic effects of clozapine include significant weight gain (gains of over 20 pounds are not uncommon), hypersalivation, and seizures, especially at higher doses. Because of sedation and hypotension, it must be started at a very low dose, followed by very gradual upward dosage titration.

Clozapine also can increase serum lipid levels, increase peripheral insulin resistance, and even contribute to the development of frank diabetes. While increased insulin resistance may occur secondarily to weight gain, it occurs in some patients who have not gained significant weight, suggesting that it also exerts independent effects on glucose regulation. Patients with schizophrenia already tend to eat poorly, 70%–90% of them smoke cigarettes (versus 25% of the general population), and most of them receive little or no preventive health care. Given this, the increase in cardiovascular risk associated with side effects such as weight gain, increased serum lipid levels, and impaired glucose tolerance is a significant consideration.

The greatest concern with clozapine is bone marrow suppression, particularly the 1% risk of agranulocytosis, which can lead to life-threatening infections. While the peak incidence occurs between 2 and 6 months after the initiation of treatment, it can occur at any time. In the United States, clozapine is available only through a system that requires that weekly white blood cell counts be obtained prior to each week's medication being dispensed. This is cumbersome, expensive, and demands a high degree of cooperation on the part of a difficult patient population.

The pharmaceutical industry has made a major push to develop other "atypical" agents that are "clozapine-like" in their therapeutic effects but lack clozapine's toxicity. Largely, they have succeeded, although clozapine remains unique in having demonstrated efficacy in patients refractory to conventional antipsychotic agents. Fortunately, the agranulocytosis associated with clozapine doesn't appear to be due to any of its above-mentioned receptor effects.

Several new agents have been introduced, and more are on the way. These new agents represent a dramatic advance in the biological treatment of schizophrenia as they offer the promise of dramatically improved side-effect profiles (diminished parkinsonism and akathisia without anticholinergic side effects, along with greatly decreased risks of TD and NMS) as well as the possibility of greater efficacy in treating negative and cognitive symptoms.

Unlike the conventional antipsychotic agents, which have very similar receptor affinities, all of the newer drugs have very different chemical structures and receptor affinities. Given, this, it remains unclear just what makes them all "atypical." Their greatest area of commonality is that they all cause little or no EPS. The term "atypi-

cal" also has been applied to antipsychotic agents that possess serotonin antagonism, but some conventional agents also possess serotonin antagonist properties but still cause EPS. Further, drugs with very high selective affinities for the $5HT_2$ receptor and no affinity for the D_2 receptor have failed to demonstrate significant antipsychotic effects in clinical trials. All antipsychotic agents to date possess at least some degree of D_2 antagonism, and some commentators suggest that what therefore is most important is the *ratio* of serotonin to dopamine antagonism.

For example, risperidone, at doses below 6 mg per day, causes little EPS. However, at doses above this it causes rates of EPS similar to haloperidol, a high-potency typical agent. (Fortunately, the average maintenance dose of risperidone for schizophrenia is between 4 and 5 mg per day.) Risperidone's affinity for the $5HT_2$ receptor appears to be greater than its affinity for the D_2 receptor. Therefore, at lower doses, it has nearly saturated the $5HT_2$ receptors while D_2 receptor occupancy remains low. However, at higher doses, D_2 occupancy increases and there isn't any further "room" for compensatory increases in $5HT_2$ blockade. EPS becomes evident and the drug begins to appear more "typical."

Finally, the atypical antipsychotic agents may exert effects on other neurotransmitter systems, particularly the glutamate system. For example, they all have been found to block the cellular and behavioral effects of NMDA antagonists, despite the fact that they themselves don't appear to bind to glutamate receptors. Given this, atypical antipsychotic drugs may boost glutamate activity indirectly, through effects on dopamine, serotonin, or other receptors.

Table 8–10 lists the atypical antipsychotic agents currently available in the United States. Which of these is the "best" or the "safest" has become the subject of intense pharmaceutical marketing campaigns. All of them appear to be effective in treating positive symptoms of schizophrenia and all demonstrate only modest efficacy in treating negative and cognitive symptoms. Their side-effect profiles vary, and the most important considerations are their extrapyramidal effects, effects on prolactin level, degree of associated weight gain, their ability to impair glucose metabolism, and their effects on cardiac conduction.

Table 8–10. Atypical Antipsychotic Agents, Dosing, and Extent of the Most Common Side Effects

Drug	Average Adult Daily Dose (mg)	Cytochrome Metabolism	Sedation	Avg Weight Gain (in kg) at 10 weeks, and % of Patients with >7% Weight Increase (per Package Insert)	Increased Glucose	Increased QTc Interval (ms)	Increased Prolactin	Other
Clozapine (Clozaril)	75–900	1A2, 2E1, 3A4	High	4.5 N.A.	Most common	N.A.	None	Potential increased efficacy; agranulocytosis risk necessitates WBC monitoring; dose-related seizure risk; orthostatic hypotension; hypersalivation
Olanzapine (Zyprexa)	10–20	1A2, glucuronidation	Moderate	4.2 30%	Possible	7	Mild	Smoking decreases blood levels; some patients require 20–40 mg/day
Risperidone (Risperdal)	2–6	2D6, 3A4	Moderate	2.1 20%	Lower risk	12	High	Higher rate of EPS than ≥6 mg/day
Quetiapine (Seroquel)	400–800	3A4	High	N.A. (2 kg at 6 wk) 25%	Lower risk	15	None	BID dosing; requires titration due to sedation; cataracts in beagles (slit-lamp exam?)
Ziprasidone (Geodon)	80–160	3A4, aldehyde oxidase	Moderate	0.04 10%	Lower risk	20	None	BID dosing; weight neutral at 1 yr; contraindicated where increaesd risk of prolonged QTc

Olanzapine (Zyprexa) is the closest to clozapine in its polyreceptor affinities. It is a more potent D_2 blocker than clozapine, and it has fewer anticholinergic and α-adrenergic effects. While it is better tolerated than clozapine, it does have a greater propensity to cause EPS than does clozapine, especially at higher doses. (Typical doses range from 10 to 20 mg per day, but some refractory patients are treated with doses of up to 40 mg per day and generally tolerate this well.)

Olanzapine is antihistaminergic and therefore relatively sedating, although this effect resolves during the first few weeks of treatment. Olanzapine causes mild, dose-related increases in prolactin levels, but these are less than the increases seen in association with conventional agents or with risperidone. An intramuscular form of olanzapine has been approved by the Food and Drug Administration, which should facilitate its use in acute psychotic episodes. Olanzapine also has been approved for use as a mood stabilizer in treating manic episodes. It appears to have antidepressant properties as well, and it has been used as an augmenting agent in major depressive disorder, even in patients without psychotic symptoms.

Treatment with olanzapine is associated with significant weight gain, almost as high as that associated with clozapine therapy. The extent of weight gain tends to be greatest during the first 6 weeks, and it then continues more slowly, leveling out by about 10 months. (If the patient has not gained weight by 6–8 weeks, she is unlikely to do so after this.) Of note, antipsychotic-induced weight gain is not a dose-related phenomenon, and one therefore should not attempt to mitigate it by lowering the medication dosage, since it probably won't work and increases the risk of relapse.

Like clozapine, olanzapine treatment is possibly associated with an increased rate of impaired glucose tolerance and even with the production or worsening of diabetes mellitus. Further research is necessary to determine whether this is in fact the case.

Risperidone (Risperdal) is a more "pure" $5HT_2/D_2$ antagonist, with little antihistaminergic effect. Risperidone causes less weight gain than clozapine or olanzapine, although a bit more than quetiapine or ziprasidone (on average, about 5 pounds). As noted above, because it is a more potent D_2 antagonist, risperidone is more likely to cause EPS, especially at doses greater than 6 mg/day. It also causes elevations in prolactin levels as high as those seen with conventional antipsychotics, making it unique in this regard among the atypical antipsychotics. Tardive dyskinesia and NMS appear to be less common with risperidone than with conventional antipsychotics, but have been reported. It also is associated with mild increases in the QTc interval, but no cases of torsades de pointes have been reported.

Quetiapine (Seroquel), like risperidone, has higher binding affinity for $5HT_2$ receptors than for D_2 receptors. It also has strong antihistaminergic properties, making it relatively sedating and necessitating gradual upward dosage titration. It is associated with mild weight gain (to about the same degree as risperidone). Beyond this, the benefits of quetiapine include a very low rate of EPS (no greater than placebo, even at high dosages) and an absence of prolactin elevation. The medication has a relatively short half-life (6–7 hours), and the manufacturer therefore recommends twice daily dosing, although anecdotal experience suggests that some patients do well with single daily dosing at bedtime. Treatment with quetiapine has been associated with cataract formation in beagles, but not in humans, and the package insert recommends an eye examination either at the initiation of treatment or shortly thereafter, followed by repeat examinations every 6 months.

Ziprasidone (Geodon) has a strong affinity for both the D_2 and $5HT_2$ receptors. In addition—and unlike the other atypical agents—it has serotonin and norepinephrine reuptake inhibitory effects. Despite its high dopaminergic affinity, it does not produce significant EPS and does not significantly increase prolactin levels. Further, ziprasidone is the only atypical agent that does not produce significant weight gain, having been found to be "weight neutral" during courses of treatment lasting over 1 year. It also does not appear to increase glucose or lipid levels.

However, treatment with ziprasidone has been associated with moderate increases in the cardiac *QT interval*. This interval describes the time that it takes for the ventricles to depolarize and then repolarize. The duration varies inversely with the heart rate, such that it is more useful to use a formula to "correct" the QT for heart rate, producing the QTc. Normal QTc intervals are around 400 milliseconds (ms), and values lower than 440 ms are considered normal. While the QTc can be affected by a variety of factors (including eating or drinking, athletic training, sleeping, and diurnal rhythms), more significant prolongations (those associated with a QTc interval of greater than 500 ms) are cause for concern.

This degree of prolongation—which most commonly occurs either congenitally, as a result of ischemic heart disease, or in association with antiarrhythmic medication—has been associated with an increased risk of developing polymorphic ventricular tachycardia (also called **torsades de pointe**), an arrhythmia that can lead to sudden death.

Ventricular depolarization results from the rapid influx of sodium through selective sodium ion channels, while repolarization involves calcium, sodium, and potassium channels. Drugs that cause torsades de pointe generally bind to one particular potassium channel, the *potassium rectifier channel*. For example, tricyclic antidepressants block the sodium channel involved in depolarization, thereby causing both a widened QRS interval and an increased QTc interval. However, while this causes them to be potentially dangerous for patients with bundle branch disease or severe ischemic heart disease or who take an overdose, they remain generally safe in healthy adults who take them in usual dosages. In contrast, thioridazine and haloperidol, which bind to the potassium rectifier channel, can cause sudden death even in otherwise healthy individuals.

At peak blood levels, ziprasidone increases the QTc by 20 ms on average. This is less that what is associated with thioridazine (36 ms) but more than what is associated with haloperidol (5 ms). Also, more significant QTc increases occurred in patients with low baseline QTc; patients with higher baseline QTc's were less likely to develop significant increases. In fact, out of 7875 patients taking ziprasidone, only three ECG tracings showed a QTc greater than 500 ms. Two of these tracings were from the same patient and the third was from a patient who was switched to thioridazine due to insufficient clinical response. Only after this switch did the patient experience a QTc of greater than 500 ms. Clinical trials have re-

vealed no evidence of an increased incidence of arrhythmias or sudden death in association with ziprasidone, and the Food and Drug Administration did not make a specific recommendation for patients to receive routine ECGs or cardiac examinations.

It also is fortunate the ziprasidone exhibits few drug–drug interactions. While other drugs are metabolized primarily by the cytochrome P450 system, about two-thirds of ziprasidone's metabolism is mediated by *aldehyde oxidase*. Cytochrome 3A4 does play a minor role in its metabolism, but in one pharmacokinetic study neither the potent 3A4 inhibitor ketoconazole nor the 3A4 inducer carbamazepine exerted significant effects on serum ziprasidone levels or on the QTc interval.

As a precaution, though, one still should not prescribe ziprasidone in patients with a history of QTc prolongation, a recent acute myocardial infarction, or uncompensated heart failure. It also should not be combined with other drugs known to prolong the QT intervals (which are listed on the drug's package insert). In older patients, especially those with known heart disease or who are taking medications known to prolong the QT interval, one should obtain a pretreatment ECG.

As can be seen, while the atypical antipsychotics appear to offer efficacy as good as (if not better than) conventional antipsychotics, usually without causing EPS, they are not benign. Each of them has its own side-effect profile that should be considered in light the patient's health status and potential sensitivity to particular side effects.

Clozapine may offer the highest efficacy, but it also has the most significant side effects, including bone marrow suppression (necessitating weekly monitoring of the white blood cell count), significant weight gain, and impaired glucose and lipid metabolism. Olanzapine is better tolerated than clozapine, but weight gain and possibly impaired glucose and lipid metabolism remain potential problems. Risperidone causes only mild weight increases and has not been associated with hyperlipidemia or hyperglycemia but is the most likely of the atypical agents to cause EPSs and it can be associated with prolactin elevation. Quetiapine offers little or no EPSs and only mild weight gain, but it requires titration to high dosages, can cause orthostatic hypotension, and can be more sedating. Ziprasidone also causes little EPS and also does not appear to cause weight gain, hyperlipidemia, or hyperglycemia. However, it prolongs ventricular repolarization to a greater extent than do the other agents. While to date it has proven to be safe and effective in large numbers of patients, caution is appropriate.

Given their greater out-of-pocket expense, some states have placed limitations on how much of the annual budget will be allotted to cover the cost of atypical antipsychotic medications. Similarly, some managed care organizations require documentation that the patient has "failed" one or more trials of a conventional agent before they will approve the prescription of an atypical agent. However, pharmacoeconomic research reveals that such strategies are shortsighted. Treatment with the atypical agents (even the most expensive one, clozapine) *ultimately* allows for significant savings compared to treatment with conventional agents when one considers costs to the *total* healthcare system.

For example, with the use of atypical agents, the length of inpatient hospital stays are reduced. Patients tend to be less assaultive, resulting in less money being spent on additional staffing and treatment of injuries. Patients remain more compliant with medication in the outpatient setting, thereby decreasing the risk of relapse and the need for rehospitalization. Lastly, it is conceivable that—if these agents can be initiated early enough in the course of schizophrenia—they may prevent patients from becoming permanently disabled. This might spare patients from having to depend on lifelong public assistance.

SCHIZOAFFECTIVE DISORDER

Phenomenology

Schizoaffective disorder is diagnosed when patients don't easily fit into the category of either schizophrenia or mood disorder. They experience episodes of illness that meet the full diagnostic criteria for a depressive, manic, or mixed episode. However, in between these episodes, and in the absence of prominent mood symptoms, they also experience hallucinations and delusions, the latter being more consistent with a diagnosis of schizophrenia.

Not surprisingly, the specific diagnostic criteria for schizoaffective disorder have changed over the years in response to changes in the diagnostic criteria for mood disorder and schizophrenia. In the early 1900s, after Kraepelin distinguished between bipolar disorder and schizophrenia, cases of schizoaffective disorder were considered to be closer to bipolar disorder since these patients didn't tend to have a deteriorating course. From about 1930 to about 1970, when Bleuler's broader conception of schizophrenia predominated, such cases were considered to be "atypical" or "better-prognosis" forms of schizophrenia. Similarly, *DSM-II* listed the diagnosis as a subcategory of schizophrenia.

In about 1970, lithium carbonate was demonstrated to be a specific, effective treatment for bipolar disorder; it also was shown to be effective in some cases of schizoaffective disorder. At about the same time, the U.S.–U.K. study demonstrated that U.S. psychiatrists tended to overdiagnose schizophrenia in cases of psychotic illness. Therefore, the pendulum has swung back toward Kraepelin, with patients who have some features of mood disorder (whether a manic or depressed mood) but who also have mood-incongruent psychotic features being diagnosed more often with bipolar disorder.

Many clinicians simply diagnose schizoaffective disorder when they aren't sure about the diagnosis. As we have noted, mood symptoms, including depression and irritability or agitation, commonly occur in schizophrenia but tend to be brief relative to the overall course of the patient's illness. *DSM-III* took this position and didn't even include diagnostic criteria for schizoaffective disorder.

DSM-IV has attempted to clarify this situation, as illustrated in Table 8–11. It states that patients should be diagnosed with bipolar disorder unless there have been some periods of psychotic symptoms that occur in the *absence* of prominent mood symptoms. These periods shouldn't be brief in relation to the overall course of illness. (The *DSM* specifies that they should last for at least 2 weeks.) Similarly, the patient should be diagnosed with schizophrenia unless there have been *extended periods* where she has displayed prominent mood symptoms (thereby distinguishing these symptoms from the prodromal or postpsychotic mood symptoms that can commonly occur in schizophrenia).

Table 8–11. *DSM-IV-TR* Criteria for Schizoaffective Disorder

A. An uninterrupted period of illness during which, at some time, there is either a major depressive episode, a manic episode, or a mixed episode concurrent with symptoms that meet criterion A for schizophrenia. (Note: the major depressive episode must include criterion A1: depressed mood)

B. During the same period of illness, there have been delusions or hallucinations for at least 2 weeks in the absence of prominent mood symptoms

C. Symptoms that meet criteria for a mood episode are present for a substantial portion of the total duration of the active and residual periods of the illness

D. The disturbance is not due to the direct physiological effects of a substance (e.g., a drug of abuse, a medication) or a general medical condition

SPECIFY TYPE

Bipolar Type

If the disturbance includes a manic or a mixed episode (or a manic or a mixed episode and major depressive episodes)

Depressive Type

If the disturbance only includes major depressive episodes

Source: Reprinted with permission from the *Diagnostic and Statistical Manual of Mental Disorders, Fourth Edition, Text Revision.* Copyright 2000 American Psychiatric Association.

Schizophrenia researchers have noted that the presence of a prominent "mood component" in schizophrenia confers a somewhat better prognosis; similarly, bipolar disorder researchers have noted that persistent mood-incongruent psychotic features confer a poorer prognosis in bipolar disorder. In clinical practice, patients who fit into one of these two groups (i.e., better prognosis schizophrenia, poorer-prognosis bipolar disorder) tend to be diagnosed with schizoaffective disorder.

Because of these changing criteria, the epidemiology of the disorder remains unclear. While it is probably less common than schizophrenia, it appears to be prevalent in inpatient settings. The age of onset is typically in late adolescence or the early 20s.

Etiology

It remains unclear whether schizoaffective disorder actually is a type of schizophrenia, a type of mood disorder (either bipolar disorder or major depressive disorder), a simultaneous expression of the genes for both conditions due to combined heredity, or a third form of psychosis that is distinct from both mood disorder and schizophrenia. (A final possibility is that Kraepelin was wrong and that there is a *continuum of psychosis*, with schizophrenia on one end, mood disorder on the other, and mixtures of the two conditions in between. However, the majority of the data still supports Kraepelin's scheme.)

As might be expected, family studies also have been difficult to interpret. Schizoaffective probands have fewer relatives with schizophrenia than do probands with schizophrenia, but also fewer relatives with mood disorder than do probands with mood disorder. There appears to be an increased prevalence of schizophrenia among relatives of probands with the depressive type of schizoaffective disorder, but not among relatives of those with the bipolar type. This is consistent with the hypotheses that schizoaffective disorder is either a heterogeneous group or that it results from shared genetic diatheses toward both schizophrenia and depression.

To illustrate the latter hypothesis, let us assume that a small number of patients have a *very high genetic predisposition* toward developing schizophrenia. These individuals go on to develop schizophrenia no matter what occurs in their lives. A much larger number of persons might have *progressively smaller genetic loadings* for the schizophrenia diathesis. These latter individuals might only develop self-limited symptoms during times of extreme stress (leading to a diagnosis of brief psychotic disorder or schizophreniform disorder). The largest group of individuals will have a *very small risk* of developing schizophrenia. They will only demonstrate mild (or subclinical) forms of the illness, such as schizotypal personality disorder.

If an individual with a "mild diathesis" for schizophrenia (the middle group) also carries a diathesis for mood disorder, going through a manic episode or major depressive episode might be enough of a stressor to "push" the patient into a schizophrenic episode as well. The presence of a lighter genetic load toward schizophrenia might help explain why these patients' prognosis tends to be better than patients with "pure" schizophrenia. This model also might explain why larger numbers of patients with schizoaffective disorder are identified clinically than might be predicted by a model that requires that patients to have clear family histories of *both* schizophrenia and of mood disorder if they are to develop schizoaffective disorder.

Treatment

Patients with a bipolar-type presentation usually are treated with lithium or an anticonvulsant agent along with a concomitant antipsychotic agent. When conventional antipsychotic agents are used, one usually attempts to gradually taper their dosage. The advent of the atypical agents has made clinicians more likely to continue with full dosages of the antipsychotic drug, particularly since these agents also appear to possess both antidepressant and antimanic properties. For patients with the depressive-type presentation, a similar strategy is used. Similarly, patients with the depressive-type presentation usually are treated with a combination of an antidepressant and an antipsychotic medication.

DELUSIONAL DISORDER

Phenomenology

Patients with delusional disorder experience circumscribed "nonbizarre" delusions, which are not accompanied by social disability beyond that which is caused by the delusional beliefs themselves. Similarly, patients' moods are normal, beyond what might be expected due to their holding the delusional beliefs. The diagnostic criteria for delusional disorder are listed in Table 8–12.

Delusional disorders are difficult to study since patients rarely present voluntarily for psychiatric treatment. These patients may be encountered only after a violent episode has occurred or after their family or friends have convinced them to come in. In the case of the so-

matic type, they may be referred by their primary care physician. This condition appears to be rare, with a prevalence in the United States of about 0.03%. The age of onset is later than what is seen in bipolar disorder or schizophrenia, with a mean age of onset of about 40 years, although some cases have been described with ages of onset as young as the teenage years and as old as the 90s.

People with *erotomanic-type delusional disorder* hold the delusional belief that another person (usually someone of higher status) is in love with them. Protestations to the contrary are only taken as confirmations. This condition may be more common in women, although men are more prone to violence and therefore they may be more likely to be referred by courts for treatment.

A 23-year-old woman is brought to the emergency room by the police, who had been called to the home of the patient's graduate school professor. The patient described having fallen "passionately" in love with her professor, and she was convinced that he shared her feelings, despite his being married and having made no explicit statements to this effect. The professor ultimately had called the police upon her having sat on the front steps of his home for 12 hours. She had refused to leave despite his coming to the door, yelling at her, even forcibly attempting to move her. When asked during the evaluation whether she took these behaviors on his part as signs that he didn't share her affection, the patient smiles and states, "He only acted that way because his wife was there."

She adds that she could tell from the way he had made eye contact with her while saying these things that in actuality he was trying to convey to her, "I'm just saying these things for show. Don't give up." She displays no signs of formal thought disorder or of significant mood changes. While she ultimately agrees to come in for outpatient psychiatric care, she adamantly refuses to take medication. After two outpatient sessions, she is lost to follow-up. Her harassment of the teacher continues. He obtains a restraining order and she is banned from the college campus. She is arrested for violating the restraining order. Her parents—who live out of state—persuade the judge to suspend her sentence provided that she move back home with them. Following this, she is not heard from further.

People with *grandiose type delusional disorder* typically believe that they have made an important discovery, one that is unappreciated by those

Table 8–12. *DSM-IV-TR* Criteria for Delusional Disorder

A. Nonbizarre delusions (i.e., involving situations that occur in real life, such as being followed, poisoned, infected, loved at a distance, or deceived by spouse or lover, or having a disease) of at least 1 month's duration

B. Criterion A for schizophrenia has never been met. (Note: tactile and olfactory hallucinations may be present in delusional disorder if they are related to the delusional theme)

C. Apart from the impact of the delusion(s) or its ramifications, functioning is not markedly impaired and behavior is not obviously odd or bizarre

D. If mood episodes have occurred concurrently with delusions, their total duration has been brief relative to the duration of the delusional periods.

E. The disturbance is not due to the direct physiological effects of a substance (e.g., a drug of abuse, a medication) or a general medical condition

SPECIFY TYPE (BASED ON THE PREDOMINANT DELUSIONAL THEME)

Erotomanic Type

Delusions that another person, usually of higher status, is in love with the individual

Grandiose Type

Delusions of inflated worth, power, knowledge, identity, or special relationship to a deity or famous person

Jealous Type

Delusions that the individual's sexual partner is unfaithful

Persecutory Type

Delusions that the person (or someone to whom the person is close) is being malevolently treated in some way

Somatic Type

Delusions that the person has some physical defect or general medical condition

Mixed Type

Delusions characteristic of more than one of the above types but no one theme predominates

Unspecified Type

Source: Reprinted with permission from the *Diagnostic and Statistical Manual of Mental Disorders, Fourth Edition, Text Revision.* Copyright 2000 American Psychiatric Association.

around them. They may seek to contact important figures or newspapers to spread the word. There may be a religious content to the delusions, and they may even become charismatic cult leaders.

A 30-year-old graduate student is referred for psychiatric evaluation by the dean, following his having made threats against his department chairman. His professors describe his work as organized and quite voluminous, but as always relating to the same theme. He is argumentative, has no friends in the department, and tends to "blame the department for all of his problems." The patient reports having been a graduate student in two other departments prior to enrolling in his current program. He ultimately left in each case because the faculty had "been threatened by my ideas." He states that his current department is "keeping me down," trying to prevent him from graduating, because they fear becoming obsolete once his own theories at-

tain general acceptance. He ultimately was referred after he sent a long, rambling letter to his department chairman in which he repeatedly addressed him on a first-name basis and concluded with the comment that this man should "watch his back." During the evaluation, the patient laughs when confronted with quotes from his letter, stating that he can't believe how comments like this one could have been "misconstrued." He refuses any treatment with antipsychotic medication but does reluctantly agrees to psychotherapy in the face of pressure from his department. (He repeatedly comments that it is unfair that *he* should be the one being forced to get treatment and not *them*.) He dominates sessions with long commentaries about literature and is offended whenever the psychiatrist attempts to change the subject. He ultimately drops out of treatment after three sessions.

Jealous-type delusional disorder (also called "conjugal paranoia" or "Othello syndrome") appears to be more common in men. It can be difficult to distinguish from nondelusional "pathological jealousy." Often these men are referred to treatment by the court or on civil commitment due to their having engaged in violence toward their partners. They may follow their partners in an attempt to prove presumed infidelity, tape record their partner's telephone conversations, search their partner's belongings for "evidence" of infidelity, and repeatedly threaten their partners. While their symptoms may remit during strictly enforced separation, they often recur in the setting of subsequent relationships.

Persecutory-type delusional disorder is the most common type of delusional disorder. Patients may claim that they are being spied upon, that their phones are being tapped, or that they have been dealt some injustice. In the last case, they may engage in "querulous" behavior such as filing frivolous lawsuits or waging extensive letter-writing campaigns. They can become furious at people who they consider to have treated them unfairly. At times it can be difficult to distinguish this condition from paranoid personality disorder, and the two conditions in fact may be genetically linked. (Consider, for example, the case presented in Chapter 2 of the man with persecutory "overvalued ideas" referred for a child custody evaluation.) Many highly publicized cases of workplace violence likely take place in the setting of persecutory delusional disorder, paranoid personality disorder, and/or schizoid personality disorder. These people may be more prone to violence than are patients with chronic paranoid schizophrenia, since they are not hindered from acting on their delusions by negative symptoms or by cognitive disorganization.

Somatic-type delusional disorder (formerly known as monosymptomatic hypochondriacal psychosis) can take several forms. The most common form is *delusions of infestation*—for example, with bacteria or parasites. These patients may be encountered most often by internists or dermatologists. For example, they might present with flecks of skin that they have collected in a vial as evidence of "larvae" that they have found on their skin. In Chapter 2, an example was presented of an otherwise high-functioning individual who has a delusional belief that he is infected with a severe venereal disease. Another form of somatic-type delusional disorder is *dysmorpho-*

phobia, which is the delusional belief that a person's nose, breasts, or some other body part is misshapen. This can become a source of severe disability. These patients are more likely to present to plastic surgeons than to psychiatrists. Most plastic surgeons attempt to avoid surgery when they recognize the disorder, since these patients are rarely satisfied with the results. They may even believe that they have been even *further* disfigured by the surgery and might threaten lawsuits or violence.

A 35-year-old man is brought to the emergency room by the police after threatening to burn his mother's house down. His mother reports that he has been preoccupied for 10 years with the belief that he has "severe acne." He refuses to leave the house, or even to leave his bedroom most of the time. His mother leaves prepared food for him outside of his bedroom door. He does leave the house late at night to walk the dog, knowing that others can't see his acne in this setting. While his mother always has supported him financially, she notes that she is getting older and "won't be able to do that forever." She repeatedly has encouraged him to look for work, but he has consistently refused to do so. When she decided to have the house repainted, the patient offered to do this. His mother told him that he had no painting experience and that she would prefer to hire a professional. He replied, "Fine, I finally offer to do something for a living, and now you don't want me to. I should just burn the house down." His mother reports that while she knows that he wouldn't actually have started a fire, she felt that this might be her only opportunity to get him a psychiatric evaluation. On examination, the patient has only very mild acne scars, hardly noticeable, and no signs of inflammation. He adamantly refuses any psychiatric intervention but repeatedly asks for a prescription for Accutane. He comments that he has visited multiple dermatologists and plastic surgeons over the years but that they all "have refused to treat me." He refuses offers of outpatient psychiatric follow-up.

A third form of somatic-type delusional disorder is *olfactory reference syndrome*, in which patients are convinced that they are exuding a foul odor. They may be seen by dermatologists or allergists for this complaint. Despite this conviction, the patient may deny having ever noticed the smell himself. Some patients benefit from antipsychotic medication when they can be persuaded to take it, but they may insist that this benefit resulted from anticholinergic side effects—that is, from their sweat glands no longer secreting the foul odor.

It can be difficult to distinguish somatic-type delusional disorder from **body dysmorphic disorder (BDD)**. The latter condition listed in *DSM-IV* under the category of the *somatoform disorders* (discussed in Chapter 13), is characterized by a *preoccupation with an imagined defect in one's appearance*. Sometimes, a slight physical anomaly actually is present, but the person's concern is markedly excessive. Individuals with BDD usually focus on "flaws" involving the face or head such as thinning hair, acne, wrinkles, scars, vascular markings, facial asymmetry or disproportion, facial hair, and the shape or size of various facial features (nose, eyes, eyelids, ears, mouth, etc.). Less commonly, they become obsessed with the size or shape of other bodily regions (genitals, breasts, buttocks, abdomen, extremities, etc.).

In contrast to delusional disorder, the beliefs in BDD are considered to be severely *overvalued ideas*. In other words, patients with BDD do not hold their convictions with "delusional intensity" or "delusional conviction." The distorted body image in BDD resembles the pervasive and excessive concern expressed by patients with anorexia nervosa that they are fat despite their being in a state of emaciation. In fact, some bodybuilders who have BDD become so preoccupied with muscle mass and definition that it becomes the center of their existence. They work out for hours even in the face of severe physical injuries and abuse protein and steroid supplements. (This condition has been colloquially called "bulkorexia.")

In practice, though, distinguishing between excessive, distorted, overvalued ideas and delusions sometimes is quite difficult. Over the course of time, patients may cling to their beliefs with varying *degrees of tenacity* and with varying *degrees of insight* such that these two conditions might actually exist along a dimensional continuum of severity. When the presentation seems to alternate between these two conditions over time, both diagnoses are assigned.

One-third of individuals with BDD become housebound due to phobic concerns about the possibility that they might be ridiculed in public

about their bodily appearance. Up to one-fifth of individuals with BDD attempt suicide. Not surprisingly, comorbid mood disorders and anxiety disorders are common.

While antipsychotic agents are effective in treating some cases, in other cases they actually might exacerbate patients' symptoms. To date, the most effective agents have been the SSRIs, even in cases where beliefs are held with delusional intensity. This pharmacologic selectivity has led some researchers to suggest that BDD, and even delusional disorder of the somatic type, may be part of an *obsessive–compulsive disorder spectrum of disorders*. In other words, these patients' somatic preoccupations may be closer to severe *obsessions* than to delusions, although—in contrast with obsessive–compulsive disorder—most patients with BDD do not retain insight into the *irrationality* of their fears.

Treatment

In all of these cases, the first goal of treatment is to persuade the patient to participate in treatment. Patients can become resentful if their delusional convictions are challenged; however, one doesn't want to *reinforce* their delusions by endorsing their veracity. In general, clinicians try to walk a fine line, agreeing with the patient that he appears to be very upset about his current situation, offering to help try to ease the suffering associated with these experiences, but avoiding implicitly or explicitly endorsing the patient's delusions. Patients with delusional disorder often are distrustful, and one goal is to be consistent and fair, such that the patient agrees to cooperate with treatment based on the strength of the therapeutic alliance even when he "doesn't see any point" to the treatment.

Antipsychotic medications may be less effective in the treatment of delusional disorder than they are in other psychotic disorders. When the medication is effective, patients often continue to lack insight into ever having had a psychotic illness. They may simply feel that things have "worked themselves out" coincidentally with their having entered into treatment.

It is important to assess the potential for violence in all of these cases. Further, one should assess for the presence of comorbid psychiatric conditions such as mood disorders, anxiety disorders, and substance-related disorders. On the one hand, these conditions can complicate delusional disorder, but on the other hand, they also might be more responsive to psychiatric intervention than the delusional disorder itself. Since many of these patients refuse psychiatric evaluation or follow-up, psychiatrists sometimes find themselves treating these patients "by proxy," by offering advice to primary care physicians and family members.

SHARED PSYCHOTIC DISORDER

Shared psychotic disorder—also known as shared paranoid disorder, induced psychotic disorder, *folie a deux*, or double insanity—is likely a rare condition. The literature consists of sporadic case reports. Here, a delusion is "passed on" from a person with a longstanding delusion to another person in the context of a close relationship. The latter person tends to not be psychotic so much as impressionable, willing to accept the delusional belief of the more dominant partner. The most common relationships are sister–sister, husband–wife, and mother–child, but other combinations have been described. Almost all cases involve members of a single family. The couple or family typically live in relative isolation. Treatment usually involves treating the "primary" case as well as separating the affected partners. With enforced separation, delusional beliefs often resolve spontaneously in the "secondary" case.

SUMMARY

Schizophrenia is a chronic, disabling psychotic illness. It affects about 1% of the population but strikes in adolescence and young adulthood (ages 15–30) and accounts for a very high percentage of worldwide functional and occupational disability.

In most cases, the diagnosis is readily apparent to clinicians. Despite this, the development of reliable and valid diagnostic criteria has been hindered by the diversity of clinical symptoms associated with schizophrenia. Whether it constitutes a single disease process with varying presentations or a constellation of disease processes with similar "downstream" symptoms remains unknown. Core symptom domains include positive symptoms, negative symptoms, and cognitive disorganization.

Mood symptoms also commonly occur in schizophrenia, particularly depression. These can occur as a prodrome to relapse, during the active phase of illness, or in the post-psychotic convalescent period. In some cases, a patient's overall course of illness overlaps with that seen in major depressive disorder or bipolar disorder. In schizoaffective disorder, symptoms meeting the criteria for a mood episode are present for a substantial portion of the total duration of the patient's illness, but during other periods the patient demonstrates schizophrenic symptoms in the absence of mood symptoms.

In delusional disorder, patients present with circumscribed, nonbizarre delusions in the absence of negative symptoms or cognitive disorganization. Apart from the impact of the delusions or their ramifications, functioning is not markedly impaired and the patient's behavior is not obviously odd or bizarre. Delusional disorder, along with "odd" personality types listed under Axis II in the *DSM-IV* scheme (schizoid personality disorder, schizotypal personality disorder, paranoid personality disorder), appear to be genetically related to schizophrenia and may reflect a spectrum of severity of the clinical phenotype.

High-resolution structural neuroimaging and neuropathological studies reveal schizophrenia to be associated with decreased sizes of the cortical limbic structures (including the amygdala, the hippocampus, and the parahippocampal gyrus), the prefrontal cortex, the thalamus, and the cerebellum. In prefrontal cortex, there is a reduction in axonal and dendritic arborization and in synaptic connections. All of these areas likely function along a circuit that coordinates perceptions, thoughts, and behavior and filters out background noise.

Failures in this circuit probably contribute to impairments in one's ability to distinguish internal from external reality (leading to hallucinations and delusions), to coordinate one's stream of thought (leading to cognitive disorganization and thought disorder), and to symptoms of apathy and impaired social relatedness (negative symptoms). Patients predisposed to develop schizophrenia likely begin life with a lesser degree of synaptic density due to a combination of genetic vulnerability and perinatal insult. Normal (or perhaps excessive) synaptic pruning during childhood and adolescence may contribute to the development of negative symptoms and ultimately of positive symptoms.

Negative symptoms and disorganization in schizophrenia may reflect hypofunction in the prefrontal cortex and associated regions, including the cerebellum. Functional neuroimaging reveals decreased frontal metabolic activity that becomes especially apparent in comparison to control subjects when patients and controls both perform cognitive tasks that tax this region. Dopamine activity is decreased along the mesocortical tract, which innervates this region. In contrast, positive symptoms likely reflect limbic system hyperactivity. The mesocortical and mesolimbic tracts are linked by pathways mediated by glutamate. These pathways run from the frontal area to the limbic region via the thalamus, thereby providing "negative feedback" that possibly acts as a "filter" and protects the cortex from excessive stimulation. This region also is innervated by dopamine fibers, and the loss of negative feedback to both these limbic structures and to the dopaminergic neurons themselves in the brain-stem ventral tegmental area may contribute to increased limbic activity and the appearance of positive symptoms. Dysfunction of the N-methyl-D-aspartate (NMDA)-sensitive glutamate receptor also may play a role in mediating psychosis, particularly since glutamate plays a key role in synaptic pruning, in the modulation of synaptic architecture in response to life experience, and in excitotoxicity.

Conventional antipsychotics are dopamine antagonists. They are effective in the treatment of psychotic symptoms and agitation, and to a lesser extent in treating negative symptoms. Dopamine blockade also accounts for their most significant side effects, particularly extrapyramidal symptoms such as parkinsonism, akathisia, tardive dyskinesia, and neuroleptic malignant syndrome. Atypical antipsychotics exert weaker dopamine antagonist effects, more rapidly dissociate from the dopamine receptor, and have serotonin antagonist properties. All of these factors may contribute to their markedly reduced tendency to cause extrapyramidal symptoms. They also may act through direct and indirect effects at the level of the NMDA glutamate receptor.

Treatment of schizophrenia requires more than the prescription of antipsychotic medication. Steps also should be taken to help the patient adapt to life in the community, to enhance the patient's compliance with treatment, to facilitate continued reductions in symptoms, and to help maximize the patient's quality of life in general. Psychotherapy, case management, and vocational rehabilitation efforts attempt to help the patient reach such goals while simultaneously offering psychological and social support. The latter is particularly important since undue stress also could trigger a relapse.

Chapter 9

Anxiety Disorders

We all have experienced anxiety, just as we all have experienced sadness. Particular life situations are especially likely to lead to anxiety, and some people are more prone to become anxious than others. Given this, the anxiety disorders—like the mood disorders—are easier to describe than to explain. Consider the following example:

A 40-year-old woman is referred for evaluation of anxiety. She describes herself as having been a "worrier" for most of her life, although the anxiety became much worse at age 17 following the death of her mother. At that time, she was seen in weekly psychotherapy for a year. She feels that the therapy helped her to cope, but she continued to worry about matters that she recognized were minor. She has tended to view her problems as being due to "not knowing where I am going in my life" and to difficulties in her interpersonal relationships. She describes herself as prone to self-doubt and rumination. She is perfectionistic, "expects the worst" even when she is putting forth her best efforts, and often worries about "what other people must think of me."

Her anxiety has always become more intense when starting at a new job. At these times, she has difficulty concentrating and finds herself constantly wondering if she is "passing the grade." Over the past two decades, she intermittently has received further psychotherapy, and ultimately has seen five therapists for weekly psychotherapy, with each course of therapy lasting for 1–2 years. She has never taken psychotropic medication and expresses fear about the potential for medication side effects, given that she has experienced side effects with almost every medication she has ever taken, including antibiotics and over-the-counter decongestants.

She has been at her current job for the past 3 years but her anxiety hasn't abated. Every day, she feels tense and restless, fatigues easily, and feels "exhausted" by the end of the day. She is irritable, with a "short fuse." It generally takes her 2 hours to fall asleep at night, and she therefore tends to stay awake "until I finally just drop." She also describes frequent nights when her sleep is fitful and when she wakes up the next morning "feeling as tired as when I went to bed." She experiences diffuse muscle aches, especially in her neck and shoulders, with occasional myoclonic jerks. Her dentist commented recently that she shows evidence of teeth grinding and prescribed a dental guard for her to wear at night.

During periods of increased anxiety, her vision feels "blurry," and she experiences hot and cold flashes, dry mouth, sweaty palms, and the urge to urinate more frequently (as often as once per hour). A urinalysis has shown no evidence of a urinary tract infection, and sexual and thyroid hormone studies also are normal. She has tachycardia and palpitations several times per week, especially when lying awake at night trying to fall asleep. Sometimes this is be accompanied by a "choking" sensation. However, she denies discrete panic attacks and denies having developed phobic fears.

She endorses chronic feelings of sadness, social isolation, and mild anhedonia, but she denies other vegetative symptoms of depression.

Her medical history is notable for past diagnoses of chronic fatigue syndrome, irritable bowel syndrome, and "noncardiac chest pain" by various physicians.

Her family history is notable for her father and brother both drinking alcohol heavily. Her mother "was an anxious person, just like me" as well as "a hypochondriac," who often consulted physicians with medical complaints for which no biologic cause was determined.

During inquiry into her social history, the patient recalls having had a history of "school phobia." When she first began kindergarten, she refused to get on the school bus. This behavior continued for a few weeks, but she ultimately was able to attend school without difficulty. She majored in accounting in college and graduate school and currently works as a CPA. She has been in three long-term relationships, each lasting from 4 to 5 years. None of these progressed to marriage, and following each breakup she has felt "alone in the world." She currently lives alone. She denies any history of alcohol or drug use, as she prefers to "remain in control." However, she does report drinking about eight cups of coffee over the course of a day.

On mental status examination, the patient appears moderately anxious and tense, and she fidgets throughout the interview. She speaks a great deal. There is a pressured quality to her speech, but no evidence of flight of ideas. She frequently asks the psychiatrist what he "thinks about her condition," and when asked for details about her life history she offers frequent interpretations, making for a lengthy interview. She describes her current mood as being "kind of low, kind of anxious, my usual self." She denies having ever experienced hallucinations, delusions, obsessions, compulsions, or phobias. Her Mini-Mental State Examination score is 30 out of a possible 30, suggesting grossly intact cognitive function.

Does this woman have a "mental illness"? If so, it is a common one. Many Americans experience similar anxiety, and benzodiazepines and alcohol are among the most commonly used (and abused) drugs in the country. Perhaps her symptoms aren't symptoms of a "disease" but manifestations of underlying psychological issues that need to be empathically understood. This always has been the patient's impression; it also has been the impression of her five psychotherapists.

However, while psychotherapy has helped her learn to live with chronic anxiety, the symptoms have persisted.

We can describe aspects of this patient' clinical presentation from each of the four perspectives, with each perspective provides different insights. From the *life-story perspective*, we might wonder about what the patient's life was like growing up, especially given her father's history of alcoholism. We might take note of how her symptoms first became severe enough to require clinical intervention following the death of her mother, about her inability to form sustained interpersonal relationships, and about her powerful feelings of failure and abandonment following breakups.

The *dimensional perspective* helps us to appreciate how the patient has features consistent with several possible "cluster C" personality disorders, including obsessive–compulsive personality disorder and dependent personality disorder (see Chapter 10). Her anxiety appears to be brought on by certain typical experiences, such as starting a new job. She even shows evidence of having experienced a similar state of apprehensive expectation when faced with her first "job," kindergarten.

From the *behavior perspective*, we might wonder to what extent the patient's anxiety has been "conditioned" from early childhood on, perhaps "modeled" on her mother's anxious–somatic behavioral style. Further life experiences may have reinforced the patient's behavioral style. For example, she may have made a mistake at work and been criticized for this, leading to significant autonomic arousal and subjective feelings of anxiety. Subsequently, whenever she fears that she is failing at something, she may experience this same autonomic response. More introverted, obsessional people appear to be particularly vulnerable to such behavioral conditioning.

From the *disease perspective*, we might suspect that this patient has an underlying mood disorder, especially dysthymic disorder, given her low-grade but chronic feelings of sadness, anhedonia, low energy, poor concentration, and low self-esteem. However, her anxiety appears to be her most prominent symptom, and this appears more severe than what is seen in an isolated dysthymic disorder. She fulfills the *DSM-IV* diagnostic criteria for having a generalized anxiety disorder. However, one would only make this diagnosis after having excluded the possibility of her having an anxiety disorder due to a general medical condition or a substance-induced anxiety disorder. For example, one medical condition associated with anxiety is hyperthyroidism, although in this case thyroid studies were normal. An example of a substance that might be contributing to her anxiety is caffeine. Excessive coffee intake or intermittent caffeine withdrawal might contribute to her headaches, gastrointestinal symptoms, and her symptoms of autonomic hyperarousal. Table 9–1 lists some other medical conditions and substances sometimes associated with anxiety.

In this chapter, we will first discuss "normal" anxiety and the neurobiological pathways and neurotransmitter systems associated with anxiety. We will then discuss the *DSM-IV* anxiety dis-orders: generalized anxiety disorder, panic disorder, phobic disorder, obsessive–compulsive disorder, and post-traumatic stress disorder (PTSD). All of these disorders include prominent anxiety as one feature, but beyond this their presentations vary quite a bit, likely reflecting different underlying pathologies and etiologies.

NORMAL ANXIETY

While the patient in the above example might have a psychiatric disease, she might simply be demonstrating variation along a physiologic dimension. This latter view was the common conception of anxiety in medical writings until the mid-1800s. Simply stated, some people are inherently more anxious than the average person, and others are less anxious than the average person.

Why do people become anxious if this is such an unpleasant emotion? Anxiety serves important functions. It alerts a person to impending danger while also helping her to mobilize resources for either "fight or flight." A *little* anxiety can be a good thing. For example, if a person had *no* anxiety the night before an exam, she might simply watch television instead of studying. However, when the level of anxiety is *too* high, it can impair performance—for example, by interfering with attention and memory. Thus, a graph of performance in response to increasing anxiety demonstrates an inverted U-shaped curve, with initial improvement in performance

Table 9–1. Some Medical and Substance Use Disorders Potentially Associated with Anxiety

NEUROLOGICAL DISORDERS

Brain tumor
Brain trauma
Cerebrovascular disease
Subarachnoid hemorrhage
Migraine
Encephalitis
Neurosyphilis
Multiple sclerosis
Wilson's disease
Parkinson's disease
Huntington's disease
Epilepsy

SYSTEMIC DISEASES

Pituitary disease
Thyroid disease
Parathyroid disease
Adrenal disease
Pheochromocytoma
Hypoglycemia
Paraneoplastic syndrome
Premenstrual hormonal changes
Porphyria
Uremia
Systemic lupus erythematosus

CARDIOPULMONARY DISEASE

Cardiac ischemia
Cardiac arrhythmia
Hypoxia
Reactive airway disease
Anemia

SUBSTANCE USE

Alcohol and drug withdrawal
Amphetamine intoxication
Sympathomimetic agents and vasopressors (including decongestants and asthma medications)
Caffeine and caffeine withdrawal
Antibiotics

accompanying mild anxiety, followed by maximum benefit, followed by a steep decline in performance as anxiety levels becomes more severe.

During normal anxiety occurring in response to a discrete stressor, a person experiences increases in blood pressure, heart rate and respiratory rate, as well as in skin conductance, muscle tension, and the plasma levels of epinephrine, norepinephrine, growth hormone, cortisol, and prolactin. While the subjective sensation of anxiety is in part related to the perception of this state of physiologic arousal, the sensation of anxiety is further mediated at the synaptic level by at least three different neurotransmitters: gamma-aminobutyric acid (GABA), norepinephrine, and serotonin.

In Chapter 4, we discussed the "fear circuit" illustrated in Figure 4–2, which centers on the amygdala. This circuit is just one component of a complex network of interrelated neural systems. Different systems within this network modulate memory, anxiety, pleasure, mood, executive function, and attention. These systems are dynamic in that they respond to threats and rewards in the surrounding environment through both acute responses and more chronic adaptations in brain neurophysiology.

Systems regulating emotions such as anxiety, pleasure, and sadness by necessity are linked to other systems that regulate memory, planning, and judgment. In some cases, the same response governs both. For example, the "emotional memory" of dangerous or stressful situations may be stored in the amygdala, and the "emotional memory" of pleasurable experiences may reside in the nucleus accumbens and related structures. In contrast, declarative memories likely are stored more diffusely in cerebral cortex, despite the subjective sense of emotional and declarative memories being seamlessly integrated.

A "stress thermostat" modulates all of these neurobiological systems. It encompasses a variety of chemical mediators, including glucocorticoids, neurotrophic factors, monoamine systems (norepinephrine, serotonin, and dopamine), and excitatory and inhibitory neurotransmitters (such as glutamate and GABA). The brain's responses to potentially harmful or pleasurable circumstances, while adaptive under most circumstances, can become maladaptive and a source of pathology under other circumstances.

The latter is particularly likely to be the case when individuals either are: *(1)* faced with *more extreme circumstances* (excessive chronic stress, acute trauma, bereavement), *(2)* affected by a *medical illness or neurological condition* that affects bodily levels of glucocorticoids, monoamines and other neurotransmitters or that causes direct injury to relevant brain regions, *(3)* ingesting *substances* (such as drugs of abuse) that directly stimulate brain reward centers, thereby bypassing this indirect linkage between environment and brain physiology, or *(4)* rendered more vulnerable to developing impaired affective or cognitive regulation due to *genetic factors* (the stress-diathesis model).

BENZODIAZEPINES

Given these interrelationships, it is not surprising that the patient in the above example appears to have several overlapping conditions. Her lifelong temperament has been characterized by a tendency toward lower-grade anxiety and sadness, and she more acutely experiences excessive anxiety and depression that place her at greater risk of developing phobic behaviors (such as her childhood "school phobia"). Depressive and anxiety disorders, while distinct in some ways, are probably related at the genetic level, and they share many features, as illustrated in Table 4–3.

Monoaminergic medications such as the antidepressants and antipsychotics work by modulating the activity of serotonin, norepinephrine, and dopamine. They act on all of the above neural networks and are efficacious in the treatment of both depression and anxiety. The onset of their clinical effects is delayed, however, suggesting that they act only indirectly by prodding the brain to respond to altered monoamine homeostasis through changes in the activity of second messenger systems.

Another class of medications, the **benzodiazepines**, works quite differently. Benzodiazepines modulate the activity of GABA. As discussed in Chapter 4, benzodiazepines are positive allosteric modulators of the GABA channel—that is, they amplify the effects of GABA. This mechanism of action allows for a rapid onset of clinical effect—that is, after the first dose.

Benzodiazepines attenuate the cognitive and somatic symptoms of anxiety that occur in the anxiety, depressive, and psychotic disorders as well in "normal" anxiety. While they are not effective in directly treating mood or psychotic symptoms, their general anxiolytic properties make them useful as *adjuncts* in the treatment of major depressive episodes, manic episodes, and schizophrenia exacerbations. Since all benzodiazepines act through the same mechanism, they all have anticonvulsant, muscle relaxant, sedative–hypnotic, and amnestic effects in addition to anxiolytic effects.

Benzodiazepines have been the anxiolytics and hypnotics of choice since they first were released in 1960, given their greater margin of safety and lower risk of addictive potential than the barbiturate drugs that preceded them. They have little effect on either respiratory drive or cardiac activity; given this, even in large overdoses the risk of death is low unless unless the patient has taken them in conjunction with another depressant agent (especially alcohol).

The various benzodiazepines and their pharmacokinetic properties are listed in Table 9–2. The various agents are distinguished from each other by their *potency, rapidity of onset of effect, and half-life*. While this makes some of them more useful than others for particular indications, categorizations based on clinical indications are related as much to marketing as to biochemistry.

All of the benzodiazepines are reliably absorbed orally. Only **lorazepam (Ativan)** and **midazolam (Versed)** are reliably absorbed intramuscularly. *Lorazepam* is useful as a parenteral agent (administered either intramuscularly or intravenously) in cases of acutely psychotic agitation, given its rapid and reliable absorption. It can be administered either alone or in combination with an antipsychotic agent. Advantages of the latter strategy include synergistic sedative effects and the fact that lorazepam helps to combat extrapyramidal symptoms such as akathisia that the antipsychotic drug might cause. *Midazolam* has a very short half-life, leading to greater amnestic effects and also allowing patients to be able to recover more rapidly from sedation. These two properties account for its popularity as a sedative during short surgical procedures.

Table 9–2 only shows in vitro comparisons of binding potency at the BZ receptor. Other factors may be important in vivo, including how *lipophilic the agent is* (and therefore how readily it crosses the blood–brain barrier) or *other receptor binding characteristics*. For example, **alprazolam (Xanax)** rapidly binds to the BZ receptor but also dissociates from the receptor sooner than many agents. Despite it having a long serum half-life, as listed in Table 9–2, patients often report that they can feel alprazolam "wear off" after only several hours. They also may experience withdrawal symptoms between doses, necessitating frequent dosing (three to four doses per day).

Patients taking a benzodiazepine for relief in the midst of an acute anxiety attack or patients using a benzodiazepine at bedtime as a hypnotic require an agent with a rapid onset of effect. Fur-

Table 9–2. Most Common Benzodiazepines, Listed in Order of Their Relative In Vitro Potency

Benzodiazepine	Dose Equivalent (mg)	Onset of Effect	Active Metabolites	$T_{1/2}$ of Metabolites (Hours)
Triazolam (Halcion)	0.1	Rapid	None	2
Clonazepam (Klonopin)	0.25	Medium	None	34
Alprazolam (Xanax)	0.5	Rapid	α-hydroxyalprazolam, 4-hydroxyalprazolam	12
Lorazepam (Ativan)	1	Medium	None	15
Diazepam (Valium)	5	Rapid	Desmethyldiazepam, oxazepam	100
Quazepam (Doral)	7.5	Rapid	2-oxoquazepam, N-desalkyl-2-oxoquazepam, 3-hydroxy-2-oxoquazepam, glucoronide	100
Clorazepate (Tranxene)	7.5	Rapid	Desmethyldiazepam, oxazepam	100
Temazepam (Restoril)	10	Medium	None	11
Oxazepam (Serax)	15	Slow	None	8
Flurazepam (Dalmane)	15	Rapid	Desalkylflurazepam, N-I-hydroxyethylflurazepam	100
Chlordiazepoxide (Librium)	25	Medium	Desmethylchlordiazepoxide, demoxopam, desmethyldiazepam, oxazepam	100

ther, a medication taken at bedtime as a hypnotic also should last long enough to help the patient sleep until morning. However, it should not cause either "rebound" anxiety or amnesia (both of which are more common with shorter-acting agents) or residual daytime sedation (which occurs more commonly with longer-acting agents). Finally, patients using a benzodiazepine during the daytime as an anxiolytic prefer one with a sustained duration of action and with minimal sedative or amnestic effects.

Flurazepam, temazepam, quazepam, and **triazolam** are marketed as hypnotics, and not surprisingly they all have a relatively rapid *onset* of effect. They differ in whether they have active metabolites and therefore in their overall *duration* of effect. Flurazepam has a long half-life, and patients taking this drug are more likely to experience daytime sedation or mild cognitive impairment the next day; it also can accumulate over a period of several days.

In contrast, triazolam has the shortest half-life. While it is less likely to cause residual daytime sedation, its shorter half-life makes it more useful for patients with initial insomnia than for those with middle or terminal insomnia. Also, because of its short half-life, it is more likely to cause amnesia and behavioral changes (confusion, agitation, or hallucinations), particularly at higher dosages. (The manufacturer of triazolam now recommends against taking it at either higher-than-recommended doses or for greater than 10 days.) Amnesia also may be more of a problem in situations where triazolam is taken to induce sleep while traveling, such as during an airplane flight, as the person may awake before the clinical effects of the drug have subsided ("traveler's amnesia").

The most common side effect of benzodiazepines is *excessive sedation,* which occurs in about 10% of patients. Patients should be advised to exercise caution when driving, especially when the medication is first started or when the dosage is being increased. Fewer than 2% of patients experience *dizziness or ataxia. Mild cognitive impairment* can occur, and these drugs therefore should be used with caution in the elderly. A greater rate of *falls leading to hip fractures* has been described in elderly patients taking benzodiazepines when compared to elderly patients not taking benzodiazepines, even when

these patients don't subjectively experience impaired coordination. Physicians also should use caution in prescribing agents with active metabolites and/or cumulative effects to elderly patients or to patients with hepatic disease. All benzodiazepines suppress REM sleep and also stages 3 and 4 sleep. As noted in Chapter 4, the novel agents **zolpidem (Ambien)** and **zaleplon (Sonata)** do not.

In cases where the patient is taking concomitant medications that inhibit *cytochrome P450 microenzymes,* particularly enzyme 3A4 (e.g., nefazodone, cimetidine, ketoconazole, and erythromycin), one should be particularly cautious about prescribing alprazolam or triazolam, since their serum levels may be increased. However, since all benzodiazepines are metabolized by the liver, one should be cautious in general when prescribing them for *elderly patients* (who have decreased hepatic function), or for patients with *liver disease* (including alcoholic patients who present for detoxification with benzodiazepines but who may have cirrhosis). In such cases, it is prudent to use agents that lack active metabolites, such as lorazepam, oxazepam, or temazepam.

Because they can potentially cause physical or psychological dependence, benzodiazepines are listed under schedule IV of the U.S. Controlled Substances Act. With longer-term usage (e.g., after several weeks), some patients develop *tolerance* to these agents. In other words, they require greater doses over time to maintain the same effect; they may also have difficulty discontinuing the medication without experiencing *withdrawal symptoms.*

Risk factors for a patient developing benzodiazepine dependence include having a *personal or family history of alcohol dependence,* taking a *higher-potency agent,* taking the drug for an *extended period of time* (months to years), and taking an agent with a *more rapid onset of CNS effects* (relating both to the drug's rapidity of gastrointestinal absorption and its lipid solubility). In addition, agents with *shorter half-lives* (necessitating more frequent dosing to prevent interdose withdrawal) may be more behaviorally reinforcing.

Thus, diazepam (Valium), despite its long half-life, is prone to cause dependence due to its rapid onset of clinical effects. The patient is more likely to feel the drug "kick in" with diazepam, thus making it more behaviorally reinforcing. Alprazolam (Xanax), a high-potency agent with a rapid onset of effect and a short duration of effect, appears to be particularly reinforcing. Alprazolam also can be difficult to taper as it can be associated with a greater degree of withdrawal symptoms. (Sometimes an alprazolam taper can be facilitated by switching the patient over to clonazepam, since the latter agent has a slower onset of effect and a longer half-life; however, some patients demand to switch back to alprazolam since it feels like it "works better" than clonazepam, likely due to its more rapid onset.) In patients with a history of long-term benzodiazepine use, it is essential to taper benzodiazepines slowly, perhaps even over a period of weeks to months. The most difficult part of the taper occurs toward the end of it, and at this point the taper should be slowed even further. For example, a patient taking 40 mg per day of diazepam may have little difficulty cutting the dosage to 20 mg per day but may have extreme difficulty cutting the dosage from 15 mg per day to 10 mg per day.

Despite these caveats, the rate of benzodiazepine abuse by patients chronically prescribed them for legitimate purposes is very low. On their own initiative, many patients cut down on their standing dosage or switch to "as needed" dosing as their anxiety improves. A 1990 survey showed that 8% of the adult U.S. population had used an anxiolytic medication during the previous year and that 2.5% had used a hypnotic medication. In terms of benzodiazepine anxiolytics, over 50% of patients who took them did so for under a month and 25% took them for longer than 12 months. In terms of hypnotics, 70% took them for under a month and 14% used them for longer than 12 months. Other surveys have found only 1.5% and 2.5% of the population to have used benzodiazepines for nonmedical indications.

It's true that substance abusers who use other drugs also have a high rate of benzodiazepine abuse. For example, up to half of methadone clinic patients have urine drug screens that are positive for benzodiazepines. However, these individuals usually report that they are using the benzodiazepine to self-medicate for other types of drug withdrawal rather than to "get high" from the benzodiazepine itself. Heroin abusers use benzodiazepines to treat the insomnia and anxiety associated with opioid withdrawal, while cocaine abusers use them to treat either the anxiety associated with acute cocaine intoxication or the dysphoria associated with a cocaine withdrawal (a "crash").

However, benzodiazepines can augment the euphoric effects of alcohol. In addition, moderate-to-heavy drinkers experience a greater euphoric response to a single dose of alprazolam than do control subjects. Finally, alcoholic subjects report experiencing increased cravings for alcohol after they are administered benzodiazepines. Given this, while some alcoholic patients who also take benzodiazepines may be "self-medicating" to prevent alcohol withdrawal or to treat an underlying anxiety disorder, others may be abusing the drug and in doing so are reinforcing their alcohol dependence. Benzodiazepines should therefore be prescribed with caution in this population.

This is not to say that one should *never* prescribe benzodiazepines to patients with histories of substance abuse. One first should consider the use of alternative anxiolytic medications, including SSRIs, other antidepressants (venlafaxine, nefazodone, or mirtazapine), buspirone, and anticonvulsants (such as valproate or gabapentin). However, some patients with underlying anxiety disorders are unable to tolerate or fail to respond to alternative medications. If they are appropriately compliant with close monitoring, they may be better able to maintain sobriety from alcohol or other drugs once their anxiety disorder is under better control, and this ultimately may necessitate the use of a benzodiazepine. The search continues for BZ-receptor *partial agonists* that might retain the anxiolytic benefits of the benzodiazepines without carrying as high a risk of physical or psychological dependence.

While dependence does not occur in most patients prescribed benzodiazepines, in most cases one still should not prescribe benzodiazepines indefinitely. Periodic attempts should be made to taper the dosage, using psychotherapy when feasible to help the patient develop better ways of coping with anxiety. As the dosage is being tapered, it is not uncommon for patients' anxiety symptoms to increase. In such cases, it may be difficult to determine whether this reflects benzodiazepine withdrawal or a recurrence of the original anxiety disorder. In the former case, the symptoms usually subside gradually; in the latter case, they typically persist and necessitate upward titration of the benzodiazepine dosage.

As safer antidepressant medications with fewer side effects have become available, these have been gradually replacing the benzodiazepines as the medications of first choice for most of the anxiety disorders, including generalized anxiety disorder, panic disorder, posttraumatic stress disorder, and social phobia. They appear to have specific efficacy in obsessive–compulsive disorder that other agents, including the benzodiazepines, lack. An additional advantage of relying primarily on antidepressant medications rather than benzodiazepines to treat anxiety disorders is that the former also are efficacious in treating commonly occurring comorbid conditions, particularly major depressive disorder. Also, while benzodiazepines are useful in the acute treatment of generalized anxiety disorder and panic disorder, they are less useful than antidepressants in treating other anxiety disorders such as post-traumatic stress disorder, obsessive–compulsive disorder, and social phobia.

Therefore, the use of antidepressants as the "first-line" strategy in most cases, reserving benzodiazepines for shorter-term or adjunctive use in most cases, is appropriate. Since antidepressants can require several weeks to take effect, benzodiazepines often are used in the interim (e.g., for about 4 weeks) and are then tapered over the next few weeks. Longer-term administration of benzodiazepines still should be considered for patients who do not fully respond to or cannot tolerate antidepressants.

GENERALIZED ANXIETY DISORDER

Phenomenology and Epidemiology

Prior to *DSM-III*, there were no specific anxiety disorders—only "anxiety neurosis," which included personality disorders characterized by prominent anxiety (such as what are now called obsessive–compulsive, avoidant, and dependent personality disorders) as well as generalized anxiety disorder and panic disorder. (obsessive–compulsive disorder was treated as a rare, separate condition.)

DSM-III, introduced in 1980, distinguished between these conditions. It also recognized that some individuals are extremely anxious but do not experience panic attacks and do not appear to have simply a major depressive disorder with prominent anxiety. These patients were considered to have **generalized anxiety disorder (GAD)**. The *content*, or *focus*, of the anxiety was not specified since many patients merely described "free-floating" anxiety—that is, a vague sense of nervousness, unease, or apprehension. Other patients describe worry about a variety of minor matters that is difficult to control. The *DSM-III* also emphasized the presence of associated *physical symptoms*, including *motor symptoms* (e.g., shakiness, restlessness, sore muscles, headache), *autonomic symptoms* (e.g., shortness of breath, sweats, shakes, palpitations, gastrointestinal symptoms), and *vigilance (cognitive) symptoms* (e.g., irritability, fatigue, difficulty sleeping, difficulty concentrating). GAD remained a diagnosis of exclusion, though, since anxious patients who demonstrated more *specific* symptoms attributable to another mood or anxiety disorder (e.g., major depressive disorder, panic disorder, obsessive–compulsive disorder) would be diagnosed with the latter rather than with GAD.

The conceptualization of GAD has evolved through *DSM-IIIR* and into *DSM-IV*. *DSM-III-R* increased the duration criterion from 1 month of symptoms to 6 months in an attempt to increase reliability, and it placed greater emphasis on a specific type of anxiety—that is, unrealistic or excessive *worry* about particular life circumstances, such as work-related matters, finances, or the health of oneself or of family members. It also added a list of 18 somatic symptoms, of which patients had to exhibit at least six to qualify for the diagnosis. *DSM-IV* maintained this emphasis on worry (rather than vague apprehension or free-floating anxiety) and narrowed the list of associated physical symptoms from 18 to six (restlessness, fatigue, concentration difficulties, irritability, muscle tension, and sleep disturbance), from which patients only had to exhibit at least three. Again, the diagnosis would not be made if the anxiety occurs exclusively in the setting of another anxiety or mood disorder. The current diagnostic criteria are listed in Table 9–3.

Table 9–3. *DSM-IV-TR* Criteria for Generalized Anxiety Disorder

---

A. Excessive anxiety and worry (apprehensive expectation), occurring more days than not for at least 6 months, about a number of events or activities (such as work or school performance)
B. The person finds it difficult to control the worry
C. The anxiety and worry are associated with three (or more) of the following six symptoms (with at least some symptoms present for more days than not for the past 6 months). Note: Only one item is required in children
   1. Restlessness or feeling keyed up or on edge
   2. Being easily fatigued
   3. Difficulty concentrating or mind going blank
   4. Irritability
   5. Muscle tension
   6. Sleep disturbance (difficulty falling or staying asleep, or restless unsatisfying sleep)
D. The focus of the anxiety and worry is not confined to features of an Axis I disorder, e.g., the anxiety or worry is not about having a panic attack (as in panic disorder), being embarrassed in public (as in social phobia), being contaminated (as in obsessive–compulsive disorder), being away from home or close relatives (as in separation anxiety disorder), gaining weight (as in anorexia nervosa), having multiple physical complaints (as in somatization disorder), or having a serious illness (as in hypochondriasis), and the anxiety and worry do not occur exclusively during post-traumatic stress disorder
E. The anxiety, worry, or physical symptoms cause clinically significant distress or impairment in social, occupational, or other important areas of functioning
F. The disturbance is not due to the direct physiological effects of a substance (e.g., a drug of abuse, a medication) or a general medical condition (e.g., hyperthyroidism) and does not occur exclusively during a mood disorder, a psychotic disorder, or a pervasive developmental disorder

---

Source: Reprinted with permission from the *Diagnostic and Statistical Manual of Mental Disorders, Fourth Edition, Text Revision.* Copyright 2000 American Psychiatric Association.

It isn't clear that the *DSM-IV* criteria are a significant improvement over the older criteria. In emphasizing *worry* about life circumstances while deemphasizing associated *autonomic and motor symptoms* (sweats, tremor, muscle tension, headaches, irritable bowel symptoms, palpitations, etc.), they place a greater emphasis on *trait anxiety* than on *state anxiety*. Given this, there now is a greater degree of overlap between GAD and the "cluster C," or "overanxious," personality disorders (i.e., dependent, avoidant, and obsessive–compulsive personality disorders, discussed in Chapter 10).

Under the current diagnostic scheme, patients with these personality disorders who also demonstrate chronic, excessive worry and a few non-specific physical symptoms during periods of increased stress might be diagnosed with both the personality disorder diagnosis on Axis II and GAD on Axis I. Under the older scheme, evidence of chronic, pervasive *state* anxiety was required before one would assign a GAD diagnosis on Axis I. The current *international* classification scheme, the *ICD-10*, has retained this older conceptualization in that it continues to emphasize the presence of free-floating anxiety associated with multiple physical manifestations of anxiety.

The above discussion is of more than academic significance. GAD is a common condition, with a lifetime prevalence in the general population of 5% using the current *DSM* criteria (6.5% using the slightly broader *ICD* criteria). It is the leading cause of workplace disability in the United States and is the most commonly encountered anxiety disorder in the primary care setting. (Only about a third of patients with GAD present to psychiatrists.) GAD also is a particularly frequent finding among patients noted to be high utilizers of medical care (as illustrated in Chapter 7, Table 7–5).

Given this, and given that GAD often responds to specific interventions, it is essential that clinicians know how to *recognize* it. Fewer than 20% of GAD patients encountered in the primary care setting present with the psychological complaints emphasized in *DSM-IV*. Rather, the vast majority of GAD patients present for treatment of *somatic symptoms.* The most common presenting complaints are muscle pain, headache, irritability, insomnia, fatigue, and restlessness. This is not to say that these patients don't *experience* psychological symptoms; they just don't *emphasize* them. They might complain of feeling "stressed," and this should prompt the clinician to probe for the presence of chronic and excessive worry. For example, around 90% of individuals diagnosed with GAD answer "Yes" to the question: "During the past 4 weeks, have you been bothered by feeling worried, tense, or anxious most of the time?" Very few of those who don't have GAD respond positively to that question.

Physicians are less likely to diagnosis GAD when patients also have a "physical diagnosis" such as diabetes or Crohn's disease because in such cases the anxiety appears to be "justified." However, like depression, GAD can worsen the prognosis associated with a coexisting physical condition if it goes untreated. Hospitalization and emergency room visits for coexisting medical conditions also are more common in patients with GAD. The medical specialists most commonly consulted by patients with GAD are gastroenterologists, and 50% of patients with irritable bowel syndrome also have GAD. In such cases, patients should be treated for both disorders.

A tendency toward anxiety may be present during childhood, where it can be associated with childhood phobias or other behavioral problems (as discussed in Chapter 19). It also is the most common anxiety disorder to first present in late life. However, the most notable increase in incidence occurs roughly in the age range of 35 to 45. The severity of symptoms tends to wax and wane over the course of a patient's lifetime, punctuated by intervening periods where the patient may have another condition such as depression. The spontaneous remission rate is around 20% to 25%, suggesting that not all patients require chronic psychotherapy or psychotropic medication.

As is the case for other psychiatric disorders, including major depressive disorder, substance use disorders, and panic disorder, GAD is associated with considerable comorbidity. The most common comorbid condition is major depressive disorder, which occurs in about 80% of patients with GAD at some point. Patients who have *both* depression and GAD are more likely than patients who are depressed but aren't anxious *(1)* to experience functional disability, *(2)* to experience a chronic course of illness without periods of remission, and *(3)* to attempt suicide or commit suicide. In just over half of these "mixed anxiety–depression" cases, the GAD symptoms

precede the onset of a major depressive episode, suggesting the importance of continually monitoring for depressive symptoms over time while treating patients with anxiety disorders.

Obviously all of the anxiety disorders are associated with worry and with somatic symptoms of anxiety. The key distinction between GAD and these other conditions is the *focus* of the worry. For example, patients with *panic disorder* commonly develop excessive worry about the possibility of having another panic attack (often leading to agoraphobia). Patients with *obsessive–compulsive disorder* fear a wide variety of things, such as contamination, the oven being left on, doors being left unlocked, etc. Patients with *social phobia* worry about being embarrassed in public. Further, anxiety and worry aren't unique to the anxiety disorders. For example, the patient with *anorexia nervosa* who constantly worries about the possibility of gaining weight or who becomes acutely anxious after having eaten "too large" a meal would not be diagnosed with GAD. In GAD, in contrast to all of these other conditions, there is more generalized worry about *everyday or real-life problems*. Only when patients express this latter type of anxiety *in addition* to the more specific worries that typically accompany these other psychiatric disorders would both diagnoses be assigned.

Pathology and Etiology

It is unclear whether GAD represents a categorically distinct disease entity, or an extreme along a continuous dimensional measure of a particular biological propensity, or an alternative phenotypic presentation of a biologic diathesis that it shares with major depressive disorder.

The *DSM-IV* attempts to distinguish GAD from "normal" anxiety by underscoring how it differs from normal anxiety in *form*. In GAD, the severity and duration of the patient's anxiety along with the associated social morbidity are all greater than might be expected under similar circumstances for the average person. However, in contrast to what is the case for psychotic symptoms in schizophrenia, all of us have experienced the symptom of anxiety. Given this, early theorists emphasized the *function* of anxiety over the form of anxiety in their attempts to understand what lies behind "anxiety neurosis." They suggested that the anxiety experienced by patients with GAD is identical to the anxiety we all intermittently experience in the face of a discrete anxiety-provoking situation, but that in the former case, a psychological conflict (whether conscious or unconscious) has contributed to the anxiety becoming more pervasive and more detached from current life circumstances.

Psychoanalytic Theories

The earliest theories of anxiety were *philosophical* ones. Free-floating anxiety (*angst*) was interpreted as being a reflection of existential dread. It was seen as occurring when an individual recognized the fact that there is no inherent "meaning" in life and that, in the end, all of us must die. Treatment was aimed at helping the patient to make her peace with these inescapable aspects of the human condition.

Sigmund Freud suggested that *anxiety* could be distinguished from *fear*. *Fear* is an emotion that arises in response to the threat of harm from some discrete external object or event. In contrast, in GAD and panic disorder there *isn't* a clear object of the fear, just the subjective emotion of anxiety. Freud suggested that there actually *was* an object to the patient's fear but that it must have been unacceptable to the patient, who therefore escaped this knowledge of it by *repressing* it from conscious awareness. (Note the similarity here to Freud's formulation of *clinical depression*. In that case, he postulated that depression resembles *grief*, but that in the latter case sadness arises in response to some clear external loss, while in the former case no lost object is readily apparent. Given this, in clinical depression there must have been an earlier loss, whether actual or symbolic, that was unacceptable to the patient and therefore had been repressed from conscious awareness.)

At the turn of the century, Freud coined the term "anxiety neurosis" and hypothesized the existence of two distinct types of anxiety: the first was a diffuse sense of worry and dread; the second was an overwhelming sense of panic accompanied by autonomic symptoms. Thus, Freud distinguished between GAD and panic disorder.

Freud initially postulated that the anxiety that occurred in GAD reflected *unconscious wishes* that were so unacceptable to the patient that they were kept repressed, bottled up outside of conscious awareness. He believed that this led to an excessive "buildup" of unconscious tension or energy, and that the latter must be relieved, either by *discharging* it in the form of anxiety, or by displacing it (symbolically expressing it) into conversion symptoms such as hysterical paralysis, or into apparently "senseless" obsessive-compulsive symptoms or phobic fears. The goal of psychoanalytic treatment was to uncover the unconscious wishes, thereby alleviating the patient's anxiety. In contrast, Freud considered panic attacks to be more biologically determined. He attributed panic anxiety to the use of *coitus interruptus* as a form of contraception, which led to the damming up of libidinal energies that ultimately are released through an acute, autonomic discharge.

By the 1920s, though, Freud had created a new model of the mind, the *structural model*. Under this model, mind consists of three primary entities: the id, the ego, and the superego. He now considered *both* types of anxiety to result from unconscious conflict between the id and the superego. The *id*, the body's primal animal urges, seeks sexual and aggressive pleasures. The *superego* (or "conscience") develops during childhood socialization and represents an internalization of parental and societal standards. It threatens disapproval (leading to guilt) should the patient act on the id's unacceptable impulses. The *ego* (or "self") mediates this conflict. It comes up with suitable compromises between primal urges and societal/parental standards, all the while repressing the fact that this conflict is taking place from conscious awareness in order to protect the individual.

However, when repression begins to fail, unacceptable, unconscious desires threaten to reach conscious awareness. Anxiety (in the form of either generalized anxiety or an acute panic attack) emerges as a warning signal. This *"signal anxiety"* puts the ego on alert to mobilize defenses such as stronger repression. If this strategy fails, the ego next resorts to converting the conflict into more palatable conscious forms through *displacement* into various psychiatric symptoms. These symptoms allow for open, but symbolic, expression of the conflict. For example, a man who unconsciously wishes to hit or even to kill his son may suddenly find that his arm is "paralyzed." This symbolically *expresses* his unacceptable urge and simultaneously *prevents* him from acting on it. Similarly, since individuals' defenses presumably are lower during sleep, unconscious conflicts might be expressed in the form of *dreams*, albeit disguised in more acceptable forms through the use of dream symbolism.

As Freud's developmental model evolved, he postulated that failures to resolve conflicts that characteristically arise during *specific stages of early development* could explain the *different forms of anxiety* experienced by patients during adulthood. For example, patients who have failed to achieve autonomy from their parents during early childhood (i.e., in the "pre-oedipal stage") might develop *separation anxiety* during childhood, followed by excessive dependency needs and fears of loved ones abandoning them later in life. Patients who fail to resolve castration fears during later childhood (during the "oedipal period") may develop *castration anxiety*—that is, phobic fears that one will suffer physical injury if one experiences or expresses "unacceptable" wishes. During the adolescent years, an individual can develop *superego anxiety*. Here, a patient becomes anxious when he feels unable to live up to his "ego ideal"—that is, his sense of how he "should be living" based on his internalized image of what his parents were like. In other words, there is a sense of guilt and anxiety related to the sense that one isn't "measuring up" to one's internal standards.

Cognitive–Behavioral Theories

Freud proposed that free-floating, generalized anxiety in actuality represents a *fear* of some dangerous situation, although the situation is an internalized, unconscious one. In contrast, while behavioral theorists also propose that anxiety starts out as a fear, they suggest that this fear is of an actual, external danger. The fear response subsequently becomes *generalized* as a result of *conditioning*, such that the fear response ultimately can be triggered by relatively innocuous stimuli that are distinct from the original circumstances.

For example, if a rat receives an electric shock (an *unconditioned stimulus*) it will become anxious (an *unconditioned response*). However, if a bell is routinely rung (i.e., presenting the rat with a *conditioned stimulus*) just before the shock is

delivered, the rat ultimately will become anxious whenever the bell is rung, *even in the absence* of the original, unconditioned stimulus (the electric shock). In other words, the rat's anxiety has become not just an unconditioned response but also a *conditioned response*, since it now can be elicited by the conditioned stimulus in addition to the unconditioned stimulus.

Similarly, humans may become more generally anxious later in life as a result of early childhood experiences such as traumatic separations or losses. These early traumas could act as unconditioned stimuli that trigger an unconditioned response (i.e., anxiety). Current life stressors, even relatively innocuous ones provided that they sufficiently resemble the initial trauma, could act as conditioned stimuli, triggering the conditioned response, anxiety. When these situations can be avoided, the anxiety diminishes temporarily, but this also reinforces the anxiety response since patients come to increasingly avoid a variety of situations and their repertoire of available choices becomes increasingly narrowed.

A significant difficulty with this theory is that in GAD it often is difficult to locate either present-day conditioned stimuli or past unconditioned stimuli. Often, patients simply report that they have been anxious "for their entire lives," and their parents sometimes describe them as having been anxious even during their very youngest years. Further, to return to our example of the rat, if we repeatedly rang the bell *without* delivering an accompanying electrical shock, the rat eventually would "unlearn" the conditioned response, a phenomenon known as *extinction*. In contrast, in GAD the patient's anxiety often persists throughout the course of a lifetime, or even develops later in life, without evidence of extinction.

A modification of these behavioral theories that emphasizes the contribution of patients' *thought processes* rather than simply their conditioned behavior is Aaron Beck's *cognitive theory*. This approach, originally developed to explicate and treat depression, later was extended to the anxiety disorders.

We have discussed cognitive theories of depression in Chapter 7. In brief, cognitive theory proposes that in different psychiatric disorders there are characteristic distortions in how patients process information. Inappropriate emotions flow from inappropriate thoughts, and not simply vice versa. Because these are "automatic" thoughts (pervasive assumptions taken for granted by the patient), patients pay much more attention to the *emotions* that these thoughts engender than to the thoughts themselves.

The typical cognitive distortions seen in anxiety disorders overlap to an extent with those seen in depressive disorders, but there also are some important differences, as listed in Table 9–4. Both types of cognitions feature negative self-appraisals and a decreased perception of personal effectiveness. However, "depressive" cognitions tend to overstate *past failures*, while "anxious" cognitions tend to overstate *the risk of future failure* or to overstate the *severity of the consequences* that would result from a future failure.

Anxious individuals also express several characteristic *automatic thoughts*, all of which emphasize the threat of future harm or danger, along with an anticipated lack of control or incompetence in one's attempts to deal with these situations. The four most common cognitive distortions in GAD are: *(1)* overestimates of the likelihood of a feared event taking place, *(2)* overestimates of the severity the event, *(3)* underestimates of one's personal coping abilities, and *(4)* underestimates of the help that others can offer.

Complicating matters, patients' distorted views about life circumstances (e.g., their physical health, finances, and family concerns) become coupled to persistent *autonomic over-*

arousal. Treatment therefore also attempts to teach the patient to distinguish bodily sensations of anxiety from anxiety-laden cognitions and to address these bodily sensations through relaxation techniques such as deep breathing and muscle relaxation.

These automatic thoughts stand in contrast to those expressed by depressed patients, whose automatic thoughts center on *current hopelessness, low self-worth,* and *failure.* Depressive thinking also tends to be more *absolutist* ("I am a total failure"), whereas anxious thinking tends to emphasize *uncertainty* about one's ability to cope. ("What if I totally fail?") In common to both conditions, however, is an overall predominance of *automatic thinking, cognitive distortions,* and *impaired problem-solving ability.* As noted above, many patients are both anxious and depressed. In such cases, one can observe a mixture of both types of thinking. The cognitive techniques used to treat anxiety disorders are similar to those employed to treat depression, but they are directed toward different cognitive distortions.

Anxious patients also tend to display *attentional biases* as they respond to potentially threatening stimuli. They are more likely than nonanxious people to *preferentially attend* to aspects of the environment that might pose a potential threat than to more benign aspects of the environment, to *unrealistically interpret* benign environmental situations as being more dangerous than they actually are, and to demonstrate *enhanced recall* for memories associated with

Table 9–4. Pathologic Information Processing in Depressive and Anxiety Disorders

Predominant in Depression	Common to Both Depression and Anxiety	Predominant in Anxiety
Hopelessness	Demoralization	Fears of harm or danger
Low self-esteem	Self-absorption	High sensitivity to information about potential threat
Negative view of environment	Heightened automatic information processing	Automatic thoughts associated with danger, risk, uncontrollability, incapacity
Automatic thoughts with negative themes	Maladaptive schemas	Overestimates of risk in situations
Misattributions	Reduced cognitive capacity for problem-solving	Enhanced recall of memories for threatening situations
Overestimates of negative feedback		
Enhanced recall of negative memories		
Impaired performance on cognitive tasks requiring effort, abstract thinking		

Source: Adapted, with permission, from Wright JH, Beck AT: "Cognitive Therapy." *American Psychiatric Press Textbook of Psychiatry*, 3rd edition, Washington, DC, American Psychiatric Press, 1999.

past threatening situations or anxiety states. Given this, one can appreciate why they become anxious so much more easily than does the average person.

Biological Theories

Family and twin studies suggest the possibility of a *genetic component* to the disorder. However, genetic contributions appear to be relatively mild. GAD appears to be unrelated genetically to panic disorder, but it might be genetically linked to major depressive disorder.

Biological theories about GAD hinge primarily upon the putative mechanisms of action of those pharmacologic agents that demonstrate efficacy in treating GAD. For example, since SSRIs and buspirone effectively treat GAD, *serotonin* may play a role in its etiology. Similarly, benzodiazepines are effective in treating the autonomic, motor, and cognitive symptoms of GAD, while flumazenil (a benzodiazepine antagonist) is anxiogenic in GAD patients. This suggests a role for the *GABA system* in its etiology. Perhaps in GAD there is a functional deficiency of GABA, a deficiency of an as-yet-unidentified "endogenous benzodiazepine," or an excess of an as-yet-unidentified endogenous benzodiazepine antagonist or inverse agonist.

Tricyclic antidepressants (TCAs) also are effective in treating GAD. Treatment with imipramine, when compared to treatment with alprazolam or diazepam, has been associated with a slower onset of clinical effect (with the benzodiazepines being superior during the first 2 weeks) but with greater efficacy after 2 weeks, particularly with regard to *psychological symptoms* such as worry and nervousness. *SSRIs and venlafaxine* also have been found to be useful in decreasing psychological symptoms, even when prescribed in low dosages.

One possibility is that these agents' noradrenergic modulating effects (direct effects in the case of the TCAs and venlafaxine, indirect effects in the case of the SSRIs) help decrease somatic symptoms of anxiety (i.e., *state anxiety*), while their serotonergic modulating effects decrease psychological symptoms of anxiety (i.e., *trait anxiety*). As described in Chapter 4, the "fear circuit" (centering on the amygdala), the "pleasure circuit" (centering on the nucleus accumbens), and the "attention–motivation" circuit (centering

on the prefrontal cortex) overlap with each other. Given this, serotonin-mediated reductions in *anxiety* also might contribute to reductions in *pleasure and motivation*, which can be side effects of the SSRIs (particularly when prescribed at higher dosages). In contrast, treatment with noradrenergic and dopaminergic medications (such as methylphenidate and the amphetamines) can be associated with improved motivation, attention, and pleasure but also can cause anxiety.

Treatment

Milder cases of GAD often are amenable to psychotherapy, typically with either a psychodynamic or cognitive approach. Many patients with GAD also respond to treatment with buspirone or an antidepressant (such as an SSRI, a TCA, venlafaxine, or nefazodone). Venlafaxine, paroxetine, and buspirone are approved by the Food and Drug Administration for the treatment of GAD, as their manufacturers have demonstrated their clinical efficacy through large, randomized, placebo-controlled clinical trials, but most antidepressants also are likely effective.

However, all of these agents may initially exacerbate patients' complaints of anxiety. Perhaps this is due to their causing an initial surge in serotonin and/or norepinephrine *prior* to neuroadaptation and receptor downregulation. Some patients have difficulty getting past this initial hurdle. A good rule of thumb in treating patients with anxiety disorders is to "start low and go slow," since they often are exquisitely sensitive to medication side effects. The clinician should educate patients about the possibility that their anxiety might seem to get a bit worse at first and also should let them know not to expect rapid, dramatic results.

Interestingly, while the antidepressants have little direct effect on muscle tension or on autonomic nervous system activity, patients' *subjective* perceptions of bodily sensations don't always correspond to their *objective* bodily states. For example, one study of patients with GAD treated with imipramine found that the patients reported less muscle tension and fewer cardiovascular symptoms after 6 weeks of imipramine therapy, despite the fact that over the course of treatment their muscle tension (measured by electromyography, EMG), heart rate, and blood pressure actually *increased*. Given this, it may be that patients with anxiety and mood disorder *excessively attend to relatively minor bodily cues* and that treatment of their psychiatric condition leads to an overall improvement in perceived bodily functioning. (Not surprisingly, an overlap between anxiety and mood disorders and **somatoform disorders** also has been described. This will addressed in much greater detail in Chapter 13.)

Until recently the benzodiazepines were considered the drugs of first choice in GAD. However, given their potential to cause both physiologic dependence and cognitive side effects, given the current availability of alternative agents, and given the high degree of comorbidity of GAD with other mood and anxiety disorders that respond preferentially to antidepressants, many clinicians have consigned benzodiazepines to a secondary role. Since they provide more rapid relief than do antidepressants, it is reasonable to initiate treatment with a benzodiazepine either before or while initiating antidepressant therapy, followed a few weeks later by an attempt to taper the benzodiazepine once the patient is more stable.

Some patients require chronic psychotherapy or pharmacotherapy, but other patients require only brief counseling without further intervention after this. The symptoms of GAD tend to diminish when life stressors aren't as prominent. Therefore, resumption of psychotherapy during periods of increased stress often is helpful. The effects of psychotherapy and pharmacotherapy can be synergistic, such that once medications have helped patients to get their anxiety under better control, they can participate more meaningfully in psychotherapy and even make major life decisions that they previously had avoided addressing due to their excessive anxiety. Over the course of treatment, many patients also learn to tolerate higher levels of anxiety without unnecessarily "becoming anxious about becoming anxious."

PANIC DISORDER

Phenomenology and Epidemiology

A **panic attack** is a discrete period (usually lasting less than an hour) in which there is the sudden onset of intense apprehension, fearfulness, or terror, often associated with feelings of impending doom. During these attacks, symptoms such as shortness of breath, palpitations, chest pain or discomfort, choking or smothering sensations, and fear of "going crazy" or losing control are present. A detailed list of the symptoms that can occur in a panic attack is presented in Table 9–5.

The somatic symptoms associated with panic attacks can be mistaken for those associated with a variety of other medical problems. These include acute myocardial infarction, asthma attack, temporal lobe seizure, hypoglycemia, hyperadrenal state related to pheochromocytoma, acute hyperthyroidism ("thyroid storm"), and drug/alcohol intoxication and drug/alcohol withdrawal. Whenever a patient presents to the emergency room with new complaints of acute anxiety, one also should assess for these other conditions.

Many individuals in the general population have experienced one or two panic attacks in the setting of more acute stress. Panic attacks also occur in the context of specific types of situations in anxiety disorders other than panic disorder. For example, a patient with PTSD may have panic attacks when exposed to reminders of the original traumatic situation, a patient with obsessive–compulsive disorder (OCD) may have attacks when trying (but failing) to resist engaging in a compulsion, and a patient with specific

Table 9–5. *DSM-IV-TR* Criteria for Panic Attack

A discrete period of intense fear or discomfort, in which four (or more) of the following symptoms developed abruptly and reached a peak within 10 minutes:
1. Palpitations, pounding heart, or accelerated heart rate
2. Sweating
3. Trembling or shaking
4. Sensations of shortness of breath or smothering
5. Feeling of choking
6. Chest pain or discomfort
7. Nausea or abdominal distress
8. Feeling dizzy, unsteady, lightheaded, or faint
9. Derealization (feelings of unreality) or depersonalization (being detached from oneself)
10. Fear of losing control or going crazy
11. Fear of dying
12. Paresthesias (numbness or tingling sensations)
13. Chills or hot flushes

Source: Reprinted with permission from the *Diagnostic and Statistical Manual of Mental Disorders, Fourth Edition, Text Revision.* Copyright 2000 American Psychiatric Association.

phobias may have panic attacks upon confrontation with the feared object or situation.

In contrast, the hallmark of **panic disorder** is that the patient has repeated *spontaneous* or *unexpected* panic attacks. *DSM-IIIR* specified that patients diagnosed with panic disorder should have experienced a minimum number of attacks over a minimum period of time (e.g., four attacks within 4 weeks). However, the *DSM-IV* committee considered these criteria to be overly restrictive. The *DSM-IV* criteria, listed in Table 9–6, do not require a minimum number of panic attacks but do require that at least some of the attacks have been *unexpected* and that the attacks have contributed to the development of significant worry about the possibility of having another attack (*anticipatory anxiety*). As discussed in Chapter 2, some patients with panic disorder also develop anxiety about being in places or situations from which escape might be difficult or embarrassing, or where help may not be readily available (*agoraphobia*). Such fears typically involve characteristic types of situations, particularly those involving being outside of the home alone, being in a crowd, standing in a line, being on a bridge, or traveling in a bus, train, or car. Such situations either are avoided, or are endured with great anxiety, or are only attempted when a companion is present.

Major depressive disorder co-occurs in 50%–65% of individuals with panic disorder. In one-third of individuals with both disorders, the major depressive disorder precedes the onset of the panic disorder, while in the remaining two-thirds, the opposite is the case or the two disorders have a coincident onset. Patients with comorbid panic disorder and major depressive disorder demonstrate a more limited response to treatment and are more likely to remain chronically ill. They also have about twice the risk of committing suicide as patients with either panic disorder alone or major depressive disorder alone (14% versus 7% and 8%, respectively).

Patients with panic disorder are at risk for developing a comorbid *substance-related disorder* due to attempts to "self-medicate" their anxiety with alcohol or illicit drugs. Another common comorbidity is *another anxiety disorder*. Social phobia occurs in 15%–30% of panic disorder patients, obsessive–compulsive disorder in 8%–10%, specific phobia in 10%–20%, and generalized anxiety disorder in 25%.

The prevalence of panic disorder is about the same in every country that has been studied to date, about 1.5%–3.5%. The diagnosis is two to three times more prevalent in women (although it also may be underdiagnosed in men). It is equally common in all races. Most often, the first panic attacks occur in one's mid-20s, although the illness can have its onset at any age. Community surveys have found that between one-third and one-half of individuals with panic disorder also have agoraphobia, and the rate of agoraphobia is even higher among individuals who present for clinical care.

Table 9–6. *DSM-IV-TR* Criteria for Panic Disorder with (and without) Agoraphobia*

A. Both 1 and 2:
   1. Recurrent unexpected panic attacks
   2. At least one of the attacks has been followed by 1 month (or more) of one (or more) of the following:
      a. Persistent concern about having additional attacks
      b. Worry about the implications of the attack or its consequences (e.g., losing control, having a heart attack, "going crazy")
      c. A significant change in behavior related to the attacks
B. The presence (or absence) of agoraphobia
C. The panic attacks are not due to the direct physiological effects of a substance (e.g., a drug of abuse, a medication) or a general medical condition (e.g., hyperthyroidism)
D. The panic attacks are not better accounted for by another mental disorder, such as social phobia (e.g., occurring on exposure to feared social situations), specific phobia (e.g., on exposure to a specific phobic situation), obsessive–compulsive disorder (e.g., on exposure to dirt in someone with an obsession about contamination), posttraumatic stress disorder (e.g., in response to stimuli associated with a severe stressor), or separation anxiety disorder (e.g., in response to being away from home or close relatives)

---

*The only difference between the criteria for these two disorders is whether agoraphobia is present under criterion B.
Source: Reprinted with permission from the *Diagnostic and Statistical Manual of Mental Disorders, Fourth Edition, Text Revision.* Copyright 2000 American Psychiatric Association.

There appears to be a genetic component to panic disorder. First-degree relatives of individuals who have panic disorder are seven times more likely to also have panic disorder than are members of the general population. Further, the concordance rate for panic disorder in monozygotic twins is greater than that seen in dizygotic twins, also suggesting an important role for genetic factors. However, as with the mood disorder and schizophrenia, the fact that the concordance rate for monozygotic twins isn't 100% suggests that environmental factors also must play a role in converting genotypic vulnerability into phenotypic illness.

The course of panic disorder may be self-limited, but more often is chronic. At long-term follow-up, 30%–40% of patients are symptom-free, 50% of patients still have mild symptoms that they have learned to accommodate, and 10%–20% continue to experience significant symptoms. The disease can be lethal in that it is associated with an increased risk of the patient attempting or committing *suicide*. In the Epidemiologic Catchment Area (ECA) community survey, the lifetime rate of suicide attempts among individuals with panic disorder was 7%, which was comparable to the 8% rate for individuals with major depressive disorder. While patients with panic disorder are more prone to also developing major depressive disorder and alcohol dependence (which themselves are associated with a higher rate of suicide), the suicide rate remained high even when these comorbid diagnoses were controlled for, suggesting that the presence of panic disorder itself was an independent risk factor.

Pathology and Etiology

Psychodynamic Theories

Classic psychoanalytic theories about the etiology of panic disorder already have been described. More recent theories recognize the biological underpinnings of panic disorder while maintaining an emphasis on the role of life events and unconscious conflict as *triggers* for the onset of illness and subsequent panic attacks.

Patients with panic disorder tend be dependent, avoidant, and fearful people to begin with, and such personality traits can be exacerbated by the experience of having panic attacks. Sensitive parenting likely assists many anxious, avoidant children to learn to compensate for their temperamental vulnerabilities and to develop a greater sense of self-esteem. However, many panic disorder sufferers recall their parents as having been critical, overprotective, and controlling. This combination of a preexisting, nervous disposition and early injuries to self-esteem might contribute to patients developing a personality structure that is characterized by "weak" internal representations of themselves and "powerful" internal representations of others (particularly authority figures).

Patients often describe their first panic attack as having been preceded by some more acute life situation where they felt trapped or abandoned, leading to feelings of helplessness and resentment. Examples of such situations include relationship breakups; unhappy current relationships; perceived unfair treatment by employers, family members, friends, or lovers; and severe dissatisfaction with one's job.

Psychodynamic theory proposes that while patients with panic disorder often feel angry, helpless, and overwhelmed in the face of these situations, they have great difficulty assertively *expressing* their emotions and needs. Their feelings therefore come to the surface in the form of anxiety attacks that might appear to be "spontaneous" but in fact are psychologically meaningful. The goal of psychodynamic therapy is to help patients gain a greater sense of control through a combination of empathic listening and interpretations designed to help them gain some insight into the nature of their interpersonal difficulties.

Cognitive Theories

Like psychodynamic theories, cognitive theories also propose that panic attacks aren't as "spontaneous" as they might appear to be. However, these theories emphasize the role of unrecognized cognitive distortions and automatic thoughts rather than the role of unconscious intrapsychic conflict. Like contemporary analytic theorists, modern cognitive theorists recognize that the propensity to experience repeated panic attacks is grounded in neurophysiologic vulnerability. However, they emphasize that a key feature of panic disorder is presence of irrational and exaggerated cognitions that come to be associated with the panic attacks. Most notably, patients with panic disorder come to overestimate the significance of their physiological states and come to hold irrational fears of imminent disaster. For example, during a panic attack, an individual usually perspires and breathes more rapidly, and her heart begins to pound. The individual takes note of these changes and begins to fear that she is having a heart attack, is about to die, or is about to lose control in public and embarrass herself. These fears then engender further somatic arousal, ultimately leading to a vicious positive feedback loop between a state of autonomic hyperarousal and catastrophic cognitions. These cognitions ultimately persist in between attacks, leading to more chronic physiologic arousal and phobic avoidance in the form of anticipatory anxiety and agoraphobia.

Cognitive therapy seeks to break this feedback loop, not by blocking the autonomic arousal (as anxiolytic medications do), but by drawing attention to and revising faulty cognitions. For example, many patients aren't even aware that what they are having are panic attacks and know little about panic disorder. Despite multiple emergency room visits and medical workups, they may only have been told that "there doesn't appear to be anything wrong with your heart" or that their symptoms are "due to anxiety." Patients often experience great relief simply learning that there is an explanation for their symptoms and that treatment is available. Next, the therapist might acknowledge how truly uncomfortable the patient's panic attacks are, but might ask the patient whether—despite having had over 20 such attacks in the past year—she ever has lost control in public or had any health complications during an attack. Most commonly, patients have been so caught up in their overwhelming *fears* of a catastrophic outcome that they haven't been able to objectively think about the low *likelihood* that such an outcomes ever would occur.

After a course of cognitive therapy, many patients report that they continue to experience some panic attacks but now are better able to "talk themselves down from them." For example, they might tell themselves during an attack: "I'm just having a panic attack. It isn't going to kill me. These always go away within an hour or so. The best thing that I can do at this moment is to focus on slowing down my breathing and on relaxing my muscles."

Cognitive therapy often is paired with *behavioral techniques* such as *relaxation training* and *respiratory control*. These techniques attempt to interrupt the positive feedback loop by teach patients to address their state of physiological arousal. Behavioral techniques such as *guided imagery,* followed by *graded exposure* to increasingly anxiety-laden situations, are especially important in helping patients learn to combat anticipatory anxiety and agoraphobia.

First, patients are educated about relaxation techniques. Then, while they are in a relaxed state and feel "safe," they might be asked to imagine themselves in a crowded public place. Ultimately, patients are encouraged to go out of the home, at first accompanied by a family member or friend, ultimately by themselves. Some patients will already have devised similar behavioral strategies without any medical guidance in their attempts to combat agoraphobia. However, explicit education about the nature of phobic avoidance and assistance in designing graded exposure plans increase the likelihood that they will be successful.

Cognitive–behavioral therapy can be combined with medication therapy without difficulty. While medication therapy alone may prevent patients from having further panic attacks, patients typically continue to experience significant anticipatory anxiety and agoraphobia, which are then amenable to cognitive and behavioral interventions.

Biological Theories

The family and twin studies cited above suggest that panic disorder has biological underpinnings. Many biological theories are based upon findings from "challenge studies" in which patients with panic disorder and control subjects are exposed to substances found to induce panic attacks more frequently in the patients than in the control subjects.

The earliest theory was that panic attacks result from a massive *peripheral autonomic discharge*. However, while infusions of isoproterenol (a sympathomimetic drug that doesn't cross the blood–brain barrier) are associated with increased sensations of arousal and anxiety in patients with panic disorder, it doesn't appear to trigger a full-blown panic *attack*. Similarly, while β-adrenergic receptor antagonist agents ("β-blockers") blunt the peripheral manifestations of panic attacks, carefully designed studies have not found them to offer significant prophylactic benefits in panic disorder.

Later theories have focused on the role of *central (brain) norepinephrine* as opposed to peripheral norepinephrine and epinephrine. As described earlier, electrical stimulation of the locus ceruleus in animals triggers a marked anxiety response, while ablation of the locus ceruleus is associated with attenuation of the fear response associated with the presentation of a threatening stimulus. Similarly, in humans, the infusion of *yohimbine* (an α-2 antagonist that increases presynaptic noradrenergic output) provokes anxiety, while *clonidine* (and α-2 agonist that decreases presynaptic noradrenergic output) decreases anxiety. Finally, we have discussed how *SSRIs* (which effectively block panic attacks) *indirectly* decrease norepinephrine output, since serotonergic projections from the brain-stem raphe region to the locus ceruleus region are generally inhibitory.

When yohimbine is infused intravenously into patients with panic disorder, they experience both a greater increase in anxiety and a greater increase in circulating plasma levels of MHPG (3-methoxy-4-hydroxyphenyl glycol—a major metabolite of norepinephrine) than do control subjects who don't have panic disorder. This suggests that the patients with panic disorder have a more sensitive noradrenergic system, perhaps with a "hair trigger."

However, this theory doesn't appear to fully account for the features of panic disorder. For example, *sodium lactate* is an important panic-inducing substance, but sodium lactate doesn't cross the blood–brain barrier. When sodium lactate is infused intravenously into patients with panic disorder, attacks are triggered that closely resemble spontaneously occurring attacks. These attacks don't occur when intravenous saline rather than lactate is infused. More importantly, control subjects given intravenous sodium lactate *don't* experience panic attacks. Finally, medications known to be effective in prevent panic attacks, including TCAs and SSRIs, can prevent panic disorder patients from experiencing attacks in response to lactate infusion.

Does sodium lactate simply trigger uncomfortable physical sensations that make panic disorder patients so anxious that they ultimately experience a panic attack, or does the lactate itself somehow act as a specific trigger? The latter appears to be the case for other "panicogenic" substances, including *fenfluramine*, which is known to stimulate the presynaptic release of serotonin (suggesting a possible role for central *serotonin hypersecretion*), and *flumazenil*, a benzodiazepine antagonist (suggesting a possible role for *GABA hypoactivity*).

One important finding is that panic attacks also can be induced by *carbon dioxide inhalation*. Despite the common belief that panic attacks can be caused by hyperventilation (which lowers carbon dioxide levels) and that "hyperventilation syndrome" can be treated by having a patient breath into a paper bag (which raises carbon dioxide concentrations), in actuality hyperventilation *doesn't* trigger panic in most vulnerable patients, while inhaling CO_2-enhanced air actually *triggers* panic attacks. Add to this the fact that lactate is peripherally metabolized to bicarbonate, which in turn is metabolized to carbon dioxide (which *does* cross the blood–brain barrier) and that *bicarbonate infusion* also triggers what appear to be true panic attacks in patients with panic disorder, and one begins to wonder if *carbon dioxide hypersensitivity* represents a "final common pathway" in panic disorder.

One theory, proposed by Donald Klein, is that carbon dioxide crosses the blood–brain barrier and produces transient cerebral hypercapnia. This in turn triggers brain-stem chemoreceptors for carbon dioxide. Perhaps panic disorder patients have *overly sensitive chemoreceptors* such that even mild increases in carbon dioxide trigger a *false sense of suffocation*, leading to the classic "smothering sensation" described by patients with panic disorder, to hyperventilation, and to feelings of panic.

This "false-suffocation" condition might be the opposite of what is seen in a rare childhood illness called "Ondine's Curse." These children stop breathing during deep sleep and die. They therefore must be kept out of deep sleep through the use of an electrical stimulator. They likely have *insensitive* carbon dioxide chemoreceptors such that when respiratory drive decreases during deep sleep and carbon dioxide builds up, they don't compensate by increasing their respiratory rate. In contrast, in panic disorder, *hypersensi-*

tive chemoreceptors may trigger hyperventilation and a smothering sensation when they are exposed to even mild increases in carbon dioxide.

The false-suffocation theory also might explain the phenomenon of *nocturnal panic attacks*. One might expect such attacks to occur during REM sleep in response to anxiety-laden dreams. However, they occur not during REM sleep but during *deep non-REM sleep*. This is the phase of sleep where respiration slows and carbon dioxide levels increase. Similarly, panic attacks also occur *premenstrually*, and they occur spontaneously during periods when the patient is *relaxing*. Panic disorder patients tend to hyperventilate chronically without being aware of it, but their respiration slows during these periods.

In contrast, panic attacks *don't* occur frequently during either pregnancy or childbirth. One might have expected just the opposite, since these events can be very stressful. However, placental maturation requires high levels of progesterone, and progesterone is also a strong respiratory stimulant. Carbon dioxide levels therefore remain very low throughout the entire course pregnancy and drop to even lower levels during childbirth. Shortly after this, however, carbon dioxide levels increase, as does the frequency of panic attacks.

There are some problems with the false-suffocation theory, however. For example, studies of the most sensitive measure of physiological response to carbon dioxide inhalation—the ratio of change in minute ventilation to change in end-tidal carbon dioxide concentration—have yielded conflicting results, with some investigators finding evidence of receptor hypersensitivity using this measure and others finding patients with panic disorder to fall within the normal range. Also, this theory doesn't explain the effects of the multiple other "panicogenic" substances.

What isn't clear from studies using either pharmacologic probes that trigger anxiety attacks or pharmacologic agents that block panic attacks is whether these agents are acting *directly* on the primary pathology, *indirectly* (by making the patient feel so uncomfortable that an attack ensues), or at only *one node within an extensive neural network*. Current research suggests that the last possibility is likely the case. For example, benzodiazepines, SSRIs, and cognitive therapy all effectively decrease the frequency and intensity

of panic attacks, despite their different mechanisms of action. Used together, they may have synergistic effects. It is likely that they each act at different nodes within the central nervous system *fear circuit* discussed in Chapter 4 and illustrated in Figure 4–2.

This circuit—which centers on the *amygdala*—includes "upstream" afferent input from the *sensory cortex* (relayed relatively directly via the *thalamus*, thereby allowing for a rapid response to immediate environmental threats) from the *prefrontal cortex and sensory association cortex* (thereby allowing for modulation of this thalamic input through higher-level cognitive processing) and from the *hippocampus* (thereby allowing for modulation of the thalamic input by analysis of relevant contextual data). The amygdala in turn acts as a gatekeeper. It triggers a wide variety of "downstream" effects via efferent projections to the brain stem and hypothalamus.

These "downstream" effects include: *motor activation* (mediated by the striatum), *escape and defensive behaviors* (mediated by the periaqueductal gray region), *sympathetic arousal* (mediated by lateral hypothalamus and locus ceruleus, with noradrenergic output), *cognitive manifestations* of anxiety (mediated by the raphe nuclei, with serotonergic output), *increased attention* (mediated by ventral tegmental area, with dopaminergic output), and hypothalamic and extrahypothalamic secretion of *corticotropin-releasing factor* (which in turn activates the stress thermostat, as discussed in Chapter 4).

The anxiety circuit may become abnormally sensitized in vulnerable individuals, reflecting the influence of both genetic and early environmental factors. In such individuals, "panicogenic" triggers—be they noxious substances (such as lactate and carbon dioxide) or noxious situations (such as closed in spaces or heights in a phobic individual)—may induce panic attacks by activating the entire circuit rather than one particular brain-stem region. Interindividual differences in the strength of afferent projections from the amygdala to various "downstream" regions, along with preferential reinforcement of one or more of these pathways over time, may explain why the autonomic and neuroendocrine manifestations of a panic attack vary between two different patients or over the course of time for any given patient.

Psychotherapy may modify this hyperactive fear response by acting "upstream" from the amygdala at the level of the prefrontal cortex and hippocampus. Education and support allow patients to modify their tendencies to misinterpret relatively benign sensory input from the environment or from their own bodies as representing "threats." *Behavioral interventions* also can help patients modify the contextual associations that have formed between panic attacks and various environmental settings (such as being in cars, on bridges, or in other situations where help might not readily be available). In contrast, *pharmacologic interventions* may act "downstream" from the amygdala. For examples, *SSRIs* appear to modulate not only the serotonergic component of the fear circuit but also the noradrenergic, glucocorticoid, and periqueductal systems, since afferent serotonergic output from the doral raphe exerts inhibitory effects on each of these latter systems.

Treatment

The first step in the treatment of panic disorder is to recognize that it is present, especially in the primary care setting. Between 50% and 60% of patients with psychiatric illness are diagnosed and treated exclusively in the primary care setting, and anxiety disorders have been listed in surveys of primary care physicians as the most common psychiatric problem seen in their clinical practice. Primary care physicians write 80% of all prescriptions for benzodiazepines.

However, like major depressive disorder, panic disorder is underdiagnosed and undertreated in the primary care setting. This contributes to both unnecessary psychiatric morbidity and extensive (often unnecessary) medical workups and diagnostic testing. As noted in Chapter 7 (Table 7–5), 22% of "distressed high medical utilizers" turn out to have a lifetime history of panic disorder.

Unfortunately, 90% of panic disorder patients don't present with complaints of "anxiety" but rather with nonspecific somatic complaints. On average, these patients have seen ten or more physicians and have spent over a decade in the health system before being correctly diagnosed with panic disorder. They report an average of 13 different symptoms: 40% of patients report cardiac symptoms (especially chest pain, tachy-

cardia, and palpitations), 30% report gastrointestinal symptoms (especially epigastric pain relieved with antacids, diarrhea, and "irritable bowel" symptoms), 40% report neurologic symptoms (especially headache, dizziness, and syncope or pseudoseizures), and 10% report pulmonary and "asthma" symptoms.

Many younger patients unnecessarily receive extensive cardiac workups when positive findings are unlikely. In one study, 40% of patients presenting to an emergency room with chest pain were found to have panic attacks; in another study, 90% of patients at a chest pain clinic were found to have panic disorder. (Among those patients with negative cardiac workups, 98% were found to have panic disorder.) Similarly, in a gastroenterology clinic, 30% of patients with well-characterized irritable bowel syndrome also met the diagnostic criteria for panic disorder; symptoms of both conditions improved when the patients were treated for their panic disorder.

The routine medical workup should include a social history, medical history, psychiatric history, and physical examination. Questioning also should be directed more specifically at symptoms consistent with panic attacks, agoraphobia, and depression. A detailed medication and drug history (including alcohol, caffeine, and over-the-counter agents) is essential.

In the course of the diagnostic interview, one should attempt to distinguish between life-long, multiple, unexplained medical complaints from hypochondriacal fears that have arisen only in the wake of acute anxiety attacks. The former would be consistent with a diagnosis of **somatization disorder** or **hypochondriasis**, as discussed in Chapter 13. With regard to the latter, up to 70% of patients with panic disorder express enough symptoms to also qualify for a diagnosis of somatization disorder, but in contrast to somatization disorder, their physical symptoms tend to be of more recent origin and also tend to improve when their panic attacks have been treated.

One also should attempt to distinguish between symptoms due to panic disorder and those due to **complex partial seizures**. In both cases, patients may complain of anxiety, derealization (feelings of unreality), and depersonalization (feelings of being detached from oneself). In complex partial seizures, however, patients are more likely to also experience confusion, bizarre behavior, and a change in the level of consciousness. In some cases, patients also describe amnesia, episodes of incontinence, or generalization to tonic–clonic (grand mal) seizures. In complex cases, an EEG or even continuous EEG monitoring helps to confirm or disconfirm the diagnosis of a seizure disorder.

In patients over age 40, it is reasonable to routinely obtain an electrocardiogram as part of the diagnostic workup. The ECG is unlikely to be abnormal in patients younger than this. A complete blood count, a chemistry and electrolyte panel, and a thyroid function panel help to assess whether anemia, electrolyte or metabolic disturbances, or hyperthyroidism is responsible for the patient's symptoms. Other tests, such as an echocardiogram or an electroencephalogram, are rarely indicated. While echocardiograms might reveals nonspecific "abnormalities" such as mitral valve prolapse in 30%–50% of panic disorder patients, the degree of prolapse is typically mild and is rarely of clinical significance.

In cases where panic attacks are less severe or are relatively infrequent, educational therapy and specific cognitive–behavioral instructions may suffice. However, some patients will report that these techniques are effective for dealing with their "minor" attacks but not their "more severe" attacks. Prophylaxis against attacks can be attempted with a variety of agents. *Benzodiazepines* often are prescribed initially, either on an as-needed or a standing-dose basis. Concomitantly, longer-term therapy can be initiated with an SSRI or a TCA. As in GAD, these agents don't take effect as rapidly but are as effective for longer-term prophylaxis and are not associated with physical or psychological dependence.

For many clinicians, SSRIs have become the first-line agents. One should start at low doses and titrate up slowly, since patients may experience an increase in anxiety when these agents are first taken. Sometimes the clinician will elect initially to use both an SSRI and benzodiazepine, as the benzodiazepine is more rapidly effective and may help combat the nervousness that can be associated with initiation of SSRI treatment. Other agents such as clonidine and β-blockers have been used, but with much less success.

After several months to a year of therapy, a gradual medication taper can be attempted. However, a significant percentage of patients will turn out to have a chronic illness that necessitates ongoing prophylactic treatment at full pharmacologic doses. Psychotherapy offers significant benefits not only in the acute phase of treatment but also in the longer-term maintenance phase. Cognitive–behavioral therapy can be associated with a success rate as high as that associated with medication therapy in controlled clinical research. Psychodynamic approaches have been described as being successful in smaller case series but have not been studied in randomized, controlled trials using validated outcome measures.

PHOBIC DISORDERS

Phenomenology and Epidemiology

The phenomenology of the various types of phobias—including specific phobia, social phobia, and agoraphobia—has been discussed in Chapter 2 and is detailed in Table 2–7.

To reiterate, **phobias** are marked and persistent fears cued by the presence or anticipation of specific objects or situations. Exposure to these objects or situations almost invariably provokes an immediate fear response, sometimes even a panic attack. This fear response occurs despite affected individuals usually recognizing that the fear is unreasonable or excessive.

Specific phobia can be subtyped as *situational type phobias* (fear of tunnels, bridges, heights, driving, flying, closed-in spaces, etc.), *natural environment type phobias* (such as fears of storms, heights, or water), *blood–injection–injury type phobias* (fears of seeing blood or an injury or fear of injections or medical procedures), *animal type phobias*. Having one type of phobia increases the likelihood of having another phobia of that same type (e.g., fear of cats and snakes), and some patients have phobias of several types.

Agoraphobia is fear of, or avoidance of, places or situations either where help may not be available or where escape might prove difficult or embarrassing. Many patients with agoraphobia previously have experienced spontaneous panic attacks. The panic attacks become associated with various situations, leading to the development of anticipatory anxiety and multiple situation-type phobias. More rarely, agoraphobia occurs in the absence of panic disorder. For example, a patient who has experienced severe migraine headaches or back pain in public also might develop anticipatory anxiety and phobic avoidance, triggered by a fears of pain rather than a fear of panic attacks.

In **social phobia**, patients experience marked and persistent fears of social or performance situations where they might be embarrassed. Typical situations include public speaking, eating in public places, using public restrooms, or attending parties or job interviews. In such situations, they tend to experience autonomic symptoms such as sweating, blushing, and dry mouth. While some patients continue to function despite these fears, others become socially isolated and suffer from severe vocational and social disability similar to what is seen in agoraphobia.

DSM-IV has made it clear that while panic *attacks* can occur in the setting of phobic disorders, generally when patients are faced with exposure to their particular phobia, a comorbid diagnosis of panic *disorder* only is assigned when the patient also experiences *spontaneous* panic attacks in the absence of such exposure. When this occurs, it next becomes important to distinguish between *social phobia* and *agoraphobia*, both of which are associated with social isolation. Patients with severe, generalized *social phobia and secondary panic attacks* usually are willing to leave their homes alone provided that they don't run into other people. Patients with *panic disorder with agoraphobia* usually prefer to be accompanied when they go out, since they fear having a panic attack and being helpless.

> A 30-year-old male presents for treatment of "panic attacks," which most commonly occurred in the supermarket. He is treated with imipramine for panic disorder but fails to show a clinical response. Subsequent interviews reveal that his panic attacks are invariably preceded by fears that other shoppers at the supermarket are "staring at him." His anxiety subsides when he leaves the supermarket. He is much more comfortable shopping late at night when the supermarket is nearly empty. He denies having experiencing spontaneous panic attacks when home alone. He is rediagnosed with social phobia and responds well to treatment with paroxetine and graded exposure therapy.

Pathology and Etiology

It should again be emphasized that each psychiatric illnesses can be viewed from each of the four perspectives discussed in Chapter 3, although one perspective may prove to be more useful than the others in particular situations. The phobic disorders provide an excellent example of this.

From the *disease perspective*, it is notable that there appears to be a strong genetic component to all of the phobias. *Specific phobia* tends to run in families. This is particularly the case for the blood–injection–injury type, which—unlike the other specific phobias—is accompanied not only by anxiety but by a tendency to experience vasovagal reactions. Seventy-five percent of people with a specific phobia have a first-degree relative who has a specific phobia. (Usually, the specific phobia in the relative is even in the same subtype.) In contrast, specific phobias only occur in the first-degree relatives of 30% of control subjects without specific phobias. At this point twin studies have not been conducted, so the relative contributory roles of genes versus shared environments remain to be more fully elucidated. Social phobias demonstrate a similar picture, with first-degree relatives of probands being three times more likely to have social phobia than are those of probands without social phobia.

The *dimensional perspective* also is useful here, particularly in the case of social phobia. *DSM-III* had a strict definition of social phobia that emphasized problems with public speaking or eating in public but excluded more generalized phobic avoidance of almost any social situations. In the latter case, the individual would have been considered to have **avoidant personality disorder**. (The diagnostic criteria for this disorder are presented in Chapter 10 in Table 10–13.)

However, this distinction wasn't based on empirical evidence. Later research demonstrated that many patients with social phobia also had more generalized social fears and that these difficulties responded to treatment with an MAO inhibitor. To label this more extensive social avoidance as solely reflecting a personality disorder might steer clinicians away from potentially effective cognitive–behavioral and pharmacological treatments. Therefore, *DSM-IV* has recommended that clinicians consider diagnosing *both* avoidant personality disorder and social phobia in more generalized cases where features of both disorders are present.

Most individuals with social phobia also have an anxious, avoidant temperament. They tend to be hypersensitive to criticism or rejection, have great difficulty being assertive, and have low self-esteem and feelings of inferiority. They also tend to have limited social skills and "under-achieve" in school or work situations because they avoid speaking up in classes or in confer-ences and experience severe "test anxiety." They tend to have limited social support networks and are less likely to marry. In the most severe cases, they may drop out of school, fail to interview for jobs, fail to date, and live at home with their par-ents in relative isolation.

The *life-story perspective* has been used to ex-plain phobias ever since Freud's discussion of Little Hans, a 5-year-old boy with a specific pho-bia concerning horses. Little Hans irrationally feared that horses would bite him. Freud hy-pothesized that the boy's fear of horses resulted from unconscious anxiety related to sexual long-ings for his mother and fears of retaliatory cas-tration by his father. Hans defended against this castration anxiety by *displacing* it onto horses. When repression isn't successful, signal anxiety may result (in the form of panic attacks), but the anxiety also might be discharged if it can be ex-pressed publicly in more "acceptable," symbolic ways, such as through obsessions or compul-sions, conversion symptoms, or phobias.

In psychoanalytic theory, specific phobias in-volve previously neutral objects or situations onto which the patient has displaced unaccept-able anxiety. Once the patient has done this, he can avoid experiencing anxiety provided that he avoid the object. However, when he can't do so, his defenses begin to break down and the un-conscious anxiety again begins to surface, thereby leading to a panic attack. For example, Hans became anxious because of a conflict: he loved his father but also feared assault by his fa-ther in retaliation for Hans competing against him for Hans's mother. By displacing this anxi-ety onto horses, Hans could again have a rela-tionship with his father. Things were fine so long as Hans never went around horses: when he did so, he became inexplicably anxious.

The *behavior perspective* is perhaps the most useful perspective when dealing with phobias be-cause in contrast to spontaneous panic attacks or chronic, generalized anxiety, *phobias are defined by their behavioral features*, by how the patient *acts*. Clearly, genetically determined constitu-tional and biological factors play an important *role* in the pathogenesis of the avoidant behav-ior, but only by focusing on the *behavior itself* does it become clear that the biological contrib-utors are quite nonspecific. For example, a person with a biological tendency toward vasovagal re-sponses and a personality temperament charac-terized by avoidance of potential harm still might never develop a blood–injection–injury phobia. However, following one frightening experience in which she becomes dizzy or faints while hav-ing her blood drawn, she may develop this spe-cific phobia. One cannot understand the nature of the phobia without understanding *behavioral conditioning*, and one can't treat phobias with-out understanding *behavioral deconditioning*.

The classic demonstration of how phobias can be classically conditioned took place in 1920 when John B. Watson was able to instill a spe-cific phobia in an 11-month-old boy named Lit-tle Albert. Watson presented Albert with a white rat (the *conditioned stimulus*). Albert wasn't afraid of it. Watson then presented the rat at the same time as a loud noise (the *unconditioned stimulus*). This made Albert very anxious (the *conditioned response*). After a few such pairings, Albert not only feared and avoided the white rat but also feared and avoided distantly related ob-jects, such as cotton wool and sealskin. This is an example of *stimulus generalization*, where stimuli that are similar to the original conditioned stimulus also gain the ability to elicit the condi-tioned response (although usually in attenuated form).

The behavior perspective focuses on moti-vated behaviors, such as eating and sleeping. These are biologically driven but are subse-quently shaped by personality, family and peer influence, the surrounding culture, and life ex-perience. Behaviors can become disabling when they become excessive and when they become more autonomous and self-reinforcing. In the case of the phobias, a defining theme is the fear of either *anticipated harm or loss of control*. Given this, individuals with inherited tempera-ments that render them more prone to excessive worry and to autonomic reactivity may be pre-disposed to develop phobias.

In simple phobia, such individuals may have

been exposed to particular anxiety-provoking situations (being in a car accident, being trapped on an elevator, seeing a scary movie, or simply looking down from a high place). This anxiety then generalizes to similar circumstances. Finally, the pattern of phobic avoidance itself becomes self-reinforcing, since the individuals' anxiety increases when they enter frightening situations and decreases when they exit them, thereby reinforcing the fear even when no harm has occurred.

Social phobia may be somewhat different in that the biological vulnerability may have to do more with an innate tendency toward *behavioral inhibition*. Psychologist Jerome Kagan has studied 18-month-old children who are brought into an unfamiliar room by their mothers and then left there. In the room are other people and a variety of toys. Seventy percent of the children routinely explore the room. Of the remaining children, 15% are *very exploratory*, while 15% are *very shy and behaviorally inhibited* and engage in little or no exploration.

This third group demonstrates the trait of behavioral inhibition. It appears to be a stable trait that persists through at least the first decade of life. As they age, behaviorally inhibited children begin to demonstrate personality traits consistent with a diagnosis of avoidant personality disorder and behavioral signs of social phobia. Not surprisingly, the parents of these children also tend to be anxious, and many of them have panic disorder. When these childrens' predisposition toward anxiety and social avoidance is combined with anxious, overly protective parenting and then they are exposed to some frightening experience (e.g., having to speak in front of one's classmates), one can see how the behavioral syndrome of social phobia might develop.

Variation along this dimensional continuum—from introversion and behavioral inhibition on one end of the spectrum to extroversion and active exploration on the other end—also occurs in other animal species. Both primates and wolves form social systems in which there are more dominant males and more submissive males. Biological underpinnings of this dimensional variation may include an important role for dopamine, a neurotransmitter involved in motivation and drive. For example, rats bred for shyness have lower brain levels of dopamine. MAOIs may be more effective in treating social phobia than

TCAs are, perhaps due to their ability to increase not only norepinephrine and serotonin levels but also dopamine levels. However, none of the typical indirect measures of dopamine function (such as serum prolactin levels) has been found to be abnormal in social phobia.

We discussed in Chapter 7 how MAOIs also might be more effective than TCAs in cases of "atypical depression," a syndrome that includes not only sadness but "rejection sensitivity." This latter symptom might be indicative of a neurobiological link between this type of depression and the tendency to develop social phobia. Whether a patient presents in one fashion or another might reflect variation in her upbringing or life story. For example, early loss might contribute more to the development of major depressive disorder, while exposure to an anxiety-laden trauma might contribute more to the development of social phobia. Many individuals develop both disorders.

Treatment

As with other conditions best approached from the behavior perspective (such as substance dependence, eating disorders, and sexual disorders), treatment of phobic disorders ultimately involves some form of behavioral modification, with other modes of therapy often playing ancillary roles. The most commonly employed behavioral technique in the treatment of phobias is *graded exposure*, in which the patient is encouraged to gradually expose himself to situations that more and more closely approximate the feared situation. This might be accompanied by *relaxation training*, *breathing exercises*, and *cognitive therapy* to help the patient recognize irrational fears while in the phobic situation.

Even Freud recognized that while insight-oriented therapy might help patients understand the *origin* of their phobias, patients improved most when they subsequently exposed themselves to feared situations but remained there rather than retreated (*exposure and response prevention*). Similarly, cognitive–behavioral therapy seeks to help patients recognize the *irrationality* of their fears through cognitive techniques and then utilizes the behavioral techniques to help them break the association between particular circumstances and the biological fear response.

Biologic therapies attempt to attenuate autonomic hyperactivity. Following this, patients again should attempt to expose themselves to the feared stimuli. The most commonly employed ancillary medications in specific phobia are *β-adrenergic blockers*, although when the condition is associated with panic attacks, *antidepressant* or *benzodiazepine agents* might be employed. In Social phobia, *MAOIs* may be more effective than other agents, although *SSRIs* can also be useful and these drugs are used more frequently than MAOIs given their greater margin of safety.

POST-TRAUMATIC STRESS DISORDER

Phenomenology and Epidemiology

Our understanding both of **post-traumatic stress disorder (PTSD)** and of the role of trauma as a predisposing factor for psychiatric illness in general has greatly expanded since the *DSM-III* first "created" the PTSD diagnosis in 1980. In the late 1800s, psychiatrists such as Freud noted that trauma, particularly trauma occurring early in life, could predispose individuals to develop psychiatric symptoms later in life. Freud initially postulated that hysterical phenomena (currently called conversion symptoms and discussed in Chapter 13) reflected individuals' unconscious attempts to deal with painful, repressed memories of childhood trauma (leading him to state that "hysterics suffer mainly from reminiscences"). However, Freud later concluded that many of the traumatic memories that his patients described to him over the course of psychotherapy reflected childhood fantasies or fears rather than true memories. He decided to place less emphasis on analyzing how individuals respond to childhood trauma and more on how they resolve conflicting psychological conflicts. Freud's shift in emphasis was to exert a significant influence on both psychiatry and on our culture in general.

During periods of war, though, it remained obvious that the experience of traumatic stress left many individuals with significant psychological problems. During the American Civil War, Jacob DaCosta described a syndrome of severe cardiac and autonomic symptoms without organic explanation that he called "irritable heart"

(later it was called "soldier's heart" or "DaCosta's syndrome"). During World War I, military doctors observed a similar syndrome. The British called it "disordered action of the heart." The Americans called it "shell shock." (The latter term reflected the prevailing theory, which was that these patients' symptoms were related to brain trauma caused by the explosion of shells.) After World War II, some veterans experienced anxiety symptoms which were labeled "combat neurosis."

Beyond the symptoms noted in World War II veterans, several events in the 1940s brought attention to the role of trauma in the civilian setting. Many survivors of the Nazi concentration camps were observed to have persistent, intrusive, painful recollections of their experiences there, along with symptoms of anxiety, motor restlessness, hypervigilance, insomnia, nightmares, and phobic avoidance of situations that resembled their traumatic experience. This constellation of symptoms, labeled "concentration camp syndrome," occurred in such a large percentage of survivors (75%) that it had to be concluded that it represented a response to the trauma itself and was not simply a "neurotic" response exhibited by more psychologically vulnerable individuals. At about this same time, similar symptoms were described both among survivors of the 1941 Coconut Grove nightclub fire and among many Japanese civilians who had survived the atomic bombings of Hiroshima and Nagasaki.

Based upon these findings, when the *DSM-I* was published in 1952, it included the diagnosis of "gross stress reaction," with specifiers of either "civilian type" or "combat type." It was considered to be a self-limited condition: it was believed that if symptoms persisted, the individual must have another underlying disorder. However, by the time that the *DSM-II* was published in 1968, this diagnosis had been dropped. Severe reactions to a trauma simply were considered to be another form of "adjustment reaction" and received little further clinical or research attention.

However, after the Vietnam War, a large number of veterans were found to be suffering from a characteristic syndrome that included anxiety symptoms, a state of emotional "numbness," and painful and intrusive reexperiencing of traumatic events, either in recollections, nightmares, or "flashbacks." Many of these veterans petitioned for benefits but did not fit into a formal diagnostic category. At about this same time, society also became more aware of the traumatic effects of assault and rape on women. These women demonstrated a similar constellation of symptoms.

Organized psychiatry therefore included PTSD in the *DSM-III* in 1980. The diagnosis was placed in the anxiety disorders category, although clearly anxiety is but one feature of this syndrome, and some commentators have argued that we would be better off going back to the *DSM-I* formulation of PTSD as a "stress-related" disorder. The current *DSM-IV* criteria for PTSD are listed in Table 9–7.

The symptoms of PTSD can be grouped into three main categories: (1) *reexperiencing of the traumatic event* through intrusive images, nightmares, flashbacks, phobic anxiety when exposed to thoughts or situations relating to the trauma, and physiologic reactivity when exposed to such thoughts or situations; (2) *avoidance of stimuli associated with the trauma and emotional numbing*, and (3) *increased arousal and autonomic hyperactivity*, with symptoms similar to GAD. It is the reexperiencing symptoms that are the hallmark of the disorder, since the other symptoms are relatively nonspecific and can occur in a variety of other anxiety and depressive disorders.

If symptoms are noted within a month of the trauma, a diagnosis of **acute stress disorder** is assigned rather than PTSD, since in many cases these symptoms resolve over a period of weeks. PTSD is diagnosed if the symptoms persist be-

---

Table 9–7. *DSM-IV-TR* Criteria for Post-Traumatic Stress Disorder

A. The person has been exposed to a traumatic event in which both of the following were present:
   1. The person experienced, witnessed, or was confronted with an event or events that involved actual or threatened death or serious injury, or a threat to the physical integrity of self or others
   2. The person's response involved intense fear, helplessness, or horror
B. The traumatic event is persistently reexperienced in one (or more) of the following ways:
   1. Recurrent and intrusive distressing recollections of the event, including images, thoughts, or perceptions. Note: in young children, repetitive play may occur in which themes or aspects of the trauma are expressed
   2. Recurrent distressing dreams of the event. Note: in children, there may be frightening dreams without recognizable content
   3. Acting or feeling as if the traumatic event were recurring (includes a sense of reliving the experience, illusions, hallucinations, and dissociative flashback episodes, including those that occur on awakening or when intoxicated)
   4. Intense psychological distress at exposure to internal or external cues that symbolize or resemble an aspect of the traumatic event
   5. Physiological reactivity on exposure to internal or external cues that symbolize or resemble an aspect of the traumatic event
C. Persistent avoidance of stimuli associated with the trauma and numbing of general responsiveness (not present before the trauma), as indicated by three (or more) of the following:
   1. Efforts to avoid thoughts, feelings, or conversations associated with the trauma
   2. Efforts to avoid activities, places, or people that arouse recollections of the trauma
   3. Inability to recall an important aspect of the trauma
   4. Markedly diminished interest or participation in significant activities
   5. Feeling of detachment or estrangement from others
   6. Restricted range of affect (e.g., unable to have loving feelings)
   7. Sense of a foreshortened future (e.g., does not expect to have a career, marriage, children, or a normal life span)
D. Persistent symptoms of increased arousal (not present before the trauma), as indicated by two (or more) of the following:
   1. Difficulty falling or staying asleep
   2. Irritability or outbursts of anger
   3. Difficulty concentrating
   4. Hypervigilance
   5. Exaggerated startle response
E. Duration of the disturbance (symptoms in criteria B, C, and D) is more than 1 month
F. The disturbance causes clinically significant distress or impairment in social, occupational, or other important areas of functioning

Source: Reprinted with permission from the *Diagnostic and Statistical Manual of Mental Disorders, Fourth Edition, Text Revision.* Copyright 2000 American Psychiatric Association.

yond this acute period. About 50% of people exposed to a severe ("criterion A") stressor experience acute stress disorder, but after a few weeks about 50% of them no longer qualify for the diagnosis of PTSD. In the remainder, symptoms typically persist but do not worsen. Thus, about a quarter of people exposed to a severe, traumatic stressor go on to have PTSD. About half of individuals who progress to PTSD fully recover by 3 months post-trauma, but for many patients the symptoms persist beyond a year and become more chronic and disabling. "Delayed" PTSD (i.e., PTSD arising only after several months or years, in the absence of symptoms of acute stress disorder symptoms) is quite rare. It tends to appear following catastrophic events, such as an earthquake, rather than after more common events, such as assault.

PTSD and the response of people in general to trauma were initially studied in clinic populations. However, these individuals may not be typical, since have presented seeking help. Epidemiologic research reveals that up to three-quarters of the population has been exposed to a significant traumatic event at some point in their lives.

For example, consider victimization through crime or sexual abuse. In one community sample of women, 75% reported having experienced at least one victimization through crime, and most had been victimized multiple times. A quarter to a half of the surveyed women also reported having been sexually assaulted. Similarly, a nation-wide survey of college women revealed that half had been sexually victimized in some way, and the experience of 15% of the women would meet the legal definition of rape. In one telephone survey, 27% of women and 15% of men reported having a history of childhood sexual abuse. When one also includes other traumatic experiences (such as exposure to a tragic death, robbery, or severe motor vehicle accidents) one can see why a person is fortunate *not* to have been exposed to some traumatic event.

While the overall lifetime prevalence of PTSD in a person who has been exposed to a specific traumatic event is about 25%, the rate in the *general* population is estimated to be lower, between 1% and 3%, with an additional 5%–15% of individuals in the general population having experienced some symptoms of PTSD without meeting the full diagnostic criteria.

Of course, many victims of trauma experience psychiatric complications *other* than PTSD. In one survey, the prevalence of major depressive disorder, alcohol abuse or dependence, drug abuse or dependence, and phobic disorders occurred at least twice as often in victims of sexual abuse as in the general population. Similarly, traumatic events occurring early in life, especially repeated trauma, place an individual at risk for developing a personality disorder, especially borderline personality disorder. Not surprisingly, when PTSD does occur, it rarely occurs alone: the above comorbid conditions are diagnosed in up to three-quarters of patients.

The most common traumatic event for men is combat experience, while the most common event for women is physical and/or sexual assault. Note that PTSD is unique among *DSM-IV* diagnoses in that it requires individuals to have been exposed to a discrete event of one particular type for them to qualify for the diagnosis. One cannot diagnose PTSD unless this *A criterion* has been met.

The description in *DSM-IV* of the A criterion stressor represents a change from that which was listed in *DSM-III* and *DSM-IIIR*. In those editions, the stressor had to be one that was "outside the range of usual human experience" and that "would be markedly distressing to almost anyone." (Examples given in *DSM-IIIR* included "serious threat to one's life or physical integrity; serious threat or harm to one's children, spouse, or other close relatives and friends; sudden destruction of one's home or community; or seeing another person who has recently been, or is being, seriously injured or killed as the result of an accident or physical abuse.")

One problem with this definition of a "traumatic event" is that some traumatic events are very traumatic but—unfortunately—are not all that uncommon, including sexual assault. Further, two individuals might react very differently to the same event, and ideally the definition would take this into account. Given this, the *DSM-IV* definition of a "traumatic event" attempts to shift the emphasis away from the rarity of the event in question and toward the objective *nature of the event* and also toward the individual's *subjective experience of the event*. More specifically, the individual must have "experienced, witnessed, or been confronted with an event or events that involved actual or threatened death or serious injury or a threat to the physical integrity of the individual or to others." Further, the individual must have experienced "intense fear, helplessness, or horror."

This last element plays an important role in whether the individual develops PTSD. Milder, more chronic types of stress—such as job loss, divorce, or chronic illness—can contribute to individuals developing an anxiety or depressive disorder, but they don't appear to cause PTSD. The more severe the stressor, the greater the proportion of people who will develop PTSD. However, since many people exposed to extreme stress *don't* develop PTSD, the presence of a severe traumatic stressor appears to be *necessary but not sufficient* for symptoms of PTSD to occur. It is likely that when PTSD occurs following exposure to a *very severe* traumatic event, biological or personality vulnerabilities play a smaller contributory role, while when it occurs following exposure to "less severe" traumas (relatively speaking), innate dispositional factors play a more important role.

The *DSM-IV* definition of a stressor also attempts to limit the scope of the A criterion in a deliberate attempt to minimize the inappropriate use of this diagnosis in civil litigation. For example, some individuals sue their employer for having harassed them in the workplace, leading to symptoms of depression and anxiety. If an employee claims that his employer's unprofessional behavior ultimately led to his developing a major depressive disorder, the employer might respond that—since depression is a biological illness that can be caused by a variety of factors—it is unlikely that the employer's behavior "caused" the individual's depression. Given this, the employer would argue that he should not be forced to compensate the employee for either the treatment of his depression or for the problems that have arisen in his life due to depression.

If, however, an individual claims that her employer's harassing behavior led her to develop PTSD, the causal "link" between the employer's harassing behavior and the employee's symptoms is taken as more of a "given." Sometimes, the fact that an individual is experiencing PTSD symptoms is even offered as "proof" that a traumatic injury occurred. This is because in PTSD—unlike any other psychiatric illness—

symptoms are presumed to be "caused" by exposure to a particular life event. Because the diagnosis is "incident specific," it is particularly favored in civil litigation. Alan Stone, a forensic psychiatrist, has commented (1993): "No diagnosis in the history of American psychiatry has had a more dramatic and pervasive impact on law and social justice than posttraumatic stress disorder." Clearly, there are individuals who experience PTSD as a result of having been injured, and in many of these cases it is appropriate for the party that injured them to provide compensation. However, it is a misuse of psychiatry if a diagnosis is invoked as "proof" in itself of legal causation.

Despite the restrictions that the American Psychiatric Association has placed on what constitutes a traumatic event, some critics still argue that PTSD is a "political diagnosis." For example, in 1980, the Veterans Administration authorized compensation and service-related benefits for veterans with delayed-onset PTSD. The Veterans Administration rapidly was flooded with claims from uninsured veterans. Some of these veterans presented for their psychiatric evaluations obviously quoting every classic PTSD symptom from the *DSM*. Unfortunately, beyond the A criterion, all of the *DSM* criteria are based upon the self-report of subjective symptoms.

Therefore, assessing whether the veteran in fact even was exposed to a particular traumatic stressor becomes relevant. Such an evaluation typically includes a review of military records (to insure that the claimant really was at the battles he described during the clinical interview) as well as attempts to interview family members (both to verify the claimant's account of good psychological functioning prior to the traumatic experience and to verify that his currently claimed symptoms have been observed by others). Civil considerations apply during evaluations conducted in the context of private disability evaluations or personal injury suits.

Pathology and Etiology

In PTSD, a severe traumatic stressor (an unconditioned stimulus) is presented in association with intense feelings of fear, loss of control, and a powerful autonomic response (the unconditioned response). This response then generalizes to other stimuli in the patient's current environment. It is subsequently reinforced both by ensuing behavior patterns such as phobic avoidance and by reexperiencing phenomena. Over the longer term, pathological changes in mood also occur, including depression, emotional numbing, anxiety, and autonomic hyperarousal.

Certain situations are more likely to trigger PTSD, even within the group of criterion A stressors. Further, some people appear to be more vulnerable to developing the subsequent neurophysiologic and behavioral response, likely due to a combination of genetic factors, developmental factors, and current life factors.

With regard to the *traumatic experience* itself, circumstances leading to perceptions of powerlessness are particularly likely to be associated with subsequent psychological symptoms. For example, combat veterans are more likely to experience PTSD when they have been exposed to situations where they have been placed in greater danger, have witnessed the death or dismemberment of friends, have witnessed or participated in atrocities, or have suffered a physical injury leading to permanent disability. Among rape victims, those exposed to physical force, the display of a weapon, or a physical injury have a greater risk of developing PTSD. In both cases, physical injuries can serve as ongoing reminders of the original trauma and also can cause further trauma in the form of repeated hospitalizations, reconstructive surgeries, and/or chronic pain.

Some *characteristics of the victim* also are associated with a greater likelihood of developing PTSD after a trauma. For example, victims with a previous history of exposure to domestic violence or to physical or sexual abuse are more likely to develop PTSD. Some of them have experienced trauma-related symptoms earlier, for which they had successfully compensated, only to have these feelings "reactivated" by the more recent trauma. Perhaps people who have experienced earlier traumas also are "sensitized" at the neurophysiologic level such that they experience a more profound stress response in the future following objectively "less severe" traumas (similar to the "kindling" hypothesis proposed for mood disorders).

Further, trauma that has occurred earlier in life, particularly trauma that has been repeated throughout the course of childhood development, may contribute to the victim having developed a significant personality disorder, such as borderline personality disorder. These individuals already have an inconsistent view of the world, difficulty trusting others, a fragile sense of self-esteem, and heightened vulnerability to becoming depressed or anxious in response to life events. Given this, they likely are more prone to feeling helpless in the face of a new traumatic event, more prone to developing a subsequent depressive or anxiety disorder, and more prone to experiencing an exacerbation of their baseline personality vulnerabilities.

The victim's *current environment* also can serve to either facilitate or impede recovery. Family members and friends may provide a sense of security and solace, but they also may feel poorly equipped to deal with the trauma. For example, the husband of a woman who has been raped may be hindered from providing full support to his wife by his rage at the rapist or guilt about not having been there to protect his wife. Some victims also isolate themselves from family and friends, erecting a "trauma membrane." Sometimes they do allow people who themselves have either "have been through it themselves" (in the case of rape victims) or "were actually there" (in the case of Vietnam veterans) through the "membrane." Given this, group therapy for trauma survivors can play an important role in treatment. Of course, mental health professionals who attempt to facilitate such groups but aren't themselves "survivors" may be met with distrust or hostility by some members of the group.

Biological factors also appear to play a substantial role in heightening one's vulnerability to developing PTSD. For example, family studies suggest that genetic factors account for a significant percentage of the variance in whether Vietnam veterans exposed to trauma did or did not develop PTSD.

One theory is that *limbic kindling* plays a role in PTSD. Either repeated traumas or a single, severe trauma could cause excessive sensitization of the memory, anxiety, and pleasure circuits discussed in Chapter 4 and illustrated in Figures 4–2 and 4–3. Excessive activity by stress response systems (which includes the glucocorticoid, excitotoxic, and neurotrophic systems) may contribute to hyperactivity and even neurotoxicity along these circuits.

The hippocampus is particularly sensitive to such injury, and it is notable that both major depressive disorder and PTSD, conditions triggered or exacerbated by stress and associated with memory complaints, are associated with significant losses of hippocampal volume when the brains of patients with these conditions are compared to those of control subjects using volumetric magnetic resonance brain imaging.

Coordinated activity along these circuits is normally adaptive, in that it allows the organism to rapidly respond to current potential threats or rewards based on past experience. However, this network can become maladaptive when these emotional responses become autonomous and/or excessive. In the case of PTSD, neurons within these circuits may develop lower firing thresholds, such that stored traumatic memories are "replayed" either spontaneously or in response to stimuli that resemble the original trauma.

Chronic symptoms of *autonomic hyperarousal* also are present in PTSD patients. These include higher resting heart rates and blood pressure and higher urinary norepinephrine levels than those that are seen in control subjects. All of this suggests *increased noradrenergic activity* at the level of the locus ceruleus. One possibility is that heightened activity along pathways linking the locus ceruleus to the hippocampus and amygdala contributes to symptoms such as arousal, flashbacks, and nightmares.

Another possible mediator of these symptoms might be *excessive endorphin release* occurring in response to the trauma. Perhaps individuals with PTSD become "addicted" to the traumatic event, similar to the person who uses large amount of cocaine or heroin and then develops powerful withdrawal symptoms. These latter symptoms include sympathetic arousal, anxiety, psychological numbness, and dysphoria. Such people also can experience intrusive "emotional memories" of the intoxication experience along with psychological cravings, and these sensations may be analogous to the flashbacks and nightmares experienced by individuals with PTSD.

This theory might help explain the increased prevalence of substance abuse among individuals with PTSD. It also might explain why some Vietnam survivors seek out higher-risk jobs such as driving ambulances or flying airplanes, per-haps in an attempt to experience greater arousal and thereby combat psychological numbness. One empirical study consistent with this hypothesis found that Vietnam veterans with PTSD had decreased sensitivity to painful stimuli while watching a war video. Another study found that subjects with PTSD administered placebo injections were more likely to experience a placebo response than were control subjects and that this response could be blocked by the opiate antagonist naloxone (Narcan).

Not surprisingly, the norepinephrine and endorphin systems appear to be closely connected. For example, clonidine, an α-2 autoreceptor agonist that decreases neuronal norepinephrine release, helps to decrease autonomic symptoms associated with opiate withdrawal.

The closest animal model to PTSD is the *learned helplessness* paradigm. Animals administered repeated, inescapable electrical shocks ultimately develop a characteristic behavioral syndrome that includes passivity, diminished responsiveness to environmental stimuli, and an inability to act on opportunities presented to them to escape from the shocks. Of note, the propensity to develop this syndrome varies among different strains of mice raised under the same circumstances, suggesting the importance of genetic factors.

Animals placed in the learned helplessness scenario demonstrate *initial hypersecretion of brain norepinephrine* followed by *subsequent depletion of brain norepinephrine*. Learned helplessness behavior improves when animals are treated with tricyclic antidepressants, which raise brain norepinephrine and serotonin levels. In addition, animals with this syndrome develop increased analgesia that is blocked by naloxone, again suggesting that they are experiencing excessive endorphin activity.

Another biological abnormality noted in patients with PTSD is *dysregulation of the hypothalamic–pituitary–adrenal axis*. With *acute stress*, cortisol is released and enhances vigilance, physical exertion, and increased endurance. However, with *chronic stress*, cortisol secretion declines overall, along with exaggerated responsiveness of the cortisol system.

As with the other anxiety disorders, the role of *serotonin* is unclear. Serotonin activity is linked to norepinephrine activity at the level of the locus ceruleus and also is linked to regulation of mood and motivation. Decreased activity along serotonergic pathways therefore might be linked to both anxiety symptoms and symptoms of numbing, social withdrawal, and depression.

Putting these elements together, severe stress appears to alter the nervous system, leading to impairment in the normal regulation of emotions and memories. Preexisting biological and psychological conditions likely contribute to some individuals having an enhanced vulnerability to develop such dysregulation, but in the face of a severe-enough stressor, the majority of people likely experience these symptoms. Symptoms are self-limited in most cases, but in a minority of cases the syndrome progresses to the point of causing chronic disability. Superimposed on the these hormonal, chemical, and neurophysiologic changes are behavioral patterns that likely interact with the biological changes in a positive feedback loop. The goal of treatment is to interrupt this cycle, ideally at multiple points.

Treatment

Treatment of PTSD typically is multimodal. In acute but uncomplicated situations, the condition may be self-limited and intervention may not be required. For example, many individuals experienced profound feelings of anxiety and numbness along with unsettling reexperiencing phenomena (nightmares, flashbacks, and intrusive memories) in the wake of the World Trade Center tragedy. These symptoms gradually improved over time in the absence of psychiatric treatment for the majority of these individuals.

The next level of intervention is supportive psychotherapy. Patients are encouraged to process the traumatic event and to "work through" the trauma, since the symptoms of PTSD reflect in part a failure of adaptive coping mechanisms. The patient with PTSD is encouraged to "relive" the experience in a safe, controlled setting, often through mental imagery. The goal is to help the patient develop a greater sense of mastery both over the traumatic memories and over the physiologic responses associated with them. Behavioral techniques such as graded exposure to reminders of the trauma or even to the actual site of the original trauma are sometimes useful (This is the rationale for returning wounded soldiers to the front as soon as possible and for some

rape victims to later revisit the scene of their rape.) Such therapy may be supplemented by relaxation techniques or by hypnosis.

One recently described supplemental technique is *eye movement desensitization and reprocessing (EMDR)*. Here, the patient recreates the trauma through mental imagery, attending to the accompanying cognitions and sensations of arousal while also tracking the therapist's rapidly moving finger. This process is repeated until the anxiety decreases, at which point the patient is instructed to generate a positive thought and to associate it with the scene while moving his or her eyes. Case reports of this technique have been encouraging, although outcomes in controlled studies have been less impressive.

Medications also can play an important adjunctive role in treatment. However, as is typical for psychiatric disorders with a significant behavioral component, they rarely are effective when used in isolation. In studies involving patients with severe and chronic PTSD, most patients still meet the diagnostic criteria for PTSD at the conclusion of the drug study period, including those who have demonstrated a degree of symptomatic improvement.

TCAs and MAOIs are useful in treating mood and anxiety symptoms, hypervigilance, and reexperiencing phenomena. Unfortunately, they have much less effect on social withdrawal and emotional numbing. This also has been the case for treatment with *clonidine, naltrexone,* and *propranolol*.

Given the "kindling" hypothesis, *lithium and carbamazepine* have been prescribed for veterans. They do appear to help with anger outbursts, but not with the other symptoms of PTSD.

Benzodiazepines must be used with caution because they can lead to behavioral disinhibition and also to addiction (particularly in cases already complicated by substance abuse). In addition, they have little effect on numbing and reexperiencing symptoms, suggesting that these symptoms don't simply reflect a state of generalized anxiety.

SSRIs can lessen not only depression and anxiety but also reexperiencing phenomena and emotional numbing. They may be more helpful in the civilian than in the veteran population, though. Some patients are unable to tolerate the increased arousal that can be associated with these agents. These symptoms may be minimized by starting with low doses and only gradually titrating the dosage upward.

Even when these medications aren't fully effective in treating some aspects of PTSD, they may be effective in treating comorbid psychiatric conditions. They also can facilitate psychotherapy and behavioral interventions. Treatment of comorbid alcohol and substance abuse also is an essential part of treatment when these conditions are present.

OBSESSIVE–COMPULSIVE DISORDER

Phenomenology and Epidemiology

We discussed the typical symptoms of **obsessive–compulsive disorder (OCD)** in Chapter 2. The prevalence of OCD in the community is probably about 2%–3%, but the prevalence in psychiatric clinics may be as high as 10%, making it the fourth most common psychiatric diagnosis after phobias, substance-related disorders, and major depressive disorder. Comorbidity is common in OCD, with recurrent major depressive disorder occurring in up to 80% of individuals with OCD. Social phobia occurs in about 25% of affected individuals. Other anxiety disorders and alcohol or substance dependence also occur in many patients.

There appears to be a clear genetic component to OCD given that 35% of first-degree relatives of individuals with OCD also have OCD. Also, there is a significantly higher concordance rate in monozygotic twins than in dizygotic twins. However, as with the mood disorders and schizophrenia, the concordance rate in monozygotic twins is not 100%.

Whether OCD actually constitutes an anxiety disorder (beyond the fact that attempting to resist obsessions can be associated with significant anxiety) is unclear. Biological studies reveal a high prevalence of decreased REM latency, nonsuppression on the Dexamethasone Suppression Test, and decreased growth hormone secretion following clonidine infusion, all of which suggests that OCD may have more in common with major depressive disorder than it does with the other anxiety disorders.

OCD has been linked to **Tourette's disorder**, a neuropsychiatric condition characterized by vocal and complex motor tics, many of the latter being essentially indistinguishable from compulsions. About two-thirds of patients with Tourette's disorder meet criteria for OCD, and about 5% of OCD patients meet criteria for Tourette's disorder. The two conditions may be genetically linked; for example, they might be phenotypic variants of a similar genotypic vulnerability.

OCD typically becomes apparent at a young age; the mean age of onset is in the early 20s. Over half of the patients present by age 25 and three-quarters present by age 30. Cases have been described in children as young as 2 years of age. Among younger patients, there is a greater preponderance of males; however, by adulthood the ratio of males to females has equalized, suggesting that females may simply have a later age of onset.

No specific personality type has been linked to OCD. A clear distinction should be made between OCD and **obsessive–compulsive personality disorder**, despite their similar names. OCD can occur along with any personality disorder or in the absence of personality disorder. One study, using *DSM-III* criteria, found that only 6% of patients with OCD also had an obsessive–compulsive personality disorder, while a study using the broader *DSM-IIIR* criteria for obsessive–compulsive personality disorder found a prevalence of 25%. Obsessive–compulsive personality disorder is not characterized by the presence of true obsessions or compulsions; rather, it describes a lifelong pattern of pervasive preoccupation with orderliness, perfectionism, and control. If an individual manifests symptoms of *both* obsessive–compulsive disorder and obsessive–compulsive personality disorder, both diagnoses are assigned.

Pathology and Etiology

Freud postulated that OCD is caused by regression to the anal stage of psychological development, thus explaining patients' preoccupations with cleanliness and difficulties controlling sexual or aggressive thoughts. He postulated that three defense mechanisms are used against primal sexual or aggressive impulses. *Isolation* involves separating an unacceptable impulse from its associated affect such that the affect is repressed and only the (now seemingly "sense-less") impulse remains. *Undoing* occurs when isolation isn't fully successful. The patient attempts to "undo" the unacceptable obsessional impulse symbolically through compulsive behaviors. *Reaction formation* refers to the formation of obsessive–compulsive character traits, again as a defense. These traits are often the *opposite* of the underlying urges. For example, a person who has aggressive urges might present as fastidious and overly controlled.

However, clinical studies suggest that these psychodynamic theories aren't especially useful in the treatment of OCD. Psychodynamic psychotherapy might provide patients with some insights into their interpersonal functioning, but they don't decrease obsessive thoughts or compulsive behaviors.

A key aspect of OCD is that it responds preferentially to serotonergic medications—that is, the *SSRIs* and *clomipramine*. This indicates that OCD is not simply a different presentation of major depressive disorder. In major depressive disorder, noradrenergic medications such as desipramine and bupropion demonstrate efficacy equal to that associated with the SSRIs. In OCD, while noradrenergic medications are effective in treating superimposed comorbid depression, they have little effect on the OCD itself.

When patients with OCD are given m-chlorophenylpiperazine (mCPP), a 5HT agonist, OCD symptoms become worse; this effect doesn't occur in patients currently being treated with clomipramine or an SSRI. This finding is consistent with there being an upregulation of 5HT receptors in OCD, with successful treatment being associated with downregulation of these receptors. Similarly, electroconvulsive therapy isn't particularly effective in OCD, perhaps because ECT leads to downregulation of norepinephrine receptors but to *upregulation* (rather than downregulation) of serotonin receptors.

Functional neuroimaging in patients with OCD reveals a pattern of increased metabolic activity in the *orbitofrontal lobes, the caudate, and the anterior cingulate gyrus* These findings stand in contrast to those associated with conditions such as major depressive disorder and schizophrenia, since these other conditions are associated with *decreased* frontal activity and with associated impairments in "executive func-

tion"—that is, symptoms such as impaired motivation and self-care, decreased mental flexibility, and difficulty planning for the future. In contrast, patients with OCD can't *stop* engaging in such behaviors, especially when they are associated with the avoidance of potential future harm. Thus, patients with OCD almost appear to have too *much* executive function.

One theory posits that in OCD a *positive feedback loop is established between the frontal lobes and the basal ganglia*, perhaps reflecting an injury to pathways that normally serve to regulate or dampen this activity. Consistent with this hypothesis are volumetric CT and MRI studies revealing a loss of volume in the *caudate nucleus* in OCD patients. Animal models have demonstrated the presence of multiple such modulatory "loops" or "networks" in the extrapyramidal system. Thus, different frontal–basal ganglia pathways may be involved in major depressive disorder, schizophrenia, and OCD.

A subgroup of prepubescent youngsters has been identified in whom the onset of OCD symptoms occurs abruptly (with parents often able to identify the exact day of onset), in the setting of a **group A β-hemolytic streptococcal upper respiratory infection**. In these cases, the OCD symptoms may be caused either by a toxin or by an autoimmune reaction (with antibodies formed against the streptococcus ultimately becoming *antineuronal* antibodies which in turn bind preferentially to the caudate). In these children, OCD symptoms are but one of a spectrum of symptoms that can occur, part of what has been called the syndrome of "pediatric autoimmune neuropsychiatric disorders associated with streptococcal infection," or **PANDAS**. Other potential clinical manifestations include the abrupt onset of Sydenham's chorea, emotional lability, hyperactivity, oppositional behavior, tics, and/or "soft" neurologic signs.

Children who develop acute obsessional symptoms should receive a pharyngeal examination and a throat swab for a streptococcal rapid antigen detection test and/or culture. In about one-fourth of cases, the initial swab will be negative, but children should be retested in 72 hours, since it often becomes positive by then. When treated acutely, a 10-day course of antibiotics eradicates the organism and eliminates the OCD symptoms in an average of 14 days. Early recognition is essential, however, since antibiotics appear to have no effect on children with long-standing PANDAS. (The latter may reflect a "kindling" effect, in which longer-term exposure to a toxin or autoantibody ultimately leads to a permanent alteration in neuronal function.)

Dopamine also may play a role in OCD. Up to 40% of patients don't respond to SSRI therapy. Sometimes, adding an antipsychotic agent (i.e., a dopamine antagonist) helps to augment the response to an SSRI. This is consistent with a reciprocal relationship between dopamine and serotonin, as postulated in Chapter 8. For example, high doses of dopaminergic drugs (e.g., amphetamine, bromocriptine, or L-dopa) can cause stereotyped behaviors that resemble behaviors seen in OCD. Similarly, cocaine and amphetamine can worsen the symptoms of OCD and can exacerbate vocal and motor tics in Tourette's disorder, while antipsychotic agents can suppress these tics.

Our evolving understanding of OCD and its underlying pathology has led some investigators to postulate that may be a "spectrum" of obsessive–compulsive phenomena that encompasses disorders falling under a variety of *DSM-IV* diagnostic categories. What all of these disorders have in common is either *an obsessive concern or preoccupation with some aspect of bodily functioning or appearance* (e.g., body dysmorphic disorder, depersonalization disorder, anorexia nervosa, hypochondriasis), *or stereotyped, compulsive or impulsive behaviors* (Tourette's disorder, trichotillomania, paraphilias, or impulse control disorders such as pathologic gambling, kleptomania, pyromania, or self-injurious behavior). Another potential area of overlap is with neuropsychiatric conditions such as epilepsy, autism, and Huntington's disease. Many of these potential "OCD spectrum conditions" demonstrate at least a partial response to SSRIs and also may respond to cognitive and behavioral strategies similar to those used to treat OCD.

Treatment

The cornerstones of current OCD therapy are *pharmacotherapy with serotonergic antidepressants* and *behavior therapy*. While meta-analytic studies comparing different pharmacologic treatment trials have found a slightly greater antiobsessional effect to be associated with clomi-

pramine than the SSRIs, studies involving direct comparisons have found the therapeutic efficacy of all of these agents to be about the same. It is likely that since clomipramine was the first antiobsessional agent to be studied that some patients who enrolled in later trials involving the SSRIs had a more refractory illness that had not responded to earlier treatment with clomipramine, thus falsely suggesting SSRIs to be less effective.

Most clinicians initiate treatment with an SSRI since clomipramine has significant anticholinergic and antihistaminergic side effects that can make it difficult to tolerate. Compared to SSRI therapy for major depressive disorder, higher dosages and longer durations of therapy tend to be required in treating OCD. For many patients, symptom improvement may not be noted for 6–10 weeks, and symptoms may continue to improve over a period of 3 months.

Unfortunately, only about 60% of patients respond to SSRIs, and the response is usually only partial (i.e., up to about a 40% reduction in symptom severity). Failure to respond to one SSRI does not necessarily predict a failure to respond to a different SSRI. Given this, if a patient shows no response to the first medication trial after 10–12 weeks, clinicians could try switching to another SSRI. OCD is a chronic condition, and virtually all patients who discontinue the medication relapse within weeks even if they have maintained a successful response to the agent for over a year.

If an alternative SSRI or clomipramine isn't successful, or if the patient attains only a partial response, one might try adding a second agent as an augmenting strategy. Potential augmenting agents include *buspirone* (a serotonin partial agonist) or *fenfluramine* (a serotonin agonist). Unfortunately, while early case reports supporting these strategies were encouraging, placebo-controlled studies have been disappointing. Adding an *antipsychotic* agent is sometimes helpful, especially when a comorbid tic disorder such as Tourette's disorder is present.

Behavior therapy involves two major components: exposure and response prevention. *Exposure* forces patients to come into contact with feared situations while *response prevention* forces them to avoid engaging in their characteristic compulsions. In vivo exposure is more effective than exposure through imagery. For example, a patient who fears contamination might be given the assignment to touch a toilet seat (exposure). He then would not be permitted to wash his hands (response prevention).

During such an exercise, the patient's anxiety level initially increases. However, as he remains in this situation over an extended period of time, his anxiety level ultimately declines. As the exercise is repeated over the course of days and weeks, anxiety levels experienced in the course of the exercise ultimately decline to levels below those that were experienced even in the absence of having touched the toilet seat prior to the initiation of treatment.

Behavior therapy's beneficial effects tend to be more sustained than those associated with pharmacotherapy, although periodic "booster sessions" still may be required. The primary limiting factor is patient motivation and compliance with what can be a quite demanding form of treatment. With proper guidance, about 75% of patients can comply with such a program, and there is up to a 90% response rate when behavior therapy is used in combination with pharmacotherapy.

Pharmacotherapy and behavior therapy aren't mutually exclusive. In fact, pharmacotherapy may prove to be necessary in order to allow for successful behavior therapy. Pharmacotherapy doesn't decrease behavior therapy's effectiveness, since OCD symptoms typically are reduced in intensity but not eliminated by pharmacotherapy. Neuroimaging studies of patients with OCD reveal that both pharmacotherapy and behavior therapy are associated with similar changes in brain activity, with reductions being seen in right caudate metabolic activity. This finding suggests that at least some types of "psychological" interventions do affect brain activity and that psychotherapy is not simply handholding.

For the most refractory and disabling cases of OCD, neurosurgery remains an option. Decades ago, frontal lobotomies were found be effective for patients with OCD, but the procedure was associated with excessive morbidity as a result of extensive frontal lobe injury. However, highly selective, accurate stereotactic procedures now are available. The most common of these procedures are anterior cingulotomy, subcaudate tractotomy, a combination of these two interventions called limbic leucotomy, and anterior capsulo-

tomy. One retrospective study reviewed 379 cases of OCD treated with these procedures. It found that 88% of patients were either "symptom-free" or "much improved" or "improved" following the procedure. Some of these patients still required medication, but they had been converted from "nonresponders" to "responders." Complications, including cognitive side effects, were rare and tended to be very subtle.

SUMMARY

Anxiety disorders are extremely common. Because the somatic manifestations of anxiety are so diverse, clinicians from every specialty encounter patients with anxiety disorders but they sometimes focus on one or another particular symptom cluster while failing to address the anxiety disorder itself.

The anxiety disorders force us to deal with conceptual ambiguities that are more complex than those encountered in patients with delirium, dementia, or schizophrenia. We have not all experienced cognitive decline or psychosis, but we all have experienced anxiety. Therefore, where one draws the lines dividing "normal" anxiety from "pathologic" anxiety, dividing chronic "trait" anxiety from acute "state" anxiety, or dividing "autonomous" anxiety from "conditioned" anxiety isn't always clear.

This should not be surprising. While anxiety is an unpleasant sensation, it nonetheless is biologically adaptive and necessary for survival. It arises out of a complex interaction between primal biological survival mechanisms, a memory of past stressful or dangerous experiences, our current circumstances, our personality traits, conditioned behaviors, and our attitudes about whether the world in general is a safe or a dangerous place.

The anxiety disorders are a heterogeneous group of conditions. They range from a condition that may represent an exaggeration of the normal physiologic fear response (generalized anxiety disorder) to a condition that perhaps should be placed in another category (obsessive–compulsive disorder). However, what all of these conditions have in common is excessive anxiety, the presence of intrusive and anxiety-laden worries or memories, and secondary phobic behaviors.

In *generalized anxiety disorder*, both the physiologic manifestations of the anxiety response and cognitive expectations of future harm are exaggerated, leading affected individuals to experience significant distress when confronted with relatively minor life stressors. In *panic disorder*, an acute fear response occurs either spontaneously or following exposure to a relatively mild provocation. In *specific phobia*, *social phobia*, and *agoraphobia*, relatively benign stimuli have become associated with an excessive fear response, usually triggering avoidance behaviors. In *post-traumatic stress disorder*, exposure to a severe, fear-inducing stimulus ultimately triggers a constellation of symptoms including intense arousal, emotional numbing, intrusive "emotional memories." In *obsessive–compulsive disorder*, fears of particular types of potential harm become unduly amplified, leading to the development of excessive, irrational fears and compensatory behaviors.

All of these disorders are associated with biological vulnerabilities that become amplified in response to life stressors and that unfortunately come to be associated with behavior patterns that are useful in the short term but maladaptive in the longer term. Avoiding or leaving a feared situation does allow one to escape from painful, acute anxiety but it also reinforces the pathological pattern and allows the anxiety disorder to become self-perpetuating.

In the vast majority of cases, effective treatments are available. Pharmacologic therapy is a useful adjunct, but the treament of anxiety disorders typically requires more. Clinicians should educate patients about the nature of anxiety in general and about their pattern of anxiety in particular. They should explore which unpleasant somatic symptoms, thoughts, or life situations tend to reinforce their anxiety and then should attempt to help the patient discover ways in which he or she might learn to *cope* with them, even *challenge* them, rather than avoid them.

Patients with anxiety disorders demonstrate maladaptive thoughts and behaviors, but these all have arisen in response to anxiety and out of attempts to decrease this very unpleasant emotional state. Asking patients to deliberately avoid using the tools that they have come to rely upon over the years is asking a lot of them. The clinician, in proposing that patients reject their current strategies and try using new and unfamiliar ones such as medications and cognitive–behavioral interventions, are asking a lot of the patient. Patients may not follow the clinician where he or she wants the patient to go in the absence of a trusting therapeutic alliance. The clinician needs to be honest with the patient in saying that change may not come easily and that the anxiety may seem to get worse before it gets better. Patients are more likely to "stay the course" when the rationale and goals of the treatment plan are clear, both to the patient and to the clinician.

Chapter 10

Personality Disorders

Chapter 3 introduced the concepts of personality and personality disorder. Unlike the term "disease," the term "personality" doesn't describe a condition that a person *has*. Rather, it describes what a person *is*. In defining personality disorder and demarcating this diagnosis from "normal" personality, one can use either a *categorical approach* (i.e., personality disorder is distinct from normal personality) or a *dimensional approach* (i.e., personality disorder differs from normal personality only in the degree to which it deviates from what is average in the population, similar to variations in height or weight).

As might be expected for a group of disorders defined by variation along a dimensional continuum, the personality disorders are extremely common in the general population, with a prevalence of between 10% and 18% in various surveys. The prevalence is even higher in the clinical setting: 30%–50% of psychiatric outpatients have a personality disorder and 15% of inpatients are hospitalized primarily for problems attributable to personality disorder (with as many as half of the remaining inpatients having a comorbid personality disorder). Comorbid personality disorders are important to recognize, as they increase the likelihood that the other psychiatric illness will be more refractory to treatment. This is particularly true for the treatment of comorbid mood dis-

orders, anxiety disorders, and substance-related disorders.

DIMENSIONS AS FORMS

Clinicians diagnose personality disorders by noting salient aspects of patients' social histories as well as by directly assessing their interpersonal styles over the course of the diagnostic interview. They compare their impressions with the *DSM-IV*'s descriptive criteria for the various personality disorders and attempt to determine whether or not a given patient's "life picture" is close enough to the diagnostic manual's "classic picture" to be considered a "match." The investigator also must decide if a patient's personality features are so severe, maladaptive, or inflexible that it would be appropriate to assign the diagnostic label of personality disorder.

When clinicians diagnose personality disorder in a patient, they typically consider that individual to have one particular type of personality disorder. While they appreciate that the patient has a wide variety of traits, they attempt to identify one or more *prevailing themes*, such as excessive narcissism or excessive perfectionism. In contrast, research involving individuals without personality disorders reveals that most people have prominent attributes of several *different* personality types. Similarly, many patients with personality disorders, when assessed with standardized diagnostic scales, are found to actually fulfill the diagnostic criteria for *more than one* personality disorder.

Note the differences here from the process of diagnosing a condition such as dementia. In the present case, the categorical distinctions are more awkward. First, the diagnostic criteria are *disjunctive*. In other words, they are linked by the word "or" rather than the word "and." Given this, two patients with very different presentations both might be diagnosed with the same personality disorder diagnosis. Second, the *boundaries* between "normal" and "abnormal" are less clear here, particularly for cases that fall near the "margins."

Despite these limitations, typological reasoning is a powerful way of understanding people as individuals. Only by using such reasoning do we begin to understand why *particular people* might be expected to act *particular ways* when placed in *particular situations*, while other people might be expected to act very differently under the same circumstances.

Trait Theory

The building blocks of personality are **traits**. Traits are an individual's abiding, consistent tendencies to react to particular circumstances in particular ways. **Personality** reflects the overall pattern, the sum total, of all of a person's individual traits. From the dimensional perspective, every individual has every trait; although she expresses each particular trait to a greater or lesser degree than do the people around her. Expressing a particular trait to a different degree than other people may confer some protections in life, but it also may confer some vulnerabilities, depending on the particular trait in question and also one's current situation.

Just how many traits are there? If the answer turns out to be a large number, which traits are the "most relevant" ones? Over the years, trait theorists have attempted to answer these questions through empirical research and statistical analysis. One common-sense approach is to simply go to the dictionary, the repository for every natural language adjective our culture has used to describe people. In 1936, Gordon Allport and Henry Odbert combed through an unabridged English dictionary and found 18,000 descriptive words that could be meaningfully applied to people. Of course, not all descriptive words are particularly useful (e.g., "great," or "annoying"), and Allport and Odbert were able to winnow the list down to about 4000 terms.

Is it really necessary for clinicians to evaluate patients for 4000 traits? Most likely, some of these terms either are synonyms or only differ from each other in subtle ways. Two traits might be *so* similar that they probably reflect a single underlying factor. For example "dependent" people are also likely to be "needy." Other terms might overlap for some cases but not others. For example, many "volatile" people also might be described as "aggressive," but probably not all of them.

In 1946, Raymond Cattell took the list of 4000 traits and grouped together what he took to be either synonyms or near-synonyms, thereby cutting the list down to 35 personality variables. He tested his list by asking research subjects to fill out self-report questionnaires that assessed for these 35 variables. He then used a statistical tool called *factor analysis* to identify which terms appeared together ("covaried") to such an extent that they likely reflected a single underlying factor. By doing so, he was able to distill his list even more, down to 16 factors. He then devised an instrument to assess for these factors which he called the *16 Personality Factor Questionnaire (or 16PF)*, a tool that remained in use for decades.

This still sounds like a lot of factors. Obviously, one can be a "lumper" or a "splitter" with regard to how many traits one believes should constitute the "right" number. For example, a lumper might decide that there really are only two types of people, optimists and pessimists. We might even be able to assign people reliably into two groups based on this distiction. However, in doing so, we would obscure many other important aspects of personality (i.e., those aspects that aren't particularly related to whether one is an optimist or a pessimist).

In 1947, Hans Eyesenck came up with a smaller number of traits. He began with ratings provided by psychiatrists of 39 personality trait terms in 700 neurotic military men. Using factor analysis, he was able to distill this number down to two primary factors. He called these "introversion–extraversion" and "neuroticism–

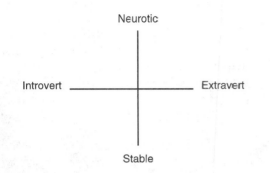

Figure 10–1. Eyesenck's two-factor model of personality

stability." These two factors formed the basis of a measure called the *Eyesenck Personality Inventory (or EPI)*, which also has been used extensively since then.

Figure 10–1 illustrates Eyesenck's two-dimension model. One can imagine each line as a bell curve rising out of the page. The majority of the general population will fall somewhere toward the center of both lines. However, some individuals will fall more toward one extreme or the other extreme of one factor, or of the other factor, or of both factors.

The trait of *neuroticism* describes a person's degree of emotional reactivity. Some people are quite stable, even to the point of appearing "bland" or "emotionless." (For example, the character of Mr. Spock from the television show *Star Trek* is a good example of an individual who would have an extremely low score on the neuroticism scale.) Other people are extremely emotional, even to the extent that relatively minor stressors cause them to become quite depressed, anxious, or angry. (The character of George Costanza from *Seinfeld* is a good example of an individual who would have an extremely high score on the neuroticism scale.)

People who are less emotionally stable have a greater risk of developing diseases such as mood disorders and anxiety disorders, as well as of developing behavioral problems such as an eating disorder or substance-related disorders. In contrast, greater personality stability confers a degree of protection. This observation could reflect the greater tendency for emotionally unstable individuals to feel overwhelmed by their circumstances, since stress can trigger or exacerbate Axis I disorders. Alternatively, it could reflect shared underlying biological diatheses toward Axis I and Axis II conditions.

Not surprisingly, the bulk of patients encountered in clinical practice have higher neuroticism scores. In other words, they would fall above the horizontal line in Figure 10–1. For clarification, the term "neuroticism" is something of a misnomer. It is easily confused with the outdated notion that psychiatric illness reflects underlying "neuroses." In fact, emotional reactivity is a normal part of personality functioning. Most people with higher degrees of neuroticism do *not* require psychiatric care, despite their having a greater *risk* of developing a psychiatric disorder.

Even among people who are very "emotional," there are differences. The characters portrayed by Woody Allen and by Robin Williams in some of their films, while both emotional, would hardly be mistaken for each other. The Woody Allen characters tend to be neurotic introverts, while the Robin Williams characters tend to be neurotic extraverts.

Individuals who score higher on the trait of **introversion** are more self-critical, more future-oriented, more bothered by uncertainty, more likely to have difficulty relaxing, more prone to worrying about minor matters, and slower to warm up to new situations or relationships (although they tend to be more persistent once they *do* finally commit to a job or a relationship).

In contrast, individuals who score higher on the trait of **extraversion** are more impulsive, more easily bored, and more interested in seeking novelty and excitement. They tend to live "in the moment" rather than worrying about what lies down the road if they make one choice rather than another. They tend to say whatever happens to be on their minds without much worry about what others might think of them.

More severe introverts and more severe extraverts both tend to experience difficulties in their lives, but the types of situations that cause problems for them are different. Introverts typically experience difficulty during periods of transition or uncertainty or where they fear that they aren't performing to the high standard that they have set for themselves. At such times, they are prone to fall into self-criticism, avoidance, anxiety, or depression. In contrast, extraverts typically experience life difficulties because of their poor impulse control and low frustration tolerance.

Since Eyesenck's EPI, other scales have been designed based upon the results of factor analysis. The number of traits that are assessed by these scales ranges between about 2 and 16. In an effort to achieve greater consensus, some investigators have administered a number of these scales to the same research subjects and then have used factor analysis to determine the extent to which the factors measured by one scale correlate with the factors measured by other scales. Several investigators have independently reached the conclusion that there are five major dimensions of personality. In addition to neuroticism and extraversion, three additional factors have been delineated: openness, agreeableness, and conscientiousness. Each dimension of personality varies relatively independently from each of the others.

Openness describes the extent to which a person takes an interest in exploring new ideas or having new aesthetic experiences (such as trying out new restaurants or traveling abroad). **Agreeableness** describes the extent to which a person tends to think the best of others, trusts others, behaves selflessly, defers to others rather than pushing his or her own agenda, and experiences sentimental feelings. **Conscientiousness** describes the extent to which a person values achievement, is self-disciplined and organized, and plans ahead.

Within each of the five major factors of personality are "subfactors." While these subfactors covary with each other in the general population viewed as a whole, particular individuals can demonstrate variation between subfactors. For example, neuroticism describes the general tendency of a person to experience *powerful emotions* (e.g., to become more angry, more depressed, and more anxious than the average person when under stress). However, there are some neurotic individuals who are much more likely to become sad than to become angry when under stress, while there are other neurotic individuals for whom the opposite is the case.

How does this *dimensional trait* model relate to the *categorical typology model* employed by *DSM-IV*? *DSM-IV* delineates *10 specific personality disorders*. Each disorder is defined by a mixture of characteristic attitudes and specific behaviors. *DSM-IV* only considers a person who expresses such attitudes and behaviors to have a **personality disorder** if the person *also* demonstrates the following features:

- There should be a characteristic pattern of difficulties in multiple areas of functioning, including *cognition* (i.e., how one perceives and interprets oneself, other people, and events), *affectivity* (i.e., the range, intensity, lability, and appropriateness of one's emotional responses), *interpersonal functioning*, and *impulse control*.
- The pattern of difficulties should be *inflexible and pervasive* across a broad range of personal and social situations.
- The pattern of difficulties should lead to *clinically significant distress* or to *impairment in social, occupational, or other important areas of functioning*.
- The pattern should be *enduring*—that is, it should follow a stable pattern and should be of long duration, with its onset traceable back at least to adolescence or early adulthood.
- The pattern should not be better accounted for as a manifestation or consequence of another mental disorder (e.g., mood disorder, anxiety disorder, or schizophrenia), and it should not be due to the effects of a substance or a general medical condition such as head trauma.

Table 10–1 schematically illustrates some hypothetical correlations between *DSM-IV* personality disorder diagnoses and variations along different domains within the five-factor model. For example, patients with histrionic personality disorder tend to have high scores on openness and agreeableness. In contrast, patients with obsessive–compulsive personality disorder tend to have low scores on openness (i.e., they are rigid) but extremely high scores on conscientiousness (i.e., they are deliberate and achievement-oriented).

The *DSM-IV* criteria for each personality disorder essentially consist of lists of particular types of traits that tend to covary. Each item from the list is only considered to be "present" when the trait that it describes is severe enough or inflexible enough to interfere with the patient's life. For example, here is the first trait criterion for obsessive–compulsive personality disorder (see Table 10–13): "is preoccupied with details, rules, lists, order, organization, or schedules to the extent that the major point of the activity is lost." An individual cannot be diagnosed with a personality disorder unless he or she "accumulates" enough of these items.

Table 10–1. The Five-Factor Model and Hypothetical Relations to *DSM-IV* Personality Disorders

Domain	*Facets*	*High*	*Low*
Neuroticism (N)	Anxiety Hostility Depression Impulsivity Vulnerability	Most Axis I and II disorders	Increased resilience?
Extroversion (E)	Warmth Gregariousness Assertiveness Activity Excitement seeking Positive emotions	Histrionic Narcissistic	Avoidant Schizoid
Openness (O)	Fantasy Aesthetics Feelings Actions Ideas Values	Schizotypal Histrionic Narcissistic	Schizoid
Agreeableness (A)	Trust Straightforwardness Altruism Compliance Modesty Tender-mindedness	Dependent Histrionic	Paranoid Antisocial Narcissistic Borderline
Conscientiousness (C)	Competence Order Dutifulness Achievement striving Self-discipline Deliberation	Obsessive-compulsive	Antisocial Borderline

Source: Adapted from data in Costa PT, Widiger, TA. *Personality Disorders and the Five-Factor Model of Personality,* second edition. Washington, D.C., American Psychological Association, 2002. Copyright © 2002 by the American Psychological Association. Adapted with permission.

However, from the dimensional perspective, it can be readily appreciated that there are far more people in the community who meet one or two of these criteria than there are who accumulate enough of them to qualify for a diagnosis of personality disorder. For example, when the Epidemiological Catchment Area (ECA) study was conducted, one research site recruited a large number of subjects from the community who agreed to submit to an extensive diagnostic interview that lasted up to 3 hours. Over the course of the interview, the evaluator assessed for each of the criteria for each of the *DSM-III* personality disorders.

For example, Figure 10–2 demonstrates the prevalence of each diagnostic criterion for obsessive–compulsive personality disorder in the general community. While 20% of people in the community have one trait that is severe enough

to count as being "present," the percentage rapidly falls off as we assess for the prevalence of people who have larger numbers of obsessive–compulsive traits. Only 12% of people had two such traits, and ultimately only 1%–2% of individuals had enough maladaptive traits for them to qualify for the diagnosis of obsessive–compulsive personality disorder.

This is essentially the procedure that most clinicians use to diagnosis personality disorder in clinical practice. They first think dimensionally about whether various traits are severe enough to consider them to be "present," and they then tally up these traits and consider whether the patient's overall degree of impairment is severe enough for patient to qualify for a personality disorder diagnosis. However, given that the average clinical interviews is largely unstructured, whether or not a maladaptive trait is recognized

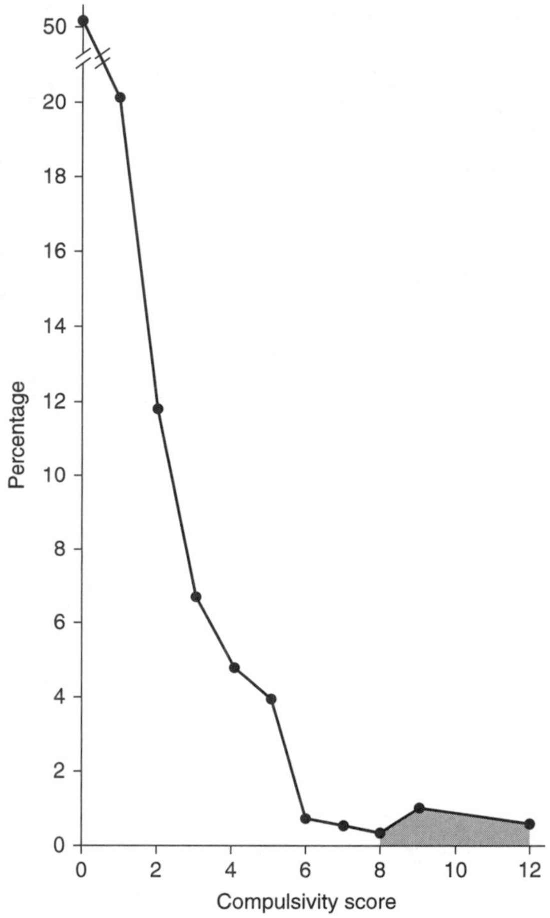

Figure 10–2. Prevalence of obsessive–compulsive traits in the community. The shaded area represents those individuals who meet the *DSM-III* criteria for obsessive–compulsive personality disorder. Nestadt G, Romanoski AJ, Brown CH, et al: "DSM-III Obsessive-Compulsive Disorder: An Epidemiological Survey." *Psychol Med* 21:461–471, 1991. Reprinted with the permission of Cambridge University Press.

depends upon a variety of factors, including what information is elicited from the patient, the patient's behavior during the interview, and the interviewer's own biases.

Consequently, the interrater reliability associated with the personality disorders is lower than that associated with most Axis I conditions, while psychological test instruments designed to generate categorical *DSM-IV* diagnoses are less reliable than scales that merely quantify different dimensional factors. For example, a *dimensional* instrument might indicate that a person who is prone to becoming acutely depressed or

anxious when her needs are frustrated scores high in neuroticism. However, it is more difficult for a *diagnostic* instrument to accurately distinguish between patients who have narcissistic personality disorder and those who have borderline personality disorder since both of these disorders are characterized by the tendency to experience excessive emotionality.

Diagnostic reliability improves considerably when we group together personality disorders that share some features. For example, we can group together narcissistic and borderline personality disorder since both conditions share the feature of excessive emotionality. The *DSM-IV* divides personality disorders into three such clusters. Table 10–2 lists the specific personality disorders within each cluster along with their key defining features.

Cluster A is comprised of individuals who often appear to be "odd or eccentric." **Cluster B** is comprised of individuals who often appear to be "dramatic, emotional, or erratic." (This group corresponds to Eyesenck's "extraverts.") **Cluster C** is comprised of individuals who often appear to be "anxious or fearful." (This group corresponds to Eyesenck's "introverts.") Specific personality disorders within each cluster differ from each other primarily in the particular *ways* that the individual expresses these predispositions.

Biological Aspects of Personality

To *describe* a person's traits and to determine where he falls along a continuum of severity doesn't *explain* how the person "got that way." How is personality formed? While several factors contribute to personality development, none is solely responsible.

Genetic factors play an important role. Strikingly, studies of monozygotic twins who have been reared separately reveal them to be as similar to each other as are identical twins who have been reared together. The twins not only have similar temperaments as measured by formal personality tests, but they tend to have adopted similar occupations, leisure activities, and social attitudes. Further, the concordance rate for personality disorder among monozygotic twins is greater than the concordance rate for dizygotic twins, which also suggests a role for genetic factors.

Table 10–2. *DSM-IV* Personality Disorders
Grouped by Diagnostic Clusters

CLUSTER A: ODD

Paranoid Personality Disorder

Distrust and suspiciousness such that others' motives are interpreted as malevolent (although not of delusional severity)

Schizoid Personality Disorder

Detachment from social relationships and a restricted range of emotional expression

Schizotypal Personality Disorder

Acute discomfort in close relationships, cognitive or perceptual distortions (although not so severe that these would be considered hallucinations), and eccentricities of behavior

CLUSTER B: DRAMATIC

Antisocial Personality Disorder

Disregard for, and violation of, the rights of others

Borderline Personality Disorder

Instability in interpersonal relationships, self-image, and affects, and marked impulsivity

Histrionic Personality Disorder

Excessive emotionality and attention seeking

Narcissistic Personality Disorder

Grandiosity, need for admiration, and lack of empathy

CLUSTER C: ANXIOUS

Avoidant Personality Disorder

Social inhibition, feelings of inadequacy, and hypersensitivity to negative evaluation

Dependent Personality Disorder

Submissive and clinging behavior, related to an excessive need to be cared for by others

Obsessive-Compulsive Personality Disorder

Preoccupation with orderliness, perfectionism, and control

While personality disorder diagnostic criteria often specify that the individual should have engaged in specific characteristic *behaviors* (e.g., self-injurious behavior, substance abuse, or behavior that violates the rights of others), much of the variation between individuals involves dimensions related to temperament. **Temperament** refers to biologically based aspects of personality such as shyness, impulsivity, intensity of one's emotions, or novelty-seeking.

A person's characteristic temperament becomes evident at a very young age, even during infancy. As discussed in Chapter 4, temperament likely reflects variations in neurotransmitter concentration, in neuroreceptor density, and in neuroreceptor configuration. These variations confer upon each of us at birth a unique "neurochemical identity," or "neurochemical fingerprint."

This is not a new idea. Genetic researchers working in the 1920s and 1930s suggested that genetic factors play a major role in determining not only one's personality but also one's predisposition toward developing mental illnesses such as schizophrenia. Unfortunately, genetic research ultimately became associated with the "eugenics" movement, which aimed to improve the genetic quality of humanity by encouraging the breeding of more genetically "fit" individuals while placing restrictions on the breeding of more "unfit" individuals (those with mental retardation, criminal records, or mental illness, for example). Eugenic theories were later relied upon by the Nazis to justify Holocaust atrocities.

After World War II, organized psychiatry largely lost interest in the field of genetics. It rejected these deterministic theories in favor of *psychoanalytic* theories, which treated infants more as "blank slates." The infant expressed pure biological *drives*, which were then shaped over the course of childhood development, through interactions with significant others (especially parents). An individual's final "personality structure" was a reflection of whether or not that individual had learned over the course of development to *channel* these basic drives in socially appropriate ways—through the use of mature, rather than immature or neurotic, defense mechanisms.

However, in a radical departure from their peers, Stella Chess and Alexander Thomas initiated the New York Longitudinal Study in the 1950s. They followed 123 children from birth through early adulthood. Over the course of the study, they identified nine different types of behavioral styles that could be identified reliably even in infants: activity level, rhythmicity (i.e., the regularity of biological functions), approach to or withdrawal from new situations, distractibility, adaptability to altered situations, sensory threshold of responsiveness to situations, quality of moods, intensity of mood expression, and attention-span/persistence. Based upon these nine categories, children in the study segregated into three main clusters.

The "easy" child demonstrated good regularity, had a positive approach to new stimuli, showed high adaptability to change, and had expressions of mood that were only mild to moderate in intensity, with positive emotions predominating.

The "difficult" child demonstrated a lack of rhythmicity, withdrew from new stimuli, exhibited slow adaptability to change, and had expressions of mood that were of high intensity, with negative emotions predominating. These children essentially fell at the opposite end of the spectrum from the "easy" child.

The "slow to warm up" child demonstrated slower adaptability and withdrawal responses to novel stimuli or changes in situation. The intensity of their responses was mild but was mostly negative when they were placed in new situations. This child, typically characterized by involved adults as being "shy" or "inhibited," corresponds to the child with high behavioral inhibition mentioned in Chapter 9 in the discussion of social phobia and its relationship to avoidant personality disorder.

Chess and Thomas found that these clusters could be identified by the time that a child was 3 years old. They usually persisted through young adulthood. "Easy children" became "easy adults." Similarly, "difficult children," while fewer in number (comprising only 10% of the sample at age 3) were far more likely to run into difficulties later in life; 70% of them would develop clinically significant behavior problems in their early to middle childhood years.

However, constitutional temperament did not appear to be the sole factor that predicted whether or not a "difficult" child went on to develop such behavioral problems. Another important factor was the interaction between their temperament and the expectations and demands of the adults around them. Chess and Thomas termed this interaction "goodness of fit." (This theory continues to provide the foundation for most self-help books on "how to raise your child.")

Given that biological factors play such an important role in determining one's personality, it is not surprising that in some cases it can be difficult to distinguish between a severe Axis II personality disorder and a chronic, subtle Axis I disorder (e.g., a mood disorder, anxiety disorder, or even a psychotic disorder). In fact, family studies involving probands with clear Axis I disorders find that many of their relatives have milder-"spectrum" conditions. While many of these relatives have never required clinical care, they often express the same biological markers as the proband. For example, relatives of probands with major depressive Disorder may fail to suppress cortisol secretion during the Dexamethasone Suppression Test, while relatives of probands with schizophrenia may demonstrate impaired smooth-pursuit eye movements.

How does the interaction between environment and biological predisposition determine whether an individual develops an Axis I disorder, an Axis II disorder, or no disorder at all? While we currently lack a detailed answer to this question, it is noteworthy that most of the same neurotransmitters that have been associated with the major symptoms of Axis I disorders (such as depression, anxiety, cognitive disturbances, and psychosis) also have been associated with the major symptoms of Axis II disorders (such as mood lability, impulsiveness, novelty-seeking, and aggressiveness). Dopamine and norepinephrine appear to be more "activating," while serotonin and GABA appear to be more "inhibitory."

For example, low cerebrospinal concentrations of the serotonin metabolite 5-hydroxyindoleacetic acid (5-HIAA) have been associated with a variety of impulsive and aggressive behaviors, including violent crimes, recurrent firesetting, and violent suicide attempts. Subtle early birth injuries and brain anoxia may further increase the likelihood that some persons will become violent. Violent criminals (who often meet the diagnostic criteria for antisocial personality disorder) who have engaged in repeated acts of violence also are more likely to demonstrate "soft" (i.e., subtle and nonspecific) neurological signs and are more likely to demonstrate nonspecific EEG abnormalities.

Several theorists have attempted to discern the connection between between Axis I and Axis II disorders by examining potential areas of overlap in their dimensional phenomenology and in their associated biomarkers. For example, Table 10–3 presents one such theoretical model.

It also is noteworthy that association cortex in the frontal, parietal, and temporal regions does

Table 10-3. Proposed Correlations between Some Axis I and Axis II Disorders, Including Potential Neurotransmitter and Other Biological Markers, Characteristic Traits, and Characteristic Coping Strategies

Dimension	Axis I	Axis II	Transmitters	Other Biological Indexes	Characteristic Traits	Defenses and Coping Strategies
Cognitive/perceptual organization	Schizophrenia	Cluster A ("odd")	Dopamine	Smooth-pursuit eye movement dysfunction, impaired executive function	Disorganization, psychotic-like symptoms	Social isolation, detachment guardedness
Impulsivity/aggression	Impulse disorders	Cluster B ("dramatic")	Serotonin, norepinephrine	Galvanic skin response	Readiness to action, irritability, aggression	Externalization, dissociation, repression
Affective instability	Mood disorders	Cluster B ("dramatic")	Norepinephrine, ? acetylcholine	REM latency	Environmentally responsive, rapid affective shifts	Exaggerated affectivity, "manipulativeness," "splitting"
Anxiety/inhibition	Anxiety disorders	Cluster C ("anxious")	GABA, norepinephrine	Heart rate variability, orienting responses, response to lactate infusion	Autonomic arousal, fearfulness, inhibition	Avoidant, compulsive, and dependent behaviors

Source: Adapted by permission from Siever LJ, Davis KL: "A Psychobiological Perspective on the Personality Disorders." *Am J Psychiatry* 148: 1647–1658, 1991. The American Psychiatric Association; http://ajp.psychiatryonline.org.

not become fully myelinated until the third or fourth decade of life, while apoptosis and synaptic "remodeling" continue to occur through young adulthood. Given this, circumstance and "goodness of fit" likely interact with one's underlying temperament in complex ways. For example, the parents of a "difficult" child may become overwhelmed as they attempt to deal with the child's problematic behaviors. (They may themselves be predisposed toward low frustration tolerance if they share their child's personality vulnerabilities.) The already-difficult child therefore may experience inconsistent nurturing, neglect, or abuse. The child, already endowed with an unstable temperament, may therefore develop the unstable sense of identity that characterizes the more severe personality disorders. The child also is at risk of developing a mood disorder, anxiety disorder, or substance-related disorder due to the combination of genetic vulnerability and childhood loss or trauma.

Similarly, the "slow to warm up" child, if reared by equally anxious and overly protective parents, may be more vulnerable to developing not only an Axis II avoidant personality disorder but also an Axis I generalized anxiety disorder or phobic disorder. This outcome may be mitigated if the child's parents consciously try to "tone down" their own disproportionate concern for their child's well-being, since that concern could reinforce the child's innate tendency to retreat from new or frightening situations.

DIMENSIONS AS FUNCTIONS

The preceding discussion has attempted to examine personality variation using the *approach from form*. First, we *delineated and labeled specific traits* as being of particular clinical interest (e.g., "aggressiveness," "novelty-seeking," and "extraversion"). Then, we *compared individuals* with regard to the extent to which they expressed these traits. In comparing them, we used two different approaches. When we compared them using a *categorical approach*, we attempted to divide them into groups (i.e., those whose traits could be labeled "maladaptive" and who therefore "have" a personality disorder versus those whose traits are "not maladaptive" and who therefore do not "have" a personality disorder). In contrast, when we compared them using a *di-*

mensional approach, we emphasized the *degree* to which different individuals expressed various traits and to what extent the variation was so far from the average that it contributed to impaired adaptive functioning.

However, personality also is something that can be appreciated *as a function*, a reflection, of an individual's meaningful attempts to deal with internal and external circumstances. By analogy, consider the example of two chairs: one chair is a large, red, fluffy beanbag chair; the other is a small, brown, wooden desk chair. Using the approach from form, these two chairs would appear to have very little in common. However, using the approach from function, they turn out to be very much the same, despite their superficial differences. Once one gains an appreciation of the function—the *purpose*—of a chair (i.e., to be something on which one can sit), their structural differences can be seen as mere matters of style. Similarly, while the approach from form might view the shy, self-deprecating person with avoidant personality disorder as the polar opposite of the aggressive, self-aggrandizing person with narcissistic personality disorder, the approach from function might lead us to see them as fundamentally the same. We might begin by asking, "*Why* do these two individuals act the way that they do? What purpose does such behavior serve?" The answer might be that perhaps both of them lack a consistent, stable sense of *self-esteem*. The avoidant person deals with this deficit by retreating from any challenges and by excessively relying on the help of other, more confident people. The narcissistic person deals with this deficit by constructing a fantasy that he is better than other people, exaggerating his achievements while denigrating those of anybody around them whom he fears might "outshine" him. However, following even a minor perceived failure or criticism, he may "inexplicably" become acutely despairing and full of self-loathing, suggesting that his fantasy has been constructed on a very shaky foundation.

Psychoanalytic theory defines personality in this manner. Patients' attitudes and behaviors are explored not for the sake of assigning some diagnostic label but in an attempt to discern what lies *behind* them. An individual's personality is considered to be the reflection the "defenses" or "coping skills" that she employs in order to deal with conflict or stress. The traditional goal of longer-term psychoanalytic therapy has been to help the patient to examine which defenses she is using, to gain insight into their nature, and to replace more "neurotic" or "immature" defenses with more "mature" defenses.

For example, some men fly into jealous rages whenever their wives speak to any other male. They may beat their wives in order to feel more in control of their lives—in order to guarantee that their wives will never abandon them or stop loving them. Psychotherapy in such a case might attempt to help them explore their anger, their lack of trust, and their excessive need for control. It might try to help them learn to empathize with their spouses rather than control them and to think ahead about the long-term consequences of their impulsive and aggressive behaviors. If an individual such as this can learn to change his attitudes and adjust his behaviors, then—by definition—he has "restructured" his personality.

Obviously, this is a very different conceptualization of "personality" than the one provided by trait theory. However, these two schools of thought are not incompatible with each other so long as one recognizes that they use the same term—"personality"—to refer to different constructs. Longitudinal studies indicate that the personality traits of individuals who have reached adulthood essentially remain stable over their remaining life span. However, one's traits are not one's destiny. While a person's underlying affective and cognitive *temperament* remains stable over the years, individuals can still "change" as a result of having examined and adjusted various preconceptions and having worked to change self-defeating patterns of behavior.

Even when these changes are relatively minor, they still can contribute to major improvements in an individual's interpersonal functioning. For example, simply helping a rigid, obsessional patient come to appreciate that there may be "more than one way to skin a cat" might allow her to feel a bit less angry and threatened when family members or coworkers fail to do things the way that *she* likes them to be done.

Similarly, one can accept the notion that an individual's behavior is strongly influenced by genetics, biochemistry, and neurophysiology without rejecting the idea that his behavior also may be serving various *psychological purposes* be-

yond his conscious awareness. For example, the last column in Table 10–3 lists some characteristic defenses and coping strategies employed by individuals of various dimensional or biological personality "types."

The notion of that there are "more mature" and "less mature" types of coping strategies was proposed by George Vaillant, based on findings from a study of 268 Harvard undergraduates followed up longitudinally from 1939 through the next several decades. Vaillant found that as people matured, the types of coping strategies that they utilized tended to shift from more immature or neurotic ones toward more mature ones. Various definitions of defenses have been proposed, and the definitions presented here rely primarily on the *DSM-IV* and on the writings of Glen Gabbard.

Mature defenses are appropriate, realistic ways of dealing with painful feelings brought on either by emotional conflict or by stressors (whether internal or external):

Altruism. The individual deals with conflict or stress through dedication to meeting the needs of others. Unlike the self-sacrifice that sometimes characterizes *reaction formation*, in this case the individual receives gratification either vicariously or from the response of others. Note that altruism isn't always used as a "defense"; research in humans and animals suggests that the drive to engage in altruistic behavior has biological roots and likely contributes to the preservation of the species as a whole.

Anticipation. The individual deals with conflict or stress by anticipating possible future adverse events, considering potential responses, and "priming herself" to experience appropriate emotions. For example, a woman who has discovered a lump on her breast and is now anxiously awaiting the results of a breast biopsy might think about what emotions she likely would feel were she to be informed that the test did in fact reveal cancer. She also might think about how she would break the news to her family and about the effect that having cancer would have on her life.

Humor. The individual deals with conflict or stress by emphasizing amusing or ironic aspects of the situation. The use of "gallows humor" by medical interns and residents in discussing critically ill patients is one example of this phenomenon.

Sublimation. The individual deals with conflict or stress by channeling potentially maladaptive feelings or impulses into socially acceptable behavior. For example, some people find that strenuous exercise or contact sports provide them with outlets for angry, anxious, or competitive impulses.

Suppression. The individual deals with conflict or stress by intentionally avoiding thinking about disturbing problems, wishes, feelings, or experiences. For example, a person who is upset about a problem that she is having at work might avoid dwelling on it all evening by reading a book or by watching television.

Affiliation. The individual deals with conflict or stress by turning to other people for help or support. This essentially is "getting by with a little help from your friends." While this involves sharing one's problems with others, it does not imply that the individual is trying to burden other people with the responsibility of solving his problem for him.

Most adults, at some points in their lives, also rely on **neurotic defenses**, particularly during periods of high stress when more mature defense mechanisms are not sufficient. However, people with personality disorders tend to rely on neurotic defenses more *frequently*, even when they are under lesser degrees of stress. Examples of neurotic defenses include the following:

Displacement. The individual deals with conflict or stress by transferring negative feelings about one object onto another, usually less threatening, substitute object. For example, a man who is furious at the way his boss treated him earlier in the day may—shortly after arriving home—become enraged over some minor behavioral infraction by his child. The anger directed at the child is extreme and inappropriate; the true object of the anger is his boss, but since the child is available and is less threatening to him, he displaces the anger he feels at his boss onto his child.

Externalization. The individual deals with conflict or stress by blaming all of one's problems on the actions of other people, rather than by taking personal responsibility. Individuals who consistently view the world in this manner are considered to have an "external locus of control." Externalization is a more general term than *projection*; the latter is an even more immature defense.

Intellectualization. The individual deals with conflict or stress by relying excessively on abstractions or generalizations or by focusing the majority of her attention on minor details in order to maintain some distance from the painful emotions associated with thinking about the situation as it "really is." One specific type of intellectualization is *rationalization,* where an individual deals with painful feelings by coming up with reassuring, self-serving, but ultimately incorrect explanations for why she is experiencing difficulties.

Dissociation. The individual deals with conflict or stress through a breakdown in the usually integrated functions of consciousness, memory, sensory–motor behavior, and perceptions of self and of the environment. Dissociation can range from mild feelings of unreality such as derealization or depersonalization (e.g., time may seem to "slow down" or perceptions may become muted during a car accident or in the midst of a combat situation) to severe dissociative fugue states or even dissociative identity disorder. Dissociation is discussed in more detail in Chapter 14.

Repression. The individual deals with conflict or stress by expelling disturbing wishes, thoughts, or experiences from conscious awareness. For example, a man who discovers that his wife has been having an extramarital affair may clearly appear to an outside observer to be in a state of rage, despite his protestations that he feels "no anger at all toward my wife or her lover." Sometimes in repression the associated *emotion* remains conscious, despite the unacceptable thoughts having been repressed. In such cases, the individual may express genuine bewilderment as to why he is feeling so angry, anxious, or sad. Repression is a less mature defense than *suppression*. In suppression, the individual is *aware* of having disturbing thoughts but *consciously* elects to avoid dwelling on them by seeking distractions. In contrast, the individual who uses repression unconsciously refuses to acknowledge his problems.

Reaction formation. The individual deals with conflict or stress related to unacceptable thoughts or feelings by substituting *diametrically opposed* thoughts or feelings. This typically usually occurs in conjunction with *repression* of the unacceptable thoughts or feelings. An example would be "hypocritical" behavior, such as publicly condemning homosexuals while privately engaging in "closet" homosexual behavior. Another example would be a minister who publicly preaches against sexual promiscuity and adultery while privately seeking out prostitutes. The loud public behavior that appears to "protest too much" might be a defense against their feelings of private personal guilt. Surprisingly, the patient might not even recognize the incongruity between his public and private behavior.

Immature defenses are used by people with more severe personality disorders. They include the following types:

Denial. The individual deals with conflict or stress by simply refusing to acknowledge some aspect of external reality or subjective experience that is readily apparent to other people. For example, the mother of a death-row inmate might refuse to accept explicit evidence of her son's guilt, insisting that her son "has always been a good boy" and that this "is all just a mistake." Similarly, an alcoholic patient whose wife and children have just left him, who has just been fired from his job, who has been arrested for driving while intoxicated, and who currently is experiencing active symptoms of alcohol withdrawal (such as a gross tremor and diaphoresis) might only admit to "having an occasional drink" while literally seeing no connection between his current difficulties and his drinking. The difference between denial and *repression* is that in the latter case the unacceptable thoughts or feelings are *internal and unconscious* (e.g., incestuous wishes, homicidal fantasies, etc.). That a patient is repressing unacceptable thoughts or feelings is something that a therapist must *infer* through the interpretation of other symptoms (such as physical complaints, compulsive behavior, or phobias). In contrast, *denial* involves ignoring an obvious, objective life situation. Denial therefore is considered an even more "immature" defense than repression.

Autistic (schizoid) fantasy. The individual deals with conflict or stress through excessive daydreaming, which acts as a substitute for engaging in human relationships or working toward solving one's problems. People with this style tend to frustrate those around them because they appear to be chronic underachievers who refuse to "make anything of their lives."

Passive–aggressive behavior. The individual deals with conflict or stress by indirectly and unassertively expressing feelings of aggression toward others. A facade of overt compliance masks covert resistance, resentment, or hostility. Examples include chronic tardiness, "forgetting" to do unappealing jobs, and frequently calling in sick due to vague somatic complaints.

Passive–aggressive individuals may be constantly amazed that family members or coworkers are upset with them, unaware that their behavior is such a source of frustration.

Acting out. The individual deals with conflict or stress by engaging in inappropriate actions rather than by thinking things through. Acting out not simply a synonym for "bad behavior," although it is often misused in this way. Rather, to label a behavior "acting out" requires that one have some evidence that the patient's inappropriate behavior relates to underlying conflicts or needs. For example, a patient with borderline personality disorder who also experienced childhood abuse may have powerful, contradictory urges to be both cared for and punished. On the psychiatric inpatient unit, she may superficially cut her arms, throw furniture, or engage in other severe, "manipulative" behaviors. These ultimately lead to the staff both restraining her and initiating "every 15-minute checks for safety." Therefore, she has not only replayed, or "acted out," her underlying psychological conflicts, but she has been successful in forcing the hospital staff to take part in her drama as well (with the staff taking on the role of the nurturing/punitive parent).

Splitting. The individual deals with conflict or stress by compartmentalizing opposite affective states. An individual engaging in splitting has difficulty integrating positive and negative qualities—either of himself or of other people—into a single, cohesive image. Therefore, his internalized images vacillate between opposite polar extremes: he sees himself or those around him either as "all good" (loving, powerful, worthy, nurturing, kind, etc.) or as "all bad" (hateful, angry, destructive, rejecting, and worthless, etc.). Note the difference between splitting and having ambivalent feelings or being in a "love–hate" relationship. In the latter situations, individuals are *aware* of experiencing multiple feelings at the same time, whereas individuals engaging in splitting can only oscillate between "all good" and "all bad" and may not even be aware that they are doing so. Sometimes, the term "splitting" is used inappropriately to refer to attempts by inpatients with borderline personality disorder to "split the staff against each other" (i.e., some staff members end up angry at the patient, while other staff members end up defending the patient). In actuality, these patients likely are "splitting" in the way that they view each *individual* staff member, and this then leads to the staff becoming divided in their individual reactions to her, leading to conflict between the staff members. (This scenario, viewed as a whole, is an example of *projective identification*.)

Projection. The individual deals with conflict or stress by falsely attributing to another person or organization his or her own unacceptable feelings, impulses, or thoughts. While the persecutory *delusions* expressed by individuals with psychotic disorders such as delusional disorder also traditionally have been considered to reflect projection by psychoanalytic theorists, *nondelusional* forms of projection are commonly encountered in individuals with more severe personality disorders. For example, a person with paranoid personality disorder might project his fears of being violated onto the U.S. government or onto a neighbor, insisting that the problem "isn't with me, it's with *them*. You just can't trust them."

Projective identification. This is a process that requires *two* people. The first individual (usually a patient) engages in *projection*, dealing with conflict or stress by falsely attributing to the second individual (either the therapist or other significant figures in her life) her own unacceptable feelings, impulses, or thoughts. However, in this case, the recipient *accepts* this projected image (usually unconsciously) and in turn projects it *back* to the patient, thereby confirming the patient's "world view." This process typically occurs with patients who have borderline personality disorder. It accounts for many of the difficulties that they encounter sustaining relationships with their lovers, employers, and therapists. It often occurs in combination with the defense of *splitting*.

For example, a patient who was abused as a child might come to see herself as being unloved and unlovable. She assumes that "nobody cares about me and nobody ever will." She then projects this attitude in all of her significant relationships. She is unable to trust, due to her belief that all this will lead to is rejection and abandonment. In her therapy sessions, she repeatedly insults and challenges the therapist. The therapist in turn begins to see the patient as an extremely frustrating and annoying person. He essentially *accepts* the image of herself that she has been projecting and begins to act toward her in ways that convey this. He might express frustration with the patient and suggest to her that if she finds so little value in his attempts to help her perhaps she would be better off seeking treatment with another therapist. This of course *confirms* the patient's "all bad" image of

herself as somebody who nobody cares about and who will just be abandoned by anybody who she allows herself to trust. Throughout this process, she also engages in *splitting* with regard to the therapist, variably seeing him as a caring, near-perfect person or as a harsh, rejecting person (but never as what he likely is, a caring but imperfect human being).

In the above example, note that the patient not only has engaged in splitting with regard to the therapist but also has *transferred* feelings from earlier relationships onto her relationship with the therapist. **Transference** describes a process whereby an individual unconsciously assigns to current significant others (including a therapist) feelings and attitudes originally associated with earlier important life figures (such as parents and siblings). One goal of psychoanalytic psychotherapy is to help the patient *recognize and examine* transference feelings as they arise in the course of therapy sessions.

Transference is most obvious when a patient's attitudes or behavior toward the therapist appear to be extreme or unrealistic. The patient might excessively idealize the therapist, seeing the therapist as a "genius"; alternatively, the patient might become severely offended by even minor slights. In the above example, note that the therapist, in *identifying* with the patient's transference feelings and *acting* on them, was expressing **countertransference** feelings and behaviors. (Such attitudes may reflect the influence of the therapist's *own* earlier relationships, since we all carry "baggage" from earlier in life that sometimes bias our attitudes in our current relationships to excessive or inappropriate degrees.) It is normal for doctors or therapists to have countertransference feelings, but—ideally—they strive to *recognize* them for what they are as they arise and try to avoid letting these feelings interfere with their ability to work with the patient in an objective, professional manner.

CLUSTER A
PERSONALITY DISORDERS

Paranoid Personality Disorder

Presentation

Paranoid personality disorder is characterized by pervasive distrust and suspiciousness of oth-

Table 10–4. *DSM-IV-TR* Criteria for Paranoid Personality Disorder

A. A pervasive distrust and suspiciousness of others such that their motives are interpreted as malevolent, beginning by early adulthood and present in a variety of contexts, as indicated by four (or more) of the following:

  1. Suspects, without sufficient basis, that others are exploiting, harming, or deceiving him or her
  2. Is preoccupied with unjustified doubts about the loyalty or trustworthiness of friends or associates
  3. Is reluctant to confide in others because of unwarranted fear that the information will be used maliciously against him or her
  4. Reads hidden demeaning or threatening meanings into benign remarks or events
  5. Persistently bears grudges, i.e., is unforgiving of insults, injuries, or slights
  6. Perceives attacks on his or her character or reputation that are not apparent to others and is quick to react angrily or to counterattack
  7. Has recurrent suspicions, without justification, regarding fidelity of spouse or sexual partner

B. Does not occur exclusively during the course of schizophrenia, a mood disorder with psychotic features, or another psychotic disorder and is not due to the direct physiological effects of a general medical condition

Note: If criteria are met prior to the onset of schizophrenia, add "premorbid"—for example, "paranoid personality disorder (premorbid)."

Source: Reprinted with permission from the *Diagnostic and Statistical Manual of Mental Disorders, Fourth Edition, Text Revision.* Copyright 2000 American Psychiatric Association.

ers (Table 10–4). Kraepelin recognized this condition, distinguishing it from schizophrenia and other psychotic disorders but theorizing that it existed along a spectrum with them and sometimes presaged the later development of delusional disorder.

Virtually every psychiatric classification scheme in the past 200 years has recognized paranoid personality disorder and has described it using similar terminology. While it has been estimated to affect between 0.5% and 2.5% of the general population, it is rarely encountered in psychiatric outpatient clinics and is diagnosed in only 1% of psychiatric inpatients.

Perhaps its low prevalence in the clinical setting reflects the fact that these individuals typically do not enjoy talking to doctors (especially psychiatrists) and also do not see their behavior as being problematic. Often, when they *do* present for a psychiatric evaluation, they have been coerced into doing so by employers concerned about their antagonistic workplace behavior or by spouses concerned about their pathological jealousy. During the evaluation, these individuals usually minimize or rationalize these concerns, perhaps even expressing surprise that anybody would have seen a need for them to be evaluated by a psychiatrist. They tend to present themselves as being fully "in control."

Paranoid personality disorder is distinguished from *schizophrenia* by the absence of clear hallucinations or delusions, despite the patient's suspicious attitude. During times of stress, however, their paranoid ideas can become more intense and more pervasive, making it more difficult to distinguish them from paranoid delusions. Paranoid personality disorder is distinguished from *schizotypal personality disorder* by the absence of the "odd" or "magical" thinking seen in the latter condition.

Etiology

Form. Paranoid personality disorder likely shares a genetic diathesis with schizophrenia, since the prevalence of paranoid personality disorder among relatives of individuals with schizophrenia is higher than that encountered in the general population. Paranoid personality disorder is even more common in the relatives of patients with delusional disorder, suggesting that all of these conditions are related and fall along a spectrum.

Function. Classic psychodynamic theory posits that the primary coping strategies engaged in by individuals with paranoid personality disorder are *externalization* and *projection*. They act in an openly hostile manner that alienates themselves from almost everybody around them, but they just don't seem to recognize this quality in themselves. Instead, they see themselves as merely responding to *other* peoples' hostile behavior toward *them*. Some writers have theorized that perhaps these individuals have repressed feelings of inadequacy that lead them to externalize all of their difficulties. They blame others for their problems whenever things go wrong in their lives rather than taking personal responsibility for their problems and ending up feeling like a failure.

Treatment

While there are isolated case reports of patients with paranoid personality disorder responding to psychotherapy, most of them refuse to engage in the therapy process, either out of a lack of motivation or a lack of trust in the therapist's intentions. The ultimate goal of psychotherapy is to help the patient learn to become more trusting. In working with such patients, therapists must try to avoid acting either overly intimate with the patient or overly challenging of the patient's beliefs. Either type of behavior may inflame the patient's paranoid tendencies. The patient may challenge the therapist, claiming, for example, that the therapist wrote down the wrong appointment date or made insulting comments at the last session. At these times, the therapist may attempt to address such issues in a straightforward manner, acknowledging that the patient is upset, apologizing if he is at fault, but also trying to avoid being overly defensive. Anecdotal experience suggests that low doses of antipsychotic medication are sometimes useful, but there is little empirical literature in this area.

Schizotypal Personality Disorder

Presentation

Schizotypal personality disorder, described in Table 10–5, affects about 3% of the general population. It is characterized by a pervasive pattern of social withdrawal and an impaired ability to form interpersonal relationships, along with bizarre or "magical" ideas that are eccentric but not clearly delusional. For example, these patients may have *ideas of reference* (beliefs that everyday neutral occurrences carry unique, personal significance) that are less firmly held than delusions of reference. It is the presence of such beliefs that distinguishes schizotypal personality disorder from *schizoid personality disorder* (which also is characterized by a restricted affect and social withdrawal) and from *paranoid personality disorder* (with also is characterized by suspiciousness).

This pattern of behavior may first become apparent to their family or peers during childhood or adolescence. Common features include solitariness, poor peer relationships, social anxiety, underachievement in school, hypersensitivity, peculiar thoughts and language, and bizarre fantasies. Their "odd" or "eccentric" manner may have made them chronic targets for teasing by their peers. Later in life, they continue to have very few friends. They may appear disheveled and their behavior may be socially inappropriate. For ex-

---

Table 10–5. *DSM-IV-TR* Criteria for Schizotypal Personality Disorder

A. A pervasive pattern of social and interpersonal deficits marked by acute discomfort with, and reduced capacity for, close relationships as well as by cognitive or perceptual distortions and eccentricities of behavior, beginning by early adulthood and present in a variety of contexts, as indicated by five (or more) of the following:
  1. Ideas of reference (excluding delusions of reference)
  2. Odd beliefs or magical thinking that influences behavior and is inconsistent with subcultural norms (e.g., superstitiousness, belief in clairvoyance, telepathy, or "sixth sense"; in children and adolescents, bizarre fantasies or preoccupations)
  3. Unusual perceptual experiences, including bodily illusions
  4. Odd thinking and speech (e.g., vague, circumstantial, metaphorical, overelaborate, or stereotyped)
  5. Suspiciousness or paranoid ideation
  6. Inappropriate or constricted affect
  7. Behavior or appearance that is odd, eccentric, or peculiar
  8. Lack of close friends or confidants other than first-degree relatives
  9. Excessive social anxiety that does not diminish with familiarity and tends to be associated with paranoid fears rather than negative judgments about self
B. Does not occur exclusively during the course of schizophrenia, a mood disorder with psychotic features, another psychotic disorder, or a pervasive developmental disorder.
Note: If criteria are met prior to the onset of schizophrenia, add "premorbid"—for example, "schizotypal personality disorder (premorbid)."

Source: Reprinted with permission from the *Diagnostic and Statistical Manual of Mental Disorders, Fourth Edition, Text Revision.* Copyright 2000 American Psychiatric Association.

ample, they may talk to themselves or strike up overly familiar conversations with strangers.

Etiology

Form. Like paranoid personality disorder and delusional disorder, schizotypal personality disorder is likely a "schizophrenia spectrum disorder." Again, among relatives of individuals with schizotypal personality disorder, there is a greater prevalence of *schizophrenia* than would otherwise have been expected, and vice versa. Many of these individuals also have the typical "biological markers" of schizophrenia, including increased cerebral ventricular size, eye-movement abnormalities, and deficits in "executive functioning" that become more apparent during formal neuropsychological testing.

While this personality has been described in patients with schizophrenia prior to their having their first "psychotic break," and while 10%–20% of individuals with schizotypal personality disorder do go on to develop schizophrenia, most patients with schizotypal personality disorder remain stable over time.

Function. Analytic theory postulates that individuals with schizotypal personality disorder engage in defensive strategies similar to those discussed for paranoid personality disorder and for schizoid personality disorder.

Treatment

As with individuals with other cluster A personality disorders, these individuals typically do not present for treatment voluntarily and do not express interest in establishing a therapeutic relationship. They ultimately may agree to treatment if they are brought in by their families for a superimposed acute illness such as a depressive or brief psychotic episode. They most often present for treatment of *depression*, and clinicians may miss the underlying personality disorder, suspecting instead that the odd beliefs are signs of a subtle depression with psychotic features. A more detailed developmental history and information from collateral informants can help the clinician make this distinction. These patients also might benefit from low doses of antipsychotic medication, but this is not well established.

Schizoid Personality Disorder

Presentation

As described in Table 10–6, individuals with **schizoid personality disorder** demonstrate a pervasive, long-standing pattern of detachment, social withdrawal, and restricted emotional range. They are typically described as "reserved," "cold," "aloof," "quiet," and "detached." They may find occupational success in solitary jobs that require little social interaction. While they might appear lonely to others, they typically deny being so. They may live with their parents through adulthood, seeking little company from others, spending hours in their room engaged in solitary activities such as reading or doing crossword puzzles.

Table 10–6. *DSM-IV-TR* Criteria for Schizoid Personality Disorder

A. A pervasive pattern of detachment from social relationships and a restricted range of expression of emotions in interpersonal settings, beginning by early adulthood and present in a variety of contexts, as indicated by four (or more) of the following:
  1. Neither desires nor enjoys close relationships, including being part of a family
  2. Almost always chooses solitary activities
  3. Has little, if any, interest in having sexual experiences with another person
  4. Takes pleasure in few, if any, activities
  5. Lacks close friends or confidants other than first-degree relatives
  6. Appears indifferent to the praise or criticism of others
  7. Shows emotional coldness, detachment, or flattened affectivity
B. Does not occur exclusively during the course of schizophrenia, a mood disorder with psychotic features, another psychotic disorder, or a pervasive developmental disorder and is not due to the direct physiological effects of a general medical condition

Note: If criteria are met prior to the onset of schizophrenia, add "premorbid"—for example, "schizoid personality disorder (premorbid)"

Source: Reprinted with permission from the *Diagnostic and Statistical Manual of Mental Disorders, Fourth Edition, Text Revision.* Copyright 2000 American Psychiatric Association.

Some community surveys have revealed a prevalence of schizoid personality disorder of as high as 7%. Based on personal experience, one wouldn't expect such a high prevalence, and yet these people often go unnoticed. They are rarely encountered in psychiatric practice, since they don't tend to complain of depression or anxiety; rather, they are detached from life, almost emotionless. They may be brought for evaluation by their parents, who may voice concern at their grown child's failure to leave home, marry, or otherwise establish an independent life. They also may present for treatment of a comorbid psychiatric condition, such as major depressive disorder.

Etiology

Form. The condition resembles the negative symptoms of schizophrenia in the absence of overt positive symptoms. While some family studies have suggested a possible genetic association with schizophrenia, the genetic links appear to be weaker than those observed between schizophrenia and paranoid personality disorder and schizotypal personality disorder. Dimensionally, these patients (along with patients with schizotypal and avoidant personality disorder) score high on *introversion*, and this trait does demonstrate significant heritability.

Function. Psychoanalytic theory has emphasized the defense mechanism of *autistic fantasy*— that is, turning inward as a retreat from external reality.

Treatment

As with the other cluster A personality disorders, these patients often see little value in establishing a therapeutic relationship. They may be willing to accept medication or psychotherapy for treatment of a superimposed depression but may also express a preference to keep the treatment "limited to this." Sometimes writing assignments or exercises may help "break the ice" in establishing a therapeutic relationship, as these patients may otherwise shy away from intimacy. Similarly, while the therapist may suggest group therapy as a means of helping the patient learn to interact appropriately with others, these patients generally are uninterested in joining a group. Conceivably, low doses of an atypical antipsychotic agent may be helpful, but there is little empirical research to guide the clinician in this regard.

CLUSTER B
PERSONALITY DISORDERS

Antisocial Personality Disorder

Presentation

Like paranoid personality disorder, **antisocial personality disorder** (described in Table 10–7) has been recognized by every major psychiatric diagnostic scheme over the past two centuries, although it has repeatedly confounded clinicians' attempts to fully understand it. Individuals with

Table 10–7. *DSM-IV-TR* Criteria for Antisocial Personality Disorder

---

A. There is a pervasive pattern of disregard for and violation of the rights of others occurring since age 15 years, as indicated by three (or more) of the following:
   1. Failure to conform to social norms with respect to lawful behaviors as indicated by repeatedly performing acts that are grounds for arrest
   2. Deceitfulness, as indicated by repeated lying, use of aliases, or conning others for personal profit or pleasure
   3. Impulsivity or failure to plan ahead
   4. Irritability and aggressiveness, as indicated by repeated physical fights or assaults
   5. Reckless disregard for safety of self or others
   6. Consistent irresponsibility, as indicated by repeated failure to sustain consistent work behavior or honor financial obligations
   7. Lack of remorse, as indicated by being indifferent to or rationalizing having hurt, mistreated, or stolen from another
B. The individual is at least age 18 years.
C. There is evidence of conduct disorder . . . with onset before age 15 years
D. The occurrence of antisocial behavior is not exclusively during the course of schizophrenia or a manic episode

---

Source: Reprinted with permission from the *Diagnostic and Statistical Manual of Mental Disorders, Fourth Edition, Text Revision.* Copyright 2000 American Psychiatric Association.

antisocial personality disorder rarely commit to psychiatric treatment in more than a superficial and self-serving way, and the inclination of clinicians is to allow the legal system to deal with them. However, the courts tend to recognize that something appears to be "wrong" with many of these individuals, especially when the disorder first presents in childhood or adolescence, and they may therefore refer them for psychiatric care. Thus, these individuals sometimes bounce back and forth between the medical system and legal system.

The major feature of antisocial personality disorder is disregard for and violation of the rights of others. Early descriptions emphasized a striking absence of "morality" in these individuals, to the point where their behavior can seem to have little logical purpose. For example, an individual might impulsively lie, just for the sake of getting away with it. Given this, in the 1800s the disorder was called "moral insanity."

In the 1940s, Hervey Cleckley reported detailed case histories of several such individuals and in doing so suggested that in these individuals a superficial veneer of composure and normality concealed considerable disorganization as well as a lack of self-control or direction. Cleckley considered people with antisocial personality disorder (or, as he called them, "psychopaths") to have only a "mask of sanity." He described how these individuals didn't appear to have empathy for others and didn't even appear to have a "conscience," despite being able to engage in facile, superficial displays of affection when it served their purposes. He also emphasized their glib charm and their lack of remorse for their antisocial behavior.

DSM-I and *DSM-II* were heavily influenced by Cleckley's formulation. However, the authors of the *DSM-III* criteria were primarily interested in diagnostic reliability. Given this, they were concerned that "lack of empathy" was simply too subjective and vague a criterion to reliably assess. The *DSM-III* criteria therefore emphasized particular antisocial *behaviors*, As a result, antisocial personality disorder became a disorder characterized by repeated episodes of lying, stealing, arrests, substance use, and socially irresponsible behavior. In consequence, the *DSM-III* did achieve significant reliability. For example, antisocial personality disorder was the only personality disorder assessed for in the ECA study. It wasn't clear how to assess for other personality disorders using a standardized "yes–no" interview.

Unfortunately, in emphasizing antisocial *behavior*, the *DSM-III* (and later the *DSM-IIIR*) criteria may have been too broad, including many individuals who lied or stole in order to support a drug habit but who lacked the core "sociopathic" features described by Cleckley. Similarly, there may be many "psychopaths" who succeed in life in spite of (perhaps even as a result of) these personality features. These individuals perhaps may fail to meet many of the behavioral criteria, perhaps due to greater intelligence or self-control. For example, they may have become successful salesmen or politicians rather than career criminals.

In other words, the *DSM-III* criteria may have achieved reliability at the expense of construct validity. *DSM-IV* attempted to at least partially rectify the situation by adding back a criterion specifying that these individual may "lack remorse" for their antisocial behavior.

There are some areas of overlap between antisocial personality disorder and *narcissistic personality disorder*, including superficiality and lack of empathy, and these conditions may reflect a similar underlying genetic diathesis. However, individuals with antisocial personality disorder tend to be more impulsive and are more likely to have a history of violence and criminal behavior. In addition, they don't seem to place as much of a premium on achieving the affection and admiration of others as do individuals with narcissistic personality disorder.

According to the ECA study, the prevalence of antisocial personality disorder in the community is about 3% for men and 1% for women. There is a higher prevalence in lower socioeconomic urban populations. Half of the prison population has antisocial personality disorder. While the prevalence is about 2% in the clinic population, in drug treatment or probation program settings the prevalence is closer to 20% of men and 10% of women. It may be that the condition is underdiagnosed in women due to diagnostic gender bias. (For the same reason, borderline personality disorder may be underdiagnosed in men.)

Antisocial personality disorder is lifelong. By definition there must be signs of a childhood *conduct disorder*, with onset before age 15. However, in some individuals, the temperamental features of impulsiveness and aggression may decline with age. Their period of highest risk for engaging in violent crime is the late teens and early 20s. People with high levels of "psychopathy" tend to continue to display a high degree of criminality until about age 40. After this point, there is a decline in the overall rate of recidivism, although it should be noted that half of all individuals with antisocial personality disorder continue to be convicted of crimes after age 40. The ECA study found that, in the community, the prevalence of antisocial personality disorder is lower among people in their later years. However, it isn't clear whether there are fewer older people with antisocial personality disorder because the tendency toward psychopathy declines with advancing age or because individuals with antisocial personality disorder demonstrate early mortality as a result of their greater tendency to engage in a high-risk behaviors or get into violent altercations.

Etiology

Genetic factors appear to play an important role in antisocial personality disorder. The prevalence of antisocial personality disorder is greater among first-degree relatives of probands with the disorder than it is in the general population. The risk to biological relatives of females with the disorder tends to be higher than the risk to biological relatives of males with the disorder. This suggests that females may require a greater "genetic load" if they are to develop the disorder. There appears to be a higher concordance rate in monozygotic than in dizygotic twins, again consistent with a genetic contribution.

Biological relatives of persons with this disorder also are more likely than the average person to have *somatization disorder* and *substance-related disorders*, indicating possible shared temperamental dispositions. Gender appears to influence the presentation: if a family has one member with antisocial personality disorder, the males in that family more often have antisocial personality disorder and substance-related disorders, whereas the females more often have somatization disorder. Perhaps females with this temperament are more likely than men to complain of medical symptoms, while men with this temperament are more likely to engage in criminal behavior. (Of note, however, in these families there is an increase in the prevalence of all of these disorders in *both* males and females compared with the general population.)

Adoption studies indicate that both genetic and environmental factors contribute to the risk of developing this group of disorders, but they do confirm a strong genetic factor, in that adopted-away children resemble their biological parents more than they resemble their adoptive parents. The greatest degree of conduct problems is found in adopted-away children of a biological parent with antisocial personality disorder who are then unfortunate enough to be placed into yet another "disturbed" household (i.e., the adoptive parents also have problems with drugs, alcohol, or the law). However, children with a parental history of antisocial personality disorder who are placed in a "stable" household demonstrate a lower degree of conduct problems and aggression. Finally, adopted children with no history of antisocial personality disorder in the biological parents have a low incidence of conduct problems even when they are placed into a "disturbed" adoptive household.

There is also evidence that some patients with antisocial personality disorder have certain distinctive electrophysiological responses, such as decreased galvanic skin response and a diminished cortical EEG response to novel stimuli. Perhaps these findings are due to superimposed attention-deficit hyperactivity features, but they raise the question as to whether people with antisocial personality disorder require more stimulation than other people, thus accounting for their low threshold for becoming bored and their constant search for excitement and risk.

Therefore, in antisocial personality disorder there appears to be an underlying biological temperament that is further shaped by exposure during childhood to an erratic parenting, abuse or neglect, attention-deficit hyperactivity disorder, poverty, early substance abuse, or growing up in a large family with limited structure. It is also likely that at least in some cases, antisocial personality disorder may arise solely out of such an environmental background.

Treatment

No particular psychological or biological treatment has been found to be especially helpful. Patients may present for treatment as a condition of probation for a criminal offense or they may present to the inpatient unit on a civil commitment order after threatening violence against others. They may present voluntarily for alcohol or drug treatment. Psychotherapy often is hindered by these individuals' lack of desire to change. However, psychotherapy may still be helpful for selected individuals who do have some capacity for empathy (since this, too, varies along a dimension of severity) or who recognize how their antisocial behavior has hindered them from achieving more in life. SSRI medications may be useful adjuncts to treatment, since they can decrease irritability or impulsive aggression; however, their use in antisocial personality disorder hasn't been systematically studied. A similar case could be made for anticonvulsant medications, lithium, and atypical antipsychotic medications. It should be noted that medications may be useful in decreasing *impulsive* aggression, but they are not likely to decrease the risk of patients engaging in *premeditated* aggressive acts.

Borderline Personality Disorder

Presentation

A 32-year-old woman with borderline personality disorder is admitted to the inpatient unit after overdosing and superficially cutting her wrists. On the second night of her hospital stay, she attempts to cut her wrists with a plastic knife and then repeatedly slams herself against the door to the unit. She is placed in four-point restraints to protect against further self-injurious behavior. The next morning the patient is in tears over the way that she was treated by the nursing staff who had been working the night shift. She attributed having been placed in restraints to their punitive, uncaring attitude. After speaking with the patient on morning rounds, the treating psychiatric resident confronts the nurse who initially placed the patient in restraints, seeing the action as excessive and hostile. The nurse defends her actions and goes on to criticize the resident for repeatedly undermining the authority and credibility of the nursing staff in their attempts to work with the patients on the unit. This conflict ultimately reaches the level of the attending psychiatrist, who calls a team meeting to "process" this conflict.

Questioning by the attending reveals that on the day of the patient's admission, during the patient's intake interview, the resident felt that he and the patient had developed a strong working alliance. The patient seemed to him like a sympathetic person who had been through several very traumatic life experiences but appeared to be "psychologically minded" and very motivated to examine these issues. While the resident usually didn't have much time on the busy inpatient service to engage in one-to-one psychotherapy, he thought that this case would demand it. He also thought that he could learn a lot about psychotherapy from working with the patient. Finally, he thought that it was likely that after a few sessions the patient would start to feel much better, given that she already appeared to have benefited just from having had this initial opportunity to discuss her problems. The patient had commented at the end of the interview that she had been to many physicians, but that the resident had been the first one to really understand her current difficulties.

On the day after admission, the patient approached the resident after he had led the morning psychotherapy group to say that this was the best group that she had attended in some time and that she really appreciated the way that he had put some of the patient's issues into better perspective. She then asked if she could talk to him about something that she hadn't been able to tell anyone, since she felt that she could trust him. He brought her to his office, where she related an extensive history of childhood sexual abuse by her father. This turned into a lengthy session. Afterwards, the resident was emotionally drained but felt that he and the patient had made "real headway."

The patient's old charts arrived on the unit, and they were extensive. Her history included multiple admissions, and she had been treated by at least six different local therapists over the past several years. Despite this, the resident wondered whether he might pick up the patient as an outpatient after she was discharged, since—given the progress that they are making—"this time it might be different."

On the night in question, the patient came to the nursing station and demanded to sign out of the hospital following an argument on the telephone with her boyfriend. She entered the nursing station and was informed by charge nurse that she wasn't allowed into the nursing station. She was asked to sit outside the nursing station and was informed that her nurse would meet her there shortly. The patient at this point yelled that she wanted to talk to somebody, "Right now!" The nurse reiterated, "Sit outside the nursing station and I will call for your nurse. Right now she's giving medication to another patient." The patient then pulled out a plastic knife (which she previously had concealed in her shoe), cut her wrist, and began banging on the locked doors of the unit, ultimately throwing herself against them. She then was placed in restraints and at that point began yelling at the charge nurse, "You bitch! You bitch!" She also attempted to spit on the nurse. She calmed in about a half-hour, but the nursing staff kept her in restraints for another 2 hours as she remained overtly hostile and her behavior potentially placed herself, other patients, and the staff at risk.

The next morning she complained about this "punitive" treatment to the resident, saying that the nurses could "at least have given me a chance out of restraints." The resident felt that the patient already had suffered extensive victimization throughout her life and was now again being victimized, only this time by hospital staff rather than by her father.

What is going on in the above case example? From the psychodynamic perspective, this scenario offers examples of the use of several defense mechanisms. From the outset of treatment, the patient engaged in "splitting," which is a hallmark feature of borderline personality disorder. She idealized the psychiatry resident as being "all good," different from all of her previous therapists. The resident in turn responded by falling into *countertransferential* "rescue fantasies."

This is also an example of "*projective identification.*" Here, the patient views herself as a lost waif and the resident as her rescuer. The resident *identifies* with this image, both of the patient and of himself, and he begins to offer comfort and solace rather than more detached, clinical concern. He projects his own image of their relationship back to her, and she in turn accepts this image. He doesn't recognize how he has been subtly *led* into this relationship. (Incidentally, one can also see how patients with borderline personality disorder are at high risk of entering into inappropriate sexual relationships with their therapists during the course of treatment. Typically, the relationship has evolved into an intensely emotional one, with a gradual erosion of treatment "boundaries." The sexual relationship typically represents the culmination of this process, despite it often seeming to both the patient and the therapist that it "just happened one day.")

The patient has engaged in a similar process with the nursing staff. She sees herself as being "abused" by the nurses, just as she has been abused by earlier authority figures. Again this is "splitting." In contrast to the resident, who was seen as "all good," in this case the nurses are seen as being "all bad." The patient also acts differently around the nurses than she acts around the resident: around the nurses, she isn't a fragile waif but a "problem patient," hostile and belligerent, believing herself to be entitled to more attention than any of the other patients on the unit.

Not surprisingly, the nursing staff, like the resident, begins to respond to the patient, in turn, by becoming angry and resentful. Again, this is an example of projective identification. Here the patient projects the "problem patient" image to the staff, who in turn accept this image and convey back to the patient (through their negative attitudes) that this is exactly how they see her as well. The ultimate example of this process is patient's severe act of violence when frustrated by the staff, leading to the staff physically restraining her. Thus, the patient has gotten people to act toward her in a way that confirms the negative view she has of herself. She feels that she is unstable, and the staff treats her as if she is unstable; she feels that people don't like her, and the way the staff treats her confirms this. However, what she doesn't see is the role she herself has played in orchestrating the behavior of those around her.

Note that this patient also displays *rapidly shifting moods* and *extremely poor impulse control*. Over the course of several hours, she has shifted from appearing to be "psychologically minded" and a "good therapy candidate" to becoming so severely agitated that she had to be restrained. She also has an *unstable self-image*, acting differently around different people, even feeling differently about whether she deserves to live or die over the course of several hours.

These all are hallmark features of **borderline personality disorder**. Individuals of this personality type demonstrate a pervasive pattern of instability in their interpersonal relationships, self-image, and moods, as well as marked impulsivity (Table 10–8). Borderline personality disorder occurs in 2%–3% of the general population but it is overrepresented in the clinical pop-

Table 10–8. *DSM-IV-TR* Criteria for Borderline Personality Disorder

A pervasive pattern of instability of interpersonal relationships, self-image, and affects, and marked impulsivity beginning by early adulthood and present in a variety of contexts, as indicated by five (or more) of the following:

1. Frantic efforts to avoid real or imagined abandonment. Note: Do not include suicidal or self-mutilating behavior covered in criterion 5
2. A pattern of unstable and intense interpersonal relationships characterized by alternating between extremes of idealization and devaluation
3. Identity disturbance: markedly and persistently unstable self-image or sense of self
4. Impulsivity in at least two areas that are potentially self-damaging (e.g., spending, sex, substance abuse, reckless driving, binge eating). Note: do not include suicidal or self-mutilating behavior covered in criterion 5
5. Recurrent suicidal behavior, gestures, or threats, or self-mutilating behavior
6. Affective instability due to a marked reactivity of mood (e.g., intense episodic dysphoria, irritability, or anxiety usually lasting a few hours and only rarely more than a few days)
7. Chronic feelings of emptiness
8. Inappropriate, intense anger or difficulty controlling anger (e.g., frequent displays of temper, constant anger, recurrent physical fights)
9. Transient, stress-related paranoid ideation or severe dissociative symptoms

Source: Reprinted with permission from the *Diagnostic and Statistical Manual of Mental Disorders, Fourth Edition, Text Revision.* Copyright 2000 American Psychiatric Association.

ulation, where it is the most common personality disorder encountered. Twenty percent of psychiatric inpatients meet the criteria for borderline personality disorder.

Borderline personality disorder has been recognized as a discrete diagnosis only over the past few decades. The label itself only first appeared in the *DSM-III*. The diagnostic label unfortunately is misleading and an anachronism. A better label might be "unstable personality disorder." The term "borderline" reflects early psychoanalytic conceptions—that this personality disorder straddled the "border" between neurosis and psychosis. However, subsequent research has not confirmed this conceptual model. What these early commentators appear to have been noticing was that there appears to be a particular type of patient who appears at first glance to be high-functioning but who can rapidly regress over the course of more intensive psychotherapy. While these patients can become very disorganized, they are not "psychotic" in the traditional sense.

The characteristic problems that these individuals encounter with their therapists parallel the difficulties that they encounter with other important figures in their lives. They alternate between overidealizing and devaluing them, and their relationships therefore tend to be both intense and unstable. They make frantic efforts to avoid real or imagined abandonment. They also have an unstable sense of self, with no sense of

"direction." While they frequently complain of "depression," most often the emotions that they are describing are "anger," "loneliness," "emptiness," or "boredom" rather than "sadness." (This overall emotional state has been called "dysphoria.")

Like their moods and their views of themselves and others, their behavior also is intense and unstable. They are prone to engage in impulsive behavior in multiple realms (spending, sex, substance abuse, driving, binge eating), and they also are prone to engage in impulsive self-injurious behaviors. They may make suicidal threats or engage in milder suicidal "gestures."

During times of stress, these patients even may experience so-called "micropsychotic episodes" where they become very regressed, display paranoid thinking, and complain of dissociative symptoms (such as amnesia) or of hearing "voices" that tell them to hurt themselves. In contrast to more common psychotic phenomenon such as those that are encountered in schizophrenia, these symptoms usually appear to be more self-serving. They often have the quality of pseudohallucinations, and the patient may appear to be remarkably intact when observed outside of the context of the *clinical interaction.* (For example, the patient may appear to be fine when she is unobtrusively observed talking on the telephone just a few minutes after she appeared withdrawn, distraught, and psychotic during a clinical interview.) "Bizarre" thinking, such as that which is seen in schizotypal personality disorder or in schizophrenia, is notably absent.

Etiology

Form. There appears to be genetic contribution to borderline personality disorder: family studies reveal the disorder to be five times more common among first-degree relatives of probands with the disorder than it is in the general population. Substance-related disorders, mood disorders, and antisocial personality disorder also are more common in members of their extended family. However, one small study found no difference in concordance rate in monozygotic versus dizygotic twins. Patients with more severe forms of borderline personality disorder, who engage in self-injurious behaviors and who are more prone to rage and affective instability, appear to have lower levels of cerebrospinal fluid (CSF) serotonin metabolites. This suggests that low serotonin activity may be a biologic correlate. Patients with more severe forms of the disorder also sometimes demonstrate neurologic "soft signs."

Function. The major defense mechanisms employed by individuals with borderline personality disorder are *splitting* and *projective identification*. Theories of the psychological roots of borderline personality disorder have focused on the role of early childhood interactions, especially with parental figures. The most influential theory has been based on Margaret Mahler's theories of separation–individuation.

This theory postulates that individuals with borderline personality disorder have failed to develop *emotional object constancy* during the *rapprochement phase* of development, which occurs at around age 2. During this phase, the child develops autonomy through the recognition that her parents remain available even when the child is "out on her own." Doing this requires the child to have previous established an ability to trust her parents to behave toward her in a reliable manner. In contrast, when a child's parents have been unavailable or punitive, the child may develop a profound lack of confidence in herself and in the availability of significant others, along with profound fears of being abandoned.

Unfortunately, studies in children have failed to provide empirical support for this theory. While this process may occur in some families, difficulties at this stage of development appear to be neither necessary nor sufficient to explain the occurrence of borderline personality disorder. Other theories have emphasized more generally how—*throughout* these individuals' childhoods—their parents have been either inconsistent or unavailable. This may reflect either of their parents having engaged in a similar interpersonal style. (For example, when the patient as a child became angry at her parents, as all children routinely do, one parent may have reacted by thinking, "If you don't want anything to do with me, I don't want anything to do with you." This in turn may have encouraged the patient to develop pathological attitudes such as splitting— hating her parents but also loving her parents— and projective identification.)

Family studies have supported these theories, revealing that both of such patients' parents often demonstrate significant psychopathology. Mothers tend to be erratic and depressed, whereas fathers tend to be absent or uninvolved. The early family environment as a whole tends to have been chaotic, marked by violence, by the patient's parents having separated or divorced, by parental alcohol abuse, and by histories of abuse.

There appears to be a higher rate of childhood neglect and abuse, including sexual abuse, in these families. There also is a higher rate of early parental loss and/or of traumatic separation. These factors may have contributed to these individuals having developed such intense dependency and fears of abandonment. In Chapter 6, we discussed how having experienced childhood abuse or neglect can cause children to cling *more* tenaciously to their abuser. Also in support of this theory is the finding that patients with borderline personality disorder are more likely than other patients (such as those with antisocial personality disorder) to have continued to hold onto "transitional objects" (such as stuffed animals) for extended periods. (This pattern even may have persisted into adulthood. It isn't uncommon when working on an inpatient unit to encounter patients who have brought their favorite stuffed animal with them to the hospital.)

Treatment

The treatment of choice for borderline personality disorder is long-term psychotherapy. However, therapy commonly is complicated by behavioral problems and "acting out." Other patients angrily quit therapy. Goals of therapy include helping to keep patients out of the hospital and helping to keep them from committing suicide. About 10% of patients with borderline personality disorder ultimately go on to die by suicide. Sometimes they do so accidentally during what initially was intended to be a suicide "gesture." Given this, even these "gestures" need to be taken seriously.

Over the course of psychotherapy, the patient typically engages in splitting and projective identification. Ideally, the therapist recognizes that this process is occurring and avoids acting on it in kind. Rather, the therapist attempts to *modify* the patient's projected affects and to present them back to the patient in a more *appropriate* form.

For example, an *inappropriate* interaction might occur following the patient's having repeatedly stated to the therapist: "I'm a bad person and you are mad at me and want to get rid of me." The therapist might become annoyed with the patient, ultimately stating that perhaps she is right, perhaps she could be better served by a different therapist. The patient then "reintrojects" this image of herself as "a bad person who the therapist wants to get rid of."

The *appropriate* interaction would be for the therapist to recognize this projection, to also recognize his or her own rising anger, and then to state to the patient, "You know, you get me very upset and even angry when you act this way. Maybe we should look at what's going on here." As a result of this interaction, the patient might reintroject an image of herself as "a troubled person who does things that get people mad, but who needs to work on this." The therapeutic interaction therefore helps the patient to change her view of herself, of the outside world, and of her place in it. *Group therapy* can offer similar benefits, as it can allow the patient to obtain more accurate feedback as to how peers actually perceive her and of her own contributions to these perceptions.

A cornerstone of psychotherapy is the conviction that patients with borderline personality disorder are doing the best that they can with the skills that they have. The goal is to help these patients to learn new coping skills. One hopes that their way of relating to the world isn't carved in stone, but is at least slightly malleable. While their *personalities* are unlikely to change as a result of therapy, they still may be able to learn to think about their world differently or to become more attentive to the role that they play in their relationship difficulties.

Medications haven't proven to be a panacea, but sometimes they can play a very useful complementary role. SSRIs can be effective in combating affective lability, dysphoria, anger, and impulsiveness. They may have to be prescribed in higher dosages and for longer treatment trials than in major depressive disorder. Carbamazepine or lithium may also be effective in helping with modulation of anger. They also should be considered when the personal or family history suggests a diathesis toward bipolar disorder. Low doses of antipsychotics may be helpful not only to treat paranoid thinking but also to treat excessive anger and affective lability. They should be discontinued as soon as feasible due to their potential to cause tardive dyskinesia. No medications have been found at this point to be especially useful for symptoms of identity disturbance. Benzodiazepines are not especially useful in inhibiting self-injurious behaviors, and in fact sometimes lower patients' inhibitions in this regard. They also carry the potential for addiction. Therefore, benzodiazepines should be avoided if possible. (This being said, many patients with borderline personality disorder experience significant anxiety, including panic attacks, and ultimately are treated with benzodiazepines).

The clinician should continually assess for superimposed major depressive episodes, either with "atypical" features or with melancholic features. MAOIs can be helpful, but they carry the risk of causing hypertensive crises in this population, since patients with borderline personality disorder may fail to follow dietary restrictions, either to "test limits" or out of attempts to harm themselves. SSRIs therefore have become the most prescribed antidepressants in these patients. TCAs haven't proven to be as effective in this population and they sometimes are destabilizing, perhaps due to their greater noradrenergic component.

Unlike patients with schizophrenia, patients with borderline personality disorder have been described as being "stably unstable." In other words, despite their episodic crises, they don't tend to deteriorate over time. Longitudinal studies reveal that about a third of patients with borderline personality disorder achieve some greater consistency and improved ability to sustain jobs and relationships over time. Another third learn to function at a more reasonable, albeit somewhat unhappy level. They often have learned that their best course of action is to live alone and to avoid intense or romantic relationships. The remaining third continue to experience intense interpersonal difficulties, sometimes complicated by occupational disability and repeated hospitalizations. Some patients experience a decrease in anger and impulsiveness after about age 40, similar to the "burnout" that occurs in some individuals with antisocial personality disorder.

Histrionic Personality Disorder

Presentation

Histrionic personality disorder is characterized by pervasive and excessive emotionality and attention-seeking behavior. As indicated in Table 10–9, these individuals feel uncomfortable when they aren't the "center of attention," and they may sexualize relationships in order to get the attention that they crave. They have a flamboyant, dramatic way of speaking and dressing that draws attention to themselves. Over the course of treatment, they may offer the clinician gifts or excessive praise. They may call the clinician by his or her first name after a single meeting and may talk about their "friendships" with previous treatment providers. While they are emotional, their emotions often appear to be "shallow" and superficial.

During the clinical examination, these patients typically tell overly digressive stories, accompanied by a wealth of detail. Despite this, the history may remain quite vague, lacking essential details. Their overall style of perceiving the world is "impressionistic." For example, the patient's father may be described as "wonderful," or "brilliant," but the patient may be unable to provide any further details. These patients also tend to be highly suggestible. They may impulsively play hunches in making purchases rather than first looking into matters further.

Despite their outward appearance of being the "life of the party," individuals with histrionic personality disorder often have few successful interpersonal relationships. They have difficulty relating to members of the opposite sex in a non-sexualized or nonmanipulative way, and even their same-sex relationships are impaired by their constant need to be the center of attention. Like other members of the Cluster B group, they are easily bored, seek excitement, and have difficulty following through on longer-term projects. They have low frustration tolerance and can be quick to anger. Despite their sexual provocativeness, they often experience sexual dysfunction, with women often reporting anorgasmia or hypoactive sexual desire and men often reporting impotence. Thus, their sexually provocative behavior may reflect their cravings for attention rather than increased libido.

The prevalence of histrionic personality disorder in the community appears to be 2%–3%, although in the clinic population the rate can be as high as 15%. There may be similar rates for men and women in the community setting, but women appear to be overrepresented in the clin-

Table 10–9. *DSM-IV-TR* Criteria for Histrionic Personality Disorder

A pervasive pattern of excessive emotionality and attention seeking, beginning by early adulthood and present in a variety of contexts, as indicated by five (or more) of the following:

1. Is uncomfortable in situations in which he or she is not the center of attention
2. Interaction with others is often characterized by inappropriate sexually seductive or provocative behavior
3. Displays rapidly shifting and shallow expression of emotions
4. Consistently uses physical appearance to draw attention to self
5. Has a style of speech that is excessively impressionistic and lacking in detail
6. Shows self-dramatization, theatricality, and exaggerated expression of emotion
7. Is suggestible—that is, easily influenced by others or circumstances
8. Considers relationships to be more intimate than they actually are

Source: Reprinted with permission from the *Diagnostic and Statistical Manual of Mental Disorders, Fourth Edition, Text Revision.* Copyright 2000 American Psychiatric Association.

ical setting, perhaps because they are more likely than are men to seek medical attention. Gender bias may also influence the diagnosis: men who dress flamboyantly and brag about their sexual exploits are more likely to be called "narcissistic," while women who behave the same way are generally labeled "histrionic."

Etiology

Form. These patients may possess an "affective temperament" that is similar to that which is seen in patients with borderline personality disorder, but without the severe anger and identity disturbance. It is possible that individuals with borderline personality disorder have a histrionic *temperament*, with their pervasive anger and identity disturbance reflecting superimposed changes that occur following childhood developmental influences such as neglect or abuse.

Function. Analytic theory suggests that the main defenses used by patients with histrionic personality disorder are *repression* and *dissociation*. In other words, while they may appear to be very "emotional," their emotional displays are superficial and they themselves have little awareness of how they "really" feel. When pressed, they also tend to have difficulty explaining why they act the way that they do.

Treatment

These patients are more likely to benefit from psychotherapy than are patients with borderline personality disorder or antisocial personality disorder because their psychopathology is less se-vere. The goal is to help them gain insight into their true feelings and to help them learn how to achieve greater intimacy with others. Clinicians need to be aware of these patients' tendency to idealize treatment providers, especially since clinicians' own needs for love or approval may lead them to engage in countertransference behavior. This is a particular concern given these patients' tendencies to sexualize their important relationships. Medications can play an adjunctive role: antidepressants and anxiolytics can be useful in the treatment of comorbid depressive or anxiety disorders.

Narcissistic Personality Disorder

Presentation

Individuals with **narcissistic personality disorder** demonstrate pervasive grandiosity, an excessive need for admiration, and a lack of empathy for others, as described in Table 10–10. They tend to appear boastful and pretentious, exaggerating their accomplishments. They also may appear genuinely surprised or even offended when others don't recognize and praise their contributions.

Such people tend to be preoccupied with fantasies of personal success or of finding ideal love. They may feel that only other "special" people can recognize their talents and therefore may preferentially seek out only the "best" clinicians. (However, they may subsequently devalue these clinicians if they prove not to measure up to their high expectations.) Similarly, they may only

Table 10–10. *DSM-IV-TR* Criteria for Narcissistic Personality Disorder

A pervasive pattern of grandiosity (in fantasy or behavior), need for admiration, and lack of empathy, beginning by early adulthood and present in a variety of contexts, as indicated by five (or more) of the following:

1. Has a grandiose sense of self-importance (e.g., exaggerates achievements and talents, expects to be recognized as superior without commensurate achievements)
2. Is preoccupied with fantasies of unlimited success, power, brilliance, beauty, or ideal love
3. Believes that he or she is "special" and unique and can only be understood by, or should associate with, other special or high-status people (or institutions)
4. Requires excessive admiration
5. Has a sense of entitlement—unreasonable expectations of especially favorable treatment or automatic compliance with his or her expectations
6. Is interpersonally exploitative—takes advantage of others to achieve his or her own ends
7. Lacks empathy: is unwilling to recognize or identify with the feelings and needs of others
8. Is often envious of others or believes that others are envious of him or her
9. Shows arrogant, haughty behaviors or attitudes

Source: Reprinted with permission from the *Diagnostic and Statistical Manual of Mental Disorders, Fourth Edition, Text Revision.* Copyright 2000 American Psychiatric Association.

wish to marry an especially attractive spouse who admires them and reinforces their self-image. They tend to be "entitled," feeling that the usual rules don't apply to them, and they tend to exhibit low empathy for the feelings of other people. They often become impatient when other people try to talk about their own problems and concerns.

Despite this apparent exaggerated sense of self-esteem, these individuals also have been noted to have a very *fragile* self-image. This may explain their need for constant admiration. They frequently compare themselves to others and are prone to feelings of envy, which they cope with by deprecating these other people. In many cases, they haven't achieved as much in the occupational arena as one might have expected, possibly reflecting their pathological fear of failure or of being humiliated. Sometimes, a minor failure or a mild criticism by a peer overwhelms this defense strategy, leading them to abruptly plummet into a state of severe depression and self-loathing, feeling like a "complete failure." At other times, they fly into a state of rage. In other words, all it takes is a small "pinprick," a minor *"narcissistic injury,"* to pop their protective narcissistic "bubble."

These feelings often resolve within a few days: their usual defenses come back into play, their failures are rationalized or projected onto others, and they again are protected from having to face painful feelings of sadness, anger, and self-doubt. The rapidity of the mood swing and its clear relationship to a precipitating situation and to their narcissistic attitudes help to distinguish their abrupt rages from major depressive disorder and from rapidly cycling bipolar disorder.

While the prevalence of narcissistic personality disorder in the general population is 1%, the prevalence in the clinical population ranges from 2% to 16%. Between 50% and 75% of patients are male. This possible gender difference could reflect the influence of biological factors, cultural factors, or gender bias. The condition can overlap with the other Cluster B conditions, and some patients receive more than one diagnosis. In "pure cases," the excessive grandiosity is a key feature, along with an absence of the self-destructiveness, impulsivity, and abandonment concerns seen in borderline personality disorder, an absence of the antisocial behavior seen in an-

tisocial personality disorder, and an absence of the dramatic, sexually provocative behavior seen in histrionic personality disorder.

Etiology

Family and twin studies haven't been conducted for narcissistic personality disorder. However, temperamental vulnerabilities are likely similar to those for the other Cluster B conditions. Dynamic theories have centered on childhood experiences in which failure by the patient wasn't acceptable to the parents, who reacted with criticism or neglect. However, no specific type of trauma or difficulty during a specific developmental phase has been identified.

Treatment

Patients may present for treatment of symptoms of major depressive disorder, dysthymic disorder, or a substance-related disorder. Antidepressant medication can be helpful in treating depression, although blows to self-esteem will still cause significant sadness and interpersonal relationships will remain impaired. Psychotherapy sometimes helps the patient address the core difficulties of unstable self-image and impaired ability to form meaningful relationships. Debate in the therapeutic community has centered on whether one should actively *confront* narcissistic patients from an early stage about their lack of empathy for others or whether one should provide *support* for the patient's fragile sense of self-esteem. In actual practice, many therapists attempt to skillfully alternate between these strategies, attempting to gently help patients gain insight into how their grandiosity acts as a defense against low self-esteems while also attempting to avoid appearing overly critical or rejecting.

CLUSTER C PERSONALITY DISORDERS

Avoidant Personality Disorder

Presentation

Individuals with **avoidant personality disorder** desire social interaction (which distinguishes them from individuals with schizoid personality

Table 10–11. *DSM-IV-TR* Criteria for Avoidant Personality Disorder

A pervasive pattern of social inhibition, feelings of inadequacy, and hypersensitivity to negative evaluation, beginning by early adulthood and present in a variety of contexts, as indicated by four (or more) of the following:

1. Avoids occupational activities that involve significant interpersonal contact, because of fears of criticism, disapproval, or rejection
2. Is unwilling to get involved with people unless certain of being liked
3. Shows restraint within intimate relationships because of the fear of being shamed or ridiculed
4. Is preoccupied with being criticized or rejected in social situations
5. Is inhibited in new interpersonal situations because of feelings of inadequacy
6. Views self as socially inept, personally unappealing, or inferior to others
7. Is unusually reluctant to take personal risks or to engage in any new activities because they may prove embarrassing

Source: Reprinted with permission from the *Diagnostic and Statistical Manual of Mental Disorders, Fourth Edition, Text Revision.* Copyright 2000 American Psychiatric Association.

disorder, who prefer solitude) but they are *inhibited* from fully engaging in usual life activities such as intimate relationships or challenging jobs by their extreme fears of criticism or rejection. Diagnostic criteria for this disorder are listed in Table 10–11.

These individuals may function well in a restricted, protected environment. Since they often become dependent on their family and a close circle of friends, failures in this support system can lead to the development of a major depressive episode or to an anxiety disorder, particularly social phobia. The prevalence is 1% in the community but 10% in the clinic population.

Etiology

The potential biological underpinnings of childhood shyness and behavioral inhibition have already been discussed. Many anxious, avoidant children ultimately learn to compensate for these tendencies, but in other cases their traits likely are reinforced by subsequent traumatic experiences where they have been made to feel acutely humiliated or rejected. Unfortunately, these children, by virtue of their demeanor, may encourage ridicule by their peers.

Treatment

These patients may fear psychotherapy as they fear all significant relationships. Psychotherapy tends to initially be primarily supportive in orientation, with the therapist attempting to bolster the patient's fragile sense of self-esteem. Later, the focus may be able to shift to the use of more cognitive and behavioral interventions, such as encouraging the patient to challenge his expectation of failure and criticism by others, to work

on being more assertive, and to explore new experiences. These interventions might be facilitated by the use of SSRIs, anxiolytic medication, or β-blockers (the last being particularly useful for *performance anxiety*).

Dependent Personality Disorder

Presentation

Dependent personality disorder is characterized by an excessive need to be cared for by others, leading to submissive behaviors and to difficulties being alone or doing things independently, as described in Table 10–12. Often these individuals have difficulty making even simple decisions (e.g., what to wear) without first seeking guidance or reassurance from others.

Because they fear losing this support, they have difficulty expressing their own opinion or criticizing others. Their interpersonal relationships therefore tend to be unbalanced, with other people taking advantage of them. They belittle themselves as being "stupid" and are at higher risk of developing depressive and anxiety disorders.

In the community, the prevalence of dependent personality disorder may be as high as 15%, making it one of the most common personality disorders. However, dependent personality disorder is only diagnosed in 2%–3% of patients seen in psychiatric clinics. This is in contrast to most of the other personality disorders we have covered, where the prevalence in the clinic was *higher* than in the community. However, when structured interviews using *DSM* criteria are employed in the clinic setting, the prevalence is found to actually be 20%. This indicates that clinicians tend to overlook this diagnosis in the face

Table 10–12. *DSM-IV-TR* Criteria for Dependant Personality Disorder

A pervasive and excessive need to be taken care of that leads to submissive and clinging behavior and fears of separation, beginning by early adulthood and present in a variety of contexts, as indicated by five (or more) of the following:

1. Has difficulty making everyday decisions without an excessive amount of advice and reassurance from others
2. Needs others to assume responsibility for most major areas of his or her life
3. Has difficulty expressing disagreement with others because of fear of loss of support or approval. Note: do not include realistic fears of retribution
4. Has difficulty initiating projects or doing things on his or her own (because of a lack of self-confidence in judgment or abilities rather than a lack of motivation or energy)
5. Goes to excessive lengths to obtain nurturance and support from others, to the point of volunteering to do things that are unpleasant
6. Feels uncomfortable or helpless when alone because of exaggerated fears of being unable to care for himself or herself
7. Urgently seeks another relationship as a source of care and support when a close relationship ends
8. Is unrealistically preoccupied with fears of being left to take care of himself or herself

Source: Reprinted with permission from the *Diagnostic and Statistical Manual of Mental Disorders, Fourth Edition, Text Revision.* Copyright 2000 American Psychiatric Association.

of more prominent presenting complaints such as depression or panic attacks.

Etiology

Form. As with avoidant personality disorder, genetic factors may play a role. Several twin studies have shown monozygotic twins to have greater concordance for submissive tendencies versus dominance than do dizygotic twins.

Function. Innate biological tendencies are likely reinforced by the childhood environment, with some parents reinforcing the child's dependency by being overly protective. However, in some cases the child may become more dependent as a result of childhood loss, neglect, or abuse.

Treatment

These individuals often present with depressive or anxiety disorders or with somatic complaints, especially following some type of loss. Treatment is similar to that described for avoidant personality disorder, although special attention needs to be paid to the risk of the patient becoming overly dependent on the therapist or the therapist becoming overly protective of the patient.

Obsessive–Compulsive Personality Disorder

Presentation

Individuals with **obsessive–compulsive personality disorder** are preoccupied with orderliness,

perfectionism, and mental and interpersonal control, as detailed in Table 10–13. They experience a strong need to do things the "right way," and so they tend to make inefficient use of their time and they have difficulty "seeing the forest for the trees."

Such individuals tend to be future-oriented and have difficulty tolerating situations involving uncertainty, such as when they are preparing for a major exam or trip or are applying for a new job. They don't like to "waste time" and therefore have difficulty relaxing at home or while on vacation, tending to "take some work along" in case there is any "down time." They tend to hold themselves to a high personal standard and also can become frustrated or angry with other people who don't live up to these same standards. They tend to micromanage, fearing that if they delegate authority to other people, those people won't do the job as effectively as they could do it themselves.

The prevalence of obsessive–compulsive personality disorder in the community is 1%, but these individuals represent between 3% and 10% of the clinic population. This personality disorder is reported to be twice as prevalent in men as in women. Comorbidity can include avoidant personality disorder and paranoid personality disorder. Patients may initially present to the clinic for treatment of a major depressive episode, but the prevalence of depression among individual with obsessive–compulsive personality disorder isn't higher than what is seen in the general population. The same applies for the

Table 10–13. *DSM-IV-TR* Criteria for Obsessive–Compulsive Personality Disorder

A pervasive pattern of preoccupation with orderliness, perfectionism, and mental and interpersonal control, at the expense of flexibility, openness, and efficiency, beginning by early adulthood and present in a variety of contexts, as indicated by four (or more) of the following:

1. Is preoccupied with details, rules, lists, order, organization, or schedules to the extent that the major point of the activity is lost
2. Shows perfectionism that interferes with task completion (e.g., is unable to complete a project because his or her own overly strict standards are not met)
3. Is excessively devoted to work and productivity to the exclusion of leisure activities and friendships (not accounted for by obvious economic necessity)
4. Is overconscientious, scrupulous, and inflexible about matters of morality, ethics, or values (not accounted for by cultural or religious identification)
5. Is unable to discard worn-out or worthless objects even when they have no sentimental value
6. Is reluctant to delegate tasks or to work with others unless they submit to exactly his or her way of doing things
7. Adopts a miserly spending style toward both self and others; money is viewed as something to be hoarded for future catastrophes
8. Shows rigidity and stubbornness

Source: Reprinted with permission from the *Diagnostic and Statistical Manual of Mental Disorders, Fourth Edition, Text Revision.* Copyright 2000 American Psychiatric Association.

prevalence of comorbid obsessive–compulsive disorder.

Etiology

Whether there is a biological predisposition for obsessive–compulsive personality disorder is uncertain. Psychoanalytic theories have centered on fixations at the anal stage and toilet training, as issues of control are so clearly paramount in children at this age. However, from the dimensional perspective, it may be expected that premorbidly anxious, control-oriented children might have more difficulty with toilet training than other children, rather than the reverse chain of causation. Regardless of the theory, analytic notions of typical defense mechanisms—especially externalization, isolation, rationalization, displacement, and reaction formation—have been helpful in understanding these individuals' characteristic coping styles.

Treatment

Individuals with obsessive–compulsive personality disorder often present due to feeling overwhelmed by having to make a major decision but being unable to commit to a course of action. They may be acutely anxious in the face of a recent change in a stable situation, such as the loss of a job or a marriage, since they have more difficulty when their life isn't predictable. They may present because they are aware that their style of interacting with others bothers their

coworkers or family members, or they may present out of a recognition that they are working hard but still don't feel especially happy about their lives.

Psychotherapy focuses on helping them start to recognize how they "feel," not just intellectually but emotionally. Another goal is to help them start to question their need to be "in control." Paradoxically, the main stumbling block in psychotherapy may be their need to exert control over the psychotherapy itself, as well as their desire for a quick "solution" to their problems. These patients may wish to spend hours discussing their childhoods in the hopes of discovering the "answer" to their problems, while also avoiding any serious discussion of their feelings about their current relationship difficulties.

CONCLUSION

Personality disorders are prevalent in the medical setting. They complicate the treatment of both psychiatric and medical conditions, especially when they go unrecognized. Clinicians known for having an excellent "bedside manner" tend to "size up" their patients' personality styles in the course of their clinical interactions, even if they only do so implicitly or "intuitively." They then tailor their own behavior to provide the best "fit."

Ideally, more explicit training in how to recognize and address specific personality types offers profound benefits to all physicians (and not simply to psychiatrists), since it can assist them in providing more effective medical care. Physicians who hope to meet patients "where they are" must have the ability to recognize specific types of severe or maladaptive personality traits, to appreciate the characteristic life circumstances that are most often associated with acute crises, and to offer appropriate support during times of need.

Personality disorders are listed in the diagnostic manual as categorical diagnoses, discrete "conditions." However, clinicians may find the dimensional perspective more appropriate. From this perspective, personality disorders reflect variations in traits that we all possess to greater or lesser degrees. More extreme variations confer either strengths or vulnerabilities, depending upon the particular trait in question as well as the individual's life circumstances.

Psychiatrists tend to be consulted only under particular circumstances, such as when a patient's character pathology causes her to refuse needed medical care or to threaten self-harm. In less acute situations, the primary care or specialist physician acts as both the patient's doctor and the patient's therapist, even when neither the physician nor the patient appreciates the interaction in this latter light, and even when the patient's visits are brief or infrequent.

Since some of these personality disorders are associated with self-destructive behaviors, with a predisposition toward regression when under stress, and with a tendency to form inappropriate relationships with treatment providers, an additional goal of this chapter has been to help physicians learn to recognize some of the typical pitfalls that they might encounter in working with these patients.

One should not let the presence of an obvious, dramatic personality disorder blind one to the presence of coexisting Axis I conditions such as major depressive disorder, generalized anxiety disorder, panic disorder, substance-related disorders, or somatization disorder. These conditions, which more commonly occur in patients with personality disorders, may require specific treatment interventions. Further, conditions such as major depressive disorder may amplify maladaptive personality traits, such that treating the depression may greatly improve the quality of life of both the patient and the patient's friends

and family. Conversely, it is tempting for physicians to ignore a personality disorder while emphasizing comorbid Axis I conditions such as mood disorders or anxiety disorders, since these conditions may lend themselves more readily to pharmacologic interventions. However, the presence of a personality disorder can contribute to an Axis I condition being more refractory to treatment, and patients who do *not* respond to typical "first-line" interventions should be reassessed with attention paid to the possibility that there may be an underlying personality disorder.

In the primary care setting, some "clues" that the clinician may be faced with a patient with a personality disorder include an inappropriately endearing, seductive, or hostile interpersonal style on the part of the patient, repeated noncompliance with treatment recommendations, or the presence of multiple somatic complaints without associated organic pathology (i.e., "somatoform" complaints). Clinicians also can benefit from learning to monitor their own "visceral response," whether positive or negative, as they work with patients. These feelings can include strong feelings of dislike or anger, strong (even sexual) attractions, or feelings of dread upon learning that the patient is in the waiting room. Also, when the patient's various treatment providers are repeatedly coming into conflict with each other, or when a current treatment provider finds herself excessively angered at a previous treatment provider's "incompetent" care, or even when clinicians find themselves attempting to defend the patient from the "incompetence" or "uncaring attitude" of the front desk staff, one should consider the possibility that these reactions reflect a response to "splitting" on the part of the patient.

On cannot ignore the important role of the provision of *attention* by a caring, concerned, medical professional in the care of these patients. The nihilistic, pejorative attitudes that are held by many clinicians with regard to patients with personality disorders usually is unwarranted. The doctor–patient relationship may become one of the most important relationships in some patients' lives. This allows the clinician an opportunity to intervene in a manner that family members and friends cannot. Simple emotional support may offer some patients the solace and confidence that they need if they are to overcome their resistance to again making a major but nec- essary life change, such as divorcing a physically abusive spouse or quitting a stressful job.

However, the concerned attention of a med- ical professional also can become a powerful re- inforcer of *maladaptive, inappropriate behaviors* on the part of the patient. For example, some pa- tients will generate an ever-increasing list of so- matic complaints since these are the required "tickets of admission" to the doctor's examina- tion room. Other patients may even resort to self- injurious behaviors or suicidal gestures that worsen in severity rather than improve over time. In managing such behaviors, clinicians need to remain concerned for the patient's well-being but also may need to actively confront the patient and set appropriate limits. For example, the fre- quency of sessions and telephone contacts, the extent of diagnostic testing, and access to med- ications or hospital admissions may need to be limited, sometimes by explicit, written contracts.

In doing so, clinicians need to attempt to rec- ognize and resist acting on both positive and neg- ative countertransference attitudes. Most doctors went into medicine to help patients. Therefore, when their extensive attempts to "do the right thing" for a patient are unsuccessful, their natu- ral tendency often is either to try "even harder" to help the patient or to "cut bait" and give up on the patient. This is particularly the case with patients who either are excessively flattering to the doctor's self-image or are excessively hostile or dissatisfied with the doctor's care. In the ei- ther case, clinicians can become personally *overly* invested in the patient's case. When in doubt, informal consultation with a trusted col- league or even a formal referral for a second opinion can be useful.

Chapter 11

Eating Disorders

We could approach the eating disorders from any of the four psychiatric perspectives. For example, review the case presented at the outset of Chapter 3, which involves a patient who presents with anorexia nervosa. Note how, given the complexity of this presentation, no single perspective fully accounts for her illness. Clearly, anorexia and bulimia nervosa are associated with biological abnormalities and one therefore could treat them as "diseases." They also tend to occur in people who have particular personality vulnerabilities and particular types of life stories.

However, we might most fruitfully approach the eating disorder syndrome from the perspective of *motivated behavior*. In doing so, we place the emphasis squarely on the *eating behavior itself*; other elements of her presentation look different when viewed from this particular vantage point. In this case, in using the *dimensional perspective* we would have emphasized the patient's obsessive–compulsive personality features; in using the *life-story perspective* we would have focused on the stress that she felt in the gifted student program or the pressure that she felt to lose weight in her ballet class; using the *disease perspective*, we would have noted how her current symptoms meet the diagnostic criteria for a major depressive disorder.

From the vantage point of the *behavior perspective*, all of these factors remain relevant, but mainly in the sense that they all were factors that encouraged the patient to ultimately develop of a particular behavior: self-induced starvation. As the starvation behavior becomes more entrenched, more self-perpetuating, these other factors begin to fade in importance.

In clinical practice, of course, one does not use one or the other perspective in isolation. Rather, one *shifts* back and forth between perspectives. For example, one shifts from the disease perspective to the behavioral perspective when considering how the distorted self-image and rigid thinking that accompany a major depressive disorder can reinforce self-starvation behavior. One might shift back again in considering how self-starvation can cause a depletion of brain monoamines, thereby exacerbating the state of depression. One can shift from the disease perspective to the dimensional perspective in considering how major depressive disorder can exacerbate obsessional personality features. One can then shift back again, considering how the tendency toward obsessional worry predisposes individuals to develop depression.

Likewise, one can shift between dimensions and behaviors, noticing how rigid, perfectionistic, obsessional individuals are more prone to stick with a painful, restrictive diet. In shifting back, it is noteworthy that the resulting state of starvation tends to exacerbate obsessional tendencies, even in people who don't have an obsessive–compulsive personality Disorder to begin with. One can easily perform this same back-and-forth shifting process in considering the relationship between the life-story perspective and the other three perspectives.

In this chapter, we will examine the eating disorders primarily from the behavior perspective. In doing so, we introduce the concept that multidetermined disturbances of behavior can cause life difficulties that ultimately become so severe that psychiatric intervention becomes necessary. In the chapters that follow, we will apply this same approach to the substance-related disorders, the somatoform disorders, the dissociative disorders, and the sexual disorders. Finally, we will discuss two pathological behaviors that cut across the diagnostic spectrum, suicidal and violent behavior.

In each case, we will begin by reviewing the clinical phenomenology of the disorder. We then will examine the nature of the behavioral pathology in each disorder. What factors are most important in initiating the pathological behavior? What factors are most important in sustaining the behavior? (Note that the factors that sustain a behavior might turn out to be very different from those that initiated it in the first place.) Finally, how does one treat these disorders? A treatment plan that fails to address the driven, addictive quality of the patient's behaviors is much less likely to succeed, particularly in the more severe cases.

PHENOMENOLOGY

One might imagine that eating disorders are a twentieth-century cultural phenomenon forced onto American women by fashion magazine editors and Madison Avenue advertisers. In actuality, these disorders were first described centuries ago, and the presentation has changed little since then.

Perhaps the first written description of an eating disorder involved Friderada, an industrious and extremely pious serf in the ninth century AD, who first gorged and then became disgusted by food, ultimately leading her to engage in a prolonged fast that caused severe weight loss. In the thirteenth century, women starved themselves to become more acceptable to God. For example,

Catherine Benincasa starved herself to the point of severe emaciation and continued to do so even in the face of a church sanction. After eating only a mouthful of food, she induced vomiting, and continued to vigorously outwalk her companions even when she was at death's door. In both of these cases, a highly "driven" person, motivated by some "higher" goal, attempted to triumph over the physical needs of the body. This is a recurring theme in the eating disorders.

The first clinical description of an eating disorder was by Richard Morton in 1694, in *Phthisiological: or, a Treatise of Consumptions*. Morton considered anorexia distinct from other types of wasting illness (consumption) such as tuberculosis ("the green sickness") in that it was more of a "nervous" consumption. He described a girl who "fell into a total suppression of her monthly courses from a multitude of cares and passions of her mind, but without any symptom of the green-sickness following upon it." He added,

I do not remember that I did ever in all my practice see one that was conversant with the living so much wasted with the greatest degree of consumption (like a skeleton only clad with skin). . . . The causes which dispose the patient to this disease, I have for the most part observed to be violent passions of the mind. . . . This distemper, as with most other nervous diseases, is chronical, but very hard to be cured, unless a physician be called at the beginning of it. At first it flatters and deceives the patient, for which reason it happens for the most part that the physician is consulted too late. . . . Let the patient endeavour to divert and make his mind cheerful by exercise, and the conversation of his friends. For this disease does almost always proceed from sadness and anxious cares.

Morton's description includes all of the typical features of our present-day anorexia nervosa. An adolescent female ceases menstruating, becomes emaciated, and exhibits depression and anxiety. The condition becomes more entrenched the longer it persists and becomes more resistant to medical intervention. The patient herself resists medical intervention, since she is inappropriately content with her wasted state. The recommended treatment is essentially psychotherapy.

Anorexia received little further attention until 200 years later, when William Whitney Gull in England (1874) and Lasègue in France (1873) independently offered nearly identical descriptions of anorexia. Gull coined the terms anorexia nervosa, "apepsia hysterica," and "anorexia hysterica," again in an attempt to distinguish this condition from tuberculosis. Gull noted that the disease occurred mostly in young women, although he had "occasionally seen it in males at the same age. Like Morton, he was struck by the how incongruously content the patients were with their state: "The patient complained of no pain, but was restless and active. This was in fact a striking expression of the nervous state, for it seemed hardly possible that a body so wasted could undergo the exercise which seemed agreeable."

Gull also noted that the starved state itself could account for all of the patient's medical difficulties. He also had gradually come to the conclusion that the only effective treatment for anorexia was to feed the patient, by coercively means if necessary:

It will be observed that all the conditions in this case were negative, and may be explained by the anorexia which led to starvation, and a depression of all the vital functions; viz., amenorrhoea, slow pulse, slow breathing. In state of greatest emaciation one might have been pardoned for assuming that there was some organic lesion, but from the point of view indicated such an assumption would have been unnecessary. . . . The medical treatment probably need not be considered as contributing much to the recovery. . . . Food should be administered at intervals varying inversely with the exhaustion and emaciation. The inclination of the patient must be in no way consulted. In the earlier and less severe stages, it is not unusual for the medical attendant to say, in reply to the anxious solicitude of the parents, "Let her do as she likes. Don't force food." Formerly, I thought such advice admissible and proper, but larger experience has shown plainly the danger of allowing the starvation-process to go on. . . . The treatment required is obviously that which is fitted for persons of unsound mind. The patients should be fed at regular intervals, and surrounded by persons who would have moral control over them; relations and friends being generally the worst attendants.

Lasègue offered a nearly identical description of this condition and independently came to the same conclusions about its cause and its appropriate treatment. He, too, recommended psychotherapy (then called "moral therapy"), but only in conjunction with strict behavioral interventions. He concluded:

Woe to the physician who, misunderstanding the peril, treats as a fancy without object or duration an obstinacy

which he hopes to vanquish by medicines, friendly advice, or by the still more defective resource, intimidation. . . . When after several months the family, the doctor, and the friends perceive the persistent inutility of all these attempts, anxiety and with it moral treatment commences. . . . The patient, when told that she cannot live upon an amount of food that would not support a young infant, replies that it furnishes sufficient nourishment for her, adding that she is neither changed nor thinner. . . . she says that she never was better. . . . I might almost say a condition of contentment truly pathological. Not only does she not sigh for recovery, but she is not ill-pleased with her condition.

This brings us to the modern *DSM-IV* criteria for **anorexia nervosa**, listed in Table 11–1. As can be seen, the syndrome has not substantially changed. The key features are a *refusal to maintain body weight* beyond the minimum weight expected for that age and height (or in the case of children, failure to achieve normal weight gains) accompanied by a *morbid fear of fatness*, a *distorted body image*, and (in postmenarcheal females) *amenorrhea*. There are two subtypes of anorexia nervosa, the *restricting type* (in which there is no binge eating or purging behavior during the current episode) and the *binge eating/purging type* (in which the patient regularly engages in binge eating or purging behavior during the current episode).

While binging and purging can occur in association with anorexia nervosa, **bulimia nervosa** was not described as a distinct diagnostic entity until 1979, when Russell coined the term for what he considered to be an "ominous variant of anorexia nervosa." Table 11–2 lists the *DSM-IV* diagnostic criteria for bulimia nervosa. By definition, anorexia nervosa is the broader diagnosis, such that patients who meet the diagnostic criteria for both disorders would receive a diagnosis of "anorexia nervosa, binge-eating/purging type."

Patients with bulimia nervosa aren't below weight, and they therefore may have less severe body-image distortions. However, concerns about body weight and shape remain a significant cognitive component of the disorder. The defining feature of bulimia, however, is the behavior of *binge eating*. *DSM-IV* attempts to define a "binge" operationally, to allow for greater diagnostic reliability. A binge is defined as the ingestion of a *large amount of food* (i.e., more

Table 11–1. *DSM-IV-TR* Criteria for Anorexia Nervosa

A. Refusal to maintain body weight at or above a minimally normal weight for age and height (e.g., weight loss leading to maintenance of body weight less than 85% of that expected, or failure to make expected weight gain during period of growth, leading to body weight less than 85% of that expected)
B. Intense fear of gaining weight or becoming fat, even though underweight
C. Disturbance in the way in which one's body weight or shape is experienced, undue influence of body weight or shape on self-evaluation, or denial of the seriousness of the current low body weight
D. In postmenarcheal females, amenorrhea, i.e., the absence of at least three consecutive menstrual cycles. (A woman is considered to have amenorrhea if her periods occur only following hormone, e.g., estrogen, administration)

SPECIFY TYPE

Restricting Type

During the current episode of anorexia nervosa, the person has not regularly engaged in binge-eating or purging behavior (i.e., self-induced vomiting or the misuse of laxatives, diuretics, or enemas)

Binge-Eating/Purging Type

During the current episode of anorexia nervosa, the person has regularly engaged in binge-eating or purging behavior (i.e., self-induced vomiting or the misuse of laxatives, diuretics, or enemas)

Source: Reprinted with permission from the *Diagnostic and Statistical Manual of Mental Disorders, Fourth Edition, Text Revision.* Copyright 2000 American Psychiatric Association.

than the average person would eat under similar circumstances), over a *discrete period of time*, accompanied by a feeling of *lack of control* over one's eating behavior.

Patients often describe their binging episodes using language that resembles that used by patients with alcohol and drug addiction to describe their binges. For example, the binging alcoholic patient might state, "I know that I can't have one drink, because after I have that one, I just can't stop myself. I just keep drinking until I pass out." Similarly, bulimic patients often describe an *appetitive or craving phase*, a state of "tension" and powerful craving. This ultimately is followed by the *consummation phase*. During this phase, selectivity for particular types of food may be lost:

Table 11–2. *DSM-IV-TR* Criteria for Bulimia Nervosa

A. Recurrent episodes of binge eating. An episode of binge eating is characterized by both of the following:
    1. Eating, in a discrete period of time (e.g., within any 2-hour period), an amount of food that is definitely larger than most people would eat during a similar period of time and under similar circumstances
    2. A sense of lack of control over eating during the episode (e.g., a feeling that one cannot stop eating or control what or how much one is eating)
B. Recurrent inappropriate compensatory behavior in order to prevent weight gain, such as self-induced vomiting; misuse of laxatives, diuretics, enemas, or other medications; fasting; or excessive exercise
C. The binge eating and inappropriate compensatory behaviors both occur, on average, at least twice a week for 3 months.
D. Self-evaluation is unduly influenced by body shape and weight
E. The disturbance does not occur exclusively during episodes of anorexia nervosa

SPECIFY TYPE

Purging Type

During the current episode of bulimia nervosa, the person has regularly engaged in self-induced vomiting or the misuse of laxatives, diuretics, or enemas

Nonpurging Type

During the current episode of bulimia nervosa, the person has used other inappropriate compensatory behaviors, such as fasting or excessive exercise, but has not regularly engaged in self-induced vomiting or the misuse of laxatives, diuretics, or enemas

Source: Reprinted with permission from the *Diagnostic and Statistical Manual of Mental Disorders, Fourth Edition, Text Revision.* Copyright 2000 American Psychiatric Association.

the patient just eats whatever is readily available. (However, the patient may have previously "hoarded" a stash of high-calorie foods or sweets prior to the binge, similar to an alcoholic's hidden stash of vodka.) As with the alcoholic patient who "can't stop once I start," bulimic patients describe a loss of the normal sensation of *satiety*: they continue to eat until they are physically unable to continue, due to gastric distention or due to having exhausted their food supply.

Patients often describe a rush of euphoria while engaging in a binge. This is short-lived, however. Powerful feelings of guilt rapidly take its place, and these are reinforced by the somatic sensation of gastric distention and fears of becoming fat from having ingested so much food. The patient therefore at this point engages in some sort of *compensatory behavior*. Many patients with bulimia engage in more than one such behavior, but the most common is induction of vomiting, a behavior engaged in by 80%–90% of patients with bulimia presenting for treatment. The vomiting may be induced by inserting fingers down the throat to stimulate the gag reflex, and this may lead to characteristic abrasions on the knuckles ("Russell's sign"). Sometimes patients use ipecac syrup to induce vomiting. Ultimately, many patients are able to vomit at will. Other patients use other techniques to "purge," such as taking laxatives, diuretics, or (more rarely) enemas.

Although purging is the most common compensatory strategy, 10%–20% of bulimic patients compensate through *excessive exercise* or *attempts to fast*. In their attempts to lose weight through fasting, they are not as successful as anorexic patients, likely because the hunger they

experience in the course of fasting further reinforces the craving to engage in another binge. Bulimic patients ultimately remain at the same weight or even gain weight. More rarely, patients may take excessive (or unprescribed) *thyroid hormone* in an attempt to lose weight, and patients with diabetes mellitus (who may be predisposed to acquire eating disorders as a result of their chronic need to fastidiously monitor their body's metabolism) may *omit or reduce insulin doses* in order to reduce the metabolism of the food consumed during binges.

As is the case for all behavioral disorders, these behaviors exist along a continuum of severity. Given this, many individuals who clearly have a significant behavioral disturbance still will fail to fulfill all of the diagnostic criteria for the categorical diagnosis of anorexia or bulimia. Therefore, *DSM-IV* also includes a residual category, eating disorder not otherwise specified, as detailed in Table 11–3.

EATING DISORDER AS A PATHOLOGICAL BEHAVIOR

Using *DSM-IV* diagnostic criteria, clinicians can diagnose anorexia and bulimia with virtually 100% reliability. As is the case for all psychiatric illnesses, but particularly for those disorders that involve deliberate but maladaptive behaviors on the part of the patient, the remaining question has to do with the *validity*. How can we *account* for this consistency of clinical findings? What lies *behind* anorexia and bulimia?

Answering these questions has proven to be more difficult. As was the case for the disease perspective and the dimensional perspective, a

Table 11–3. *DSM-IV-TR* Criteria for Eating Disorder Not Otherwise Specified

1. For females, all of the criteria for anorexia nervosa are met except that the individual has regular menses
2. All of the criteria for anorexia nervosa are met except that, despite significant weight loss, the individual's current weight is in the normal range
3. All of the criteria for bulimia nervosa are met except that the binge eating and inappropriate compensatory mechanisms occur at a frequency of less than twice a week or for a duration of less than 3 months
4. The regular use of inappropriate compensatory behavior by an individual of normal body weight after eating small amounts of food (e.g., self-induced vomiting after the consumption of two cookies)
5. Repeatedly chewing and spitting out, but not swallowing, large amounts of food
6. Binge-eating disorder: recurrent episodes of binge eating in the absence of the regular use of inappropriate compensatory behaviors characteristic of bulimia nervosa

Source: Reprinted with permission from the *Diagnostic and Statistical Manual of Mental Disorders, Fourth Edition, Text Revision.* Copyright 2000 American Psychiatric Association.

major question in the behavioral perspective is whether pathological behaviors are best viewed as *forms* or *functions*. In other words, is the anorexic's behavior (refusal to eat) something that should be biologically *explained*, a reflection of a "broken brain," or is it something to be meaningfully *understood*, through psychological interpretation? This is more than just a philosophic distinction. Treatment strategies for anorexia nervosa based on these differing assumptions might prove to be diametrically opposed.

Theories about anorexia nervosa, along with treatment plans based on these theories, always have reflected the prevailing assumptions of the age. In the early twentieth century, anorexia was viewed primarily from the *disease perspective* as an abnormal biological form. While the exact nature of the underlying disease remained unclear, it was presumed to be an endocrine abnormality. In fact, until the 1980s, anorexia appeared in standard medical texts in the section on "endocrine disorders."

This assumption dates back to 1914, when Simmonds described "hypopituitary cachexia" (later called "Simmond's disease), a wasting condition caused by postpartum infection complicated by septic thromboemboli to the pituitary gland. The symptoms of hypopituitarism can resemble those seen in anorexia, such that one can see why anorexia continued to be treated as an endocrine disorder even after it had been distinguished from Simmond's disease. This emphasis led doctors to focus on medical treatments for the condition. Unfortunately, while medical management of secondary complications of starvation is an essential part of the overall treatment plan in anorexia, the disease model hasn't led to significant advances in the treatment of the underlying behavioral disturbance.

In the 1940s and 1950s, the *life-story perspective* came to dominate American psychiatry, and the pathological behaviors engaged in by anorexic patients were viewed as abnormal functions best approached through psychoanalytic exploration. The assumption was that if clinicians could just gain an understanding of anorexic patients' unconscious *motivations* for starving themselves, they could then assist the patients to give up these maladaptive behaviors in favor of more appropriate coping strategies.

From the life-story perspective, a patient's symptoms are viewed as functions of underlying psychological disturbances, such that a patient's particular overt symptoms are less relevant than the nature of her underlying conflicts, with the latter therefore becoming the primary focus of the treatment. For example, anorexia typically has its onset at the time of puberty and it is associated with arrested menstruation and sexual development. Further, many patients express fright or revulsion as sexual development resumes and libido increases as refeeding progresses. Given this, one prominent psychological theory proposed that the anorexic patient's refusal of food reflected an unconscious rejection of adult sexuality. The goal of therapy therefore was to help patients address these developmental issues more appropriately. Similarly, during these decades, American psychiatrists adhered to a definition of schizophrenia that emphasized unconscious defense mechanisms rather than the presence of psychotic symptoms. Not surprisingly, some patients with anorexia were considered to have milder forms of schizophrenia.

While intensive psychodynamic psychotherapy has proven to be ineffective in treating acutely emaciated patients, it may be useful during later stages of treatment, when the emphasis is on weight *maintenance*. This is particularly likely to be the case when a personality disorder or difficulties with interpersonal functioning are more prominent features of a patient's presentation.

In the 1970s, psychiatry's emphasis shifted to *family dynamics*. The patient with an eating disorder was viewed only as being the "identified" patient; the "true" patient was the dysfunctional family itself. Family therapy was seen as an essential part of the treatment, since the eating behavior couldn't be understood outside of its role in preserving a particular family dynamic. In retrospect, while this appears to be the case for *some* patients, family dynamics play only a minor role for *other* patients.

In the 1980s and onward, the focus shifted back to the brain and the *disease model*. While some attention continues to be directed toward the endocrine system, an even greater emphasis has been placed on neurotransmitter systems. Clinical research continues to examine whether psychotropic agents, particularly serotonergic antidepressants, might address at least some components of anorexia or bulimia. These agents appear to be less effective in treating acutely emaciated patients but more effective in preventing relapse in weight-restored patients as part of a comprehensive treatment program. Again, however, they are unlikely to be effective unless patients also take steps to alter their eating behavior.

From the behavior perspective, all of the above factors are still important. Although genetic and biological factors clearly contribute to pathological behaviors, the behavioral perspective doesn't postulate (as the disease perspective dose) that one can locate a biological "broken part" to which a patient's clinical phenomenology can be directly ascribed. For example, there doesn't appear to be an underlying neuropathological lesion in anorexia analogous to the plaques and tangles associated with Alzheimer's disease. Similarly, personality, interpersonal conflict, and family dynamics appear to contribute to the pathological behavior, but primarily as *initiators or reinforcers* of the abnormal eating behavior rather than as the "cause."

As discussed in Chapter 3, motivated behaviors are *goal-directed* and are *designated by their consequences*. They occur intermittently, can be selectively provoked by stimuli that are later ignored, can vary in intensity, and can be voluntarily suppressed. They are characterized by three phases: *(1)* a state of *craving* characterized by both a search for pleasure and desire for release from a state of tension, followed by *(2) consummatory behavior*, and ultimately *(3)* a *decrease in the drive and its replacement by other activities*. This last phase is followed by a return to the first phase, since the patients' drives ultimately increase again.

There is no simple demarcation between normal behavior, "problem" behavior, and "pathological" behavior. These distinctions are socially defined, disjunctive, and occasionally arbitrary. Behaviors are considered to be "pathological" either when the *object* of the drive is abnormal or the *strength* of the drive is abnormal. Motivated behaviors can be influenced by both internal and external factors. However, the factors that *initiate* pathological behaviors may differ from those that *sustain* them, and pathologic behaviors can eventually become *self-sustaining*.

How does this formulation apply to eating disorders? Clearly, the *object* of the drive is not abnormal in this case. Dieting behavior is a socially accepted behavior. In fact, the majority of Americans engage in dieting behavior at some point, with the goal of attaining thinness and diminishing a fear of becoming fat. However, in the average person, dieting is under voluntary control. In anorexia nervosa, the *intensity* of the drive becomes excessive and it becomes completely preoccupying.

About 95% of the time, anorexia nervosa begins with normal dieting. Dieting behavior is a graded phenomenon. Some people are "mild" dieters, others become "serious" dieters, and in anorexia nervosa, the dieting behavior becomes so "serious" that it becomes more *autonomous*: voluntary control is either diminished or absent. Meanwhile, secondary factors come to act as reinforcers of the abnormal behavior. For example, abdominal pain or edema can occur when patients attempt to increase their food intake, which in turn triggers thoughts that they are eating "too much" or will "become fat," and these attitudes in turn reinforce the dieting behavior. Ultimately, anorexia can become a patient's *identity*. The patient may see herself not simply as *doing* certain things, but as *being* "an anorexic." This sense of identity may become the focus of the patient's life and may prove to be very difficult to relinquish.

As might be expected in a graded phenomenon, the number of people who have the full syndrome is small compared to the number of people who have fewer or milder features of the syndrome. Figure 11–1 illustrates the percentages of young women who have various aspects of the eating disorder syndrome. The *majority* of college-age women, about 70%, "feel fat." A much smaller percentage of these women, about 10%, engage in bulimic behavior at some point. However, only about 5% of individuals go on to develop some features of anorexia nervosa, and the prevalence of individuals who ultimately display the *full* syndrome of anorexia or bulimia is even lower, about 1% and 2%, respectively. Over the decades, despite changes in social norms, the prevalence of anorexia among women in Western cultures has remained remarkably stable. Of note, the prevalence can be much higher among members of certain high-risk groups. For example, the prevalence of anorexia among ballet students is as high as 25%.

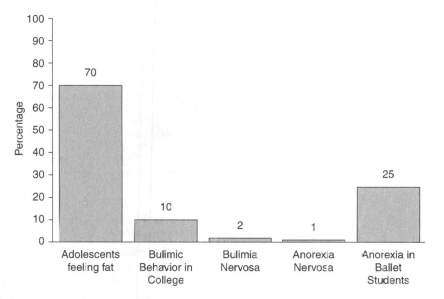

Figure 11–1. Percentages of women with an eating disorder.

Anxiety disorders (especially obsessive–compulsive disorder), mood disorders, and substance-related disorders commonly coexist in patients with eating disorders. In this regard, eating disorders resemble other behavioral disorders characterized by impaired impulse control. The latter include *self-injurious behaviors* engaged in by patients with borderline personality disorder, *impulsive violent behaviors* engaged in by patients with antisocial personality disorder, *pathological gambling*, and *pathologic shopping*. While all of these latter behavioral disorders are classified in a *DSM-IV* category that is distinct from both obsessive–compulsive disorder and the eating disorders—that is, under the rubric of the *impulse control disorders*—the distinction between disorders characterized by *compulsive* behavior and those characterized by *impulsive* behavior remains poorly understood.

Whether eating disorder and other "addictive" conditions (such as substance dependence, pathological gambling, and the sexual paraphilias) belong in one category or the other remains unresolved at this point. Interestingly, both compulsive behaviors and impulsive behaviors have been associated with lower serotonergic activity, and both types of behaviors can be attenuated by treatment with serotonin-reuptake inhibitors, suggesting that these phenomena are probably related. Low serotonergic tone might promote pathological behaviors in two ways: it could con-

tribute to a *general state of anhedonia or dysphoria* that encourages compensatory pleasure-seeking behaviors, and it could contribute to a *decreased ability on the part of affected individuals to resist cravings* to engage in the pathological behaviors.

The primary phenomenologic distinction between *obsessive–compulsive* phenomena and *impulsive/addictive* phenomena is that in the former case, cravings and resultant behaviors are viewed by the patient as unpleasant and undesired (i.e., the cravings and behavior are *ego dystonic*). Therefore, the patient attempts to resist engaging in the behavior. In contrast, in the case of impulsive/addictive disorders, the cravings and resultant behaviors (binging, ingesting alcohol or drugs, gambling, shopping, sexual activity, etc.) typically are *highly* pleasurable. Therefore, the patient usually does *not* resist acting on them (i.e., the cravings and behavior are *ego syntonic*). In fact, the behaviors may be so pleasurable that the individual rationalizes them and continues to engage in them even in the face of a multitude of negative consequences. Coercive intervention—by family, friends, employers, even the criminal justice system—may be required before the individual finally stops engaging in the behavior.

However, this distinction becomes blurred in many cases. Individuals with obsessive—compulsive disorder may at first engage in "normal, but mildly excessive" behavior, only to find themselves having to engage in the behavior with ever-increasing frequency in order to achieve the same degree of "satisfaction" or to avoid feeling anxious (perhaps equivalent to the development of *tolerance* and *withdrawal* in the "addictive" disorders). Similarly, individuals who have *recovered* from alcohol or drug use may in fact find the sensation of drug craving to be *unpleasant* and may even take active steps to resist engaging in their addictive behaviors. Therefore, the distinction between ego dystonic and ego syntonic behaviors may be more a reflection of the affected individual's (and society's) *attitudes* toward the particular behavior than it is a reflection of an underlying biological difference.

In both "compulsive" and "impulsive" conditions, behavior is reinforced and becomes self-sustaining due to two types of reinforcement. **Positive reinforcement** occurs when a given behavior leads to some *pleasant* reward (such as satiety, praise, money, or intoxication). When an individual's behavior is rewarded, he is more likely repeat the behavior in the future. **Negative reinforcement** occurs when a behavior is associated with *relief* from an *unpleasant* state. Negative reinforcement also is associated with an increased likelihood that the individual will engage in the behavior again in the future.

For example, *opioid ingestion* is associated with a sense of euphoria (mediated by dopaminergic, mesolimbic reward pathways), thereby making the opioids powerful positive reinforcers. However, individuals who experience chronic worry, anxiety, or depression may find that opioid ingestion decreases these feelings. Therefore, the opioids also are powerful negative reinforcers.

Similarly, *excessive dieting*, *strenuous exercise*, and *binging* each can become powerful positive and negative reinforcers. Further, each of these behaviors causes increased release of *endogenous* opioids (i.e., endorphins), which in turn trigger activity along the same mesolimbic reward pathways as exogenously administered drugs of abuse.

A variety of internal and external *initiating factors* may trigger the onset of anorexia and bulimia, with no single factor likely being sufficient in iself to account for the condition. While these factors also may act as *sustaining factors* once

Table 11–4. Initiating and Sustaining Factors in Anorexia Nervosa

Initiating Factors	Additional Sustaining Factors
Gender	Neurophysiologic changes
Societal pressures	from starvation
Vulnerable personality	Norepinephrine
Family functioning	Serotonin
Dieting and exercise	Endorphins
Onset of puberty	Cholecystokinin
Acute stress	Other biochemical mediators

the pathologic behavior has taken hold, additional factors (again both internal and external) begin to appear at this point. As a result, the behavior ultimately becomes self-sustaining—that is, independent of the initiating factors. The most common initiating and sustaining factors are listed in Table 11–4 and are discussed below.

INITIATING FACTORS

Gender

Eating disorders are ten times more common in women than in men. Both biological and cultural factors likely account for the substantial disparity. For example, men and women differ in how they perceive and respond to hunger. Men experience hunger that is more acute, eat earlier in day, take larger bites, and eat more rapidly than do women. Further, hormones and neurotransmitters may play different roles in appetitive behaviors for men and women, and appetite in women varies over the course of the month in response to fluctuations in hormone levels, while appetite in men does not.

We discussed above how the majority of endocrine abnormalities that occur in anorexia nervosa are caused by the starved state itself. However, this may not be the whole story. A third to a half of anorexic women had stopped menstruating or experienced irregular menses *before* they started to diet or lose weight. These menstrual disturbances could be a marker of dyregulation along the hypothalamic–adrenal–pituitary axis, perhaps constituting a biologic vulnerability toward anorexia.

Once dieting has begun, differences between the genders may be further exacerbated. Behaviorally, men and women respond differently to a perceived need to lose weight. Men's eating habits are more stable during periods of stress. When they feel overweight, they are more likely to attempt to "work it off" through increased exercise rather than initiating a diet. In contrast, women who feel stressed or depressed are more likely to gain weight and then feel dissatisfied with their bodies. They are more likely to diet than to exercise, and they are more likely to "rebound" or "yo-yo" from a diet into an episode of overeating. At the neuronal level, dieting also affects men and women differently, with serotonin and prolactin levels changing in response to dieting in women but not men.

Eating disorders tend to present differently in men and in women, perhaps reflecting the influence of cultural factors. Males who develop eating disorders tend to initially seek *muscle definition* rather than thinness, and they usually are involved in athletic activities where weight is an important factor, such as wrestling. Further, there is a higher prevalence of homosexuality and bisexuality among men with eating disorders than among women with eating disorders.

One study of 135 males with eating disorders (including both anorexia and bulimia) found the prevalence of heterosexuality to be 41% and the prevalence of homosexuality or bisexuality to be 27%. Thirty-two percent of patients identified themselves as "asexual." In contrast, the rate of homosexuality for men in the general population is about 3%, and the rate of homosexuality among women with eating disorders is about 2%. When examined by type of eating disorder, the prevalence of homosexuality/bisexuality was statistically higher in the men with bulimia (42%), while the prevalence of asexuality was higher among the men with anorexia (58%).

Asexuality (a complete lack of sexual interest for at least the past year) has been described in both men and women with anorexia. It is especially common following weight loss significant enough to cause suppression of testosterone, although psychological factors also may play a contributory role. Similarly, while the higher prevalence of homosexuality and bisexuality among men with eating disorders may reflect the influence of biological factors, cultural factors also could play a role. For example, surveys reveal that, compared to heterosexual men, homosexual men are more likely to be dissatisfied with their body weight and shape and are more likely to consider their physical appearance to be important to their sense of self. These factors therefore may make homosexual men more vulnerable to developing eating disorders.

Societal Pressures

Even a cursory glance at television and magazine advertisements demonstrates that we live in a culture that simultaneously values both high-fat, "sinful" foods and thinness. These values are passed on at a young age. Six-year-old children rate pictures of endomorphs more negatively than they do pictures of ectomorphs, and 7% of children aged 8–13 score in the "anorexic range" on a test of eating attitudes. Typical role models for young girls include ballet dancers, fashion models, gymnasts, and cheerleaders, many of whom themselves have eating disorders. Adult society also perceives thinner women in a better light than heavier women, and achievement-oriented women therefore may feel especially pressured to lose weight. For example, people looking at pictures of women manipulated to increase their bust size rated these women as less intelligent and less competent than the women in the unadulterated pictures.

Another sign that societal pressures play an important role in the etiology of eating disorders is that—in contrast to most major mental illnesses—eating disorders occur more commonly among members of industrialized nations and members of upper socioeconomic classes. Eating disorders are also more common in certain religious and ethnic groups (Jews, Italians, and Catholics). Of course, this might reflect genetic differences; however, the "culture-bound" nature of eating disorders is further suggested by the fact that members of "second-generation" minorities (African Americans, Hispanics, and Native Americans) who have achieved greater social status demonstrate a higher prevalence of eating disorders than do their parents. The same finding has been observed among natives of Arab countries who have immigrated to the West.

Vulnerable Personality

Pure restricting anorexia tends to develop in women who premorbidly are perfectionistic, rigid, socially insecure, dependent, and fear autonomy. Many of these women meet the diagnostic criteria for obsessive–compulsive personality disorder, and a few also meet the criteria for obsessive–compulsive disorder. Malnutrition further amplifies these traits. Malnutrition also causes depression, which itself also can amplify these traits.

Note that the label "anorexia" is a misnomer: while patients with anorexia nervosa do experience hunger, they *fight* the urge to eat, instead adhering inflexibly to their dietary plan. Given this, individuals with obsessive–compulsive personality features (i.e., who are perfectionistic, rigid, and driven) may be predisposed to develop anorexia nervosa.

In contrast, patients who develop either bulimia or the binging–purging form of anorexia are more likely to be extroverted, impulsive, and sensitive to rejection. In contrast to restricting anorexic patients, who most often fulfill the diagnostic criteria for obsessive–compulsive personality disorder, these patients most often fulfill the diagnostic criteria for borderline personality disorder. Further, while anorexic patients are more likely to be overly "enmeshed" with their families, bulimic patients are more likely to be *alienated* from their families. They also are more likely to demonstrate other difficulties with impulsive control, such as alcohol abuse, theft, sexual promiscuity, and impulsive suicide attempts. While anorexic patients typically demonstrate persistent depression, bulimic patients often demonstrate prominent affective instability.

Many patients with bulimia describe a different course of events leading to their initial dieting behavior. Seeing the world as a stressful and uncaring place, they turned to dieting for gratification or escape. However, they had difficulty tolerating the deprivation and the food cravings and ultimately engaged in a binge. Perhaps their unstable affect and self-image contributes to the emotional roller coaster that accompanies the typical binge–purge cycle—the initial euphoria that accompanies the binge, followed by severe guilt and intolerable anxiety, followed in turn by the purge.

Family Functioning

Family studies describe several common features in families of patients who present with eating disorders. Mothers of restricting anorexics most often are described as intrusive, dominating, overprotective, critical, socially introverted, and phobic. In contrast, fathers of restricting anorexics have been described as passive, submissive, emotionally sensitive, and withdrawn, often overshadowed or belittled by the patient's mother. As a couple, the parents tend to be overprotective and overambitious in their expectations for their children, expecting obedience and superior performance. Even when this hasn't been explicitly stated to the children, patients often recall this as having been "a given." As a family, members of such households tend to be rigidly enmeshed, lacking skills in conflict resolution, and interested in maintaining the current emotional homeostasis.

Adolescents who become anorexic may therefore be quite ambivalent about the independence that comes with reaching adulthood. This ambivalence likely results both from their underlying obsessive–compulsive personality features and from an upbringing that fostered dependence and behavioral inhibition. Rather than experimenting with different identities or making efforts to distinguish themselves from their parents ("normal" adolescent rebellion), they fear such autonomy. Self-starvation and emaciation therefore may allow the anorexic patient to simultaneously achieve two competing goals: because she is so ill, separation from her parents must be delayed; paradoxically, her starvation allows her to be assertive and aggressive, to refuse to eat despite her parents' extensive attempts to persuade or coerce her to do so.

In contrast, families of bulimic patients have been described as being less cohesive and structured, with greater expressions of overt conflict. However, high parental expectations of the children are a shared feature in the families of both anorexic and bulimic patients.

The family studies have some clear limitations. Their most obvious failing is the lack of a control group consisting of families where the children *haven't* developed eating disorders. *Many* families are "dysfunctional," and so it shouldn't be surprising that many families of patients with eating disorder also are dysfunctional. In addition, in the absence of prospective studies, it is difficult to determine to what extent family dysfunction is a *cause* of a child having an eating disorder or severe personality disorder, and to what extent it might *result* from it.

Further, these family dynamics are not unique to patients with eating disorders; for example, they also have been noted in families of patients with borderline personality disorder or somatization disorder. Most of the patients in these latter two categories also have significant behavioral problems, but they don't always have an eating disorder. Finally, every clinician has encountered patients with severe eating disorders who come from what appear to be high-functioning families.

Given this, it is likely that certain types of family dynamic encourage the development of various forms of maladaptive behavior, pathological eating behavior being one of them. It is important to explore and to attempt to address family dysfunction, especially in patients who currently live with or closely interact with their parents. While it is neither necessary nor sufficient in itself to cause an eating disorder, it is both a risk factor and potentially a perpetuating factor.

Dieting and Exercise

Up to 75% of anorexic women report having engaged in excessive physical activity *prior* to the initiation of dieting. Therefore, exercise may be more than just another way to lose weight; it may play an important role *in itself* in triggering the onset of the eating disorder.

Animal studies lend support to the theory that exercise reinforces the urge to diet as well as the ability to diet. Rats allowed only a single daily meal who are given the opportunity to run on an activity wheel predictably increase their time on the wheel and decrease their food intake even further (despite their food already having been restricted). If allowed to continue in this fashion, they continue to run and to restrict their intake until they ultimately die. In contrast, control animals who have been placed on the same restricted food schedule but who have not been given access to an activity wheel do not engage in pathological food restriction or exercise and therefore survive.

Why rats act this way isn't completely clear. One teleological theory postulates that animals in the wild (presumably including humans) whose access to food is cut off would need to be able to deal with this situation. Decreased availability of food therefore may trigger increased motor activity such as foraging or hunting. Un-

der those particular circumstances, this mechanism would be adaptive, while in anorexia it perpetuates a maladaptive behavior.

In addition, vigorous exercise likely activates the same pleasure circuit implicated in substance dependence, mediated by dopamine and other neurotransmitters and possibly including increased endorphin release. Therefore, excessive exercise can itself become self-reinforcing (leading to "exercise addiction" in these patients) in addition to perpetuating the positive feedback loop between diet and exercise. As will be discussed below, the state of starvation itself is associated with increased endorphin release. This may explain why anorexics may state that they "never felt better" and continue to engage in vigorous exercise despite being malnourished.

Onset of Puberty

Adolescence is the period of greatest risk for the development of an eating disorder. The mean age at onset for anorexia nervosa is 17. (There is a suggestion of bimodal peaks at ages 14 and 18.) It is quite rare for anorexia to have its onset after age 40 (although cases have been described).

Developmental and hormonal factors associated with puberty probably play a significant etiologic role. Another event that occurs during puberty, though, is a change in body morphology. The natural tendency of the female body is to fatten in order to prepare for the reproductive functions of pregnancy and nursing. The shift in the fat-to-lean ratio is significant: body fat increases by 120% while lean mass only increases by 40%. People predisposed toward an eating disorder who have preexisting concerns about being "overweight" may view these new bodily changes with considerable alarm, perhaps triggering dieting behavior in some cases.

Acute Stress

Many patients experience the onset of an eating disorder as well as later exacerbations of the disorder during periods of increased stress. One common scenario is the development of anorexia shortly after having left home for the first time to attend college (hence the second peak at age 18). Another scenario is the development of eating disorder in the setting of one's parents getting divorced. Because they tend to have maladaptive attitudes and difficulties in interpersonal functioning, individuals who are obsessional (often the case with anorexia) or who have borderline personality traits (often the case with bulimia) are more likely to interpret a particular situation as being "stressful" than would a person without these personality vulnerabilities.

Animal models also point to stress playing a significant contributory role in the development of pathological eating behavior. For example, rats "stressed" by having rubber bands placed on their tails continue to eat even after they should be sated. This "binging" behavior persists even after the rats have been administered amphetamine, which is normally an appetite suppressant. This finding may indicate that the bulimic patient's description of binging in order to "comfort herself" during periods of greater stress may in fact reflect a powerful underlying biological drive.

REINFORCING AND SUSTAINING FACTORS

In restricting anorexics, the state of starvation can lead to profound biochemical changes that paradoxically contribute to further starvation. For example, in one study, healthy young males without an eating disorder volunteered to starve themselves under controlled conditions. Their mood, thinking, and behavior showed striking changes. They became depressed, became preoccupied with thoughts of food, and felt hungrier after eating than they did before eating. They began to engage in bizarre "food fads" and hoarding rituals, collected recipes, cooked meals for others but not for themselves, and preferred to watch others eat. Their personalities become more obsessional and egocentric, and they behaved sarcastically when others offered help. In other words, starvation can make a person act like a person with anorexia, and not simply vice versa. What neurophysiologic factors might contribute to such profound changes in personality, cognition, and behavior?

Neurophysiologic Changes Resulting from Starvation

Structural neuroimaging studies reveal that starvation is associated with *cerebral atrophy* in 82% of patients with anorexia. This state is associated with symptoms of cognitive impairment typical of a *subcortical dementia*. While these cognitive difficulties typically resolve following weight restoration, one must always keep in mind when attempting to work with acutely ill anorexic patients that they often have subtle impairments in "executive function." These decreases in mental flexibility and judgment may exacerbate the "resistance" to psychotherapeutic interventions or to changing their maladaptive behaviors.

Functional neuroimaging studies reveal starvation to be associated with *increased caudate metabolism* (a finding that also has been observed in obsessive–compulsive disorder), which also resolves following weight restoration. The caudate is associated with vigilance, and increased caudate activity may be associated with patients have a greater likelihood of developing compulsive or driven behaviors.

Changes in *neurotransmitters and hormones* associated with starvation can make impulses more difficult to resist and also can lead to depression and cognitive impairment. Changes may occur in levels of monoamines, endorphins, cholecystokinin, and hormones associated with the "stress response" system, particularly glucocorticoids.

Finally, bulimic binging and purging behavior can cause profound metabolic changes, even in the absence of "starvation" and weight loss. Bulimic individuals consume from several thousand calories to tens of thousands of calories during a single binge, but then immediately vomit 3–4 liters of gastric contents; they might engage in several such binge–purge cycles over the course of a single day. This can lead to profound electrolyte, neurotransmitter, and endocrine changes.

Norepinephrine

Norepinephrine has been implicated in the etiology of both depression and anxiety, and depression and anxiety both can occur in association with eating disorders. Further, norepinephrine plays a more direct role in feeding behavior, influencing appetite at the hypothalamic level. For example, α-agonist drugs produce hyperphagia in animals, while β-agonist drugs inhibit feeding behavior. Starvation may lead to decreased brain norepinephrine synthesis, thereby leading to decreased anxiety and also decreased metabolism in general. The lowered metabolism may protect the anorexic by decreasing nutritional requirements.

At the pharmacologic level, *cocaine and amphetamines*, in addition to having dopaminergic effects, block α receptors and stimulate β receptors and therefore are appetite suppressants. Desipramine, a tricyclic antidepressant, has similar noradrenergic effects. When used in the treatment of bulimia, it decreases binging behavior within 2 weeks. This is sooner than the time of onset for desipramine's antidepressant effects. In contrast, *amitriptyline and marijuana* both stimulate α receptors, thereby stimulating appetite and possibly contributing to weight gain. (Amitripyline's anticholinergic and antihistaminic activity also might contribute to weight gain.)

Serotonin

Serotonin appears to play an important role in obsessive–compulsive disorder, and some researchers have suggested that the eating disorders are part of an "obsessive–compulsive spectrum" of disorders, given certain similarities to OCD. For example, patients with anorexia and bulimia have recurrent, intrusive thoughts about food and engage in highly ritualized eating behaviors. Patients with bulimia also often describe their binging–purging episodes in terms similar to those used by patients with OCD to describe their behaviors. The urge to binge is resisted, but this is followed by an increase in anxiety and tension. These feelings decrease after the patient has engaged in bulimic behavior.

A third of patients with anorexia nervosa also meet the diagnostic criteria for OCD, even when thoughts about food are excluded. Most commonly, they fear that they are not doing something "correctly," have an excessive need for symmetry and order, and fear that something terrible is about to happen. These obsessional fears often persist even after weight restoration, suggesting that they aren't simply a result of being in a starved state. SSRIs have been found to be useful in treating both OCD and bulimia, and in both cases higher dosages tend to be required than those used to treat major depressive disorder.

Serotonin plays multiple roles in the brain. In addition to mediating aspects of temperament, impulse control, mood, and anxiety, it plays a separate role in feeding and satiety. Serotonin acts on the ventromedial hypothalamus, triggering the sensation of satiety and inhibiting feeding behavior following a meal. In contrast, sero-tonin deficiency associated with dieting causes extreme hunger.

Since serotonin synthesis depends upon the dietary intake of tryptophan, the starved state that occurs in anorexia may be associated with lower CNS serotonin activity, thereby contributing to depression and increased OCD phenomena. Preliminary evidence confirms such a role of serotonin deficiency in bulimia. For example, bulimic patients who eat foods high in tryptophan control their binges rapidly, while those who eat foods without tryptophan eat until either they or their food supply is exhausted. Some research even suggests that binges in bulimia might represent attempts to stabilize mood difficulties related to a defective serotonin regulatory system. For example, family histories of depression and alcoholism are four to eight times higher in the bulimic population than in the general population.

Why, then, doesn't serotonin deficiency trigger increased hunger in the nutritionally depleted state that characterizes severe anorexia? Perhaps by this point, other biological factors assume a greater contributory role than does serotonin deficiency. However, in patients who haven't lost so much weight and who have lower serotonin and impulse control problems to begin with (such as patients with borderline personality disorder), lowered serotonin due to dieting may lead to an increased appetite, a greater drive to engage in binging behavior, and comorbid psychiatric symptoms such as depression.

Pharmacologically, **SSRIs** cause an increase in central serotonin. In anorexia, they can help decrease obsessional behaviors and depression, although they have little effect on weight gain. In contrast, in bulimia, they can increase feelings of satiety with eating, decrease cravings to binge, and decrease both depression and emotional irritability. Similarly, **fenfluramine (Pondimin)** is an agent that affects serotonin, stimulating presynaptic release of serotonin, acting on the postsynaptic serotonin receptor, and mildly inhibiting serotonin reuptake. It also inhibits binging. (Unfortunately, fenfluramine also has amphetamine-like effects on dopamine release, which can lead to abuse and even psychosis at the dosage typically required to suppress binging behavior, limiting its clinical utility.) In contrast, **cyproheptadine (Periactin)**, a serotonin receptor *antagonist*, has been shown to help some anorexic patients to gain weight, perhaps by acting on the hypothalamic feeding center to prevent serotonin-mediated satiety.

Endorphins

As noted above, starvation in anorexia may be accompanied by increased endorphin release; this could contribute to both a diminution of appetite and a feeling of elation. Among bulimics, those who vomit show increased plasma β-endorphin levels compared with bulimics who don't vomit. Perhaps increased endorphin activity contributes to the feelings of lightness and euphoria that can occur following an episode of vomiting, thereby playing a role as a positive reinforcer of the abnormal behavior.

It might seem odd that endorphin activity could be elevated in bulimia, since we've discussed how in anorexia, exercise-induced endorphin release may contribute to the appetite suppression that helps sufferers to continue to starve themselves. It turns out that the relationship between opiates and appetite is a complex one: in *nondieting* humans, exogenous opiate drugs such as morphine *increase* appetite, while naloxone (Narcan), an opiate antagonist, decreases appetite. In contrast, in *food-restricted* animals, the *opposite* is true: *opiates decrease appetite*.

Therefore, perhaps excessive endorphin release in *anorexia* helps explain the puzzling phenomenon whereby the anorexic patient no longer feels hungry after having reached a more severe point in the illness. Uncontrolled studies in anorexic patients have shown naltrexone to be mildly helpful in increasing weight gain, decreasing the preoccupation with dieting, and decreasing the exhilaration associated with weight loss.

In contrast, in *bulimia*, endorphins released during a binge might reinforce the binging behavior and also *stimulate appetite, thereby helping to trigger a subsequent binge*. As might be predicted, naloxone given to bulimic patients decreases binging behavior, perhaps due to its appetite suppressant effects in nonstarved humans as well as its ability to block the euphoria associated with the binge. (Unfortunately, naloxone usually only does this when given in doses high enough to cause hepatotoxicity; it therefore is rarely used in clinical practice.)

Cholecystokinin

Cholecystokinin (CCK) release is triggered in the ileum by medium-chain fatty acids and by some amino acids. In addition to causing the gallbladder to contract and the pancreas to release bicarbonate-rich fluid, CCK binds to vagal afferent nerves that lead to the hypothalamus, thereby contributing to the sensation of satiety. While experimental evidence hasn't suggested a role for CCK in anorexia, it may play a significant role in bulimia.

For example, when normal subjects are fed a meal, their peripheral CCK level quickly rises to about 15 units. Similarly, when they are injected with exogenous CCK while they are in the midst of eating a meal, they rapidly reported a feeling of satiety and decrease their food intake. In contrast, when *bulimics* are fed a meal, their CCK level rises only to about 3 units. They also report that they experience little sense of satiety. However, when they are injected with exogenous CCK while in the midst of eating a meal, they do experience satiety. The vagal afferent nerves also may play a contributory role in bulimia. Upon autopsy of bulimic patients who have died from acute gastric dilation and rupture, these nerves are discovered to be damaged.

Therefore, one theory is that bulimic individuals demonstrate a blunted CCK response. This in turn blunts the sensation of satiety that normally occurs in response to food intake. This may contribute to the propensity of bulimic individuals to eat to the point of becoming severely uncomfortable due to gastric distention. They then have to vomit to relieve the distention.

Neuropeptide Y and Peptide YY

Neuropeptide Y (NPY) and **peptide YY (PYY)** are both produced in the pancreas. PYY is the most potent feeding stimulator known. It is found in high concentrations in hypothalamic feeding centers, where it stimulates carbohydrate craving. In humans and animals, levels of PYY decline shortly after a meal has been ingested, thereby contributing to the sensation of satiety. Animals that have been injected with exogenous PYY eat to the point of death by gastric rupture: in other words, they experience no satiety.

In *anorexic* patients, PYY levels have been found to be normal. However, their NPY levels are elevated, and this latter abnormality resolves following weight restoration. In *bulimic* patients, the levels of both substances are normal while the patients are actively binging, but their levels significantly increase after they have ceased engaging in binging behavior. Perhaps this increase helps account for their intense cravings for food and high rate of subsequent relapse into further binging behavior. It isn't clear at this point, however, whether these alterations in normal peptide homeostasis represent a *preexisting* condition that predisposes affected individual to engage in binging behavior or whether they represent an *effect* of repetitive binging and purging.

Leptin

Leptin is a protein encoded by a gene called *obese*. Mice with a mutation to the *obese* gene that causes them to fail to make leptin rapidly grow to three times their normal weight. They lose this weight if they are administered injections of exogenous leptin.

While leptin is produced by adipocyte cells, it appears to regulate eating behavior through central, neuromodulatory effects. Another gene, called *diabetes*, codes for a leptin receptor that lies on the hypothalamus. Mice with a mutation to this gene not only become overweight; this obesity also fails to respond to exogenous leptin infusion.

Could it be that morbidly obese individuals have such difficulty losing weight because of a similar defect in one of these two genes? Leptin, along with other genetic and environmental influences, appears to be one important factor in determining a person's "settling point" (that is, the weight that an individual tends to return to, regardless of caloric intake). However, while several such gene mutations associated with abnormalities of feeding behavior have been identified in mice, no such abnormalities have been identified to date in humans.

Further, while in humans serum leptin levels do correlate with weight and with percent body fat for normal individuals for obese individuals, and for severely malnourished anorexic individuals, the amount of leptin in each of these cases is commensurate with the amount of fat that the individual is carrying. Similarly, leptin levels in patients with bulimia correlate with their body weight at the time that levels are measured. These findings suggest that altered leptin levels in patients with eating disorders follow a pattern similar to other associated endocrine abnormalities—that is, they more likely *reflect* the patient's nutritional state than cause it.

Other Endocrine Factors

Rebound hypoglycemia occurs about 2 hours after a binge–purge episode. Glucose levels of 140 to 150 can drop to levels as low as 35 to 50. Hypoglycemia is associated with not only lightheadedness, aggression, anxiety, and tachycardia but also with increased hunger. This might further exacerbate the binge–purge cycle.

Cortisol levels also are increased in bulimia. This may contribute to carbohydrate craving and weight gain given that patients treated with exogenous steroids experience these difficulties.

TREATMENT OF EATING DISORDERS

For all behavioral disorders, there are five overall stages of treatment. The first stage consists of helping the patient to *stop engaging in the behavior*. In the second stage, *medical complications* of the behavior are addressed. In the third stage, *comorbid psychiatric conditions* are addressed. In the fourth stage, *internal and external reinforcers* are addressed. In the fifth stage, patients are *maintained* in the ambulatory setting, and the goal is *relapse prevention*.

Stage 1: Address the Behavior

The treatment required for patients suffering from *disorders of motivated behavior* differs in several ways from that for patients with more "pure" diseases (i.e., those not associated with a significant behavioral component). In the latter case, the first goal is to discern the underlying pathology. The second goal is to address this pathology. For example, in treating a patient with pneumonia, we would first attempt to determine the cause of the pneumonia and then would prescribe an appropriate antibiotic.

In contrast, one faces a very different situation when attempting to treat the patient with an eating disorder. Regardless of *why* the patient with anorexia started fasting, ultimately the *behavior itself* becomes the patient's major problem, since it becomes self-perpetuating. In other words, regardless of any initial *triggering* factors, one might say that the anorexic patient starves herself today primarily because she starved herself yesterday. A failure to appreciate the central importance of addressing the behavior itself—not merely attempting to empathically understand the patient's subjective experience with the hope of addressing the underlying psychological "causes" of the disorder—may be one reason that the anorexia is associated with such a high rate of mortality. (This rate increases over time, ultimately reaching 20% for patients followed over a period of 20 years.)

In less severe cases, particularly in the outpatient setting, it is appropriate to first focus on establishing a therapeutic alliance, attempting to help the patient gain some insight into the fact that her eating behavior is a problem and to help the patient gain the motivation necessary to quit. As is the case with quitting any addictive habit, such as drinking alcohol or smoking cigarettes, some patients will be motivated to quit while others will not be motivated to do so, and the prognosis will be worse for the latter group.

Eating disorders support groups can be particularly useful in this regard, since they offer patients and their families education, motivation, and the support of peers with similar problems. Some groups are facilitated by a clinician while others are organized and run by nonprofessionals. Some are based on a 12-step addictions model. Many patients also turn to Internet Web sites or newsgroups for support. Many of these resources are very useful, but some of them perpetuate misinformation about nutrition and eating and fail to screen for or address associated psychiatric and medical comorbidity. Some peer-run groups fail to suggest or to integrate other potentially beneficial interventions, such as medication, nutritional counseling, and psychodynamic or cognitive–behavioral therapy.

In cases where the behavior is too out of control for outpatient intervention, or where the medical complications are too severe to be managed without intensive monitoring, hospitalization may be required. The goals of hospitalization are to interrupt the behavior cycle and to treat the medical complications. This treatment strategy parallels that which is employed to treat more severe cases of alcohol dependence. In treating the alcoholic patient, insight-oriented psychotherapy is of little use if the patient's con-

dition already has advanced to the point where she comes to sessions intoxicated or experiences severe physiologic withdrawal symptoms whenever she attempts to stop drinking. These more severe cases demand that detoxification be conducted in a monitored setting and that all access to alcohol be restricted.

The patient's weight in relation to ideal body weight is perhaps the best indicator of whether a patient will require inpatient treatment. Severely underweight patients (for example, those whose weight is 25%–30% below ideal body weight) are unlikely to be able to reach a healthy weight outside of an inpatient treatment program.

Within the context of an inpatient program, most patients can gain 2–3 pounds per week without significant medical complications. Some patients can be discharged before having reached 90% of ideal body weight if a transitional, intensive outpatient program is available. The closer the patient is to ideal body weight before discharge, the lower the risk of relapse.

With weight restoration, many of the classic symptoms of anorexia begin to abate, although many persist in attenuated form for years. Patients tend to obsess less about food and to broaden their range of food preferences, but distortions in body image and excessive concern with body shape tend to persist, along with the urge to exercise excessively. Apathy, lethargy, cognitive impairment, depression, and anxiety also abate with weight restoration. However, some patients remain depressed and at this point treatment with antidepressant medications may be appropriate.

In the inpatient setting, a few powerful positive and negative contingencies, along with early attempts at education, often are sufficient to change preexisting behavior patterns. For example, patients may be required to remain on bed rest until a pattern of weight gain becomes apparent. Similarly, patients may be required to sit at the meal table until their caloric intake has been sufficient. The clinician should attempt to minimize conflicts over the eating behavior by focusing not on the behavior itself but on objective weight gain. The treatment staff repeatedly confronts the patient, but it should always be with an attitude of concern.

Patients with alcohol- or drug-related disorders may be deceptive in their subjective reporting. In treating such patients, experienced clinicians rely on the motto, "Trust, but verify." They listen to their patients but also obtain random urine toxicology screens. Similarly, clinicians who treat patients with more severe eating disorders always must remain open to the possibility that their patients are "talking the talk" but not "walking the walk." They should rely more on objective measures of weight gain than on the patient's subjective reports that she is "starting to feel much better now."

Fortunately, the best objective measure of weight gain—the scale—is readily available, as are clear target weights. Several standardized tables of ideal weights for given heights are available. Some clinicians rely on weight guidelines from the Metropolitan Life Insurance Company, others on those published by the U.S. Department of Agriculture and Health and Human Services. The latter are presented in Table 11–5. In children and adolescents, growth curves should be followed. These are particularly useful since they allow height and weight to be tracked longitudinally in relation to the patient's premorbid growth trajectory. Research studies are increasingly relying on the **body mass index (BMI)**, which is calculated with the formula (weight [in

Table 11–5. Height and Weight Guidelines

Height (Inches) without Shoes	Weight (lb) without Clothes
58	91–119
59	94–124
60	97–128
61	101–132
62	104–137
63	107–141
64	111–146
65	114–150
66	118–155
67	121–160
68	125–164
69	129–169
70	132–174
71	136–179
72	140–184
73	144–189
74	148–195
75	152–200

Source: From *1995 Dietary Guidelines for Americans.* Washington, D.C., U.S. Department of Agriculture and Health and Human Services, 1995.

kg]/height [in meters]^2). Individuals with body mass indexes of less than 18.5 are considered to be underweight; body mass indexes of less than 17.5, in the presence of the other diagnostic criteria, indicate anorexia nervosa.

The goal of weight restoration in anorexia is for the patient to achieve at least 90% of ideal body weight (IBW). This weight is usually associated with a resumption of menses. Further, individuals who reach this weight have a lower likelihood of relapsing and a greater likelihood of responding to pharmacologic interventions. Unfortunately, patients can only gain 2–3 pounds per week, necessitating relatively long hospital stays. In contrast, many insurance carriers are willing to fund only acute, short-term hospital stays. Given this, many patients tend to be discharged from the hospital prematurely, leading to a "revolving door" pattern of hospital discharges and readmissions.

Stage 2: Treat Medical Complications of the Behavior

Medical complications can occur not only secondary to starvation and vomiting or laxative abuse but also as a result of refeeding. *Rapid feeding* (by nasogastric tube or by total parenteral nutrition) should be avoided, if possible, since this is more likely to produce *refeeding edema*, which can progress in rare cases to congestive heart failure, cardiac arrhythmia, or seizures. However, in severe cases where patients simply can't be fed by mouth, such interventions may prove to be lifesaving. In bulimia, correction of dehydration from the loss of gastric fluid also is essential if one hopes to correct contraction alkalosis. One also should address the electrolyte imbalances that can occur secondary to vomiting and/or laxative abuse, such as hypokalemia and hypomagnesemia. Serum phosphorus levels may precipitously drop during refeeding due to the body suddenly utilizing depleted stores of phosphorus during anabolism. Since this can be life threatening, phosphorus also should be monitored and repleted.

Patients typically enter treatment with extremely restrictive food preferences, which they are then informed they cannot adhere to on the inpatient unit. This causes considerable anxiety. A dietitian can assist the treatment team in establishing an appropriate schedule for caloric intake and also can help educate the patient about appropriate nutrition and assist the patient in making appropriate food choices that include items from each of the major food groups. Similarly, physical activity usually has to be significantly restricted early in treatment, particularly for patients who are severely underweight. Later in treatment, exercise can be reinstated, although ideally with a more appropriate emphasis on living a healthy lifestyle rather than on the rigid adherence to a fixed number of repetitions or number of hours spent at the gym.

In the outpatient setting, constant medical vigilance is necessary. One must take all physical complaints seriously, even those that have been evaluated previously. Multiple medical complications can occur in association with either malnutrition, or binging and purging behavior, or fluid–electrolyte imbalances, or refeeding. These include cardiac arrhythmia (especially bradycardia and QTc prolongation), renal complications (elevated BUN, low glomerular filtration rate, increased formation of renal calculi, hypovolemic nephropathy), tetany, grand mal seizures, gastric rupture, esophageal tears, and vitamin deficiencies.

Osteoporosis develops early in the course of anorexia and pathologic fractures are a major risk. The osteoporosis is likely multidetermined and is not caused solely by amenorrhea due to estrogen deficiency. Given this, correction of estrogen deficiency through the provision of exogenous estrogen and progesterone, while useful in treating osteoporosis in *postmenopausal, adequately nourished* women, does not appear to prevent or reverse bone loss in most patients with anorexia so long as they remain in a state of malnutrition. Given that the artificial reestablishment of menses may encourage these patients to see themselves as now being "well," many clinicians first attempt to help them achieve resumption of menses through weight restoration rather than simply prescribing hormonal replacement therapy from the outset of treatment. Improvements in bone density typically lag behind gains in weight.

Stage 3: Address Comorbid Psychiatric Conditions

Behavioral disorders such as eating disorders and substance-related disorders are frequently accompanied by other psychiatric conditions. If one doesn't attend to these, addressing the behavioral condition proves to be more difficult. For example, the patient with anorexia nervosa who currently also is experiencing severe symptoms of major depressive disorder or obsessive–compulsive disorder may have difficulty attending to a psychotherapy session or following through with treatment recommendations.

Over 1000 pharmacologic studies have been conducted on anorexia nervosa, but few have been randomized, controlled, or double-blinded. While no medication is specifically effective in treating the dieting behavior itself, about 5%–15% of patients may derive some benefit from the use of ancillary medication. Antidepressant agents, especially the *SSRIs*, have been the best studied. While they can be very useful in treating comorbid depressive and obsessive–compulsive symptoms in weight-restored patients, clinicians rarely prescribe them during the acute phase of treatment since their efficacy when used with emaciated patients is much more limited.

Further, malnourished patients may be more prone to experience side effects. For example, *tricyclic antidepressants* can cause hypotension, can increase cardiac conduction times, and can cause cardiac arrhythmia, and these side effects may be exacerbated in patients where malnutrition, dehydration, and electrolyte imbalance increase cardiac risk to begin with. When prescribing antidepressants, one should start with low doses and should avoid tricyclic agents in patients who are at greater risk for suicide or for experiencing cardiac complications. One also should avoid *bupropion*, since this is associated with a significantly increased seizure risk in purging patients.

In contrast, in patients who have achieved significant weight restoration, antidepressants may be useful not only in treating comorbid psychiatric syndromes but also in addressing the behavioral disorder itself. One study in which recently discharged patients were prescribed the SSRI agent fluoxetine at 40 mg per day found that patients who received this agent were less likely than patients who received placebo to be depressed and were better able to maintain their discharge weight and avoid rehospitalizations. Again, however, SSRIs are not a panacea, and are never a substitute for ongoing efforts to address the behavior itself. Several case reports suggest that *atypical antipsychotics* such as olanzapine also may be useful in treating both anxiety and distortions in body image.

Other agents that have been tested through clinical research include lithium, traditional antipsychotic agents, cyproheptadine, electroconvulsive therapy, and various vitamin and hormonal therapies. None has been found to offer significant clinical benefit.

Stage 4: Address Internal and External Reinforcers

As patients start to gain weight and as their cognition and mood begin to improve, they become better able to meaningfully participate in their treatment. At this point, psychotherapy assumes more a prominent role. Modalities of therapy that might be employed at this point include individual therapy (most commonly with a cognitive–behavioral orientation), group therapy, and family therapy.

Throughout this stage, one needs to continue to intensively monitor the patient's behavior. Of particular concern is the patient who expresses "empty insight," telling members of the inpatient treatment team "everything that they want to hear" in an attempt to gain earlier hospital discharge. Patients are particularly likely to experience resurgences of anxiety as they approach significant milestones, such as crossing particularly "feared" weights on the scale (e.g., 100 pounds) or packing away their "thin" clothing and having to purchase an entire new wardrobe of "larger" clothing.

We have discussed how, in addition to external reinforcers in Anorexia and Bulimia, there are internal biologic reinforcers as well. Pharmacologic interventions may prove to be useful in dampening the influence of internal reinforcers. In anorexia, SSRIs are the most commonly employed medications, particularly in cases where depression and anxiety persist following significant weight restoration.

In bulimia, several medications appear to provide efficacy in decreasing the intensity of urges to binge and purge. Again, the most widely utilized of these are the SSRIs, which also have the advantage of a greater margin of safety in this population. They have few anticholinergic or cardiac side effects and also are less sedating than the TCAs. However, they can increase glucose utilization, thereby causing hypoglycemia, and they can contribute to acute hyponatremia (a particular issue for patients who may be sodium depleted already as a result of vomiting). To date, fluoxetine is the only medication approved by the U.S. Food and Drug Administration for the treatment of bulimia.

TCAs also can help the patient to decrease binging behavior, but they can be associated with cardiac side effects, particular in patients with preexisting nutritional deficiencies and electrolyte imbalances. *Doxepin* is sometimes employed since it is a powerful H_2-receptor blocker, which can be useful in treating associated gastritis and esophagitis. *Clomipramine* also has been used since it is a powerful serotonin reuptake inhibitor that also is useful in treating associated obsessive–compulsive symptoms. However, both of these drugs are highly anticholinergic and antihistaminergic and therefore can be particularly difficult to tolerate. TCAs also carry a greater risk of being fatal in an overdose than SSRIs.

MAOIs are highly effective in bulimia, although in practice they rarely are prescribed. By definition, bulimic patients aren't discriminating about what they ingest during a binge, and they therefore may be more likely to violate a tyramine-free diet. This places them at greater risk of experiencing a hypertensive crisis. Further, these patients also are frequently volume depleted, which also can make it more difficult for them to regulate body temperature. They therefore have greater risk of experiencing hypotension, syncope, and hyperpyrexia when prescribed MAOIs.

Bupropion was found to be effective in treating bulimia during initial clinical trials. However, its use in bulimics now is contraindicated. It briefly was taken off of the market after subsequent trials demonstrated it to be associated with a high risk of seizures in particular patients, including those with preexisting seizure disorder, head injury, and bulimia. Again, massive shifts in electrolyte balance associated with active binging and purging likely play the major role in increasing the seizure risk in bulimia.

While *benzodiazepines* may be helpful in relieving anxiety, they also can carry significant risks in this population, including addiction and seizures related to benzodiazepine withdrawal. The latter is a concern since patients with bulimia have a greater risk of electrolyte imbalance and since they also may be more likely to abruptly and impulsively stop taking a prescribed medication.

Stage 5: Relapse Prevention in the Ambulatory Setting

After hospital discharge, treatment shifts toward *maintaining* these behavioral goals in a naturalistic setting. As with all of the other behavioral disorders, one's goals at this stage must, by necessity, be modest, since relapse is extremely common. In one study of hospitalized anorexic patients assessed at initial follow-up, 44% had achieved a restored weight and had resumed menses, 24% had a poor outcome (having never approached their goal weight), 28% had an "intermediate" outcome, and 5% had suffered early mortality. Even among the patients who achieve a better outcome, about two-thirds continue to have persistent morbid food and weight preoccupations and 40% still have bulimic symptoms.

While avoiding excessive nihilism, one must help patients to be "relapse-ready." In other words, they must be prepared for the possibility of "falling off the wagon" and resuming their problematic behaviors. Behavioral disorders have extremely high relapse rates since the behaviors involved are so familiar, so rewarding, and so comforting to patients, and also since they have become linked to so many internal and external reinforcers. Patients therefore should be prepared for relapse so that they don't prematurely throw in the towel and resume their previous behaviors in full force after a single misstep. Patients also need to know that the "door is always open" for a return to inpatient treatment should this prove necessary.

Patients at this stage sometimes are extremely difficult to treat. Along with weight gain, new symptoms often appear. Further, they often are unmotivated and resist forming a therapeutic alliance with clinicians. Since one goal is to help the patient to avoid premature termination of therapy, limit setting must by necessity be combined with flexibility. The art of treatment at this stage is determining the proper mix of these factors.

SUMMARY

Eating disorders are associated with significant morbidity and mortality. They are excellent examples of conditions best approached from the behavioral perspective. No single, biological "broken part" accounts for the occurrence of an eating disorder in a given individual. The condition likely arises out of the combined effects of multiple initiators (including biological factors, psychological factors, environmental factors, and the dieting behavior itself) on individuals who are at risk for developing pathological eating behaviors due to inherent constitutional vulnerabilities.

Treating these individuals requires more than simply an appreciation of the factors that led them to first engage in their pathological pattern of behavior. Behavioral disorders tend to become self-sustaining over time, and the primary intervention therefore must be to assist the patient to stop engaging in the behavior in question.

Complicating matters, patients with behavioral disorders typically don't *want* to give up these behaviors. They often refuse to adopt the "patient role," preferring to stay ill. They most often present for treatment due to the adverse effects that their behavior has had on the people around them or on their own health. Their limited insight and the difficulties associated with attempting to change established patterns of behavior are the primary obstacles to treatment.

Treatment consists of helping the patient to stop engaging in the behavior while also addressing medical complications associated with starvation and/or with binging and purging. Comorbid psychiatric conditions also must be addressed. Next, patients must be encouraged to examine those internal and external factors that are acting as behavioral reinforcers and to formulate and practice ways that they might resist acting on these reinforcers. Lastly, patients are never "cured" of behavioral disorders. Given this, a final goal in managing these disorders—even following "successful" treatment—is to continually work toward relapse prevention.

Chapter 12

Substance-Related Disorders

Substance-related disorders cost the United States in excess of $300 billion annually when one includes the costs of treatment, related health problems, absenteeism, lost productivity, drug-related crime and incarceration, and efforts at education and prevention. About 5.5 million Americans (2.7% of the population over age 12) clearly or probably need treatment for drug abuse and an additional 13 million Americans clearly or probably need treatment for alcohol abuse.

Furthermore, substance-related disorders are associated with significant morbidity and mortality, particularly among men. Substance dependence (excluding nicotine) is responsible, directly or indirectly, for 40% of all hospital admissions and for 25% of all deaths; approximately 100,000 deaths per year result directly from the use of illicit drugs or alcohol. Two-thirds of these deaths occur in individuals who are dependent on heroin or cocaine, and nearly 40% of the deaths occur in individuals between the ages of 30 and 39.

Finally, substance users exert a profound impact on the world around them. Substance intoxication is associated with about half of all highway fatalities, over half of all cases of domestic violence, and over half of all murders. These disorders also cause disinhibition and feelings of sadness and irritability, thereby contributing to many cases of attempted or completed suicide. They also significantly contribute to job absenteeism, job-related accidents, and low employee productivity. Finally, urine testing reveals that 8%–15% of all pregnant women have used a drug of abuse (excluding alcohol) shortly before their first prenatal visit.

Substance-related disorders are examples of conditions best approached from the behavior perspective. While biological factors likely help explain why one person becomes addicted to a substance while another person does not, extensive research over decades has not revealed an underlying biological "broken part" that in itself accounts for the phenomenon of addiction. Similarly, while personality and life-story variables clearly contribute to the onset of addiction, shape the clinical presentation, and influence treatment outcome, these factors in themselves are neither necessary nor sufficient to explain addiction.

The relevance of the behavior perspective becomes most obvious when we consider that substance-related syndromes are *defined* almost purely in behavioral terms. For example, whether an individual is labeled a "social" drinker, a "problem" drinker, an alcohol "abuser," or alcohol "dependent" relates solely to how he or she *behaves* with regard to the ingestion of alcohol. Similarly, the primary goal of every treatment intervention—regardless of whether it is a medication, a course of individual psychotherapy, or participation in a 12-step program—is *behavior modification*.

To review the primary tenets of the behavioral perspective, motivated behaviors are *goal-directed* and therefore are designated by their consequences. Motivated behaviors occur *intermittently*, can be *selectively provoked* by stimuli that are later ignored, and can *vary in intensity*. They also can be *voluntarily suppressed*, such that individuals retain the ability to exercise *choices*, even in the case of very powerful drives. (Of course, the more powerful the drive, the more difficulty individuals will have choosing other options.)

Individuals engage in motivated behaviors in three phases: *(1)* a *craving phase*, characterized by both a search for pleasure and a desire to achieve release from an uncomfortable state of tension; *(2)* a *consummatory phase*, wherein the individual engages in the particular behavior; and *(3)* a *satisfaction phase*, wherein the drive to engage in the behavior decreases and the behavior is replaced by other activities. Ultimately, an increase in the drive to engage in the behavior and a return of the craving phase occurs at some later point in time.

Motivated behaviors are subject to the influence of both internal and external reinforcing factors. As we have seen in the case of the eating disorders, the factors that *initiate* a problematic behavior may differ from those that ultimately come to *sustain* the behavior, and pathologic behaviors tend to become *self-sustaining*. In other words, while the initiation of alcohol ingestion may be determined by a variety of psychological and environmental factors, the severely alcohol-dependent individual drinks alcohol today largely because he drank alcohol yesterday.

Finally, there are no bright lines between normal behavior, "problem" behavior, and "pathological" behavior. These distinctions are socially defined, disjunctive, and often arbitrary. Behaviors typically are considered to be "pathological" either when the *object* of the drive is abnormal (as in bulimia nervosa or sexual paraphilia) or when the *strength* of the drive is abnormal (as in "pathological," or "compulsive," overeating, gambling, and sexual behavior).

How does this approach apply to the substance-related disorders? Whether the *object* of the drive (i.e., substance use) is "abnormal" remains a subject of intense social debate. In American society, *any* use of heroin, cocaine, or marijuana is subject to criminal penalties, because of their addictive potential and associated health risks. How-

ever, this is not the case for alcohol or nicotine, despite these *also* being potentially addictive and being associated with significant health risks.

Regardless of whether society condones or sanctions the use of particular substances, it is clear that substance-using behavior is a common phenomenon: 90% of Americans try alcohol at some point in their lives, while 50% are current alcohol users; 80% of Americans drink caffeine-containing beverages on a daily basis; 30% regularly use nicotine; 5% regularly use marijuana; almost 1% regularly use cocaine.

Not all people who engage in a particular behavior develop a behavioral *disorder*. In the previous chapter, the continuity between "normal" dieting behaviors and the more severe behaviors that characterize eating disorders was discussed. Similarly, substance use exists along a continuum of severity, with lesser severity being associated with greater prevalence.

Figure 12–1 demonstrates this phenomenon using the example of alcohol. As can be seen, 90% of the general population has *tried* alcohol. A lower percentage (40%) has experienced some *temporary social impairment* from alcohol, such as having missed work or school due to drinking or having driven while intoxicated. The lifetime prevalence of *alcohol abuse* is yet lower, 20% for men and 10% for women. Finally, the lifetime prevalence of *alcohol dependence* is 10% for men and 5% for women.

Why do some people develop a substance-related disorder while other people do not? How does the behavior perspective offer guidance in treating substance-dependent individuals? To help address these questions, we will first review the *phenomenology* of the substance-related disorders. We then will review *behavioral management strategies* for the substance-related disorders as a whole. Finally, we will review the phenomenology and neurobiology of the *specific* Substance Disorders along with associated treatment implications.

PHENOMENOLOGY

Intoxication

Substance intoxication refers to a reversible, substance-specific syndrome of maladaptive behavioral or psychological changes due to the re-

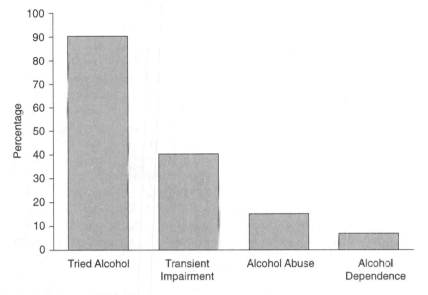

Figure 12–1. Alcohol use in the United States.

cent ingestion of, or exposure to, a substance that acts on the central nervous system.

DSM-IV defines "substance-induced intoxication" relatively narrowly. The definition excludes the CNS *side effects* that can be associated with a variety of routinely prescribed medications (such as *sedation* caused by antidepressants or an antihistamine, or *nervousness* caused by antidepressants or caffeine) since such behavioral and psychological changes aren't considered to be "maladaptive." However, if ingestion of a drug causes "maladaptive" behavioral or psychological changes—belligerence, mood lability, cognitive impairment, impaired judgment, impaired social functioning, or impaired occupational functioning—this physiologic state *could* be considered to be one of "intoxication."

The clinical symptoms of intoxication vary across different classes of drugs. *DSM-IV* offers diagnostic criteria for 11 different pharmacologic classes: alcohol; amphetamines and related agents; caffeine; cannabis; cocaine; hallucinogens; inhalants; nicotine; opioids; phencyclidine (PCP) and related agents; and sedatives, hypnotics, and anxiolytics. *DSM-IV* also includes a "residual" category, which includes a variety of other agents, including anabolic steroids and nitrous oxide.

Often, intoxication is associated with intense

pleasure or euphoria, and this emotional state becomes a powerful behavioral reinforcer. However, addiction isn't *solely* a function of drug-induced "euphoria." For example, while cocaine and heroin intoxication are associated with euphoria, alcohol intoxication more often is described as a state of increased relaxation. In further contrast, *nicotine* use is associated with a mixture of increased relaxation and increased *alertness*, and PCP intoxication may be associated with confusion, anxiety, and psychosis. However, despite these objective and subjective differences, the use of all of these agents can become *self-reinforcing*, and all of them therefore can cause substance dependence.

The specific clinical picture in substance intoxication also can vary dramatically between *individuals*. Variables that influence the clinical presentation include: the particular *substance*, the *dose* that is ingested, the *duration or chronicity* of dosing, the person's degree of *tolerance* for the substance, the *period of time since the last dose*, the *expectations of the person* as to the substance's effects, and *contextual variables* related to the surrounding environment. Short-term, "acute" intoxication states often are associated with different signs and symptoms than more sustained or "chronic" intoxication states. For example, cocaine use may initially produce gregariousness, but following repeated use over a period of days or weeks it may produce severe social withdrawal.

Note that a state of intoxication is neither necessary nor sufficient *in itself* to account for the phenomenon of substance dependence. For example, based upon the above definition, nicotine does not cause a state of "intoxication," despite the fact that using nicotine clearly is associated with pleasurable sensations and with powerful behavioral reinforcement.

Neuroadaptation

Tolerance refers to either: *(1)* the need to use a *greatly increased amount* of a substance in order to achieve the desired effect (with the effect usually being a state of intoxication) or *(2)* a *markedly diminished effect* being associated with continued use of the *same amount* of the substance.

The degree to which tolerance develops varies greatly between substances. For example, both heavy opioid use and heavy stimulant use are associated with the development of substantial tolerance, such that users ultimately can require up to 10 times the dosage that they first used (a dosage that might even be fatal for a nonuser). *Alcohol* tolerance also can be pronounced, although it usually is less extreme than what is seen for the opioids and stimulants. Many individuals who smoke *cigarettes* consume more than 20 cigarettes per day, providing them with a level of nicotine that would have produced toxic symptoms when they first started smoking. Individuals who engage in heavy *cannabis* use generally are not aware of having developed tolerance, but tolerance has been demonstrated in animal studies and in some humans. It is uncertain whether tolerance develops to *phencyclidine*.

Tolerance may be difficult to determine based on the clinical history alone since the substance in question often is illegal and often has been mixed with various diluents or with other intoxicating substances. In such situations, laboratory testing may be helpful. For example, a high serum level of a given substance, coupled with there being little clinical evidence of intoxication during the current evaluation, suggests that an individual has developed significant tolerance to the substance.

Tolerance should be distinguished from *individual variability* in one's sensitivity to the intoxicating effects of a particular substance. For example, some first-time drinkers show little evidence of intoxication after three or four drinks, whereas other first-time drinkers of similar weight experience slurred speech and incoordination.

Withdrawal is a maladaptive behavioral change, with physiological and cognitive concomitants, that occurs in an individual when blood or tissue concentrations of a substance decline following prolonged heavy use of the substance. After developing unpleasant withdrawal symptoms, individuals are more likely to take the substance again in an attempt to relieve or avoid the symptoms. This ultimately can lead to their using the substance throughout the day, beginning shortly after awakening.

Withdrawal symptoms vary greatly across different classes of substances. *Marked physiological signs of withdrawal* commonly are encountered with alcohol, opioids, sedatives, hypnotics, and anxiolytics. Withdrawal signs and symptoms often are *present but less apparent* with amphetamines, cocaine, nicotine, and marijuana. *No significant withdrawal* is observed in humans even after repeated use of the hallucinogens or phencyclidine.

Cross-tolerance and **cross-dependence** refer to the ability of one drug to substitute for another in suppressing withdrawal and maintaining a state of physiologic dependence. For example, methadone is cross-tolerant with heroin, since both substances act at the opiate receptor. Similarly, benzodiazepines and barbiturates are cross-tolerant with alcohol, since all act at the GABA–benzodiazepine receptor complex.

Neuroadaptation refers to the underlying central nervous system changes that occur following repeated administration of a drug, such that the person develops both tolerance and withdrawal phenomena. This also has been termed "physiologic dependence," a term that should not be confused with the more global term, "substance dependence." In the case of some highly reinforcing agents, *substance dependence can occur in the absence of significant neuroadaptation.*

Further, *neuroadaptation can occur in the absence of substance dependence* since neuroadaptation occurs following repeated administration of a *variety* of pharmaceutical agents, not simply drugs of abuse. For example, many antidepressants act at the antihistamine receptor and can cause sedation. This sedation tends to diminish over time, reflecting the development of *tolerance* for this effect. Also, many commonly prescribed medications (including serotonergic antidepressants) are associated with uncomfortable *withdrawal* symptoms following abrupt discontinuation but aren't self-reinforcing and don't trigger drug-seeking behaviors. (Given this, it is important to explain to patients who are taking antidepressants that they aren't "addicted" to them despite being their being at risk for experiencing either withdrawal symptoms or a depressive relapse following medication discontinuation, especially abrupt discontinuation.)

Similarly, many patients with chronic pain who are prescribed opioids for an extended period develop both tolerance (i.e., they require higher doses to obtain the same degree of analgesia) and withdrawal. However, many of them do not demonstrate compulsive drug use. In other words, while they are *physiologically* dependent on opioids, they do not fulfill the *DSM* diagnostic criteria for substance dependence, nor do they require treatment for "drug addiction."

Symptoms of *withdrawal* should be distinguished from symptoms of relapse and rebound. **Relapse** occurs when the patient has an underlying medical condition previously controlled by a medication, and the symptoms of the condition now return following discontinuation of the medication. **Rebound** is a *withdrawal* phenomenon whereby the symptoms of an underlying medical condition become *worse than they were at baseline* following abrupt discontinuation of a medication.

For example, if a patient who has been taking clonidine to treat essential hypertension gradually tapers the clonidine, he likely will experience a *relapse* of his preexisting hypertension. However, if he *abruptly* discontinues the clonidine he might experience dangerously high hypertension, a *rebound* effect. Similarly, a patient successfully taking a benzodiazepine for panic disorder might experience a *relapse* of panic attacks following a taper of the benzodiazepines. The relapse might occur days, months, or years later. In contrast, a patient with panic disorder who *abruptly* stops taking a benzodiazepine may experience *rebound* panic attacks that are even more frequent and more severe than the pretreatment attacks.

Distinguishing anxiety caused by *benzodiazepine withdrawal* from *relapse* of the underlying anxiety disorder or from *rebound* exacerbation of the underlying anxiety disorder can be difficult. Rebound and withdrawal anxiety are typically short-term phenomena that improve over a period of days to weeks. If these symptoms persist and resemble the patient's initial presentation, the patient likely has experienced a relapse of the anxiety disorder. In contrast, patients who demonstrate not only symptoms resembling those seen at initial presentation but also *new symptoms* (especially irritability, autonomic instability, or seizures) are likely in a state of benzodiazepine withdrawal.

Dependence, Abuse, and "Addiction"

Substance dependence, as defined in the *DSM-IV*, refers to more than physiologic neuroadaptation. It describes a broad neurobehavioral syndrome. In addition to neuroadaptation it includes two hallmark *behavioral* features: impaired control over the use of the substance and increased salience of the substance. Examples of *impaired control* include: taking the substance in larger amounts or over a longer period of time than initially intended, having persistent desires for the drug, and making unsuccessful efforts to cut down or control the substance use. Examples of *increased salience* include: spending a great deal of time acquiring, using or recovering from the drug; reducing or giving up important social, occupational, or recreational activities because of the drug; and continuing to use the drug despite knowledge that it is causing or exacerbating physical or psychological problems.

For years, the term *addiction* was used to describe all three aspects of pathological substance use (neuroadaptation, impaired control, and increased salience). More recently, however, the term "substance dependence" has been substituted, since "addiction" and "addict" have been applied pejoratively. The *DSM-IV* has retired "addiction" from the official nomenclature, but this term remains in common parlance, perhaps because it so much more powerfully conveys the driven quality of the cravings and behaviors associated with these agents.

Unfortunately, clinicians disagree as to whether to apply the term "dependence" narrowly (to refer only to *physiologic* dependence—i.e., neuroadaptation) or broadly (to refer the entire neurobehavioral syndrome). The problem with the "narrow" definition is that some individuals do not demonstrate "psychological/behavioral dependence" despite being "physiologically dependent," while the reverse is the case for other individuals.

DSM-IV therefore has opted for the broader definition of substance dependence. The definition is disjunctive, such that two individuals with very different symptoms both can fulfill the diagnostic criteria. The *DSM-IV* criteria for substance dependence are presented in Table 12–1. Note that criteria 1 and 2 refer to neuroadaptation, criteria 3 and 4 refer to impaired control, and criteria 5 through 7 refer to increased salience. While there isn't a separate category for physiologic dependence (neuroadaptation), the criteria require that clinicians *specify* whether this is present in a given case, given the importance of this factor in treatment planning. Also, note that the *DSM-IV* definition of substance Dependence *doesn't* include any *specific intoxica-tion or withdrawal symptoms* because the criteria are meant to apply *across all classes of substances.*

In applying these criteria, one should specify whether a patient is in **remission** (i.e., has demonstrated no symptoms for greater than 1 month), and if so, if the patient is in **early remission** (a remission of under 12 months) or **sustained remission** (a remission lasting greater than 12 months). Finally, a patient's remission can be either a **partial remission** (with the patient still experiencing intermittent or occasional symptoms) or a **full remission** (with the patient experiencing no symptoms).

Some individuals do not demonstrate evidence of tolerance, withdrawal, or "compulsive" drug use but nonetheless continue to engage in substance use despite having encountered harmful consequences. Such individuals are classified as having **substance abuse**, as described in Table 12–2. *DSM-IV* also includes substance-induced disorders that preset with symptoms from *other diagnostic categories*, including *delirium* due to substance intoxication or substance with-

---

Table 12–1. *DSM-IV-TR* Criteria for Substance Dependence

A maladaptive pattern of substance use, leading to clinically significant impairment or distress, as manifested by three (or more) of the following, occurring at any time in the same 12-month period:

1. Tolerance, as defined by either of the following:
   a. A need for markedly increased amounts of the substance to achieve intoxication or desired effect
   b. Markedly diminished effect with continued use of the same amount of the substance
2. Withdrawal, as manifested by either of the following:
   a. The characteristic withdrawal syndrome for the substance (refer to criteria A and B of the criteria sets for withdrawal from the specific substances)
   b. The same (or a closely related) substance is taken to relieve or avoid withdrawal symptoms
3. The substance is often taken in larger amounts or over a longer period than was intended
4. There is a persistent desire or unsuccessful efforts to cut down or control substance use
5. A great deal of time is spent in activities necessary to obtain the substance (e.g., visiting multiple doctors or driving long distances), use the substance (e.g., chain-smoking), or recover from its effects
6. Important social, occupational, or recreational activities are given up or reduced because of substance use
7. The substance use is continued despite knowledge of having a persistent or recurrent physical or psychological problem that is likely to have been caused or exacerbated by the substance (e.g., current cocaine use despite recognition of cocaine-induced depression, or continued drinking despite recognition that an ulcer was made worse by alcohol consumption)

SPECIFY IF

With Physiological Dependence

Evidence of tolerance or withdrawal (i.e., either item 1 or 2 is present)

Without Physiological Dependence

No evidence of tolerance or withdrawal (i.e., neither item 1 nor 2 is present)

Source: Reprinted with permission from the *Diagnostic and Statistical Manual of Mental Disorders, Fourth Edition, Text Revision.* Copyright 2000 American Psychiatric Association.

Table 12–2. *DSM-IV-TR* Criteria for Substance Abuse

A. A maladaptive pattern of substance use leading to clinically significant impairment or distress, as manifested by one (or more) of the following, occurring within a 12-month period:
   1. Recurrent substance use resulting in a failure to fulfill major role obligations at work, school, or home (e.g., repeated absences or poor work performance related to substance use; substance-related absences, suspensions, or expulsions from school; neglect of children or household)
   2. Recurrent substance use in situations in which it is physically hazardous (e.g., driving an automobile or operating a machine when impaired by substance use)
   3. Recurrent substance-related legal problems (e.g., arrests for substance-related disorderly conduct)
   4. Continued substance use despite having persistent or recurrent social or interpersonal problems caused or exacerbated by the effects of the substance (e.g., arguments with spouse about consequences of intoxication, physical fights)
B. The symptoms have never met the criteria for substance dependence for this class of substance

Source: Reprinted with permission from the *Diagnostic and Statistical Manual of Mental Disorders, Fourth Edition, Text Revision.* Copyright 2000 American Psychiatric Association

drawal, substance-induced *psychotic disorder,* substance-induced *mood disorder,* substance-induced *anxiety disorder,* substance-induced *persisting amnestic disorder,* substance-induced *persisting dementia,* substance-induced *sexual dysfunction,* and substance-induced *sleep disorder.* These conditions are discussed in the present text in the context of the "primary" forms of each of these disorders.

Reward and Reinforcement

Historically, the development of substance dependence has been ascribed primarily to neuroadaptation (i.e., to tolerance and withdrawal). Therefore, treatment has emphasized acute *detoxification.* The historical image has been of a patient "desperate to quit" but prevented from doing so by severe withdrawal symptoms, particularly autonomic hyperactivity. Detoxification usually is accomplished through a gradual taper either of the drug in question (perhaps in longer-acting forms, such as using a nicotine patch rather than cigarettes, or methadone rather than heroin), or through titration of a cross-tolerant medication (such as a benzodiazepine rather than alcohol). Sympatholytic agents such as clonidine or β-adrenergic antagonists often are prescribed to blunt sympathetic hyperarousal.

However, the observed phenomenology of substance dependence doesn't fully comport with this model. For example, if the primary factor that drives substance dependence is the fear of physiologic withdrawal, one would expect that—once out of withdrawal—patients would vow never to fall into such a predicament again and would persistently work to maintain absti-

nence. However, relapse is more the rule than the exception for most patients, even those who receive extensive drug rehabilitation following detoxification. Many of these patients report a history of multiple admissions for "detox," each of which has been followed by a resumption of drug use. Similarly, for many years, marijuana and cocaine have been thought of as more "benign" than heroin and alcohol, primarily because they are not associated with severe physical withdrawal symptoms. However, if this is the case, why do so many individuals who use cocaine and marijuana have such a hard time quitting?

The theory that withdrawal is the primary reinforcer of substance dependence also has led society (including physicians) to become very frustrated with those substance-dependent individuals who relapse despite having been "successfully" detoxified. The frustration relates to an underlying belief that these individuals were no longer physically dependent at that point and therefore "should have known better."

What these earlier theories failed to fully appreciate was the importance of *reward* in substance dependence. **Rewards** are stimuli that the brain interprets as being intrinsically positive. As such, *rewarding stimuli tend to be reinforcing*— that is, they are associated with a greater probability that behaviors paired with them will be repeated in the future.

The biochemical pathways that mediate reward appear to be distinct from those that mediate withdrawal. Substance *withdrawal* is mediated primarily by noradrenergic output from the locus ceruleus. In contrast, as discussed in Chapter 4 and illustrated in Figure 4–3, *reward—*

whether it occurs in response to natural reinforcers (such as food and sex) or in response to
direct pharmacologic reinforcers (such as addictive drugs)—relies primarily on *the pleasure circuit*. This circuit is a mesolimbic pathway centering on the *nucleus accumbens* (along with
related structures that together comprise the "extended amygdala") and primarily mediated by
dopaminergic input from the ventral tegmental
area (VTA).

Why people who have been dependent on cocaine remain prone to relapse even after months
of abstinence becomes more understandable
when seen in this light. Animal studies demonstrate that cocaine—despite being associated
with few physical withdrawal symptoms—is the
most powerful pharmacologic reinforcer known,
since cocaine is so *rewarding*. For example, rats
given unlimited access to cocaine will choose it
over food, water, or access to other animals and
continue to use it even to the point of starvation.
Lesioning a rat's locus ceruleus has no effect
on this behavior; however, lesioning a rat's
dopaminergic reward pathway has dramatic consequences. In the latter case, the cocaine loses its
reinforcing properties, and the rat can't reliably
differentiate cocaine from placebo.

Virtually all rewarding stimuli appear to exert
their effects through this pleasure circuit. *Milder*
sensations of reward in response to natural reinforcers, along with associated conditioned behavioral responses, usually are *adaptive* for an
organism. Dopamine release might help the organism to learn which events and behaviors are
more important and to pay greater attention to
such events. However, *excessive* activity along
this circuit may account for the driven, repetitive
quality of the behaviors associated with substance dependence and other "addictive" disorders. Drugs of abuse interact with this pleasure
circuit at multiple levels, as illustrated in Table
12–3. While they exert a wide diversity of initial effects, "downstream" they all either *enhance
dopamine release* at the level of the ventral
tegmental area, or *potentiate the effects of
dopamine release* at the level of the nucleus accumbens, or produce effects *similar to dopamine
release* at the level of the nucleus accumbens.

For example, **opiates** bind not only to opioid
receptors on GABAergic interneurons within the
VTA (thereby inhibiting their activity and in-

Table 12–3. Proposed Neurobiological Substrates
for the Acute Reinforcing Effects of Various
Drugs of Abuse

Drug	Neurotransmitter
Opiates	Dopamine, opioid peptides
Cocaine/amphetamines	Dopamine, serotonin
Nicotine	Dopamine, opioid peptides
Alcohol	Dopamine, GABA, glutamate, Serotonin, opioid peptides
Cannabis	Dopamine, GABA, opioid peptides
PCP	Glutamate, opioid peptides

creasing the firing of dopaminergic neurons extending to the nucleus accumbens) but also to
opioid receptors located within the nucleus
accumbens itself. (As a result of this latter, more
effect on the nucleus accumbens, opioids
continue to exert reinforcing effects even in rats
whose dopaminergic pathway has been lesioned.)

Cocaine and amphetamines act on the nerve
terminals of the VTA's dopaminergic (and other
monoaminergic) neurons, with cocaine primarily
inhibiting monoamine reuptake and amphetamine primarily increasing monoamine release.
Nicotine stimulates nicotinic receptors located
on these same dopaminergic neurons, again leading to increased output to the nucleus accumbens.

Alcohol, until recently, was believed to act primarily by intercalating itself into neuronal membranes, thereby increasing membrane fluidity
and influencing a variety of gated ion channels,
neuroreceptors, and other transmembrane proteins. While this may remain its mechanism of
action at higher doses, at lower (more clinical
relevant) doses, alcohol exerts more selective effects. Most notably, it binds both to *GABA receptors* (where it is a positive allosteric modulator, thereby amplifying the effects of GABA) and
to *NMDA receptors* (where it exerts inhibitory
effects, thereby diminishing the excitatory effects of glutamate). Various regions of the brain
differ in their sensitivity to these actions, probably reflecting regional variation both in the concentrations of these two receptors and in receptor subunit composition.

Alcohol also potentiates activity at $5HT_3$ sero-
tonin receptors, which—unlike other serotonin
receptors—are linked to a fast-acting, excitatory
ion channel. However, since these excitatory receptors are located primarily on *inhibitory* in-

terneurons, alcohol's potentiating effects contribute to an overall increase in inhibitory modulation. As if these effects weren't enough, alcohol also *elevates brain serotonin concentrations, augments the activity of opioid receptors* within the nucleus accumbens, and *raises dopamine levels* in the nucleus accumbens. The mechanism by which alcohol accomplishes these two last effects is currently unclear. It isn't known whether they reflect activity at the VTA or nucleus accumbens or whether they relate to alcohol's effects on the NMDA or GABA receptor.

Cannabinoids bind to specific cannabinoid receptors (called CB_1 and CB_2 receptors), which are widely distributed throughout the brain. Like opioid receptors, cannabinoid receptors are acted upon not only by exogenous agents but also by endogenous ligands, called **endogenous cannabinoids** (or **endocannabinoids**). Recent research suggests that endocannabinoids probably play important roles in the regulation of pain, appetite, and memory. (This may explain why cannabis use is associated with a sense of calm, with increased appetite, and with clouding of memory).

In addition to independently increasing dopamine levels in the nucleus accumbens, the cannabinoid system also probably acts indirectly through its close ties with the opioid system. For example, in animals, acute cannabinoid administration increases enkephalin levels in the nucleus accumbens, and repeated cannabinoid administration even increases opioid gene expression. Animal studies also suggest that *cross-tolerance* exists between opioid and cannabinoid agonists. In other words, morphine-tolerant animals demonstrate decreased antinociceptive responses to cannabinoid administration, and vice versa. *Cross-dependence* also appears to exist, such that the opioid antagonist naloxone precipitates a withdrawal syndrome in cannabinoid-tolerant rats, while the cannabinoid antagonist SR171416A precipitates withdrawal in morphine-dependent rats. Finally, the endogenous cannabinoid system appears to play a role in the rewarding effects of opioid agents, given that the reinforcing effects of morphine are attenuated in mice bred to lack CB_1 receptors.

Phencyclidine (PCP) (along with a related drug, **ketamine**) binds to specific sites on the NMDA glutamate receptor, where it exerts antagonist effects. It appears to exert its reinforcing effects by blocking excitatory glutaminergic input extending from the prefrontal region to the nucleus accumbens. It may also exert effects at the opioid receptor.

Reward can reinforce behavior in two major ways. **Positive reinforcement** occurs when a particular behavior *leads* to the individual receiving some *pleasant* reward, while **negative reinforcement** occurs when a behavior *relieves* the individual of an *unpleasant* physical or mental state. Both types of reinforcement are associated with an increased likelihood that the associated behaviors will occur in the future. For example, many alcohol and drug users report that, early on in their "careers," their drug of choice offered a sense of euphoria, but that this sensation diminished over time along with the development of tolerance. Despite this, and despite having experienced severe adverse social consequences as a result of their drug use (such as the loss of their job, their home, and their family) they continued to use the drug, doing so more to combat chronic apathy and dysphoria than to achieve their original "high." It therefore appears that positive reinforcement played the most important role early on, but that—over time—negative reinforcement came to play an increasingly important role.

Negative reinforcement must be distinguished from **aversive control or punishment**. In aversive control, behaviors are *less* likely to occur when they are followed by *negative consequences*. Examples of aversive control include: giving disulfiram (Antabuse) to alcoholic patients (since the threat of becoming physically ill along with alcohol ingestion may inhibit them from drinking); requiring individuals on probation for drug offenses to submit to random drug screens (along with the threat of incarceration if a test is positive); and arresting any individuals caught driving while intoxicated, carrying open liquor bottles in public, or purchasing illegal drugs.

The persistence of **craving** following the resolution of more acute withdrawal symptoms likely reflects the influence of both positive and negative reinforcement. For example, individuals dependent on alcohol, opioids, amphetamines, or cocaine who abstain from using these agents can develop more chronic psychological withdrawal symptoms that persist over a period of several weeks to several months following the resolution of more acute withdrawal symptoms. Symptoms of this state include anhedonia, general malaise, depression, decreased motivation, and decreased creativity. Some individuals report that they resumed drug use in order to "feel normal again." In other words, their chronic withdrawal symptoms acted as powerful *negative reinforcers*, thereby encouraging relapse.

It also appears likely that *positive reinforcement* also plays an important role in long-term craving. Local neuroadaptation as well as more extensive central nervous system changes (the latter resulting from increased activity along the "stress thermostat," changes in second messenger activity, changes in gene expression, even changes in neuronal morphology) may change the reward circuit's homeostatic **set point**. Given this, an individual may not be able to return to a "normal" state for quite some time following acute detoxification (perhaps, in some cases, never).

Further, since hippocampal and limbic *memory circuits* also are intimately associated with the reward circuit (as illustrated in Figure 4.3), powerful "emotional memories" of the intoxication state may persist long after physical withdrawal subsides, just as "flashbacks" of an acute trauma persist in PTSD. A multitude of environmental cues (e.g., the liquor store, images on television, a particular street corner) may trigger these "flashbacks" (**cue-induced craving**). The cues become paired with these sensations, thereby becoming positive reinforcers, despite the individual's extended abstinence. This "priming effect" appears to be associated with a *conditioned release of dopamine*. For example, rats exposed to alcohol will demonstrate increased dopamine release even *in anticipation* of receiving alcohol, while rats who have received cocaine several times through the injection route will demonstrate similar increased dopamine release even following the administration of a saline injection.

This positive reinforcement is compounded by even more powerful positive reinforcement should the individual actually give in to the craving by attempting to use the drug "just a little bit, just this one time." Exposure to the original re-

warding stimulus is even *more* reinforcing than exposure to associated environmental cues. As a result, many alcoholic patients report that they ultimately came to realize that, for them, "One drink is too many." One drink rapidly led them to fall back into the full substance-dependence syndrome. Such positive reinforcement probably assumes an increasingly important role after several months of abstinence since, by then, dysphoric symptoms associated with extended psychological withdrawal syndrome have abated.

Other components of the stress thermostat also may act as *internal reinforcers* of addictive behavior. For example, the sensitivity of the reward circuit to the reinforcing effects of addictive drugs is enhanced by the administration of **corticosteroids**. In animal models, stressful circumstances trigger both increases in corticotropin-releasing factor and cortisol and increases in drug self-administration. Perhaps, through this mechanism, relatively nonspecific life stressors (and not simply conditioned cues) may act as triggers for relapse.

Functional neuroimaging, including functional magnetic resonance imaging (fMRI), positron emission tomography (PET) and single photon emission computerized tomography (SPECT) offer useful means of exploring the neural circuits that mediate these cognitive, emotional, and motivational aspects of addiction. One study obtained functional MRI scans of individuals both with and without histories of cocaine dependence as they watched videotapes of people using cocaine. Individuals with histories of cocaine dependence demonstrated activation of their *anterior cingulate gyrus* as they watched the videotape. This activation immediately preceded the onset of the subjective perception of "craving" but it also appeared even in those cocaine-dependent individuals who denied experiencing craving. It was *not* seen in subjects who didn't have a history of cocaine use. Cocaine-dependent subjects also demonstrated decreased activation in areas of the frontal lobes as they watched the videotape. This experimental paradigm has been extended to other disorders, including pathological gambling, where similar patterns of brain activation have been observed.

In other contexts, increased anterior cingulate activity has been observed during situations where subjects either are asked to attend selectively to just one aspect of a complex stimulus or are asked to perform tasks that involve "conflicting response inclinations" (i.e., where one is forced to choose one response while actively resisting another response). This suggests that when drug-dependent individuals experience "cravings," they are faced with *powerful desires* to engage in drug use that then must be *actively resisted*. Perhaps the accompanying pattern of decreased frontal lobe activation reflects an alteration in the normal homeostasis between limbic and frontal regions that is illustrated in Figure 4–3.

Typical Presentation and Course

Patients typically present for treatment either in a state of acute intoxication, or in a state of acute or chronic withdrawal, or with substance-induced changes in mood, cognition, or behavior *Mood changes* can range from euphoria to depression, the latter perhaps accompanied by suicidal thoughts. Both intoxication and withdrawal can be severe enough to cause delirium. Even in milder cases, *cognitive changes* may be present, including shortened attention span, impaired concentration, and disturbances of thinking (including delusions) and/or perceptions (including hallucinations). *Behavioral changes* can include wakefulness or somnolence, lethargy or hyperactivity, and anxious withdrawal or belligerence.

Patients may initially present for treatment of a *comorbid psychiatric problem*, such as conduct disorder (in children and adolescents), major depressive disorder, bipolar disorder, schizophrenia, an anxiety disorder, an eating disorder, an impulse control disorder (such as pathological gambling), or a personality disorder. The symptoms and social morbidity associated with these comorbid conditions usually are exacerbated by patients' substance use and vice versa. When these *"dual-diagnosis" patients* are shuttled back and forth between mental health clinics and substance rehabilitation programs, treatment may be less effective, so *integrative, rather than parallel therapy* is the preferred treatment strategy.

Patients also may present with *medical problems related to their substance use*, such as cardiac toxicity from acute cocaine intoxication, respiratory depression or coma from severe opi-

oid overdose, and hepatic cirrhosis, pancreatitis, or gastrointestinal bleeding secondary to long-term alcohol use. Intravenous drug use can cause subacute bacterial endocarditis, HIV infection, and hepatitis. Substance use also commonly is associated with a state of malnutrition.

Substance use typically begins during adolescence or even before puberty. As might be expected from the behavioral perspective, casual users who go on to develop a substance-related disorder are not readily distinguishable at first from those who do not go on to do so. However, over time some behaviors begin to appear that are more predictive of longer-term substance dependence. These include: early onset of drug use; heavier and/or more regular use of "gateway" drugs such as alcohol, marijuana, and nicotine; early evidence of aggressive behaviors; worsening family difficulties; and forming associations with substance-using peers.

Adolescents who go on to become substance dependent also begin to distinguish themselves from their peers by their growing preoccupation with substance use, their frequent episodes of intoxication, and their use of drugs that are associated with greater dependence liability (such as opioids and cocaine). They may express a preference for more rapidly acting preparations such as methamphetamine and for routes of administration that result in a more rapid onset of effects such as injection or freebasing.

Some individuals develop a "drug of choice" while others go on to become *polysubstance* dependent. While genetic vulnerabilities or other biological factors may play a role in this process, research to date has not revealed clear associations between various biomarkers and individuals' ultimate drug preference. The influence of peers, drug availability, financial factors, and cultural fashion appear to be important contributory factors. Family history appears to be another important factor given that substance-related disorders tend to demonstrate familial aggregation (although this finding might also be explained by familial aggregation of *predisposing* factors such as antisocial personality disorder).

The substance associated with the clearest *genetic* predisposition is alcohol. Close relatives of probands with alcohol dependence have a three to four times greater risk of developing alcohol dependence than do other members of the general population. Further, individuals have a greater risk of developing alcoholism if they have a greater number of affected relatives, have closer genetic relationships to alcoholic relatives, or have affected relatives with a greater severity of alcohol-related problems. Most studies have found a significantly higher concordance for alcohol dependence in monozygotic than dizygotic twins. Adoption studies also reveal that children of alcohol-dependent parents who are adopted by nonalcoholic parents still demonstrate a threefold to fourfold increased risk of developing alcohol dependence compared to adopted-away children of nonalcoholic parents.

However, as with other psychiatric disorders, the concordance rate among monozygotic twins is not 100%, suggesting that alcoholism is not determined solely by one's genes. Environmental and experiential factors—including cultural attitudes, peer attitudes, more ready access to alcohol, expectations of the effects of alcohol on one's mood and behavior, past experiences with alcohol, and stress—all likely exert an influence on whether pathological drinking behavior ultimately develops in a vulnerable individual.

Substance dependence is a chronic condition but not a hopeless one. The highest rates of relapse occur during the first 12 months of abstinence. This might be expected, considering both the importance of negative reinforcement associated with persistent psychological withdrawal symptoms as well as the difficulties that many individuals encounter in attempting to develop alternative means of dealing with stress. During the first several years of treatment, individuals may experience remissions lasting from several months to a year or more, followed by relapses. However, those who remain in treatment often find that, over time, the frequency of these relapses declines. The *frequency* of treatment, the *intensity* of treatment, and the *duration* of treatment all positively correlate with better outcomes, regardless of the specific *modality* of treatment.

Up to 70% of substance-dependent patients who enter treatment eventually are able to abstain from substance use entirely or continue to experience brief episodes of substance use that do not progress to relapse into abuse or depend-

ence. The remaining individuals experience chronic relapses over the next two decades that require repeated intervention. Of those who can remain abstinent for 2 years, almost 90% will remain substance-free at 10 years; of those who remain substance-free at 10 years, 90% still will be so at 20 years. Clinical variables associated with a better prognosis include: a lower level of premorbid psychopathology, an ability to develop new relationships, and an ability and willingness to make use of self-help groups such as Alcoholics Anonymous and Narcotics Anonymous.

In addition, how successful substance treatment is depends upon one's definition of "success." While abstinence is an important longer-term goal, it should not be considered the *sole* end point when measuring whether a patient has benefited from treatment. Since substance dependence is a chronic neurobehavioral condition, treatment is an ongoing, longer-term process and not a "cure," and patients and their treatment providers must be "relapse-ready." Many substance users do relapse, but 1 year after the initiation of treatment, their drug use has decreased by 50% overall, their illegal activity has dropped by 80%, they are less likely to be engaging in high-risk sexual behavior, they are less likely to require emergency room care, and they are less likely to be on welfare.

In contrast, legal sanctions have not been particularly successful. Despite progressive escalations of the "war on drugs" over the past two decades, illegal substance use has persisted. The federal government now spends almost $20 billion annually on fighting drug use; two-thirds of this sum is dedicated to law enforcement and interdiction. Over the past two decades, the prison population has tripled, and most of these inmates report a history of substance abuse. However, it costs more than twice as much to incarcerate an individual as to treat him, and epidemiologic research suggests that every dollar spent on treatment saves taxpayers more than $7 in other services (primarily through reduced crime and medical fees and increased productivity). For example, one emergency room visit by a heroin abuser costs as much as 1 month in a rehabilitation program. Given these concerns, as of this writing, several states have passed or are considering measures requiring offers of treatment with probation in lieu of jail time for nonviolent drug offenders.

TREATMENT OF SUBSTANCE-RELATED DISORDERS

Since pathological behaviors ultimately become self-sustaining, stopping the behavior and working to keep it from recurring are the most important aspects of treatment. As discussed in the last chapter in the context of the treatment of eating disorder, the key steps are: to *address the behavior itself*, to *treat medical complications* associated with the behavior, to address *comorbid psychiatric conditions*, to address *internal and external reinforcers*, and to work to *maintain abstinence* from the behavior through ongoing therapy focusing on relapse prevention.

Stage 1: Address the Behavior

One cannot engage in meaningful psychotherapy when a patient arrives for sessions intoxicated. Ongoing substance abuse is such an important contributor to patients' symptoms and their social morbidity that the pathological behavior itself must be addressed as soon as possible. However, many patients—especially those presenting in the outpatient setting—may not be ready to admit that their substance use constitutes a significant problem. They may wish to "negotiate" with the clinician over how much they might simply "cut back" on their substance use. They also may be presenting for treatment only at the instigation of family, friends, or the court system without having any personal desire to address their substance use. Other individuals present requesting hospital admission for "detox" but are convinced at the time of discharge that they have no need for ongoing substance rehabilitation since they are convinced that they "will never return to drug use again."

The goal at this early stage is gentle confrontation. A therapeutic alliance, based upon empathy and honest expressions of concern over the patient's state of affairs, may become the determining factor in whether such confrontation will be successful. Patients do not have to have "full insight" into the need to stop drinking or using drugs at this point, but they at least should have what Alcoholics Anonymous calls "the desire" to stop drinking. The input of family and friends also might be enlisted at this point. Patients should be educated about the natural course of substance dependence and the need to commit to a longer-term *rehabilitation* plan given that prospective research indicates that acute detoxification in itself generally offers little long-term benefit.

Stage 2: Treat the Medical Complications

Some patients with substance dependence will not experience significant withdrawal following discontinuation of substance use and therefore can be detoxified in the outpatient setting. Other patients, while requiring an environment where their access to drugs is restricted, do not require medical or pharmacologic intervention and can be managed by a "social detoxification" program. Finally, some patients experience uncomfortable, even life-threatening withdrawal following drug discontinuation. These latter patients require inpatient detoxification accompanied by close medical monitoring and care.

Along with providing detoxification, clinicians also must *address associated medical complications* at this point. For example, alcohol dependence can be complicated by dehydration, malnutrition, subdural hematoma, dementia or amnestic syndrome, delirium tremens, seizures, pneumonia, hepatitis or cirrhosis, gastritis or ulcer, pancreatitis, cardiomyopathy, anemia, and peripheral neuropathy. Each of these conditions requires specific treatments.

How does one go about choosing the most appropriate treatment setting? Existing research only offers some general guidelines. Studies that have randomly assigned patients to different levels of treatment generally have not found significant differences in outcome. However, such conclusions must be tempered by the understanding that these studies exclude patients clearly considered to require inpatient care. Other studies suggest that successful completion of longer-term inpatient or residential programs is associated with better longer-term outcomes. Again, however, these findings may simply reflect more highly motivated patients being more likely to remain in longer-term treatment and to have better outcomes, especially since no significant differences in outcome are observed when patients are *randomly* assigned to longer-term or shorter-term inpatient programs.

Overall, since there clearly are *individual* patients who repeatedly demonstrate that they cannot maintain sobriety in less restrictive treatment settings, the setting that is most appropriate must be determined on a case-by-case basis. Commonly available treatment settings include *hospitals*, *residential treatment facilities*, *partial hospitals*, and *outpatient programs*.

Ideally, patients should be treated in the *least restrictive setting* that is likely to be *safe and to be effective*. Decisions about *which* level of care is most appropriate are made based upon consideration of several factors, including: *(1)* a patient's *willingness and ability* to engage in the therapies offered at a given location; *(2)* a patient's need for *greater structure, support, and restrictions on drug access* than what would be available in less restrictive settings; and *(3)* a patient's need for *particular types of treatment or monitoring* that would not be available in less restrictive settings.

Hospitalization is appropriate for patients who present with a drug overdose, who are at risk for more severe or medically complicated withdrawal, who have a significant comorbid medical condition that could make ambulatory detoxification unsafe, who have a history of poor compliance with or limited benefit from treatment provided in less restrictive settings, or who have a psychiatric condition such as depression with suicidal ideation that itself necessitates inpatient treatment.

Residential treatment is appropriate for patients who do not require more intensive medical or psychiatric care but whose substance dependence is so severe that they are unable to maintain abstinence in a less restrictive setting. Treatment programs lasting for 3 months or more are associated with better long-term outcome in such patients.

Partial hospitalization (i.e., hospital-based day treatment programs) can be useful for those patients who require more intensive care but also have a reasonable probability of refraining from illicit use of substances outside of an inpatient or residential setting. Partial hospital settings are frequently used as a "step down" for patients being discharged from hospitals or residential settings who remain at high risk for relapse, or as a "step up" for patients who are faring poorly in outpatient treatment, as an less-restrictive alternative to hospitalization.

Patients in alcohol withdrawal must be detoxified in a setting that allows for frequent clinical assessment and for the provision of any necessary treatments. Patients deemed to be at low risk of going into a complicated withdrawal syndrome might be able to be detoxified in a well-organized outpatient setting. However, patients with a prior history of delirium tremens or with a history of very heavy alcohol use and high tolerance, patients concurrently abusing other drugs, patients with more severe comorbid medical or psychiatric disorders, and patients who repeatedly have failed to cooperate with or benefit from outpatient detoxification generally require a residential or hospital setting that can safely provide the necessary care. Patients in severe alcohol withdrawal (delirium tremens) require inpatient hospital treatment.

Stage 3: Address Comorbid Psychiatric Conditions

Half of all people with a substance-related disorder have another comorbid mental disorder. Many patients with substance dependence present with symptoms suggesting an underlying major depressive disorder, dysthymic disorder, or Anxiety Disorder. In many cases, however, these symptoms occur secondarily to substance intoxication or withdrawal and improve over several weeks of abstinence. Given this, in many cases, patients are monitored during earlier stages of treatment and only diagnosed with or treated for comorbid psychiatric disorders later on.

However, in selected cases it might be reasonable to initiate treatment earlier on. For example, patients who express feelings of depression and are found to have either a history of major depressive disorder that predates their substance use, or a history of major depressive disorder during periods of sustained abstinence, or a strong family history of major depressive disorder are more likely to ultimately turn out to have a true comorbid condition. Prescribing anxiolytic or antidepressant medications earlier on in such cases is reasonable and might even decrease the patient's chance of relapse since anxiety and depression could be acting as internal reinforcers.

Patient with substance-related disorders, by definition, have a tendency to misuse medications, and many are prone to impulsive behavior. Therefore, one should select antidepressant and/or anxiolytic medications that carry a low potential for abuse and that are less likely to be lethal in the event of an overdose. Tricyclic antidepressants should be used with caution given the risk of poor compliance, potential interactions with alcohol, and the risk of lethality in overdose. MAOIs have been used to treat patients with atypical depressions, but recall that the "MAOI diet" includes restrictions on consumption of alcoholic beverages. The most commonly prescribed antidepressants have been the SSRIs. Patients with a comorbid bipolar disorder can be treated with lithium, valproate, or carbamazepine, but close follow-up and serologic monitoring is important given the risk of preexisting renal or hepatic injury related to alcohol and drug use.

Benzodiazepines should be prescribed to substance-dependent patients with comorbid anxiety disorders only after careful reflection given their abuse potential and also the possibility that they might induce craving in alcoholic patients through a "priming" effect. For patients with generalized anxiety disorder or performance anxiety, one might first prescribe β-blockers, buspirone, or an antidepressant since these have no cross-tolerance with either ethanol or other CNS depressants and all have minimal potential for abuse. Buspirone has also been reported to reduce alcohol consumption in patients with high levels of comorbid anxiety. For patients with anxiety disorders who prove to be refractory to other interventions, clonazepam or other long-acting benzodiazepines might be tried, with careful monitoring to ensure that patients aren't obtaining medication from multiple sources or obtaining refills too early.

Stage 4: Address Internal and External Reinforcers

Once the patient is out of acute withdrawal, medical complications have been addressed, and treatment has been initiated for comorbid psychiatric problems, longer-term rehabilitation can begin. This might be initiated in the general hospital setting through group, individual, and family therapy as well as through educational counseling and Alcoholics Anonymous meetings. In some settings, rehabilitation may only begin after hospital discharge. Outpatient rehabilitation is a cost-effective alternative to inpatient treatment, but some patients simply cannot be managed in a less restrictive environment than an inpatient or residential setting, at least during the first few weeks after acute detoxification.

Internal Reinforcers

Some medications are capable of *decreasing the positive reinforcing properties of a drug*. In the case of opioid dependence and alcohol dependence, **naltrexone (ReVia)** an opioid μ-receptor antagonist has been shown in double-blind, placebo-controlled studies to be superior to placebo in preventing relapse. In opioid dependence, it blocks the euphorogenic effects of exogenously administered opioids such as heroin, while in alcoholism it presumably acts by blocking positive reinforcing effects of alcohol mediated by the opioid system. Alcohol-dependent patients taking naltrexone typically report that alcohol no longer "feels as satisfying" and some of them report diminished cravings for alcohol. **Desipramine and SSRIs** may also have mild effects in reducing relapse even in alcoholics who are not depressed, perhaps by decreasing impulsiveness or by decreasing effects of alcohol mediated by serotonin.

Disulfiram (Antabuse) is an *aversive* treatment that has been used in the treatment of alcohol dependence. It inhibits aldehyde dehydrogenase, the enzyme that metabolizes acetaldehyde, a major metabolite of alcohol. Alcohol consumption results in the accumulation of acetaldehyde, leading to a severe toxic reaction (flushing, nausea, dizziness, and malaise, and possibly blurred vision, palpitations, shortness of breath and potentially severe hypotension) after even a single drink. Patients may even have such a response if they ingest alcohol from a sauce or use an alcohol-containing aftershave. Potentially fatal side effects can also occur (hepatotoxicity, neuropathy, respiratory depression, cardiac arrhythmia, myocardial infarction, and death).

Agonist substitution therapies substitute a longer-acting agent for a shorter-acting agent (e.g., methadone or LAAM [levomethadylacetate hydrochloride] for heroin). The longer-acting agent acts at the same receptor, thereby reducing or eliminating withdrawal symptoms and craving and decreasing negative reinforcement.

External Reinforcers

Attention should be paid to specific triggers of cravings or relapse, including particular environments, interpersonal and occupational stress, and particular emotional states.

Stage 5: Treatment in the Ambulatory Setting and Relapse Prevention

Since the goal of treatment is to modify persistent and habitual behaviors, the most effective psychotherapeutic approaches address the behavior itself. More important than the school of therapy is the *intensity* of therapy. Thus, **Alcoholics Anonymous (AA)** and other 12-step programs generally recommend daily attendance during the initial period of abstinence (e.g., "90 meetings in 90 days") and also during times of greater life stress. Similarly, in the medical treatment setting, it may be more effective to meet with a patient for 5–10 minutes daily (during which time a breathalyzer or urine drug test also might be performed) than to meet with the patient for an hour once per week.

Cognitive–behavior therapy has been adapted to substance abuse treatment through the **relapse prevention model**. The goal is to have the patient, either in individual or group therapy, direct attention to which life stressors, emotions, or environments act as "triggers" for drug craving and/or relapse. The therapist helps the patient devise better strategies to cope with these situations. If the patient has a "slip" leading to relapse, possible triggers and the thoughts and emotions that accompanied them are explored to figure out "what went wrong" so that the patient might fare better when faced with similar situations in the future. A more "client-centered" form of therapy is **motivation enhancement therapy**, which emphasizes empathic, reflective listening focused on the patient's ambivalence about giving up a problematic behavior, exploring the pros and cons of continuing versus giving up the behavior.

Behavioral strategies that can help augment compliance include **contingency management**, a form of operant conditioning. A contract is formed from the outset with defined rewards for positive behaviors or punishments for negative behaviors (relapse). The target behaviors are monitored through drug and alcohol screening tests. Rewards for negative drug tests might include vouchers or gift certificates (for movie tickets, groceries, clothing, etc.) or agreements by family members to spend time with the patient in pleasurable activities. Punishments might include notifying the family, the court, or an employer about the test results. (While this approach may appear patronizing at first glance, it should be familiar to all of us from our everyday experience. Parents use allowances or dessert to encourage their children to make their beds or eat their dinners, while employers use salaries and bonuses to reward good job performance and the threat of reprimands or suspensions to discourage inappropriate work behavior.)

Group therapy can be an extremely effective modality, as it offers opportunities to gain support from others facing similar problems, to be confronted about denial, to learn about the impact of one's substance use on others, and to practice new ways of relating to other people. The group also can offer support during periods when the patient is at greater risk for relapse.

Family therapy also can play an important role in helping patients maintain abstinence. First, it can help bolster family support for the patient. Second, it can address "enabling" behaviors on the part of the spouse or children that inadvertently have helped the patient to sustain the pathologic behavior pattern. Finally it can address situations in which a maladaptive but stable "homeostasis" has evolved within the family system while the patient was using alcohol or drugs. Unless this dynamic is addressed, family members may end up "sabotaging" the patient's recovery in order to reestablish this homeostasis.

Self-help groups often are based on the 12-step approach made popular by AA. Like group therapy, these organizations provide affiliation with like-minded others (especially for those individuals whose current peer group consists primarily of other drug users), spiritual support, the personal support of a "sponsor," opportunities to meet during high-risk periods (vacations, evenings, and weekends), and positive reinforcement for sobriety.

However, some studies suggest that while many patients who attend AA do improve, others actually deteriorate. One study of employer-referred individuals who were *actively drinking* found that referral to AA prior to professional substance intervention was either unrelated or negatively related to drinking outcome. Individuals assigned to professional treatment before joining AA had substantially better outcomes. Persons who had been abusing cocaine in addition to alcohol were particularly poor responders to the AA-only intervention.

About 50% of individuals referred to AA drop out by the fourth month of participation, and about 75% drop out by the 12th month. Some of these individuals likely stop attending because they find that they can now maintain sobriety without the program. However, other individuals reject AA and similar 12-step programs due to disagreements with their conceptualizations of spirituality, of one's powerlessness over addiction, or of addiction as a "lifelong disease." Others drop out following an excessively harsh confrontation by another group member.

Clinicians should be aware that alternative self-help groups that don't emphasize "spirituality," such as Rational Recovery, also are available, as are private rehabilitation programs that emphasize a "medical" model of addiction. They also should be aware that different AA groups have different "characters" and that patients may fare better in another group, particularly if one comprised of individuals of a similar age, occupational status, and culture as the patient. Groups also vary as to whether they consider the use of *any* psychotropic medication to be "substance abuse" or recognize and accept the need for medications in the treatment of *comorbid* psychiatric conditions such as bipolar disorder and schizophrenia. Patients who require such psychoactive medications obviously should not be referred to groups with a "no drugs at all" philosophy.

Overall, clinicians shouldn't indiscriminately refer the patient with substance problems to AA or other self-help groups without first considering the patient's total clinical picture and the patient's potential need for formal detoxification and substance treatment prior to referral to a self-help group. Further, they shouldn't adamantly demand AA attendance, particularly from patients who are reluctant to attend or who have had a bad experience with AA in the past. Finally, they always should follow up on the patient's clinical status following referral.

Throughout this final stage of treatment, patients need to be "relapse-ready." In other words, they must recognize that relapse is a common complication of behavioral disorders and that they therefore should not give up after a relapse by "throwing the baby out with the bathwater" entirely and resuming their earlier pattern of heavy substance use. The establishment of a trusting alliance with a clinician and a peer group can greatly facilitate a return to treatment after such "slips."

SPECIFIC SYNDROMES

Alcohol

Intoxication

Peak blood alcohol concentration is reached between 30 and 90 minutes after ingestion, depending on whether the alcohol was taken on an empty stomach and also on how rapidly the alcohol was consumed. Once in an individual's bloodstream, alcohol uniformly dissolves in body water and is distributed throughout the body, reaching its greatest concentrations in areas that receive the greatest amount of water. The intoxicating effects of alcohol are greater when the blood alcohol concentration is rising than when it is falling.

Alcohol is a central nervous system depressant, and intoxication symptoms can range from mild inebriation through coma and death, depending on the blood alcohol level. In people who have acquired tolerance, a blood alcohol concentration of *0.03 g/dL* is associated with mild euphoric effects and mild slowing of motor performance. Levels of *0.05 g/dL* are associated with mild coordination problems. Levels of *0.08 or 0.1 g/dL* are the legal definition of intoxication in most states. Individuals with these serum levels typically demonstrate mood lability, impaired judgement, and ataxia. Individuals with levels of from *0.2 to 0.3 g/dL* usually demonstrate nystagmus, slurred speech, and decreased levels of consciousness. Anterograde memory also can become impaired at these levels, leading to alcoholic "blackouts" (i.e., the individual has no memory later on for events that took place during the period of intoxication). Anesthesia begins at levels higher than this, and levels *above 0.4 g/dL* in nontolerant individuals can cause coma and death.

While alcohol intoxication is associated with increased ease of falling asleep (i.e., with decreased sleep latency), the sleep isn't especially restful. This reflects alcohol's suppression of REM sleep and stage 4 deep sleep, and its propensity to increase sleep fragmentation (leading to increased nighttime awakenings).

Alcohol is metabolized at a rate of about 0.15 g/dL per hour in nontolerant individuals, but may be metabolized at double this rate in tolerant individuals due to induction of the hepatic enzymes that play the greatest role in the metabolism of alcohol, *alcohol dehydrogenase (ADH)* and *aldehyde dehydrogenase*. ADH converts alcohol into *acetaldehyde*, which in turn is metabolized by aldehyde dehydrogenase. The medication disulfiram (Antabuse) competitively inhibits this latter enzyme, leading to accumulation of acetaldehyde and a severe toxic reaction.

Neuroadaptation

As noted earlier, alcohol acts at multiple sites in the CNS, including on the GABA system, the glutamate system, the dopaminergic system, the serotonin system, and the opioid system.

A variety of symptoms can occur in association with **alcohol withdrawal**. It first should be emphasized that alcohol withdrawal is related to a *relative* fall in blood alcohol levels rather than to a *total absence* of alcohol. Alcohol withdrawal therefore can occur even during continuous alcohol consumption and intoxication. As withdrawal appears to be related to neuroadaptation, it is more likely to occur in those individuals who have a history of heavier drinking over longer periods of time. Patients with combined alcohol and benzodiazepine abuse are especially at risk for experiencing more severe withdrawal. Also, patients who previously have experienced "complicated" alcohol withdrawal (withdrawal accompanied by seizures or delirium tremens) are at greater risk to experience similar difficulties during subsequent episodes of withdrawal (perhaps reflecting a "kindling effect"). In such cases, the clinician should always treat for withdrawal empirically with *standing doses* of a cross-tolerant medication such as a benzodiazepine rather than simply monitoring the patient and waiting for the appearance of signs of autonomic instability, especially since seizures may be the first sign of more severe alcohol withdrawal, preceding evidence of autonomic instability.

Uncomplicated alcohol withdrawal usually begins *several hours* after the last drink. It lasts for about a week, with or without pharmacologic management. (Milder insomnia, depression, anxiety, and irritability may continue over the next several weeks, however.) An alcohol withdrawal *tremor* often heralds withdrawal. The tremor is an exaggeration of a normal postural tremor. It begins about 6–8 hours after the last drink and peaks at about 24–28 hours. The tremor typically is accompanied by nausea, vomiting, and signs of moderate autonomic hyperactivity (such as anxiety, arousal, sweats, facial flushing, mydriasis, tachycardia, and mild hypertension).

Alcohol withdrawal seizures usually occur 8–40 hours after the individual's last drink, most commonly at about *24 hours*. (Since alcohol itself lowers the seizure threshold, some individuals experience seizures at the *peak* of intoxication, however.) Patients who present with *new-onset* seizures should receive a neurologic workup for other potential causes of seizures (e.g., hypomagnesemia, other electrolyte disturbances, hypoglycemia, or subdural hematoma), even when the seizures occur in the setting of alcohol withdrawal. For patients who experience *recurrent* seizures that only occur in the setting of alcohol withdrawal, anticonvulsants are of little prophylactic benefit.

Alcohol-induced psychotic disorder can include hallucinations or delusions, but most commonly it takes the form of auditory hallucinations ("alcoholic hallucinosis") of voices that are insulting or frightening. These symptoms usually have their onset about *8–12 hours* after the last drink. Hallucinosis can occur in patients who otherwise have a normal level of consciousness—i.e., in the absence of the broader syndrome of alcohol-withdrawal delirium. Patients may not recognize that the "voices" are hallucinations, except in retrospect, after withdrawal is completed. The symptoms often respond to treatment with benzodiazepines, although in more severe cases, treatment with an antipsychotic may be beneficial. Symptoms typically resolve within a week. However, in rare cases a more chronic hallucinosis syndrome persists despite the maintenance of abstinence. In these latter cases, one should attempt to rule out the possibility that the patient's symptoms actually reflect a comorbid psychotic illness by examining for other symptoms beyond hallucinations (e.g., disturbance of mood, formal thought disorder, negative symptoms, or cognitive decline).

Alcohol-withdrawal delirium (also called **delirium tremens**, or **DTs**) typically begins about *3 days* after the last drink. It occurs in about 5% of people hospitalized for treatment of alcohol-related disorders and sometimes occurs unexpectedly in patients hospitalized for unrelated conditions. The most commonly encountered patient is in his or her 30s or 40s and has a 5–15-year history of heavy drinking. DTs most commonly occur in the presence of some *other* predisposing medical complication such as hepatitis, pancreatitis, malnutrition, trauma, subdural hematoma, or an associated infection. DTs also occur in 30% of people who already have experienced an alcohol withdrawal seizure earlier in the hospital stay; given this, all such patients should receive adequate dosages of prophylactic medication following a withdrawal seizure.

Typically, DTs are accompanied by autonomic instability that is more severe than that seen in uncomplicated withdrawal, by changes in consciousness (ranging from lethargy to hyperactivity with agitation or terror), and by visual hallucinations (usually of insects or small animals). While DTs typically resolve in about 3 days, they can last for over a month.

The mortality of DTs in the absence of treatment is as high as 20%. Death most commonly is caused by infection, fat embolus, or cardiac arrhythmia (the latter being associated with hyperkalemia, hyperpyrexia, and poor hydration). In the modern age, and with appropriate medical care, the mortality of DTs has declined to less than 1%.

Treatment of alcohol withdrawal typically consists of giving oral or intravenous benzodiazepines, most commonly *chlordiazepoxide (Librium)*, given its long half-life and ability to be administered intravenously. *Lorazepam (Ativan)* is often used in cases where hepatic injury is suspected, as it doesn't have active metabolites that might accumulate. *Diazepam (Valium)* loading regimens have also been used to treat uncomplicated withdrawal given its long half-life.

In uncomplicated withdrawal, a patient might be administered chlordiazepoxide 25–50 mg as

needed every 2–4 hours until he or she is calm. The total dose required to reach this point then is tallied and consolidated into a standing dose that administered over a 24-hour period (along with a provision for further "as needed" dosages on top of this). The standing dose is then gradually tapered over the next several days. Alternatively, the patient might be written for a standing dose of 50 mg every 4 or 6 hours as a starting point, along with 25–50 mg to be administered "as needed" for breakthrough withdrawal symptoms. Again, the patient's total dosage requirement during the first day should be assessed, and the subsequent day's standing dosage should be increased or decreased accordingly. Patients also should be prescribed *thiamine* 100 mg by mouth twice daily for a week (with the first dose administered intramuscularly or intravenously if Wernicke's encephalopathy is suspected), *magnesium* supplementation (orally or intravenously), and a daily *multivitamin*.

In treating uncomplicated alcohol withdrawal, both *clonidine and β-blockers* have been used to block autonomic hyperactivity. In this respect, they are as effective as benzodiazepines and cause less sedation. However, they don't prevent DTs or seizures and therefore are not typically used alone in the inpatient setting. *Carbamazepine* is a promising agent; 800 mg/day is as effective as benzodiazepines both in treating autonomic withdrawal symptoms and in protecting against seizures and DTs. Carbamazepine may be particularly useful in the outpatient setting, where concerns about patients' abilities to appropriately take benzodiazepines may be a concern. However, since carbamazepine can cause blood dyscrasias, and since alcoholic patients typically present with bone marrow suppression to begin with, blood counts should be monitored. Some clinicians also have begun using *Valproate* and have found it to offer similar advantages.

Clinicians also must keep in mind that over 80% of alcoholics also are dependent on other drugs. Polysubstance dependence is particularly common in patients under the age of 30. The most commonly encountered substances, in decreasing order of frequency, are nicotine, cannabis, cocaine, benzodiazepines/barbiturates, opioids, and hallucinogens. It is important to question patients about their use of these substances, and many clinicians routinely obtain toxicology screens on all substance-abusing patients at the time of initial presentation.

As noted earlier, both *naltrexone (ReVia)* and *disulfiram (Antabuse)* have been used as part of longer-term treatment strategies. The former likely decreases drug cravings as well as the "high" associated with alcohol intoxication, while the latter is an aversive strategy.

Naltrexone is an opioid μ-receptor antagonist. When administered in combination with intensive outpatient drug treatment, its use (in comparison with placebo) is associated with a reduction of the number of drinking days, a reduction in the chance of an individual resuming "heavy drinking" (defined as five or more drinks in a single day), and an increase in the rate of total abstinence (from 31% with placebo to 54% with naltrexone). However, follow-up studies suggest that these beneficial effects may be lost following discontinuation of the drug (suggesting that longer-term maintenance therapy may be required).

In addition, these studies involved patients in the Veterans Administration system receiving an intensive form of psychosocial therapy. A subsequent study by the same investigators involving nonveterans receiving less intensive therapy revealed only minimal differences between naltrexone and placebo. However, naltrexone did appear to be superior to placebo in reducing drinking days and reducing a return to heavy drinking (although not in increasing the rate of total abstinence) specifically for those patients judged to be highly compliant with treatment. This suggests that, as with all behavioral disorders, there are no "quick pharmacologic fixes" for alcoholism and that the patient's own motivation remains an essential ingredient of successful treatment.

The most common side effects associated with naltrexone are nausea, headache, sedation, and anxiety. Hepatotoxicity is an extremely rare complication, generally associated with doses of 200–300 mg/day rather than the 50 mg/day typically prescribed for alcohol dependence. However, the drug still should not be prescribed in patients with liver disease, including alcoholic hepatitis. Patients must be assessed for opioid use within the past 7–10 days in order to to avoid precipitating acute opioid withdrawal upon initiation of therapy, and patients also must be reminded that naltrexone blocks the effects of opi-

oids such that if they require narcotic therapy for acute pain following an injury or surgery, higher dosages would be required.

Controlled trials have not demonstrated any advantage for *disulfiram* over placebo in patient's ability to achieve total abstinence, in delaying relapse, or in improving employment status or social stability. Nonetheless, it remains possible that carefully selected individuals may benefit from the addition of disulfiram therapy to their other treatment strategies. The *ideal* patient is one who is intelligent, motivated, and not impulsive, but who sometimes relapses in response to unanticipated environmental triggers. In contrast, *poor* candidates for disulfiram therapy are impulsive, exhibit poor social judgment, or are suffering from a comorbid psychiatric illness that renders them less reliable or more self-destructive (such as schizophrenia, major depressive disorder, or a severe personality disorder).

Patients taking disulfiram need to avoid all forms of ethanol (including, for example, cough syrup and aftershave). In addition, disulfiram interferes with the metabolism of many medications (including tricyclic antidepressants, chlordiazepoxide and diazepam, phenytoin, and warfarin) such that clinicians must be very careful to avoid toxicity. Disulfiram also should not be administered to patients with moderate-to-severe hepatic dysfunction, peripheral neuropathies, renal failure, or cardiac disease or who are pregnant.

Sedative–Hypnotics

Intoxication and Withdrawal

Chronic use of higher doses of benzodiazepines or barbiturates also can lead to physiologic dependence; tolerance and withdrawal syndromes similar to those observed in alcohol dependence can develop. Benzodiazepine intoxication resembles alcohol intoxication, although associated cognitive and motor impairment tends to be more subtle. Risk factors for developing benzodiazepine dependence were discussed in Chapter 9. The nearly unconditional acceptance of benzodiazepines in the 1960s has been replaced by a concern about the risk of benzodiazepine addiction that is excessive in many cases, leading some patients who might benefit from benzodiazepines to avoid taking them altogether.

Even many physicians confuse physiologic dependence—which occurs with many prescribed agents, including the benzodiazepines—with substance dependence.

Clinicians faced with a patient who has been taking benzodiazepines for some time who now presents requesting a new prescription should ask several questions: *(1)* Does the patient's medical problem justify continued use of a benzodiazepine? *(2)* Has the patient refrained from escalating the dosage inappropriately over time? *(3)* Has the patient required a reasonable dosage, and one that is not high enough to be associated with cognitive impairment or signs of intoxication? If the answer to all of these questions is "yes," one should consider continuing the medication. If the answer to one or more of these questions is "no," one should consider tapering and discontinuing the medication.

The most common mistake made during a benzodiazepine taper is proceeding too rapidly. It may take weeks to months for a taper to be completed, and the taper typically becomes most difficult when the dosage is down to about 10%–20% of the original daily dosage. Sometimes a taper of a shorter-acting agent such as alprazolam can be facilitated by switching to a longer-acting agent such as chlordiazepoxide (Librium) or clonazepam (Klonopin). When higher dosages of benzodiazepines or barbiturates are involved, inpatient detoxification may be required. For patients presenting with polysubstance dependence for whom a rapid inpatient taper of all agents is required, substitution of phenobarbital may be useful given its long half-life and cross-tolerance for a variety of substances.

Neuroadaptation

Benzodiazepine withdrawal symptoms can occur in the setting of attempts to taper even low dosages provided that the duration of therapy has been sufficiently long. The most severe withdrawal symptoms occur during the last few milligrams of the taper. These facts suggest that benzodiazepine neuroadaptation reflects alterations in the GABA receptor, such that the same dosage of a given benzodiazepine ultimately causes the chloride channel to open to a lesser degree than it previously did. This causes tolerance and the need to increase the dosage of medication yet further to obtain the same effect. When the benzodiazepine is removed, the channel may be even

more likely to shut (thereby inhibiting chloride influx) than it was in the unmedicated state, thereby leading to withdrawal symptoms. Perhaps the same phenomenon occurs in response to chronic exposure to barbiturates, but to an even greater extent, leading to the barbiturates' greater addictive potential.

Opioids

Intoxication

The opioids include *natural opioids* (such as morphine), *semisynthetics* (such as heroin), and *synthetics with morphine-like action* (such as codeine, hydromorphone, methadone, oxycodone, meperidine, and fentanyl). Medications such as pentazocine, butorphanol, and buprenorphine possess a mixture of both *opiate agonist and antagonist effects* but also are included in this class since their agonist properties produce physiological and behavioral effects that are similar to pure agonist drugs.

Opioids are prescribed as analgesics, anesthetics, antidiarrheal agents, and as cough suppressants. Heroin is one of the most commonly abused drugs of this class. It usually is injected, but it also is smoked or "snorted" when very pure heroin is available. Fentanyl is injected or supplied transdermally via an adhesive patch, whereas cough suppressants and antidiarrheal agents are taken orally. The other opioids are taken both by injection and orally.

Opioid intoxication is characterized by an initial feeling of euphoria, generally followed by apathy, dysphoria, psychomotor agitation or retardation, and impaired judgment. Intoxication is accompanied by pupillary constriction, slurred speech, impairment in attention or memory, and drowsiness (hence the colloquial term for intoxication, being "on the nod"). Individuals may demonstrate inattention to the environment, even to the point of ignoring potentially harmful events. The magnitude of the presentation depends on the dose as well as on the characteristics of the individual who is using the substance (including tolerance, rate of absorption, and chronicity of use). Symptoms usually last for several hours. *Severe intoxication* (as occurs in the setting of an intentional or unintentional overdose) can lead to unconsciousness, respiratory depression, pupillary dilation, coma, and death.

Common medical complications of intravenous opioid use include *hepatitis* (transmitted via shared needles), *dry mouth and nose* (due to decreased secretions), and *constipation*. Pupillary constriction can lead to *decreased visual acuity*. Veins can become so badly sclerosed from multiple injections that *peripheral edema* develops and individuals switch to veins in the legs, neck, or groin. When these veins become unusable, individuals may inject directly into their subcutaneous tissue ("skin-popping"), causing *cellulitis*, *abscesses*, and *circular-appearing scars* from healed skin lesions. Other, more rare complications, include *tetanus*, *bacterial endocarditis*, *HIV infection*, and *tuberculosis*. Deaths from overdose, accidents, injuries associated with buying or selling, and medical complications are relatively common (10 per 1000 per year among untreated persons).

Neuroadaptation and Withdrawal

Opioid tolerance and withdrawal commonly develop. Long-term abstinence is rare, and recidivism rates are as high as 90%. Intoxication is followed rapidly by symptoms of withdrawal (about 10 hours after the last dose of a shorter-acting agent such as heroin). Symptoms of opioid withdrawal resemble a bad case of the flu, and the symptoms are essentially the *opposite* of the intoxication syndrome: pupillary dilation, anxiety, irritability, restlessness, insomnia, muscle aches, increased sensitivity to pain, nausea or vomiting, diarrhea, lacrimation or rhinorrhea, increased sweating, yawning, and powerful drug cravings.

Later-appearing symptoms of acute withdrawal include piloerection ("goose bumps"), low-grade fever, hot and cold flashes, and cramps. This is the "cold turkey" stage of withdrawal: typically, the individual presents curled up in the fetal position (to ease cramps), with waves of gooseflesh, covered in a blanket even on a hot day (due to hot and cold flashes). Acute withdrawal symptoms for a short-acting opioid such as heroin usually peak within 1 to 3 days and gradually subside over the following 5–7 days.

These withdrawal symptoms are to a large part mediated by *norepinephrine* and can be eased with *clonidine*, an α-2 autoreceptor agonist that decreases norepinephrine release. Side effects of clonidine can include insomnia, sedation, and hypotension. In addition, clonidine does not ameliorate some symptoms of opioid withdrawal, such as insomnia and muscle pain. *Benzodiazepines, non-narcotic analgesics, and antiemetics* are commonly used to treat these symptoms. Contraindications to the use of clonidine include acute or chronic cardiac disorders, renal or metabolic disease, and moderate-to-severe hypotension.

Note that clonidine doesn't *speed up* the withdrawal process. However, under very close monitoring, clonidine has been combined with naltrexone to provide "rapid withdrawal" over a 5-day period. A variant of this is "ultrarapid withdrawal," in which even higher dosages of naltrexone are administered to patients, under general anesthesia, over a several-hour period. Whether the potential for a quicker, more comfortable detoxification justifies the increased expense and risk remains controversial. Again, there is a difference between detoxification and longer-term abstinence, and the rate of relapse associated with ultrarapid withdrawal remains very high.

After *acute* opioid withdrawal symptoms have subsided, a *prolonged abstinence syndrome* occurs in many patients. This syndrome can persist for weeks to months. Symptoms include low-grade anxiety, dysphoria, anhedonia, insomnia, and drug craving. This state likely contributes to the high rate of relapse associated with opioids, and preventing these symptoms is the rationale for *methadone maintenance therapy*.

Methadone is used as a substitute agonist that doesn't have the euphorogenic effects of the other opiates due to its slow onset and long half-life. The methadone typically is tapered over a 3–6-month period, although some patients with severe addiction have been maintained for longer than this when other treatment modalities have failed. **Levomethadyl acetate (LAAM)** is a congener of methadone with a longer half-life. Some patients prefer LAAM to daily methadone since LAAM can be dosed as infrequently as three times per week, thereby allowing for fewer clinic visits.

Methadone is started at a low dose and titrated upward over several days since the quality of street heroin can vary greatly, and too high a dose of methadone can be dangerous. If a patient presents without acute withdrawal symptoms and there are questions as to whether she really is currently opioid-dependent, one can either take a "watch and wait" approach before prescribing methadone or give a dose of intravenous naloxone. Since naloxone is an opiate-receptor antagonist, it precipitates withdrawal in dependent patient but doesn't cause such symptoms in patients already out of the acute withdrawal stage.

Methadone doesn't block the effect of street heroin, so a person could still try to get high "on top of methadone." However, given the cross-tolerance between heroin and methadone and the relative weakness of most street heroin, patients maintained on adequate dosages of methadone generally experience little reward from usual doses of heroin.

Methadone does not offer a miracle cure, but it can improve a patient's prognosis. About a third of patients do very well with methadone maintenance, while one-third do poorly (continuing to use illicit drugs and to be involved in street crime). The remaining third vacillate between these two outcomes. However this represents an improvement over the prognosis without methadone.

The FDA has set up strict criteria describing who is eligible for treatment by methadone maintenance clinics, based upon the severity and duration of their substance dependence. Methadone can be prescribed for *pain* by any licensed physician but can only be prescribed for treatment of *drug addiction* by a facility that has obtained a special state license. Some have argued that this policy has been overly restrictive, limiting access to methadone for many patients.

An alternative to methadone is **naltrexone**, an opiate-receptor **antagonist**. While methadone decreases *negative* reinforcement and drug cravings, naltrexone lessens *positive* reinforcement by blocking the ability of heroin to cause a "high." Most opioid-dependent patients, especially those who use street heroin, clearly prefer methadone to a drug that "keeps you from getting high." In fact, only 10%–15% of heroin users express any interest in trying naltrexone, and half of these patients drop out of treatment within a month.

However, some highly motivated patients prefer to utilize a longer-term treatment option that doesn't involve the administration of opioids, and these patients might do well with naltrexone

therapy. One such group is individuals who have been in sustained remission from opioid use while in prison but now are being released and fear relapse. Another group is patients with a history of prescription opiate abuse. (This group includes substance-dependent physicians, who may be ordered into treatment by their state board of medicine.) Naltrexone also appears to be moderately effective in blocking the euphorogenic effects of alcohol intoxication; it hasn't proven to be effective in blocking the powerful euphorogenic effects of cocaine, however. As might be expected, unlike methadone, it has little effect on the unpleasant symptoms associated with the sustained abstinence syndrome.

Despite the success of naltrexone in smaller, open-label studies, it has never been demonstrated in larger, double-blind trials to be more effective than placebo. However, these large studies have extraordinarily high dropout rates (with as many as 70%–80% of subjects dropping out in the first 6 months). Naltrexone therefore might be effective in more highly motivated patients as one *part* of a broader, behaviorally based treatment program.

One advantage of naltrexone is that any physician can prescribe it, since many middle-class patients are much more likely to come to their physician's private office than to a treatment clinic. Another advantage is that, since it is not a controlled substance, there is no risk of the patient becoming addicted to it. While a long-acting depot form of naltrexone may improve patient compliance and clinical outcomes, none is currently available.

Unlike naltrexone, **buprenorphine** is a *partial opiate-receptor agonist*. Buprenorphine has features of *both methadone and naltrexone*. At lower doses, it acts primarily as an opiate receptor *agonist*, similar to methadone, blocking opiate withdrawal and decreasing drug cravings. However, because it is only a *partial* agonist, there is a limit to the opiate effects that it can produce. Further, buprenorphine *antagonizes* the euphorogenic effects of other opiates in a manner comparable to naltrexone, because since it is less potent than these other opiates and is already occupying opiate receptors. Unlike agonists such as morphine and methadone, at higher doses it does not produce progressively greater opiate effects (since it essentially begins to antagonize its *own* opiate effects) and it therefore is less likely to cause respiratory depression or coma in the event of overdose. If discontinued abruptly, its withdrawal syndrome is milder than that associated with heroin and much briefer than that associated with methadone.

Buprenorphine's success rate is comparable to that of methadone. It is poorly absorbed orally and therefore is taken sublingually (holding it under the tongue for at least 3 minutes). It is only effective for 24 hours and therefore patients have to attend a drug clinic on a daily basis to receive each dose.

Cocaine

Intoxication

Cocaine is a naturally occurring substance produced by the coca plant. It is consumed in several preparations. While coca leaves can be chewed or a paste can be extracted from the leaves, both of these practices are generally limited to populations native to Central and South America, where cocaine is grown. *Cocaine hydrochloride powder* is usually "snorted" through the nostrils or dissolved in water and injected intravenously. Sometimes, cocaine hydrochloride is mixed with heroin, producing a "speedball."

Cocaine alkaloid can be separated out from cocaine hydrochloride by heating it with ether, ammonia, or some other volatile solvent to extract the *free base* (hence the term, "freebasing"). This is a dangerous process because the solvents can ignite and harm the user. The reason for separating out the alkaloid is that it has a lower volatile temperature than cocaine hydrochloride. This allows it to be smoked without destroying its psychoactive properties. A simpler process is to produce *crack cocaine*. Here, cocaine alkaloid is extracted from the powdered hydrochloride salt by mixing it with sodium bicarbonate and then allowing it to dry into small "rocks." This form of cocaine is easily vaporized and inhaled, thereby allowing for an extremely rapid onset of central nervous system effects.

Acute cocaine intoxication typically includes a feeling of euphoria and enhanced vigor, gregariousness, hyperactivity, restlessness, hypervigilance, interpersonal sensitivity, talkativeness, anxiety, tension, alertness, grandiosity, stereotyped and repetitive behavior, anger, and impaired judg-

ment. These psychological and behavioral changes may be accompanied by physical signs including tachycardia, pupillary dilation, elevated blood pressure, perspiration, chills, nausea, and/or vomiting. Weight loss, respiratory depression, chest pain, or cardiac arrhythmia also can occur. Severe cases of intoxication can include confusion, seizures, dyskinesias, dystonias, or coma. Some patients in a state of acute intoxication experience paranoid delusions, although these generally only last for a few hours and don't require treatment. *Chronic intoxication* involving high doses of cocaine can cause affective blunting, fatigue, sadness, social withdrawal, psychomotor retardation, hypotension, bradycardia, and muscle weakness.

Because the effects of cocaine are short-lived (15–30 minutes when snorted, even briefer with freebasing or crack cocaine use) individuals experience a powerful urge to use it again (leading to a "binge"). They therefore can spend huge sums of money over relatively short periods of time, leading to the devastating loss of all personal savings and property and the accumulation of large financial debts. Individuals may resort to theft or prostitution to support their drug habit.

Neuroadapatation

Cocaine blocks the neuronal reuptake of dopamine, serotonin, and norepinephrine. The dopaminergic effects appear to play the greatest role in reinforcement. Over time, *tolerance* to cocaine's acute effects develops. This may be due to decreases in reuptake inhibition, decreased release of catecholamines, or changes in catecholamine receptor sensitivity. In most cases this takes the form of **desensitization**, leading to apathy and withdrawal, although in some cases it can cause **supersensitization and reverse tolerance**—that is, an individual can experience a severe response to a dosage of cocaine that previously only caused euphoria, resulting in agitation and paranoid delusions similar to those seen in schizophrenia.

Also likely related to neuroadaptation is the *cocaine withdrawal syndrome*. Subjects note that over the course of a binge, tolerance rapidly develops; subsequent doses, even higher doses, offer little euphorogenic effect, and serve only to hold off the "crash" that accompanies cessation of use. The "crash" is characterized by dysphoria, anhedonia, fatigue, insomnia, increased appetite, vivid and unpleasant dreams, and intense drug cravings. Patients often develop an intense urge to sleep and may ingest benzodiazepines or alcohol in order to do so.

For those individuals who refrain from further use, this withdrawal state gradually declines over the ensuing several weeks, although some individuals continue to experience persistent dysphoria and cocaine cravings that are exacerbated by environmental cues (such as seeing other white powders, like sugar). This state may be mediated by increased dopamine autoreceptor sensitivity, leading to decreased dopamine release in general, punctuated by surges of dopamine in response to environmental cues. Treatment with the dopamine agonists bromocriptine and amantadine have been disappointing, however.

Patients can become suicidal while in acute cocaine withdrawal. It is generally at this point that patients also begin to realize how much money they have spent on cocaine and may present to the ER seeking inpatient admission, complaining of suicidal ideation. One New York City survey conducted in the 1990s found that one out of every five persons who completed suicide during a 1-year period had used cocaine immediately prior to committing suicide.

While small-scale studies have suggested that cocaine craving (negative reinforcement) might be reduced by various agents (including desipramine, carbamazepine, and buprenorphine) larger, placebo-controlled studies have failed to confirm the initial promise of any of these interventions. Similarly, no medications have proven effective in blocking cocaine's acute positive reinforcing (euphoric) effects. Given that dopamine appears to play such a prominent role, premedication with haloperidol has been attempted, again without success. Typically, few ancillary medications are used in treatment unless cocaine dependence is accompanied by comorbid psychiatric conditions.

Amphetamines

Intoxication

Amphetamine intoxication presents in essentially the same way as cocaine intoxication. This isn't surprising since—like cocaine—amphetamine agents inhibit the reuptake of dopamine, norepinephrine, and serotonin but exert their greatest effects by causing increased release of stored supplies of dopamine. Like cocaine, the intensity of the intoxication state depends upon the particular preparation. Unlike cocaine, amphetamines do not have local anesthetic (i.e., membrane ion channel) activity and this may account for their lower risk of inducing cardiac arrhythmia and seizures (although these still can occur at higher doses). The intoxication state typically lasts longer than that associated with cocaine, but the overall course of the disorder is similar, with extended binges or "speed runs," followed by a "crashes" into depression and anhedonia when the supply of drug ultimately becomes exhausted.

The term "amphetamines" usually includes both those agents with a phenylethylamine structure (including amphetamine, dextroamphetamine, and methamphetamine) and structurally different stimulant agents with similar actions (methylphenidate and various "diet pills"). These substances are usually taken orally or intravenously, although methamphetamine ("speed") is also taken nasally ("snorted"). "Ice" is a very pure form of methamphetamine that crystallizes and has a low vaporization point, allowing it to be smoked for a more rapid and powerful effect similar to that obtained with crack cocaine.

While cocaine is obtained illegally, amphetamines and other stimulants are often obtained by prescription for the treatment of obesity, Attention-deficit hyperactivity disorder, and narcolepsy. Prescribed stimulants have sometimes been diverted into the illegal market, often in the context of weight-control programs.

Neuroadaptation

Mechanisms of neuroadaptation likely are similar to those for cocaine. Like cocaine, no effective medications are currently available to treat drug cravings or other abstinence symptoms, nor to block the positive reinforcing effects associated with relapse. Issues related to the abuse potential of the stimulant medications used to treat attention-deficit hyperactivity disorder are discussed in Chapter 19.

Nicotine

Intoxication

Smoking tobacco has been called the most important preventable cause of death and disease in the United States. About 25% of Americans are current smokers and another 25% are ex-smokers. It is estimated that smoking tobacco is responsible for 20% of all U.S. deaths. About 45% of smokers die of a tobacco-induced disorder, including lung, oral, and other cancers; cardiovascular disease; and chronic obstructive pulmonary disease. Smoking also causes peptic ulcer disease, gastrointestinal disorders, and maternal/fetal complications. Secondhand smoke is believed to be responsible for the deaths of thousands of nonsmokers and also causes excessive morbidity in the children of smokers. Most of these associated illnesses appear to be due to the carcinogens and carbon monoxide in tobacco smoke rather than nicotine itself.

Twin studies have found that the heritability of nicotine dependence is as great as, if not greater than, that observed for alcohol dependence. There may be a genetic overlap between these conditions, and a high percentage of alcohol-dependent individuals also smoke.

The median age of initiation of smoking is 15. Within a few years of daily smoking, most smokers begin to develop physiologic dependence, with evidence of both tolerance and withdrawal symptoms. Nicotine dependence occurs regardless of the form of nicotine (i.e., cigarettes, cigars, pipes, chewing tobacco, or snuff). Half of all smokers in their 20s are nicotine-dependent. A third of adults who smoke make a serious attempt to quit each year. Unfortunately, 60% of them relapse in the first week and only 5% are successful in any given attempt. However, half of all smokers ultimately are able to quit after having repeatedly attempted to quit.

Psychiatric patients are at particular risk for nicotine addiction. Compared with the national average of 30% of individuals being smokers, 75% of schizophrenic outpatients smoke and 90% of schizophrenic inpatients smoke. Why this should be the case isn't clear. One theory is that individuals with schizophrenia are attempting to combat negative symptoms with the dopaminergic effects of nicotine. Similarly, 75% of individuals with a lifetime history of major depressive disorder have smoked, and high rates of smoking also are noted among patients with anxiety disorders.

With typical dosing, nicotine leads to an elevated mood, an overall sense of calm, enhanced concentration, and decreased appetite. Acute nicotine intoxication is rare but can occur in first-time smokers, in patients receiving too high a dose of a nicotine patch, and in those exposed to insecticides. The most common symptoms are abdominal pain, dizziness, headaches, nausea, pallor, palpitations, sweating, vomiting, and weakness. The syndrome is self-limited and no specific treatment is required.

Neuroadaptation

Nicotinic acetylcholine receptors are located on dopaminergic neurons in the ventral tegmental area, and activation of these receptors triggers dopamine release in the nucleus accumbens. Therefore, the rewarding effects of nicotine are similar to those associated with other stimulating agents such as cocaine and the amphetamines. However, the pharmacologic effects of nicotine are more complex. Unlike cocaine or the amphetamines, which produce a *sustained burst* of dopamine and a powerful sense of euphoria, nicotine produces a *biphasic effect* in which the receptors are stimulated but then quickly desensitize and become refractory to further stimulation. This limits the extent of the "rush" that occurs. After a few seconds, the receptors recover and are ready to be stimulated with the next inhalation of nicotine.

Tolerance develops rapidly. While reinforcing effects of nicotine persist over time, side effects noted upon first using nicotine (such as dizziness, nausea, and palpitations) quickly resolve. Smokers gradually increase the number of cigarettes they smoke each day over the first few years, and this finally levels off by about the fifth year. As measured by the degree to which an inhalation increases heart rate, acute tolerance occurs both in the course of smoking *each* cigarette and also over the course of the day for *multiple* cigarettes. In other words, the greatest effect from a given cigarette occurs during the first few inhalations, while greater effects are achieved from the first cigarettes smoked in the morning than from cigarettes smoked later in the day.

Nicotine withdrawal occurs within 12 hours of the last cigarette and peaks over the following 3 days. Symptoms include a dysphoric or depressed mood, irritability, anxiety, difficulty concentrating, restlessness, insomnia (with increased awakenings and vivid dreams), decreased heart rate, and increased appetite or weight gain. Craving is prominent and is triggered by environmental cues, especially the sight of other people smoking. For half of smokers, withdrawal is protracted, lasting a month or more. Nicotine craving often persists for many months.

Treatment typically involves a combination of cognitive–behavioral therapy and agonist-substitution therapy. Clinicians initially should explore with smokers the reasons that they haven't quit (the most common reasons being fears of overwhelming craving and withdrawal, fears of weight gain, and fears of failing). Patients might be asked at this point to list some positive benefits of quitting, and the clinician should reinforce these benefits. Educating patients about how half of smokers ultimately quit, but only after multiple attempts, can be beneficial, especially if patients report that they have tried to quit in the past without success.

Combination therapy with *nicotine gum* and behavioral techniques offers better results than either treatment modality alone. It is available without a prescription. Two or 4 milligrams of nicotine is bound to an ion exchange resin and mixed with sweeteners and flavoring. About half of the nicotine in each piece of gum is actually absorbed. Because nicotine is about 90% metabolized by hepatic first-pass metabolism, the nicotine must be absorbed through the oral mucosa to work properly. Users have to briefly chew the gum and then park it between cheek and gum for several minutes. The gum is discarded after 20–30 minutes. Chewing one piece every 1–2 hours on a fixed schedule is more effective than random chewing. The advantage of the gum is that it allows for "as needed" use to combat acute cravings and also offers nicotine peaks similar to those obtained with smoked nicotine. The primary side effects are mouth soreness from chewing along with gastrointestinal upset if too much nicotine is swallowed.

Transdermal nicotine patches more effectively ameliorate craving and withdrawal symptoms than nicotine gum, since fairly consistent daily blood levels of nicotine can be achieved. They are available over the counter in doses of 11 to 22 mg of nicotine per patch. With the highest-dose patch, 0.9 mg/hour of nicotine is absorbed through the skin. The patch is applied to the skin of the upper body every morning and re-moved either at bedtime or the next morning. After 4–8 weeks at the initial dose, a titration can be attempted, tapering back every 2–4 weeks. It generally is well tolerated and compliance with the nicotine patch is higher than with nicotine gum. (Of note, these two treatment modalities can be combined.) The primary risk is local skin irritation.

Other nicotine delivery routes are also available, including a *nicotine nasal spray* and a *nicotine inhaler*. They offer the advantage of nicotine gum but tend to be easier to use (although they also can cause mucosal irritation). Their disadvantage is that because they offer more rapid onset of effects and are tied to a repetitive administration ritual, they may prove to be more difficult to wean than the nicotine patch.

Bupropion (Wellbutrin) has been approved by the FDA for smoking cessation under the trade name *Zyban*. It offers success rates comparable to the nicotine patch. Presumably, bupropion's dopaminergic actions play a role in decreasing nicotine cravings. Patients generally begin taking the medication 1 week prior to their "quit day." They should take one 150 mg tablet per day for the first 3 days and then increase the dose to 150 mg twice daily after 3 days. This dosage is maintained for at least 2 months after quitting. Bupropion can be used in combination nicotine replacement therapy.

The relationship between major depressive disorder and cigarette smoking is complex. About a third of smokers have a lifetime history of major depressive disorder, a proportion that is higher than that encountered in the general population. Smokers with a history of depression are more likely to fail in their attempts to quit and also are at higher risk of experiencing a depressive relapse over the several months following smoking cessation, even if they are in remission at the time that they quit. The onset of depressive symptoms ranges from 2 days to 6 weeks after smoking cessation. It may relate to declines in monoamines. In some cases, depressive symptoms resolve with the use of nicotine replacement therapy, and antidepressants also appear to be useful.

This is not to say that smokers with a history of depression should not attempt to quit, given the significant health risks associated with continued smoking. However, they should be educated about the risk of depressive relapse and should be monitored more closely for depressive relapse in the weeks following smoking cessation. Patients in remission from depression who are considering tapering and discontinuing their antidepressant medication might best be advised to remain on them at the current dosage if they are contemplating quitting smoking in the near future.

Hallucinogens

Intoxication

This group of substances includes peyote cactus (containing **mescaline**) and "magic mushroom" (containing **psilocybin**), which Native Americans have used for years in religious ceremonies, as well as synthetic agents. The synthetics include **lysergic acid diethylamide (LSD)**, **dimethyltryptamine (DMT)**, **2,5-dimethoxy-4-methylamphetamine ("STP")**, and **3,4-methylenedioxymethamphetamine (MDMA, "Ecstasy")**. Most of these agents are taken orally. An exception is DMT, which is degraded in the GI tract and therefore is smoked, sniffed, or injected.

Despite their name, these agents only rare cause true hallucinations and typically only when they are taken at higher doses. The more typical intoxication experience is characterized by perceptual alterations (*illusions*) such as colorful geometric patterns or distortion of shapes. Colors also may appear more intense. While auditory hallucinations are seldom described, a sensation of *hyperacusis* is commonly reported. Greater *sensitivity of touch* also is regularly noticed, and sometimes *taste and smell* are altered. *Synesthesia* is frequently described (for example, with colors being "heard" or sounds being "seen"). At higher doses, one's body parts may seem larger or smaller, or one's body may appear to be blending into the surroundings. This may be accompanied by a sense of "oneness" with the world or with the universe. Time also can become distorted: time may appear to be "standing still," and past memories and present events may seem to blend together.

Emotional responses to the hallucinogens can vary markedly depending on the individual, the setting in which the drug is taken, and the form and amount of drug consumed. While many users report a calm feeling of "bliss," emotions also can be extremely labile, ranging from tearfulness to euphoria to panic. Some patients become acutely anxious and paranoid (i.e., have a "bad trip"). The perceptual disturbances and impaired judgment associated with the intoxicated state can result in injuries or fatalities from automobile accidents, physical fights, or attempts to "fly" from high places.

The intoxicated state can increase or decrease in waves over a several-hour period. With LSD, the onset of psychological and behavioral effects occurs approximately 30–60 minutes after oral administration and peaks at from 2 to 4 hours postadministration, with a gradual return to the predrug state after 8–12 hours. In contrast, DMT has a very rapid onset and a short duration of action, 60–120 minutes. (It has been called "the businessman's LSD" since one might have a brief "trip" during one's lunch hour.)

MDMA ("Ecstasy") is a "designer drug" that has been promoted as enhancing empathy and personal insight without causing severe illusions. It has become popular as a "club drug" at dance parties called "raves." Its effects last for about 3–6 hours; effects observed are similar to those seen with the stimulant drugs, including euphoria, increased libido, increased energy, and decreased social inhibitions. Acute side effects typically include tachycardia, hypertension, increased muscle tension, involuntary teeth clenching, nausea, blurred vision, rapid eye movements, faintness, and chills or excessive sweating. Some individuals experience confusion or memory loss while intoxicated, and over the next several days to weeks some individuals develop depressive or anxiety symptoms.

Of great concern is that—while most teen drug use has remained steady over the past few years—MDMA use has risen dramatically. According to one survey, 5.6% of 12th graders used it at least once in 1999, while 9.2% used it in 2000. However, MDMA is far from benign. In animals, it can cause Parkinson's disease, perhaps mediated by overstimulation and subsequent destruction of dopaminergic nerve terminals. While no evidence has been found at this point that hallucinogens cause lasting brain injury in humans when used at typical dosages, fatal overdoses have occurred, and severe cases of toxicity also have been reported. In high doses

MDMA can cause hyperthermia, dehydration, seizures, and ultimately cardiovascular and renal failure leading to coma and death. Contaminants contained in illicit MDMA also may contribute to the occurrence of such reactions.

Neuroadaptation

Hallucinogens affect multiple neurotransmitter systems, including the serotonin, dopamine, and norepinephrine systems, but their predominant effect appears to be as *serotonin $5HT_2$-receptor agonists*. Hallucinogens can cause tolerance after even a single dose: this may be due to desensitization of the serotonin receptor after such powerful stimulation.

With longer-term dependence, a syndrome with symptoms resembling the negative symptoms of schizophrenia can occur, as discussed in Chapter 8. It remains unclear whether chronic hallucinogen use *produces* a psychotic disorder, merely triggers the *onset* of psychotic symptoms in vulnerable individuals, or is a *symptom* of an already-evolving psychotic illness. The condition is treated with antipsychotic medication and counseling.

In addition, some individuals experience "flashbacks"—repeated episodes that resemble the intoxicated state but that occur spontaneously—weeks or even months after the last episode of drug use. This phenomenon appears to be unique to the hallucinogens. Its etiology is uncertain, but it likely involves neuroadaptation. Flashbacks occur in a minority of individuals and appear to decrease in intensity and frequency over time. Despite the rapid onset of tolerance, true hallucinogen withdrawal has not been described in humans.

Cannabis

Intoxication

Cannabinoids are substances derived from cannabis, a hemp plant. When the upper leaves, tops, and stems of the plant are cut, dried, and rolled into cigarettes, this product usually is called **marijuana**. The dried, resinous exudate that seeps from the tops and undersides of cannabis leaves is called **hashish**, and hashish oil is a concentrated distillate of hashish.

Cannabinoids are usually smoked, but they also may be taken orally mixed with tea or food

The cannabinoid that has been identified as primarily responsible for the psychoactive effects of cannabis is **Δ-9-tetrahydrocannabinol** (Δ-9-THC, or simply THC). The THC content of available marijuana can vary greatly. The THC content of illicit marijuana has increased significantly since the late 1960s from an average of approximately 1%–5% to as much as 10%–15%. Synthetic THC has been used for certain general medical conditions (e.g., for nausea and vomiting caused by chemotherapy in cancer patients and for anorexia and weight loss in individuals with AIDS).

Marijuana is the most commonly used illicit drug in America. A 1991 survey found that a third of the population had tried marijuana, 10% had used it in the past year, and 5% had used it in the past month. While its use among teenagers has declined since its peak in the 1970s, it is still among the most commonly used drugs at that age, along with alcohol and tobacco. Many individuals use marijuana along with another drug—for example, to compensate for the nervousness associated with cocaine or to extend or potentiate the effects of heroin or alcohol.

When smoked, THC levels reach their maximal serum levels at between 10 and 30 minutes. THC and its metabolites are very lipid soluble and accumulate in fat cells, contributing to its long half-life (approximately 50 hours). Intoxication usually lasts from 2 to 4 hours, depending on the dose. On physical examination, tachycardia, dry mouth, and conjunctival injection may be noted.

The intoxication experience can be subtle, and first-time users may not notice a "high." Typical symptoms resemble a milder LSD experience, with time seeming to slow; appetite and thirst increasing; colors, sounds, and tastes seeming clearer; increased confidence and euphoria; feelings of relaxation; and increased libido. Some individuals experience transient depression, anxiety (including panic attacks), or paranoia. These experiences are more common among early users.

Objective neuropsychological testing conducted on subjects who are intoxicated reveals slowed reaction time and motor speed and impaired cognition, including short-term memory, attention span, and concept formation. The ability to drive or perform other skilled activities remains impaired for several hours beyond the period of acute intoxication.

Neuroadaptation

Two cannabinoid receptors (CB_1 and CB_2) have been discovered. They are located in the brain and also throughout the body, particularly in the immune system. Large concentrations of these receptors are present in the cortex, the substantia nigra, the cerebellum, the limbic system, and the hippocampus, consistent with cannabinoids' effects on cognition, motor coordination, memory, and mood. These receptors are coupled through G-proteins and adenylate cyclase to calcium channels, thereby inhibiting calcium influx. They also alter membrane lipids and other membrane-associated proteins. Finally, they also are located presynaptically, where they may exert a neuromodulatory effect by reducing the uptake of GABA and dopamine, thereby potentiating their actions.

Endogenous cannabinoids (endocannabinoids) have been discovered. The first of these was named **anandamide** (after the Sanskrit word for bliss). Several other endogenous cannabinoids have been found since then, and other cannabinoid agonists and antagonists also have been synthesized. Endogenous cannabinoids likely are involved in pain modulation, control of motor activity, cognition, and memory. Cannabinoid agonists one day might be prescribed as analgesics, antiemetics, antispasmodics, or appetite stimulants. However, smoked marijuana is a crude delivery system that also delivers toxic and potentially carcinogenic substances, suggesting the need for further research into more reliable parenteral delivery systems.

Cannabis users frequently develop tolerance to its effects. A subset of users (about 10%–15%) develop more compulsive use that interferes with social and occupational responsibilities. Family or friends may fail to notice that the individual has a problem since the consequences of cannabis dependence tend to be less striking than those associated with dependence on other drugs. For example, cannabis-dependent individuals don't spend all of their money on binges or engage in embarrassing behavior while intoxicated.

However, cannabis can become a daily habit and can influence major life decisions. An "amotivational syndrome" also has been described affecting chronic, heavy cannabis users, characterized by significant social morbidity but little accompanying insight into personality changes that have gradually progressed over time.

Cannabis withdrawal is not listed in the *DSM-IV*, but can occur. The symptoms are generally milder than those encountered with other substances of abuse, reflecting cannabis' high lipid solubility and long half-life. The clinical syndrome has been characterized by restlessness, anorexia, irritability, and insomnia that begins less than 24 hours after discontinuation of marijuana, peaks in intensity on days 2 to 4, and lasts for 7–10 days. This syndrome can be abruptly precipitated by administering a cannabinoid receptor antagonist to heavy users. Detoxification and rehabilitation therefore follow a behavioral model, as no specific pharmacologic agents have been shown to be useful to date.

As with the hallucinogens, high doses of cannabis can precipitate psychosis. In substance-abusing adolescents presenting in an acute psychotic state, it can be difficult to determine whether the psychosis is secondary to drug use alone, or whether it preceded the drug use (and perhaps led the individual to "self-medicate" anxiety or agitation by using cannabis), or whether it reflects a genetic predisposition toward schizophrenia simply unmasked by drug use. Usually, psychotic symptoms are treated with antipsychotic medication and counseling. It is essential, however, for these patients to receive close longitudinal follow-up of their symptoms following detoxification, along with assessment of the need for continued treatment for an underlying psychotic illness.

Phencyclidine (PCP)

Intoxication

PCP ("angel dust") was originally synthesized as an anesthetic. It is structurally similar to ketamine, which is still used in anesthesia. PCP intoxication is associated with severe dissociative reactions, including paranoid delusions, hallucinations, anesthesia, and amnesia. The neurologic exam is notable for prominent *cerebellar symptoms*, including ataxia, dysarthria, and nystagmus (both horizontal and vertical). With *severe intoxication* due to overdose, individuals can present with symptoms resembling those seen in neuroleptic malignant syndrome: the individual is mute and catatonic, with muscle rigidity and elevated temperatures. Complications include rhabdomyolysis and seizures.

PCP had a brief period of popularity in the 1960s, which rapidly faded due to the severity of adverse reactions. However, the drug has made a small comeback more recently among post high school–aged minority males in some cities, most of whom are polysubstance abusers. Patients also may present to the emergency room having ingested PCP unintentionally, having used cannabis or LSD that was "laced" with PCP.

Intoxication typically is managed in the emergency room setting. The diagnosis may be suspected based on the neurologic findings but ultimately is only confirmed by serum or urine toxicology testing. While patients intoxicated with LSD can sometimes be talked down, this approach typically only makes matters worse when dealing with individuals intoxicated with PCP. Patients need to be protected from engaging in dangerous behaviors, although restraint alone may worsen rhabdomyolysis due to muscle injury. There is no PCP antagonist drug analogous to naloxone or flumazenil. Treatment involves giving antipsychotic or benzodiazepine agents for sedation and administering activated charcoal to help clear unabsorbed drug. In addition, acidifying the urine (with intravenous ammonium chloride followed by oral cranberry juice and vitamin C) causes PCP to be released from fat stores and increases urinary excretion by 100-fold.

Neuroadaptation

PCP appears to exert effects at both the opiate receptor and as a negative allosteric modulator of the glutamate NMDA receptor. Tolerance and withdrawal have not been demonstrated in humans, although heavy users do report powerful cravings for the drug, possibly due to the drug's potent positive reinforcing effects.

CONCLUSION

The substance-related disorders involve multiple agents, either natural or synthetic, that act at different receptors and have differing pharmacological and psychological effects. Some of these substances are illegal, some are available by prescription, and others are readily available over the counter. At the margins, the lines between use, abuse, and dependence aren't clear, consistent with these being disorders of motivated behavior with associated physiological and cognitive features.

The key feature of all of these disorders, however, is the repeated self-administration of a particular substance despite adverse physical, psychological, or social consequences. Substance dependence includes three main aspects: loss of control over the use of the agent, dramatically increased salience of the agent, and physiologic dependence (neuroadaptation). Under the current *DSM* system of classification, one can be substance dependent without being physiologically dependent, and one can also become physiologically dependent on a substance without having substance dependence. One also can fail to meet these criteria and yet still might meet the broader criteria for substance abuse when the individual's substance use is not as compulsively driven but still adversely affects social or occupational functioning.

As with other disorders of motivated behavior, an essential part of treatment is helping the patient regain control of her behavior. This may not be possible without interventions aimed at helping the patient to "detoxify" from these drugs—that is, to help the patient's brain to recover from adaptations that it has made in response to drug exposure. However, detoxification rarely is a "cure." Once a driven behavioral pattern has been established, individuals can break this cycle by attending to and resisting those factors that continue to reinforce the behavior. Reinforcers can be either internal or external, positive or negative.

Treatment takes place incrementally, first by helping the patient recognize the fact that a behavioral disorder exists and that it is important to address it. Medical interventions may be essential both in helping the patient to safely withdraw from the agent and in treating the medical complications that result either from the drug use or as a result of substance withdrawal.

Interventions after the acute detoxification phase attempt to address comorbid psychiatric illnesses, to modify other internal biological reinforcers through pharmacologic interventions (when available), and to help patients learn to recognize the biological, psychological, and environmental reinforcers of their substance use and to develop effective compensatory strategies.

Chapter 13

Somatoform Disorders

Patients present to physicians for evaluation of a wide variety of somatic complaints. Sometimes it isn't clear to what extent these complaints are physical or "psychological" in nature, especially when assessment for commonly associated physical conditions is unrevealing. Such cases frequently lead primary care physicians to worry that they are overlooking an underlying psychiatric problem; however, just as often they lead consulting psychiatrists to worry that they are overlooking an underlying medical problem.

In the some cases, it soon becomes apparent that—despite the presence of dramatic physical *complaints*—no underlying physical *pathology* is present. For example, pathological signs and symptoms might be inconsistent from one minute to the next or might not adhere to any known physiologic distribution (such as when the patient covers one eye but his complaints of "double vision" persist, or when he complains of having "triple vision"). While physicians have acknowledged the existence of such cases for over 4000 years, their cause remains just as baffling today, despite the our technological advances.

The basic question has remained the same over the years: are these patients *consciously* lying, *deliberately* feigning medical illness? In some cases, the answer turns out to be "yes." However, in many other cases, these patients appear to be genuinely devastated by their somatic symptoms. They also appear to be genuinely resentful of any suggestion that their illnesses might not be "real." This suggests that if they are in fact "pretending" to be ill, they must be doing so at an *unconscious* level. Consider the following example:

Chief complaint: A 37-year-old former nurse's aid is admitted to the inpatient neurology service for continuous electroencephalogram (EEG) monitoring to assess the nature of "spells" that were initially believed to represent temporal lobe seizures. Psychiatric consultation is requested after the patient experiences two "spells" that are found to be unaccompanied by any evidence of seizure activity on the EEG.

Psychiatric history: The patient has no previous psychiatric history. Her spells began about 3 years ago. She notes that her spells often are preceded by stressful life events or strong negative emotions. During a spell, she initially experiences an internal sensation of "shaking, a nervous feeling." This is followed by bilateral shaking of both hands, progressing to involve the head, sometimes associated with shortness of breath. A typical spell lasts for between a few seconds and a few minutes. She is fully conscious during the spell and remains able to converse. Her spells are not accompanied by incontinence or tongue biting. She feels fatigued after a spell but is not disoriented or confused. The spells have never generalized to a grand mal seizure. She has never had a spell while alone, and she has never been injured during a spell. (Rarely, she has "lost control" of her legs, but on each of these occasions her husband has been near enough to catch her before she could hit the ground.)

Medical history: Her medical history is extremely complex, although no old records are readily available for review. She recalls having had rheumatic fever as a young child, and this caused her to miss school for an entire year. She had a hysterectomy at age 25 to treat menses that were painful and associated with heavy bleeding. She states, "I would lose a huge amount of blood and then would have to stay in bed for a whole week out of each month." Since the surgery, she has experienced difficulties with hypoactive sexual desire as well as anorgasmia. She also had an appendectomy at age 27 and a cholecystectomy at age 33. (She is not aware of whether surgical pathology findings ultimately confirmed the clinical diagnoses that led to her having received these procedures.)

She reports a history of conjunctivitis "that comes and goes." She has a history of intermittent gastrointestinal bloating and nausea. Food sometimes gets "caught" in her throat, and this occasionally is associated with vomiting. She has been diagnosed in the past with "irritable bowel syndrome," as well as with "hiatal hernia," but she isn't aware of whether the latter diagnosis was based on findings from radiological studies. She has a history of chest pain which has led to multiple emergency room visits and at least two inpatient hospitalizations. During one of these hospital stays, she reportedly was told that she had suffered a "mild coronary infarction." (She is wearing a nitroglycerin patch at the time of the evaluation.) She reports frequent pain and burning with urination, which has been treated intermittently with antibiotics, although her doctor has told her in the past that her urine "looks okay under the microscope."

She reports a history of daily occipital headaches for the past 3 years, which sometimes radiate across the top of her head. Sometimes she experiences blurred vision and sees flashing lights along with the headache. She had experienced intermittent left-sided weakness for the past 3 years, sometimes associated with a "pins and needles sensation" and a sensation of "falling to the left." She reports a history of periods of either amnesia or confusion. She notes: "Sometimes I can write perfectly, but at other times I can't even write my name." She states that she sometimes has difficulty remembering her own phone number.

Eventually, some of the patient's past medical records are obtained. She has evaluated by at least nine different clinicians over the last 3 years. No laboratory tests have revealed a specific pathologic abnormality. She has visited the emergency room several times with complaints of chest pain on two occasions was hospitalized overnight for further assessment, although on both occasions she was "ruled out" for a myocardial infarction. It isn't clear who initially prescribed the nitroglycerin patch; her current primary physician simply has been refilling the prescription. She also has been prescribed a large number of medications at different points in time by different specialists, often without their having been aware that she simultaneously was visiting other physicians or receiving other prescriptions.

Family history: She denies having a family history of mental illness. She describes her father, a minister, as having been a man believed by his congregants to be witty and outgoing but who at home was a strict disciplinarian with a low threshold for anger. He enforced corporal punishment, using a belt. She recalls her mother as having been a "passive person," very subordinate to her husband, who showed little affection toward either the patient or her two brothers.

Social history: She had a normal gestation and birth. She left the household after high school to marry her husband, also a minister. She describes her husband as "extremely supportive." For example, he does all of the shopping, as she herself becomes very fatigued walking through the supermarket. (She even has had "drop attacks" in the supermarket.) They have no children, and their social life centers on the church where her husband is a minister. She describes her fellow congregants as being supportive of her. For example, they pray with her before each Sunday service, including a prayer that the patient "won't have a seizure during the service." She has never worked outside of the home. Three years ago, she trained to become a nurse's aid, but her spells began shortly after she began working and have prevented her from returning to work ever since. She denies a history of alcohol or substance use.

Premorbid personality: The patient and her husband both describe her as a caring, religious person. She is socially extroverted but despite this has few close friends. She is short-tempered and experiences rapid shifts in her mood in response to life situations. She tends to worry about the future but denies denies being perfectionistic. Her primary hobbies are reading and listening to religious music.

Mental status examination: Throughout the interview, the patient displays a resting tremor in her hands. The tremor is intermittent and disappears when she is distracted from it, for example, when she becomes more engaged in conversation. Shortly after the interview begins, she experiences a typical "spell." She begins to tremble in both hands, and this progresses to shaking of both arms and finally to shaking of her entire body. This lasts for about 5 seconds. She has two more of these episodes over the course of the interview. The psychiatrist remains calm throughout each spell. He instructs her to try to calm herself and to "take control," and he then shifts the conversation to other subjects. The patient's speech is overly inclusive of detail and "dramatic," but without evidence of formal thought disorder. She describes her mood as "relieved to be here" and denies experiencing sustained periods of depression or self-deprecation. She denies hallucinations, delusions, obsessions, compulsions, or phobias. Her Mini-Mental State Examination score is 30.

Physical exam: Vital signs are stable. The skin exam is notable for multiple surgical scars. The head, neck, and chest exam are normal, but when asked to hold her breath during auscultation for carotid bruits, she becomes "unable" to exhale for several seconds. Abdominal exam reveals mild epigastric tenderness without guarding. The neurologic exam is notable for weakness in all extremities, but with a volitional "give-away" quality. Cranial nerves are normal, as are reflexes in all extremities. Her sensory exam is notable for complaints of numbness in all of her extremities in a distribution inconsistent with normal dermatomal patterns. Her numbness also "splits the midline" in that she notes numbness across the left side of her body terminating in a straight line down the center of her face, thorax, and abdomen. She complains of severe back pain during the straight-leg raise test (which involves 90-degree hip flexion while lying supine). However, when her Babinski reflex is elicited (again by raising her legs to 90 degrees of flexion, although this time in the sitting position) she does not complain of any back pain. Her gait is mildly unstable with an inconsistent, "astasia–abasia" quality (i.e., she "loses her balance" in a dramatic way, having to lean on the wall to "catch herself").

PHENOMENOLOGY OF SOMATIZATION

The above example vividly demonstrates the difficulties posed by the patient who voices multiple somatic complaints in multiple organ systems, many of which do not appear to have a physiologic basis. The patient has been treated by a variety of physicians, including several specialists, and her medical records are not readily available. The history as she presents it isn't fully reliable. She is taking many medications, and her primary care physician has feared discontinuing several of them given her report of several significant illnesses, including a seizure disorder and ischemic heart disease with a history of two previous myocardial infarctions.

This case also demonstrates the utility of approaching a patient from all four perspectives. One must be wary of only using the disease perspective, since if all one has is a hammer, everything will look like a nail. Certainly, this patient presents for evaluation of an **illness**—that is, a *subjective* complaint of physical and/or mental distress. In contrast, **disease** is a construct employed to *explain* what objectively lies *behind* the patient's illness. (Similarly, behaviors, dimensions, and life stories also are constructs.) We all might agree that the patient described above is *ill*; the question is: does she have a "disease"?

The essential feature of this patient's presentation is that she *complains of physical symptoms* that suggest the presence of an underlying medical condition, but—ultimately—her symptoms *cannot be fully explained* by any such medical condition. Nor are they explained by the direct effects of a substance or by the presence of a mental disorder (such as major depressive disorder, panic disorder, or generalized anxiety disorder). Further, her symptoms are *so severe* that they have become a source of clinically significant distress as well as impairment in her social and occupational functioning. Finally, as far as we can tell, her symptoms are *not feigned or intentional* (i.e., they do not appear to be under her voluntary control). Using *DSM-IV* terminology, this patient has a **somatoform disorder**. More specifically, since she voices long-standing, unexplained medical complaints referable to multiple organ systems, she has the subtype of somatization disorder called **somatization disorder**.

Until the publication of *DSM-III* in 1980, this patient would have been diagnosed with *hysteria*. Many general physicians still use this term, although "hysteria" is no longer a part of the official psychiatric nomenclature. The term had sexist connotations, and it also was imprecise. It came to refer to a *behavior* (that of complaining of multiple, unexplained physical symptoms), to a *dimension of personality* (so-called "hysterical personality"), and to a psychoanalytic *theory* based on particular aspects of the patient's *life story*. In other words, the term "hysteria" was an amalgam of all four perspectives.

However, not all patients demonstrate all of these elements. For example, not every person who presents with unexplained physical complaints has a self-dramatizing or attention-seeking personality style. Conversely, most people with such a personality style do not present to doctors with unexplained physical complaints. Given this, "hysterical personality" was removed from the "hysteria" syndrome and was placed among the other personality disorders, renamed as **histrionic personality disorder**, a more gender-neutral term connoting a dramatic and attention-seeking style.

What remained of "hysteria" was the illness behavior itself, and this condition also was relabeled, now being called the **somatoform disorders** (Table 13–1). "Lumping" of a variety of manifestations of illness behavior into a single syndrome gave way to "splitting" into several syndromes, each distinguished from the others by the specific nature of the patient's complaints. It therefore should come as no surprise that these syndromes demonstrate significant overlap with each other. Under *DSM-IV*, the somatoform disorders include the following:

Somatization disorder: Multiple, unexplained physical complaints spanning multiple organ systems. The condition also should be *chronic*, with the somatic complaints beginning before age 30 and continuing over a period of at least several years. The full diagnostic criteria are presented in Table 13–1. When a patient does not meet these full criteria, he still might be diagnosed as having an *undifferentiated somatoform disorder*.

Conversion disorder: Unexplained symptoms or deficits affecting voluntary motor or sensory function that suggest a neurological or other general medical condition, but with psychological factors judged to be associated with the symptoms or deficits. Common symptoms include pseudoseizures, blindness or "tunnel vision," vocal cord dysfunction, paralysis, and anesthesia.

Pain disorder: Pain is the predominant focus of clinical attention, with psychological factors judged to have an important role in its onset, severity, exacerbation, or maintenance. The

---

Table 13–1. *DSM-IV-TR* Criteria for Somatization Disorder

A. A history of many physical complaints beginning before age 30 years that occur over a period of several years and result in treatment being sought or significant impairment in social, occupational, or other important areas of functioning

B. Each of the following criteria must have been met, with individual symptoms occurring at any time during the course of the disturbance:

   1. *Four pain symptoms*: a history of pain related to at least four different sites or functions (e.g., head, abdomen, back, joints, extremities, chest, rectum, during menstruation, during sexual intercourse, or during urination)

   2. *Two gastrointestinal symptoms*: a history of at least two gastrointestinal symptoms other than pain (e.g., nausea, bloating, vomiting other than during pregnancy, diarrhea, or intolerance of several different foods)

   3. *One sexual symptom*: a history of at least one sexual or reproductive symptom other than pain (e.g., sexual indifference, erectile or ejaculatory dysfunction, irregular menses, excessive menstrual bleeding, vomiting throughout pregnancy)

   4. *One pseudoneurological symptom*: a history of at least one symptom or deficit suggesting a neurological condition not limited to pain (conversion symptoms such as impaired coordination or balance, paralysis or localized weakness, difficulty swallowing or lump in throat, aphonia, urinary retention, hallucinations, loss of touch or pain sensation, double vision, blindness, deafness, seizures; dissociative symptoms such as amnesia; or loss of consciousness other than fainting)

C. Either 1 or 2:

   1. After appropriate investigation, each of the symptoms in criterion B cannot be fully explained by a known general medical condition or the direct effects of a substance (e.g., a drug of abuse, a medication)

   2. When there is a related general medical condition, the physical complaints or resulting social or occupational impairment are in excess of what would be expected from the history, physical examination, or laboratory findings

D The symptoms are not intentionally feigned or produced (as in factitious disorder or malingering)

Source: Reprinted with permission from the *Diagnostic and Statistical Manual of Mental Disorders, Fourth Edition, Text Revision.* Copyright 2000 American Psychiatric Association.

psychological factors may be judged to be the *sole* cause of the pain complaint or may be judged to have contributed to an *exacerbation* of pain associated with an underlying general medical condition.

Hypochondriasis: Preoccupation with the fear of having, or the idea that one has, a serious disease, based upon a misinterpretation of bodily symptoms or functions. This preoccupation persists despite appropriate medical evaluation and reassurance. The belief isn't held with delusional conviction (as in the case of *delusional disorder, somatic type*) and isn't restricted to a circumscribed concern about bodily appearance (as in *body dysmorphic disorder*), but it is preoccupying and has persisted for some time (at least 6 months). Because these fears of being ill often are intrusive, senseless, and persist despite reassurance, an overlap between hypochondriasis and *obsessive–compulsive disorder* has been postulated. Hypochondriasis is quite common in the medical clinic setting, present in about 5% of outpatients. It occurs most commonly in patients in the fourth or fifth decade of life.

Body dysmorphic disorder: Preoccupation with an imagined or exaggerated defect in physical appearance.

Somatoform disorder not otherwise specified: Somatoform presentations that do not meet the criteria for any of the specific somatoform disorders.

As can be seen, these different terms embrace different domains of discourse. For example, *conversion disorder* emphasizes patients' complaints of specific pseudoneurologic symptoms or signs, while *pain disorder* emphasizes patients' complaints of pain. *somatization disorder* constitutes a broader, supraordinate diagnosis, in that the physical symptoms tend to be more chronic and more widespread and include (but not limited to) *both* conversion symptoms and unexplained or exaggerated pain symptoms. What all three of these conditions have in common is: (1) the presence of "nonphysiologic" or "exaggerated" physical symptoms, along with (2) an excessive focus on these symptoms and an accompanying, intensely held *belief* that the person is ill and in need of medical attention.

In *hypochondriasis*, the latter belief system is present, but the focus of the patient's preoccupation is not unexplained physical or neurologic symptoms but relatively benign bodily experiences. The patient misattributes the latter experiences, considering them to reflect an undiagnosed, serious disease.

Body dysmorphic disorder was discussed in Chapter 8. While this condition also features prominent somatic complaints, here patients excessively focus on imagined or exaggerated physical defects which cause them to be "ugly," such as acne, thinning or excessive hair, or a "misshapen" appendage (nose, ears, lips, genitals, hands, etc.). They often seek treatment from dermatologists or plastic surgeons rather than from primary care physicians. Whether this condition is best considered a subtype of somatoform disorder, a variant of obsessive–compulsive disorder, or a variant of delusional disorder remains an area of active research. The condition highlights the difficulties that clinicians sometimes encounter in attempting to distinguish between *delusions, obsessions,* and *overvalued ideas.*

The diagnosis of a somatoform disorder is assigned only when a patient engages in *a particular type of behavior.* As we have seen with other behavioral disorders, such as the eating disorders and the substance-related disorders (discussed in Chapters 11 and 12, respectively), a failure to *recognize* the presence of the pathologic behavior often contributes to diagnostic confusion as well as to unintentional *reinforcement* of the aberrant behavior by well-intentioned family, friends, or physicians. Somatoform disorders also resemble these other behavioral syndromes in that comorbid psychiatric diseases, dimensional personality variation, and life stories clearly play important *contributory* roles but are neither necessary nor sufficient to account in themselves for the presence of the somatoform disorder. The *excessive behavior itself* and *the overvalued belief system that comes to be associated with the behavior* (e.g., a preoccupation with bodily appearance in the case of the eating disorders, a preoccupation with being unable to function unless one is intoxicated in the case of the substance-related disorders, and a preoccupation with physical symptoms and bodily health in the case of the somatoform disorders) are the defining features of the somatoform disorders.

The somatoform disorders should be of particular concern to physicians, since they themselves may unintentionally reinforce the patient's behavior and belief system. Understandably, perhaps, a physician's greatest fear when evaluating a patient is that he or she will fail to diagnose or will misdiagnose an underlying disease process. Therefore, patients with unexplained somatic complaints commonly receive extensive medical tests and procedures, including exploratory surgery. Certainly, some serious diseases first present with nonspecific or variable physical or mental complaints and unremarkable results on diagnostic studies. Examples of such illnesses include *multiple sclerosis, systemic lupus erythematosus, acute intermittent porphyria, syphilis, brain tumor, hyperparathyroidism, hyperthyroidism,* and *myasthenia gravis.*

Sometimes, after an initial workup is negative but the patient's symptoms persist, the physician repeats this workup in the hope that the underlying disease process will finally "declare itself." Further, new complaints on the part of the patient involving a different organ system may trigger an entirely new medical workup, along with referrals to additional specialists. This problem is further compounded by a medical system where patients see multiple physicians, sometimes misrepresenting or misrecalling what they have been told by previous physicians. Medical records of earlier evaluations typically are not readily available to current evaluators. Some physicians, responding to pressure to "make a diagnosis," assign labels such as "fiibromyalgia" or "multiple environmental sensitivity syndrome" even when there isn't clear evidence that a patient has one of these conditions. The patient may embrace such a diagnostic label, read about it in books or on the Internet, and join support groups, relieved to finally have an explanation for his suffering. However, such behavior even further reinforces illness behavior. Finally, physicians have the "power of the prescription pad" and may feel pressured by patients to prescribe a medication even in the absence of clear indications for doing so, further validating and reinforcing illness behavior.

Therefore, as with all disorders of motivated behavior, a primary goal in treating the patient with a somatoform disorder is to break an established behavioral cycle that involves the patient, treating clinicians, and members of the patient's social and occupational milieu. Since biological factors may play an important contributory role, medications can play a useful (although adjunctive) role. Medical school curricula do not place much emphasis on the diagnosis and management of patients with complex somatoform disorders. They should, though, since it is conservatively estimated that 10% of all medical services are provided to patients who have no evidence of organic pathology.

SOMATIZATION AS A DISEASE

Is somatization disorder a disease? For centuries, physicians have been most comfortable with the disease perspective. Given this, it is understandable that they repeatedly have returned to the conjecture that there must be some underlying biological dysfunction that can fully account for the bewildering diversity of physical complaints encountered in "hysterical" patients. However, since no "broken part" has been discovered, disease formulations have relied on unproven, unfounded hypotheses.

The diagnosis of "hysteria" did not initially have sexist connotations. The term itself is derived from the Greek word *hustera,* or "uterus." (This also is the root of the word "hysterectomy.") Egyptian physicians working in 2000 BC believed that hysteria was caused by a "wandering uterus," a theme echoed by Greek physicians at the dawn of the millenium.

These clinicians took note of the fact that hysteria typically occurred in women. They also were aware that the uterus was an organ that was present only in women and that—during menstruation and pregnancy—it clearly changed in size, shape, and position. Therefore, they hypothesized that the uterus, in its "wanderings," could compress against other bodily organs, thereby accounting for the diversity of clinical symptoms that occur in hysteria. The disease also was noted to occur more commonly in younger women rather than in older women, which might be accounted for by the uterus being more mobile in the former group. For example, in the second century AD, Aretaeus of Cappadocia (who also was the first person to hypothesize that mania and depression were two parts of a single illness) offered the following explanation for "hysterical suffocation":

In the middle of the flanks of women lies the womb, a female viscus, closely resembling an animal; for it is moved of itself hither and thither in the flanks, also upwards in a direct line to below the cartilage of the thorax, and also obliquely to the right or left, either to the liver or spleen; and it likewise is subject to prolapsus downwards, and, in a word, it is altogether erratic. It delights, also, in fragrant smells, and advances toward them; and it has an aversion to fetid smells, and flees from them; and, on the whole, the womb is like an animal within an animal. When, therefore, it is suddenly carried upwards, and remains above for a considerable time, and violently compresses the intestines, the woman experiences a choking, after the form of epilepsy, but without convulsions. For the liver, diaphragm, lungs and heart are quickly squeezed within a narrow space; and therefore loss of breathing and speech seems to be present. And, moreover, the carotids are compressed from sympathy with the heart, and hence there is heaviness of head, loss of sensibility, and deep sleep. (Quoted in Slavney, 1990)

For treatment, Aretaeus recommended that "cinnamon, pounded with any of the fragrant oils" be "rubbed on the female parts" or that fetid smells such as "old urine" be inhaled. The goal was coax the uterus downward, back into its proper position, either by enticement (the cinnamon) or by provocation (the urine).

In contrast, Galen believed—based on dissection studies—that the uterus could never reach up far enough to cause an arrest of respiration, fainting spells, or seizures. He noted that in pregnancy an increased respiratory rate is seen but one rarely encounters more severe physical problems. However, Galen did not reject the uterine hypothesis. Rather, he proposed that hysteria was caused by the uterus retaining *putrefied substances* that subsequently could spread through the body, accounting for these more remote symptoms:

It is generally agreed upon that this disease mostly affects widows, and particularly those who have previously menstruated regularly, had been pregnant and were eager to have intercourse, but were now deprived of all this. Is there a more likely conclusion from these facts than that in these patients the retention of menstrual flow or of semen causes the so-called uterine condition by which some women become apnoic, suffocated or spastic? And possibly, this affliction is made worse by the retention of semen. (Quoted in Slavney, 1990)

Galen's treatment involved the restoration of an active sex life or else manipulations by midwives or physicians of the affected bodily parts. Again, he did not confirm this presumed disease mechanisms through clinicopathologic correlation.

Despite this, the presumption that "hysteria" was a medical illness caused by uterine pathology persisted, essentially unchallenged, until the seventeenth century.

By that point, physicians had begun to question the uterine hypothesis. The primary difficulty with the theory was that sometimes men developed hysteria. In these cases, the organ imputed in men was the *spleen*, which lay below the diaphragm (hence the term "hypochondriasis") and also was known to sometimes become enlarged. It was assumed that in men an enlarged spleen might compress the subdiaphragmatic viscera causing symptoms similar to those involving an enlarged uterus in women. However, Thomas Sydenham doubted this theory, noting that the clinical presentation of hysteria in women and in men was nearly identical.

The focus therefore shifted from the uterus to an organ system known to connect to the entire body, the *nervous system*. If nervous system pathology caused hysteria, it might explain the association noted by many clinicians between life stress (particularly stress associated with a powerful emotional response) and the subsequent development of hysterical symptoms. The observation that hysteria occurred more often in women than in men could be accounted for by the fact that women had a "weaker" nervous system, or perhaps by a presumed interaction between the nervous system and hormonal or uterine "factors" or "molecules."

The most influential elaboration of the nervous system hypothesis was offered by the French neurologist Jean-Martin Charcot. Charcot was the chief physician at La Salpêtrière Hospital, a hospice for elderly women. He first achieved fame in France for describing clinicopathologic correlations between the symptoms that occur in multiple sclerosis and in amyotrophic lateral sclerosis and the central nervous system pathology.

Charcot achieved his greatest fame, however, for his studies of epilepsy. The epilepsy ward at his hospital contained both "pure" epileptics and so-called "hysteroepileptics." Charcot found that he could induce neurologic symptoms at will in the "hysteroepileptics" through the use of hypnosis, and physicians from throughout the world traveled to his hospital to witness this. He developed an elaborate classification scheme for hysterical symptoms, distinguishing them from "matched control" patients with neurologic diseases and identical symptoms (e.g., hysteroepilepsy versus epilepsy, hysterical paralysis of the arm versus paralysis due to stroke, etc.). He also compared the hysterics with normal subjects asked to feign (i.e., to *malinger*) having an illness and noted some differences in the these two types of presentation. This convinced Charcot that the hysterics weren't simply feigning illness but rather had a brain lesion. Since no lesion could be demonstrated, however, he postulated that they must have a "functional," or emotional lesion, resulting from an earlier, emotionally traumatic experience.

Sigmund Freud (a student of Charcot) later elaborated on Charcot's view. However, since many of Freud's patients hadn't experienced any obvious traumatic experience, Freud shifted his focus to the role of *unconscious* wishes and conflicts and also to the possible *symbolic meanings* of hysterical symptoms. In consequence, the treatment of hysteria shifted from the realm of neurology to that of psychology and psychiatry, although hysteria still was thought of as a disease. Freud was the one who coined the term "conversion" to refer to the process by which patients convert unconscious psychic anxiety into overt neurologic deficits.

The latest and clearest formulation of hysteria using the language of disease was by Purtell and associates in 1951. In order to achieve greater diagnostic reliability, these researchers first constructed a very long list of physical symptoms. In order to diagnose hysteria, a clinician had to document that the patient had a large enough number of these symptoms, each of which was medically unexplained. This list was refined by Perley and Guze in 1962 and again by Feighner and associates in 1972. The so-called "Feighner criteria" for hysteria required that the patient present with chronic or recurrent illness beginning before the age of 30, that the illness be associated with at least 25 medically unexplained symptoms out of a list of 59 symptoms, and that the symptoms span out of 10 symptom categories. These researchers still considered hysteria to be a "disease" but conceded that evidence for this conclusion remained lacking:

For the present, if we claim that hysteria is an "illness" we are forced to define "illness," itself no easy matter. We use the so-called medical model chiefly because it has provided us with practical, useful information. Some of the information from existing follow-up and family studies does tend to support the concept of hysteria as an illness or disease. It is possible that our view of hysteria will eventually evolve in a new and different direction. That will depend on the data which become available. (Feighner et al., 1972)

The advantage of applying strict operational criteria to the construct of hysteria was that it allowed the diagnosis to be assigned with greater *reliability*. Once this could be achieved, researchers could then focus on the task of attempting to *validate* the diagnosis through longitudinal, family, and biological studies.

Studies using these criteria demonstrated that the prevalence of hysteria in the general female population was 2%. (The prevalence was found to be much lower in the Epidemiologic Catchment Area [ECA] Survey, perhaps because that study utilized *nonphysician* interviewers, who may have been more uncomfortable in determining that a given physical complaint should be listed as being "unexplained".)

In addition, longitudinal study of a group of patients diagnosed according to these criteria demonstrated that hysteria was a relatively stable condition. While a physician's greatest fear may be that of diagnosing somatization disorder and "missing" an occult medical condition that subsequently becomes apparent, 90% of these patients had not been diagnosed with a new medical illness and had not deteriorated physically when they were reassessed 6–8 years later. In fact, 20% of patients even showed some *improvement* in their symptoms over that time. (Improvement, of course, also is contingent on the physician avoiding interventions that potentially might *cause* harm, especially unnecessary surgical interventions. This underscores the importance of delineating this particular group of patients.)

These criteria obviously proved to be unwieldy in real-world clinical settings. Along with changing the name of the condition to "somatization disorder," the *DSM-III* work group shorted the list of symptoms to 37 and placed greater emphasis on those symptoms from the Feighner symptom list that had best-discriminated hysteria from specific medical conditions.

Fourteen unexplained symptoms from this list were required for women to be diagnosed, and 12 for men. (A smaller number of symptoms were required for men in order to minimize gender bias given the absence of menstrual or pregnancy-related symptoms in their case.) These criteria were changed only minimally in *DSM-IIIR*. However, the criteria were dramatically streamlined in *DSM-IV*, again to allow for greater utility in the clinical setting, since few physicians carried the *DSM-IIIR* symptom list around with them.

The *DSM-IV* criteria for somatization disorder require that the patient demonstrate four pain symptoms, two gastrointestinal symptoms, one sexual symptom, and one pseudoneurological symptom, all of them unexplained, and that the complaints begin before age 30. These criteria are summarized in Table 13–1. Despite their greater simplicity, statistical analysis of these diagnostic criteria in a medical clinic population identified the same core group of patients that the much stricter Feighner criteria had identified.

SOMATIZATION AS A BEHAVIOR

Spectrum of Severity

As in the case of other behavioral disorders, it is likely that genetic and biological factors contribute to the genesis of somatization disorder. However, it is likely that most people with these underlying constitutional factors *don't* go on to develop the disorder. Biological predispositions likely are expressed in the form of behaviors through a combination of factors in the internal and external environment that initiate and sustain the behavior.

As with other traits and behaviors, the tendency toward somatization occurs in a spectrum of severity in the general population; milder forms are extremely common and more extreme forms such as somatization disorder are relatively rare, as demonstrated in Figure 13–1. About 80% of healthy individuals experience somatic complaints in any given week. One study that assessed for the prevalence of "subsyndromal" somatization (six of the *DSM-IIIR* symptoms of somatization disorder rather than the requisite 12) found that 11% of Caucasians and

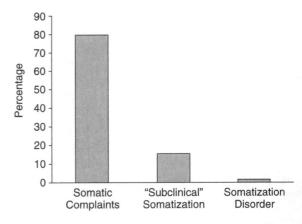

Figure 13–1. Prevalence of somatization in the general population.

Hispanics and 15% of African Americans in the United States fulfilled these criteria, while in Puerto Rico 20% of Puerto Ricans fulfilled the criteria. Other studies have found that the medical and emotional disability associated with such "subsyndromal" forms of somatization (included in *DSM-IV* as "undifferentiated somatoform disorder") remain quite high.

As might be expected, the rate of somatization is much higher in the medical setting than in the general population. Up to 50% of patients who present to physicians do so with somatic complaints for which no adequate physical cause is detected. Of course, minor or transient physical causes likely are present in many of these cases. Among all patients presenting to one academic family practice clinic, 5% fulfilled the full diagnostic criteria for somatization disorder. If this figure is accurate, then of the 50 patients seen in the average primary care clinic each day, two or three probably have somatization disorder, making it as prevalent a disorder as diabetes and urinary tract infection.

The prevalence of somatization disorder is even higher in the inpatient general hospital setting and in specialty clinics. Up to 9% of patients admitted to a medical–surgical floor have somatization disorder. Among patients presenting to specialty clinics with conditions such as irritable bowel syndrome, polycystic ovary disease, and chronic pain, the prevalence of somatization disorder is even higher, ranging from 12% to 28%. Similarly, one-third of women who receive noncancer-related hysterectomies have somatization disorder.

As we have done for other behavioral disorders, in thinking about somatization disorder we must consider both *initiating factors* and *sustaining (reinforcing) factors*. Before doing so, however, we must first consider a more fundamental question. If somatoform disorders are behavioral disorders, what is the fundamental *goal* of the behavior? In all of the previously discussed disorders, individuals engaged in the behaviors to satisfy certain *drives or cravings*. For example, the goal in eating disorder is to become more slim (a positive reinforcer) and also to diminish the fear that one is fat and unattractive (a negative reinforcer). Similarly, the goal of paraphiliac sexual behavior is to achieve sexual release (a positive reinforcer) while diminishing sexual cravings (a negative reinforcer). Seen in this light, the two questions that have preoccupied physicians for centuries are: what is the nature of the behavior, and what is the goal of the behavior?

Normal and Abnormal Illness Behavior

"Illness" is not the same as "disease." Earlier, we defined "disease" as a breakdown in the structure or function of a bodily part. Whether or not a person has a disease is determined *objectively*. In contrast, "illness" refers to the *subjective* experience of a particular patient, and the severity of illness refers to the extent to which the patient is "suffering."

The construct of "illness" has both *personal* aspects (e.g., the degree to which a patient perceives pain) and *interpersonal* aspects (e.g., whether or not a patient is able to work or to drive her children to school). Given this, different individuals with the same disease may have quite different perceptions of how "ill" they are. One individual with breast cancer may remain quite functional despite having extensive metastatic disease, while a different individual may experience overwhelming anxiety and depression despite being ostensibly "in remission."

In the 1960s, David Mechanic proposed the term **illness behavior** to encompass all of the different ways in which an individual perceives, evaluates, and acts upon (or fails to act upon)

physical symptoms. It is likely that many factors—including genetics, personality style, previous personal experience with having been ill, and family attitudes toward illness—influence a particular patient's illness attitudes and behaviors.

Another major influence on illness behavior is the extent to which the illness allows the patient to play culturally sanctioned roles. In the 1950s, Talcott Parsons, a sociologist, described how people who are ill are allowed to assume the "sick role." Assuming this role entitles them to receive certain *privileges*, such as being excused from normal social expectations and not being held to blame for being sick. For example, the ill child might be allowed to stay home from school, to stay in bed, to watch more television than usual, and (if her tonsils have been removed) to eat all the ice cream she wants. Similarly, the ill adult might be allowed to stay home from work and—in cases of more severe injury—to receive disability payments from either a private insurance carrier or from the government. Family and neighbors all may pitch in to help accommodate the affected person, since the person, after all, "is sick" and therefore is deserving of such support.

However, the individual who assumes the "sick role" also is expected to fulfill certain *responsibilities*. The individual is expected to have the desire to get well, and she also is expected to avail herself of all resources offered to her by society that might assist her to do so. Therefore, the child is expected to drink plenty of fluids and to stay in bed. The adult who receives disability payments is expected to follow the recommendations of all evaluating physicians, such as to take prescribed medications and to attend physical therapy.

While patients are free to present themselves as being ill to family or friends, only physicians are sanctioned by society to lend legitimacy to the sick role. However, patients' expectations sometimes end up at variance with physicians' expectations in this regard. In describing patients with somatoform disorders, physicians may use pejorative labels (such as "crocks," or "turkeys"), suggesting their general aversion to endorsing the sick role in patients who don't appear to legitimately "deserve" to assume the role.

Table 13–2. Pilowsky's Model of Abnormal Illness Behavior*

		Patient	
		Ill	*Not Ill*
Doctor	Ill	A	B
	Not ill	C	D

*Patient A demonstrates illness-affirming, normal illness behavior; patient B demonstrates illness-denying, abnormal illness behavior; patient C demonstrates illness-affirming, abnormal illness behavior; patient D demonstrates illness-denying, normal illness behavior.
Source: Adapted from a theoretical model presented in Pilowsky I: "A General Classification of Abnormal Illness Behaviors." *Br J Med Psychol* 51:131–137, 1978.

When doctors and patients disagree about the patient's health status, the patient can be considered to be demonstrating "abnormal illness behavior." Table 13–2 (based on a theoretical model by Issy Pilowski) summarizes the different ways that a doctor and a patient might agree or disagree about whether the patient is "ill" or is "healthy."

> *Scenario A: illness-affirming normal illness behavior.* A patient goes to her internist, complaining of feeling ill. She has been feeling very warm and also has experienced dysuria and flank pain. The clinician discovers during the physical examination that the patient has a fever and flank tenderness, and laboratory tests reveal bacteria and white blood cells in the patient's urine sample and a serum leukocytosis. The doctor informs the patient that she has good reason to feel ill, since she in fact *is* ill, with pyelonephritis. He prescribes an antibiotic and fills out a work-release slip.
>
> *Scenario D: illness-denying normal illness behavior.* A patient goes to her internist for a yearly physical, with no specific complaints. The doctor discovers no pathologic findings on either the physical exam or on basic screening tests. The patient states that she doesn't think that she is ill, and the doctor confirms her impression, telling her that he gives her a "clean bill of health." He instructs her to return next year for her next annual check-up.
>
> *Scenario B: illness-denying abnormal illness behavior.* A patient goes to her internist for a yearly physical, with no specific complaints. Her doctor discovers that she has hypertension. He informs her that she must change her diet,

exercise more, and take antihypertensive medication every day. However, the patient denies that she has an illness, repeating that she "feels fine." She says that if she did have significant hypertension she "would know it because I would have a headache, which I don't." She refuses to follow the doctor's recommendations. Such "pathologic denial" sometimes leads to a request for psychiatric consultation, depending upon the severity of the patient's medical condition, the short-term and long-term implications of the patient going without treatment, and the degree to which the treating physician is concerned about the patient's competence to understand the information that has been presented to her and to rationally compare her options.

> *Scenario C: illness-affirming abnormal illness behavior.* A patient presents to her internist with multiple somatic complaints. However, the doctor does not find any objective evidence of illness. The patient wishes to be allowed to assume the sick role, but the doctor refuses to legitimize this role. The somatoform disorders would fall into this category.

Seen in this light, all of the somatoform disorders, despite their disparate presentations, share the common feature of presenting with *illness-affirming abnormal illness behavior*, with one goal of this behavior being *to assume the sick role*. Given this, we will now examine the various factors that might help explain why some individuals engage in illness behavior more than other individuals do and the factors that serve to *reinforce* this pattern of behavior over time. These factors are listed in Table 13–3.

Table 13–3. Initiating and Sustaining Factors in Somatoform Disorders

Initiating Factors	Additional Sustaining Factors
Genetic factors	Unconscious gain
Neuropsychological and	Primary gain
physiologic factors	Secondary gain
Personality factors	Family and friends
Alexythymia	The physician
Somatic amplification	
Neuroticism	
Personality disorder	
Learned responses	
Comorbid depressive disorders	
Comorbid anxiety disorders	

PREDISPOSING AND INITIATING FACTORS

Genetic Factors

Somatization disorder runs in families: 20% of first-degree female relatives of patients with somatization disorder also have somatization disorder. Adoption and cross-fostering studies are consistent with both genetic and environmental factors playing roles in the familial transmission of somatization disorder.

Interestingly, male relatives of female patients with somatization disorder are not more likely to have somatization disorder than are other members of the general population, but they are more likely to have *antisocial personality disorder* and *alcohol dependence*. This finding suggests the possibility that somatization disorder and antisocial personality disorder are phenotypic variants of similar genetic predispositions. Perhaps the fact that men present with alcoholism and antisocial personality disorder while women present with multiple somatic complaints reflects neurobiologic differences, hormonal differences, or varying cultural expectations.

Neuropsychological and Physiologic Factors

Clinical experience suggests that individuals with somatization disorder demonstrate *selective attention* during conversations. For example, a clinician can have a conversation with the patient with somatization disorder, but at their very next meeting the patient may recount a very different version of their conversation than what the clinician recalls. For example, the patient might recall the clinician having voiced serious concerns about the patient's health, even when he had expressed the opposite opinion. Consistent with this clinical observation, neuropsychological testing in somatization disorder patients has revealed subtle *attention and memory deficits* consistent with *bilateral, symmetrical frontal lobe dysfunction*. (Interestingly, individuals with antisocial personality disorder often have similar neuropsychological findings, as discussed in Chapter 10.)

Personality Factors

One personality factor that has been associated with somatoform attitudes and behaviors is **alex-**ithymia, an inability to recognize and communicate one's emotions. Alexithymic individuals have a tendency to focus on the *somatic* manifestations of their emotional state while failing to recognize or minimizing the *affective* and *cognitive* components of their emotional state. This results in both a *misinterpretation of somatic sensations as symptoms of physical illness* and in *somatosensory amplification*.

Whether or not an individual identifies a somatic sensation as being the bodily concomitant of an emotional state depends to a large extent on how her brain processes the sensation and places it in its appropriate context. Therefore, the inherited tendency toward alexithymia may offer a potential linkage between the observed clinical features of somatoform disorders and findings from family studies that suggest the presence of underlying inherited predispositions.

Of course, inheritance is only one potential cause of alexithymia. An association also has been observed between alexithymia and childhood *emotional trauma*. Perhaps chronic alexithymia is similar to the "emotional numbing" described by patients with post-traumatic stress disorder (described in Chapter 9), although in this case the trauma may have occurred early in life, and the numbing has become an established personality trait.

A separate (although perhaps related) trait observed in patients with somatoform disorders is the tendency to engage in **somatic amplification**. Individuals demonstrate significant variability in *the degree to which they experience visceral and somatic sensations*. For example, two individuals may demonstrate significant variation in their thresholds for experiencing sensations of pain in response to the same stimulus or in their ability to tolerate the same painful stimulus. Individuals who are more sensitive to pain have been called "amplifiers" or "augmenters," while those who are less sensitive to pain have been called "minimizers" or "reducers."

While somatic amplification likely occurs to greater or lesser degrees in all individuals, one's current circumstances can influence the process. For example, one study has found that the more frequently that postsurgical patients are asked to rate the severity their postoperative pain, the higher they rate it. Similarly, in another study, subjects were asked to run on a treadmill while listening through headphones either to interesting bits of conversation or to the sound of their own breathing. The two groups did not differ in their physiological measurements but did differ in the way that they *perceived* their physiological functioning while exercising. The subjects who listened to their own breathing subjectively experienced more fatigue, palpitations, and sweating than those who listened to bits of conversation.

This suggests that the degree to which one attends to one's bodily sensations can affect one's overall perceptions of bodily health. As Barsky has noted, it isn't uncommon for someone else's cough to draw our attention to our own throats; we might even begin to note mild sensations of dryness or scratchiness in our throats that we previously had ignored. Studies specifically involving patients with somatoform disorders reveal that they are even *more* susceptible than other people to experiencing somatic symptoms of an illness that they have heard about or read about.

Patients with somatoform disorders also demonstrate several other aspects of excessive somatic amplification, including: *(1) heightened vigilance* for normal but unpleasant bodily sensations (e.g., intestinal peristalsis, postural hypotension, changes in heart rate, and the somatic concomitants of intense affect such as sympathetic arousal); *(2)* a tendency to focus on *relatively weak or infrequent sensations* (e.g., transient tinnitus, a twitching eyelid, or dry skin); and *(3)* a tendency to *mislabel visceral and somatic sensations* as being abnormal, pathological, and symptomatic of disease. Therefore, the symptoms reported by hypochondriacal individuals are not necessarily imagined or "in their heads." However, psychological processes clearly play an important role in how they attend to their bodies and perceive their bodily processes.

Somatic amplification may involve a "positive feedback loop" between heightened attention to somatic sensations and excessive concerns about one's bodily health. In other words, heightened attention to somatic sensations contributes to the development of thoughts that one is ill, and this in turn causes the individual to pay even more attention to his bodily sensations.

The trait of "amplification" may be one subfacet of the broader trait of **neuroticism** discussed in Chapter 10. Neuroticism describes an individual's overall predisposition to experience negative affects such as anxiety, depression, hostility, impulsivity, and vulnerability. Among individuals with somatic complaints, an almost "dose–response" relationship has been observed between neuroticism scores and the number and severity of somatic complaints.

Using *DSM-IV* terminology, about 60% of these patients will quality for one or more *personality disorder* diagnoses, the most common being avoidant, paranoid, and obsessive–compulsive. What these diagnoses all share is a greater tendency to be concerned with "harm avoidance." This can either be focused outward (on the potentially threatening actions of others) or inward (on the safety of one's own body). As noted above, many patients with somatoform disorders also demonstrate histrionic traits which, when combined with obsessive–compulsive traits and high neuroticism, predispose them to worry about minor physiological symptoms and then to experience and express these somatic concerns in an excessively dramatic way. In these cases, the histrionic features tend to be so obvious, so "out there," that the treating clinician may not notice the patient's obsessional features.

Learned Responses

As we have discussed in the case of personality disorders, traits reflect general *tendencies* that only become evident under particular circumstances. Thus, while an individual may be *predisposed* to develop somaticizing behavior by her predispositions toward attentional biases, neuroticism, alexithymia, and somatosensory amplification, the pathologic behavior ultimately is initiated, shaped, and sustained by particular life events.

The patient's early home environment might be especially important. Children's somatic symptoms often imitate symptoms that have been experienced by other members of the family. Adult patients with somatoform disorders also are more likely to recall their parents having subjected them to excessive attention when they expressed any physical complaints. (A caveat to this finding is that it is based solely upon the recollections of patients whose memories sometimes are biased and unreliable.)

In the case of conversion symptoms, there often is a "model," or "template," for that particular illness behavior. For example, about a third of patients with "pseudoseizures" also have an *actual,* preexisting seizure disorder. One can imagine how when a child has a seizure at home or at school it has a powerful effect on everyone around him. He might be brought to the school nurse, sent home from school early, and relieved of any immediate responsibilities. This well-intentioned behavior in response to normal illness behavior may set the stage for the child later assuming the sick role by unintentionally feigning these same symptoms during periods of emotional distress. In some cases of pseudoseizures, patients who don't have a preexisting seizure disorder recall having once *witnessed* a seizure.

Comorbid Depressive Disorders

Somatoform disorders don't appear to simply be "masked" forms of major depressive disorder. However, patients with depressive disorders clearly experience more somatic complaints than do nondepressed individuals. Further, depressive disorders are a commonly observed comorbidity among patients with somatoform disorders, occurring in about half of patients. Given this, attention should always be paid in the somaticizing patient to the possibility that an underlying major depressive disorder is a contributing factor.

It is especially important to probe for depression when examining alexithymic individuals, since they may not spontaneously state that they "feel sad." In such cases, one might consider initiating a trial of an antidepressant medication empirically. Also of note, greater degrees of alexithymia are associated with poorer or more limited responses to psychotherapy, perhaps because while psychotherapy aims to help patients recognize the links between depressive thoughts, feelings, and behaviors, alexithymic individuals often resist this process.

Comorbid Anxiety Disorders

Anxiety disorders are associated with significant visceral and somatic symptoms, and secondary hypochondriacal concerns commonly arise in these patients, especially if they haven't been educated about the nature of their disorder. In addition, patients with anxiety disorders may become sensitized to their body sensations, further encouraging somatic amplification.

Comorbidity occurs in the other direction as well. About a third of patients diagnosed with somatization disorder are found to also fulfill the diagnostic criteria for generalized anxiety disorder, and a quarter fulfill the criteria for panic disorder. As with the depressive disorders, when the distinction between a somatoform disorder and an anxiety disorder is in doubt, an empirical trial of medication may be of utility.

REINFORCING AND SUSTAINING FACTORS

Unconscious Gain

Primary gain refers to the *unconscious, intrapsychic benefit* that a patient may achieve by experiencing a particular somatic symptom, typically a conversion symptom. A prototypical example is the man who unconsciously wishes to hit his child but develops a conversion paralysis of the arm. The conversion symptom not only allows for symbolic expression of the unconscious wish but also prevents him from engaging in the feared act.

Secondary gain refers to the *external benefit* achieved by experiencing a somatic symptom. For example, the patient with a paralyzed arm may receive more attention from his family and friends, may be relieved of work responsibilities, may receive monetary compensation in a lawsuit, and may receive narcotic medication from a physician because of associated pain complaints. While this gain sometimes is conscious, in most cases it is unconscious or is minimized and rationalized.

One variant of secondary gain has been termed "disability neurosis," and describes the difficulty that many patients have in relinquishing their somatic complaints in the setting of ongoing disability litigation. For example, Ford (1986) has described what he calls the "Humpty-Dumpty syndrome," which acts as a powerful incentive to remain in the sick role:

These patients have been very hardworking persons who prematurely assumed responsibility, perhaps starting to work full-time at age 13 or 14, who married young, and who frequently have many children. They have worked long hours, usually in relatively unskilled positions. Following an industrial or automobile accident, they have their dependency needs gratified, often for the first time in their lives. The defenses, primarily reaction formation, against dependency wishes crumble, and they remain permanently dependent and disabled. Frequently complicating the situation is that the patients are reaching an age where they are no longer as physically strong and therefore a return to work spells the possibility of increasing failure.

Two important caveats about primary and secondary gain. First, most patients don't demonstrate a clear symbolic symptom. Interpretations aimed at determining whether such symbolism is present can be highly unreliable. For example, "symbolic" physical complaints have been ascribed to individuals later determined to have been experiencing a true medical disorder. Therefore, the fact that a somatic symptom may be reinforced by secondary gain shouldn't be offered as "proof" that the symptom was psychological in *origin*. Patients with obvious physical injuries also experience secondary gain that predisposes them to develop a worsening of their symptoms in the face of psychological distress. (This has been termed a "psychological overlay.")

Second, despite the long-held *assumption* that patients with ongoing personal injury or disability litigation might dramatically improve once their litigation issues have been resolved, longitudinal studies suggest that this assumption is not valid: in most cases, despite successful resolution of the litigation, the disability persists at a severe level.

Family and Friends

In the clinical example presented at the beginning of this chapter, the patient's husband and friends made significant efforts to accommodate her illness. In many cases, the family life of patients with somatoform disorders ultimately comes to revolve around their illness, just as it might around a severe "organic" illness such as cancer. In this way, patients' daily interactions with their family and friends can become powerful reinforcers of their illness behavior.

A patient's illness may come to play such an important role in family members' lives that the family members themselves may be reluctant to accept the diagnosis of somatoform disorder or to change their behavior toward the patient. (This might come as a surprise to the clinician who reasonably assumed that family members would

be *relieved* to find out that their loved one does not have a significant medical condition and has the potential to live a relatively normal life.)

For example, parents may prefer to focus their attention on their child's "illness" rather than on their own marital difficulties. Or, a wife may prefer that her previously abusive husband remain "weak" or in "chronic pain" if he hasn't engaged in any acts of domestic violence since the onset of his somatoform complaints. Family members also may reinforce abnormal illness behavior by inadvertently becoming "enablers" of the behavior. For example, in the case described above, the patient's husband always "happened to be" in a position to "catch" the patient when she had her "drop attacks" in the supermarket. Over the course of treatment, when he was told that he should ignore these "attacks" rather than reinforcing them, he asked (quite reasonably), "But what should I do if she falls down in the supermarket? Just let her lie there?"

Clearly, clinicians can't simply dispense pat advice and expect the entire social system that has evolved around a patient to change overnight: the process of therapy requires skillful mediation between the sometimes-conflicting goals of the physician, the patient, and the patient's family members and friends.

The Physician

As is clear from the above discussion, patients with somatoform disorders are prone to focus on certain physical sensations or to unconsciously feign symptoms. However, another essential reinforcer of this abnormal illness behavior is the patient's *belief* that he or she is in fact ill. This belief tends to be powerfully validated by the behavior of the patient's physician.

The physician may unintentionally reinforce particular symptomatic complaints and may even contribute to the evolution of new complaints. For example, directive questioning in the course of taking a detailed history may contribute to further illness behavior by suggesting new symptoms to the patient. The patient with pseudoseizures, for instance, who previously has remained awake and alert during her "shaking spells," may be asked in the course of an evaluation, "Have you ever lost consciousness during a seizure? Have you been confused afterward? Have you bitten your tongue?" Following this session with the physician, future pseudoseizures may evolve over time toward a more "classic" presentation, with the patient ultimately becoming uncommunicative during a spell, repeatedly biting down on her tongue, and appearing "confused" following the spell. The physician may remain unaware of her contributory role.

Patients with somatoform disorders also can be persistent and demanding. They may feel that the physician "hasn't done anything for them" if the physician hasn't offered another diagnostic test or prescribed a new medication. In the short term, the physician who wishes to avoid confrontation may feel that a patient will be "satisfied" if a diagnosis is assigned (e.g., "spastic colon," "hypoglycemia," or "environmental allergy") and a relatively benign medication is prescribed. Unfortunately, this strategy sometimes simply leads to further escalation of patient's symptoms:

A 31-year-old woman presents to a chronic pain clinic for evaluation of severe, persistent leg pain. She initially had pulled a muscle in her leg in a job-related injury, but the pain became increasingly worse over the next few weeks, spreading from her calf to her entire leg. The pain has prevented her from attending work and also becomes much worse when she attempts to have sexual intercourse with her husband, during which time she also experiences "numbness" in the affected leg. The physical examination is unremarkable save for sensory deficits in an inconsistent pattern affecting both legs. There is no evidence of temperature differences between her legs, and the affected leg shows no evidence of skin or nailbed changes, edema, or atrophy. The physician, in spite of this negative exam, feels the patient "deserves the benefit of the doubt." He tells her that that she might have a case of reflex sympathetic dystrophy. He explains the pathophysiology of the disorder to her, prescribes a low dose of a calcium channel blocker, and instructs her to return for follow-up in 2 months.

During this interval, the patient's paralysis worsens to the point where her "entire body" now occasionally becomes paralyzed (with the exception of her still being able to speak throughout these episodes). Her "RSD attacks" always occur when others are present, and her symptoms are relieved within a minute of taking a 25-mg trazodone tablet, placed in her mouth by a family member. (She had been prescribed 100 mg of trazodone at night to help with sleep.) Also during this time, she has her car outfitted with hand controls (to help ensure her

safety in case her legs should became paralyzed while driving), and she is excused from testifying in a court case out of concern that the stress of testifying might "set off her RSD," thereby causing her to become acutely paralyzed or even unable to breathe.

Physicians should attempt to avoid reinforcing abnormal illness behavior, but they also must recognize that patients with somatoform disorders do suffer greatly and are not simply "wasting the physician's time." Using standard health status assessment measures, all aspects of these patients' health—physical, social, and mental—rate in the "severely impaired" range. When compared with patients with chronic medical conditions (such as hypertension, rheumatoid arthritis, chronic obstructive pulmonary disease, and insulin-dependent diabetes mellitus), the health of patients with somatization disorder is worse. Patients with somatization disorders perceive themselves as "sicker than the sick," and this belief becomes their reality.

While patients with somatization disorder significantly overutilize health-care services, this is due as much to their physicians' reactions to them as to their own behavior. When the patient with somatization disorder repeatedly returns to her physician, her symptoms unimproved or worse since the last intervention, her physician undertakes further diagnostic interventions. She returns again, her symptoms unchanged. This cycle of complaint and response continues until both parties become frustrated and the patient finally is referred to a new physician, perhaps a specialist or subspecialist. Further tests are arranged, again to no avail. The patient, now frustrated even further, may seek care from a new set of physicians, who may begin the workup "from scratch." Breaking this cycle requires the physician to both refuse to reinforce the behavior further while also avoiding alienating the patient or discouraging her to the point where she simply seeks care from a different doctor.

Perhaps the most famous example of patients and a physician inadvertently colluding, thereby perpetuating the patients' symptoms, is that of Charcot and his "hysteroepileptic" patients. While Charcot postulated that his patients' symptoms were caused by a "psychological lesion" within their brains, his colleague Babinski astutely noted that these patients were residing on the same ward as the true epileptics. Babinski postulated that the hysteroepleptics' behavior had been shaped by their observations of and identification with these true epileptic patients. After the hysteroepileptics were moved to a different ward, their pseudoseizures dramatically improved.

Further, after Charcot's death ended his dramatic demonstrations of hysterical phenomena to visiting physicians, his former patients' symptoms improved even further. Perhaps the most impressive evidence that he himself had become a reinforcer of his patients' behavior was that— years after his death—many of his patients were symptom-free but would gladly reenact their earlier hysterical deficits for visitors upon request, especially if they were offered a bit of money.

TREATMENT OF SOMATOFORM DISORDERS

Address the Behavior

The management of somatoform disorders parallels that of other behavioral disorders. The first step is to *address the behavior*. Since multiple physicians may be involved in the patient's care and since all of them must agree about the treatment plan, somebody must be elected "quarterback." Typically, this will be the patient's primary care physician, although in the inpatient psychiatric setting it might be the attending psychiatrist. This primary physician should be person responsible for ordering all tests and consultations and reviewing the results with the patient.

At some point early on, all physicians involved in the case must agree on the diagnosis. While some members of the team may have the urge to order "just one more test" (often a test that must be sent to a lab in Minnesota packed in dry ice), it will be impossible to inform the patient that he has somatization disorder or conversion disorder unless all of the doctors have agreed that this is the case. One strategy is to have all of the specialists involved submit their "wish list" for diagnostic testing with the understanding that—if these tests come back negative—the workup will end and the patient will be informed of the somatoform disorder diagnosis.

Once the diagnosis of a somatoform disorder has been agreed upon by all concerned, the patient should be informed of the diagnosis and about its nature. This does not mean that the patient should be told that her symptoms "are all in her head" or that her symptoms are "psychological," not only because such statements trivialize the patient's very real suffering but also because they aren't accurate. It should be explained to the patient that some individuals appear to be physiologically more attuned to actual but benign visceral and somatic sensations. She should be informed that the fact that no life-threatening disease (such as cancer or stroke) has been uncovered in the course of the workup is good news rather than cause for further frustration. Rather than informing the patient that "no diagnosis can be made," she should be informed that an empirical diagnosis *has* been made—that is, a somatoform disorder. The role of stress in exacerbations of the patient's condition should be explained, and the goals of treatment should be delineated. These goals include helping the patient learn how to more effectively manage life stress and also helping her learn how to live *with* chronic somatic symptoms rather than putting important activities on hold until she can be "cured." Many patients may not have thought until this point about making substantive lifestyle changes, since their focus has been on finding the "cure" that would obviate the need to do so.

In cases of somatization disorder or conversion disorder, it might be reasonable to specifically present these diagnoses by name to the patient. Many physicians hesitate to do so, fearing that patients will be offended by the diagnosis. (For similar reasons, many physicians are reluctant to discuss the diagnosis of personality disorder with patients.) My own experience has been that when this information is presented to patients in a supportive and empathic manner, they rarely react with defensiveness or resentment. Some patients even express gratitude that somebody "is finally offering me an explanation for what I've been going through," rather than a shrug of the shoulders and comments to the effect that "the workup has all been negative." The importance of avoiding excessive testing or surgical procedures should be emphasized, and the patient should be informed of the importance of educating all future physicians about the diagnosis of somatoform disorder and of the importance of these physicians obtaining and reviewing the patient's old records rather than "reinventing the wheel."

This one-time discussion is the equivalent of an "intervention" for patients with a substance-related disorder. One major goal of this discussion is for the patient to achieve "the desire" to modify her belief system and behavior and to commit herself to making substantive life changes. However, *lasting* changes in an individual's beliefs and behaviors usually only occur over time, in response to positive reinforcement.

The primary care physician should recognize that—to the patient—*the clinic visit itself* is more important than any particular prescribed treatment. Therefore, *brief visits should be scheduled at regular intervals*. Initially, visits should be spaced at every 1–2 weeks; the interval should be gradually increased to every 4–6 weeks as tolerated. This way, the patient doesn't need to develop new symptoms as the requisite "ticket of admission" to see the physician. If the patient begins to call between visits complaining of a worsening of symptoms, this suggests that she needs a greater degree of support and that the interval between office visits again should be decreased, followed down the road by a renewal of attempts to gradually increase this interval. During the first year, the interval between visits rarely should exceed 6 weeks unless it is at the suggestion of the patient.

Obviously, patients with somatization disorder may go on to develop true somatic diseases since somatization disorder does not "immunize" the patient. Therefore, another goal of these follow-up visits is to monitor for the development of new disease processes while avoiding either reinforcing abnormal illness behavior or making "errors of commission" such as unnecessary surgery. One recommended strategy for achieving this balance is that, for any *new symptom* (i.e., one that hasn't been part of the patient's current symptom profile) the physician should take a basic history and conduct a routine workup (e.g., a focused physical examination and basic laboratory testing). This should be done with the understanding that—if this workup is negative—the new symptom will be added to list of symptoms already attributed to somatization disorder, but the physician will continue to follow closely for the development of any serious disease.

Address Comorbid Psychiatric Conditions

While one goal is to also avoid the prescription of unnecessary medications (especially potentially addictive ones), the clinician always should attempt to address *comorbid medical and psychiatric conditions* (especially depressive and anxiety disorders), preferably with conservative interventions. Antidepressant medications may be useful in treating these conditions, even when the depression or anxiety appears to be "subsyndromal."

However, a few caveats must be offered about the use of medication in this population. First, these patients may be especially prone to experience side effects or new symptoms. Therefore, one should initiate treatment with low doses and strong support. One also should be wary of having to spending the majority of one's time with the patient attempting to manage such side effects through dosage adjustments and changes to alternative agents, often at the expense of helping the patient learn to address interpersonal issues.

Second, one also should avoid "overselling" the benefits of the medication. Clinicians sometimes attempt to raise patients' expectations of relief in the hope that this will increase the strength of the placebo response. However, in the case of somatoform disorders, patients' chronic physical complaints are reinforced through multiple venues, and lasting placebo responses therefore are unlikely. Prescribing a medication is not a substitute for addressing maladaptive beliefs and addictive behaviors; rather, it is an effective way of addressing one *underlying factor* that contributes to patients having these beliefs and behaviors. Further, patients who are led to expect dramatic results and subsequently do not obtain them may prematurely discontinue the medication, failing to recognize how the medication might still prove to be useful in treating one particular *aspect* of the overall clinical presentation.

Finally, as Barsky (1996) has noted, "The hypochondriacal patient often views the prescription of medication as a paltry and unsatisfactory substitute for the personal interest and attention of the physician." Again, medications should be presented to the patient as being an *adjunct* to the *total care plan* rather than a means of hustling the patient out the door.

In complex cases, such as when psychological factors are *exacerbating* chronic pain due to a medical condition, a *coordinated interdisciplinary approach* often works best. Referral to a multidisciplinary pain treatment program also may prove to be useful.

Address Internal and External Reinforcers

During each visit, the physician should convey the implicit message that *the patient is more important than any particular symptom*. In practice, this means that extensive inquiry into chronic symptoms is avoided, and attentive listening to details of the patient's past and current life history is the norm. A supportive and optimistic attitude on the part of the physician can be essential in the case of conversion symptoms.

Conversion symptoms typically occur as a defense against some other problem in the patient's life; unless attention is paid to what that problem is, the physician is asking the patient to give up a powerful defense strategy without offering anything to take its place. This is especially likely to be the case when the patient's symptoms have persisted for some time. In acute cases (which typically arise in response to a transient stressor) support and the suggestion that the symptoms likely will resolve "on their own over the next few days" may suffice. In more chronic cases, referral for a course of physical therapy may be entirely appropriate, both to prevent disuse atrophy and contractures and also to provide a face-saving means of returning to normal activity.

As the focus shifts toward events in the patient's life, reinforcing elements in the patient's support system can be addressed, sometimes with the help of the social services system or an outside psychotherapist. *Group therapy* for patients with somatoform disorders has been demonstrated to be a cost-effective supplement to individual patient visits (although it does not constitute a complete substitute for the latter).

Since failure to return to work can be a major reinforcer of abnormal illness behavior, and

since work provides meaning and structure to peoples' lives, the patient usually should be encouraged to return to the work setting, although perhaps to a less stressful job. Vocational counselors and rehabilitation therapists may be able to provide additional assistance in this regard. However, for some patients who are chronically disabled by their condition, assistance in obtaining disability may ultimately prove to be the most appropriate intervention.

FACTITIOUS DISORDER AND MALINGERING

Patients with somatoform disorders, while engaging in behavior that either feigns or exaggerates illness, engage in this behavior *unconsciously*, and they do so for *unconscious reasons*. In contrast, patients with **factitious disorder** and **malingering** *intentionally* feign or exaggerate illness. As indicated in Table 13–4, the difference between these two latter diagnoses lies in patients' *motivations* for doing so.

The malingerer *consciously feigns having a disease* in order to obtain some *conscious external gain*, such as avoiding military service, avoiding work, obtaining financial compensation in a lawsuit, evading criminal prosecution, or obtaining a prescription for a controlled substance. *DSM-IV* does not consider malingering to be a mental disorder. It lists Malingering in a section entitled "Other Conditions That May Be a Focus of Clinical Attention." Malingering should be strongly suspected when an antisocial personality disorder is present, when the patient presents in the setting of a legal dispute, when the patient isn't fully compliant with the evaluation, or when there is a marked discrepancy between the patient's claims of disability or distress and objective findings on examination.

Factitious disorder is more commonly known

Table 13–4. Distinctions between Illness-Affirming Abnormal Illness Behaviors

Disorder	Behavior	Motivation
Somatoform disorders	Unconscious	Unconscious
Malingering	Conscious	Conscious
Factitious disorder	Conscious	Unconscious

to physicians as **Munchausen's syndrome,** so named for the Baron von Munchausen, a former Russian cavalry officer who became known for wandering from town to town giving fanciful accounts of his "marvelous travels and campaigns." Like the malingerer, the patient with factitious disorder is felt to be deliberately feigning signs or symptoms of disease. However, the patient's motivation in this case isn't to obtain some conscious external gain, since none is readily apparent. Given this, the prevailing assumption has been that the patient's primary motivation is to obtain some *unconscious psychological gain.*

To understand this gain, one must look at the behavior itself. Patients with factitious disorder seek hospital admission and extensive medical testing and treatment. They may inject themselves with insulin in order to feign hypoglycemia, may ingest anticoagulants to instigate bleeding, or may inject foreign matter subcutaneously to create an abscess or cellulitis that "just won't heal." They may submit to repeated surgeries. (One sign of this on physical examination is a "train-track" or "gridiron" abdomen, the result of multiple surgical scars.)

Given this presentation, it appears that these patients' primary motivation for engaging in such disturbing behavior is *to gain access to the sick role.* It has been difficult to assemble patients to study in more detail, since—once confronted—they usually become defensive and leave, only to seek medical care elsewhere. However, case series suggest that these patients are seeking support, sympathy, and relief from responsibility from concerned medical professionals. Personality testing often reveals a mixture of histrionic, narcissistic, impulsive, and dependent traits. They tend to be both care-seeking and care-rejecting and they have ambivalent attitudes about their bodies, their sexuality, and their relationships to authority figures. Past histories of childhood abuse and abandonment are common.

As with the somatoform disorders, treatment involves confrontation with an attitude of concern, attempts to keep the patient in the current treatment setting (sometimes this requires an initial transfer to an inpatient psychiatry unit), and exploration of possible reinforcers of the behavior (especially current interpersonal stressors). Treatment of the patient's true medical problems

as well as of the medical complications of the patient's self-injurious behavior still is required, and obviously it is important to try to distinguish the former from the latter. Since patients may continue to present unreliable histories and refuse to give consent to communicate with previous care providers, this may be extremely difficult. Also, one should attempt to treat possible coexisting psychiatric conditions (particularly mood and anxiety disorders).

One variant of this syndrome, **Munchausen's syndrome by proxy,** involves parents who induce or feign illness in *their child,* with the child then being forced to undergo multiple medical or surgical workups. While these parents appear on the surface to be long-suffering but extremely devoted "superparents," surreptitious observation (sometimes by hidden video cameras) has revealed many of these parents to be engaging in severe physical and emotional abuse of the child once they believe that they and the child are alone. Cases even have been described of children having died by "respiratory arrest" when in fact the parents actually smothered them with a pillow. In some of these cases, a previous sibling also had died under mysterious circumstances, and the death had been attributed to sudden infant death syndrome (SIDS).

In practice, unless the patient "confesses" or unless clear evidence of self-induced injury is uncovered (e.g., through biopsy of an abscess revealing fecal material, or by a syringe of insulin being found in a bedside table), making a clear distinction between a somatoform disorder, a factitious disorder, and malingering can be extremely difficult. Even in the cases of somatoform and factitious disorder, where the major gain appears to be internal and unconscious, some external gains tend to result from the patient's "illness," which also reinforce the patient's behavior, making the exclusion of malingering more difficult.

Further, patients with factitious disorder sometimes come to believe at some level that they truly are ill. They play the part so convincingly that they begin to fool themselves. Given this, some researchers have suggested that we should think of factitious disorders and somatoform disorders as *two poles* along a *continuum* of abnormal illness behaviors. At different points in time, some patients appear to fall at various positions along this spectrum, demonstrating varying degrees of insight into their own responsibility for their symptoms.

CONCLUSION

All physicians encounter "somaticizing" patients on a daily basis. An appreciation of the nature of somatization is essential for several reasons.

First, physicians who fail to recognize psychological contributors to their patients' physical complaints may have an enormous "blind spot." Opportunities for psychological intervention may be missed, and their patients may experience increased chronicity, morbidity, and disability.

Second, since many patients with somatoform disorders refuse psychiatric consultation, the primary physician typically must act as the patient's psychotherapist. Treatment is largely supportive and empathic, but more specific interventions aimed at behavioral modification may be necessary. While patients may be unconscious of the behavioral nature of their condition, one goal of the treatment is to gradually draw their attention to the role of life stressors, personality factors, emotions, and ingrained beliefs as reinforcers of an underlying tendency to experience and complain of physical symptoms.

In their ability to visit so many physicians and to receive such a plethora of diagnoses, these patients also expose the limitations of the medical system. While they frequently require the combined attention of multiple physicians, this attention must be *coordinated* if the benefits of diagnosing and treating an occult physical illness are to be appropriately balanced against the risks of reinforcing abnormal illness behavior and inadvertently *increasing* the patient's disability.

Chapter 14

Dissociative Disorders

Human consciousness, the awareness of oneself and one's environment, is an artificial construction. In a normal state of consciousness, the brain seamlessly integrates sensory perceptions, emotional states, current thoughts, and past memories. The essential feature of the various **dissociative disorders** is that these elements have become disrupted, *dissociated,* from each other. The distinctions between the different types of dissociative disorders are based on which particular *aspect* of subjective experience has become dissociated from the others.

Dissociative amnesia is characterized by *dissociation of memory.* The affected individual demonstrates an inability to recall important biographical information, usually of a traumatic or stressful nature. The memory deficit is too extensive to be explained by ordinary forgetfulness.

Dissociative fugue is characterized by an even greater dissociation of memory, such that the individual dissociates not only key historical information but also his own *sense of identity.* Affected individuals may engage in sudden, unexpected travel away from their homes or customary places of work, accompanied by an inability to recall their past, confusion about their personal identity, or the assumption of a new identity.

Dissociative identity disorder (DID, formerly called multiple personality disorder) is char-

acterized by *even greater fragmentation of personal identity.* Here, two or more distinct identities or personality states recurrently take control of the individual's behavior, accompanied by an inability to recall important personal information. Again, these memory deficits are too extensive to be explained by ordinary forgetfulness.

Depersonalization disorder is characterized by *dissociation of one's perception of oneself in relation to the surrounding environment.* The individual doesn't actually lose contact with reality but experiences a persistent or recurrent feeling of being detached from his mental processes or his body.

Over the past two decades, the dissociative disorders have received a great deal of attention and have been the subject of extensive debate within and outside of the mental health field. Some patient's presentations have been so dramatic that it is no surprise that they have become the frequent subject of talk shows and Hollywood films.

The most controversial issue has been whether these disorders, particularly dissociative identity disorder, are even valid constructs. Some commentators have argued that DID is another subtype of somatoform disorder, similar to conversion disorder. A related issue has centered on dissociative amnesia, which is a component of all of the above disorders except for depersonalization disorder. Can memories be completely dissociated from conscious awareness, only to be "retrieved" at some later point in time? This latter issue has proven to be especially relevant for those patients who have "recovered memories" of alleged childhood physical or sexual abuse, often in the context of having received psychotherapy aimed at encouraging this process.

The source of this controversy is a fundamental uncertainty about the nature of dissociation itself. Is dissociation a *disease*? When the phenomenon of dissociation is encountered in a patient, does it inevitably represent a *response to some earlier traumatic event* (especially childhood physical or sexual abuse) such that a history of abuse can be inferred even when the patient denies any current conscious recollection of the abuse? Finally, is dissociation (especially more severe forms, such as DID) most often an *iatrogenic phenomenon*, produced in highly suggestible patients by well-intentioned but misdirected psychotherapists?

While it is not typically described as such, dissociation may best be understood as a *behavior*. In other words, dissociation is something that a person *does*, even if he or she is doing so unconsciously. As we have discussed previously, individuals engage in behaviors to achieve some goal, and the behavior can't be understood unless the goal is appreciated. The goal may not always be apparent, especially when the behavior has become so extensive and self-reinforcing that the initial goal is no longer acting as one of the sustaining factors.

For example, the initial goals of the self-starvation behavior encountered in anorexia nervosa are to obtain slimness and to diminish the fear of becoming obese. These goals may not be readily apparent in the more advanced stages of the illness, when the patient has become severely emaciated but despite this continues to diet and exercise. By that point, other sustaining factors have come to play increasingly important roles. However, we still can discern the original goal by talking to the patient, who usually will readily admit to having persistent concerns that she remains overweight and to having powerful desires to reach some irrationally low target weight.

Sometimes, the goal of a behavior is more obscure, even unconscious. The patient may actually deny any desire to achieve these goals. For example, in the somatoform disorders and in factitious disorder, the major goal appears to be to gain access to the sick role, even in those patients who adamantly insist that they have no desire to be in this role and desire only to attain a state of health.

Viewed in this light, the debate over the nature of the dissociative disorders is one that centers on how best to *explain* dissociative behavior. Those who frequently diagnose dissociative phenomena, especially DID, assert that dissociative behavior is a *defense*, a coping mechanism that usually first came into play during childhood in the face of severe trauma (most commonly, repeated trauma such as ongoing physical or sexual abuse). The original goal of the behavior was to "escape" from the situation when more mature defenses were overwhelmed and proved to be ineffective. This fracturing of identity then became self-sustaining and persisted over time. The patient may not even have been aware of these separate personality states, only of the resulting social disability.

Proponents of this view have recommended specific treatment interventions. These are based on the presumption that patients only can be restored to psychological health through *integration* of the various fragmented aspects of the self. The psychotherapist attempts to bring the personality fragments (or "alters"—as in alter egos) to the fore and then encourages the alters to communicate with each other. The goal of this intervention is to help the patient break down psychological barriers that have been erected between the alters. A related treatment goal is to help the patient retrieve the original, dissociated, traumatic memories and then to help the patient face them without resorting to dissociative amnesia as a defense. This therapeutic approach is viewed as being analogous to techniques used in treating post-traumatic stress disorder, although in this case the trauma must first be uncovered (e.g., through hypnosis or drug-assisted interviews, where the patient is taken back, or "regressed," to previous points in time).

However, an alternative theoretical formulation suggests that dissociative behaviors are *conversion phenomena*: these patients are engaging in somatoform behavior in an attempt to avoid dealing with other aspects of their lives. As with other conversion phenomena, clinicians must always strive to avoid reinforcing illness behavior or creating new illness behaviors through subtle (and sometimes not so subtle) suggestion. Many patients become highly invested in their psychotherapy and in their newfound identity of being "a multiple," and psychotherapy therefore risks consolidating a maladaptive belief system rather than discouraging it.

If this latter formulation is correct, then the treatment strategy outlined by the "DID advocates" borders on malpractice. To engage in a prolonged exploration of patients' dissociative symptoms, memories, and alters over several years of therapy—in an attempt to elicit more and more of them—is to *collude* with the patient in reinforcing abnormal illness behavior. Such therapy could be seen as being tantamount to treating a patient who presented with conversion paralysis of one arm by subtly encouraging him through suggestions or implied expectations to develop a paralysis of the other arm, followed by the leg, followed by blindness, etc.

From this latter viewpoint, the more appropriate treatment approach when faced on the inpatient unit with a patient diagnosed with DID who now has been admitted by her outside therapist for treatment of a supposed "side issue" (such as major depressive disorder, or a suicide attempt) is to refuse to "enable" the pathologic behavior any further. There may be obstacles to taking such an approach. The referring therapist may wish to continue with therapy sessions two to three times per week, even while the patient is in the inpatient setting. Further, the patient may be a member of one or more dissociative disorder support groups. As was noted for the somatoform disorders, it is unlikely that treatment interventions will be successful unless *(1)* all treatment providers can work together in providing a consistent, integrated, treatment strategy and *(2)* the patient has "signed on" to the treatment approach.

Given all of these reinforcing and sustaining factors, treatment of dissociation sometimes requires *isolation* and *countersuggestion*. For example, in the last chapter we discussed how the symptoms of Charcot's "hysteroepileptics" dramatically improved after they were physically separated from the patients who had true epilepsy (and after they were separated from Charcot himself). In addition, we discussed in Chapter 8 how this same treatment strategy has been employed

in attempting to address the symptoms of the nonpsychotic partner in a relationship characterized by a *folie a deux* (shared psychotic disorder).

Similarly, in this case, patients are isolated from the reading materials, Internet sites, and support groups (and sometimes even the treatment providers) that have sustained the patient's focus on "alters." The new treating clinicians refuse to speak to the patient's "alters," requesting instead that the patient focus on present life difficulties. They advise the patient that she appears to be engaging in dissociative behavior in response to her current life stressors and emphasize that she could more effectively address these stressors if she could learn (with the clinician's assistance) more effective coping strategies.

Again, both points of view share the assumption that the patient is engaging in a particular type of behavior, dissociation. To better understand the nature of the behavior, we therefore must first explore the nature of dissociative phenomena, particularly dissociative forgetting. We then will examine specific dissociative disorders.

DISSOCIATION AS A BEHAVIOR

At any given moment, our "self" is a synthetic construct, "built up" from a myriad of perceptions of internal bodily states, current sensory perceptions (in all five modalities), thoughts, and memories. Without any conscious effort, we integrate all of these inputs into a coherent whole. At the same time, however, we also are capable of *distinguishing* between different types of mental phenomena. For example, the average person has no difficulty distinguishing between a *current* visual perception (e.g., seeing or tasting an apple), a *sensory memory* (e.g., recalling an apple seen in the past), and an *imagined sensation* (e.g., imagining a blue apple, or even a square apple). In dissociation, the ability to make such distinctions becomes impaired.

"Dissociation" represents a *spectrum* of behaviors ranging from mild, everyday experiences through severe, rarely encountered experiences. As discussed in previous chapters, behavioral pathology is multidetermined. *Initiating and reinforcing factors* can include genetic influences, personality traits, biological variation, comorbid medical and/or psychiatric conditions, and environmental influences.

Mild forms of dissociation commonly occur in the general population. For example, one study involving the general population of Winnepeg, Ontario, found that almost half of all respondents had at some point driven their car for some distance without being aware of their actions. We have all engaged in similar "absent-minded" behavior, especially when the behavior in question is a highly "overlearned" one. For example, we might drive halfway to work on a Saturday when we had initially planned to drive to the supermarket, or we might pour orange juice into our cup of coffee, having initially picked up the container of juice intending to pour it into a glass.

More *significant dissociative phenomena* occur in many individuals when they are placed in *particular conditions*, especially *sleep deprivation, fatigue, stress, or trauma*. A high percentage of accident victims, witnesses to natural disasters, soldiers in battle, and witnesses to death-penalty executions subsequently report having experienced symptoms of anxiety, depersonalization, and derealization. In most cases, these symptoms are transient, but a percentage of individuals go on to develop chronic feelings of depersonalization, along with emotional "numbing," as part of the overall syndrome of post-traumatic stress disorder.

Dissociative symptoms also can occur in many individuals when they are in *altered states of consciousness*. For example, such symptoms commonly occur during *hypnagogic or hypnopompic states*, during states of *alcohol or drug intoxication or withdrawal*, and as a *side effect of prescribed medications* (such as narcotics and anticholinergic medications). Altered states of consciousness also can occur in the context of some *general medical conditions*, especially *temporal lobe epilepsy*, where dissociative symptoms can occur during preictal, ictal postictal, and interictal states.

Dissociation also commonly occurs in individuals who have *other psychiatric conditions*, including *schizophrenia*, all of the *anxiety disorders* (especially those associated with panic attacks), and the *somatoform disorders*. With regard to the somatoform disorders, the international classification scheme (the *ICD*) emphasizes the overlap between somatization and dissociation to a greater extent than does the United States classification scheme (the *DSM*).

The *ICD-9*, published in 1978, grouped the conversion and dissociative phenomena together under the label of "hysteria" since both syndromes involved an unconscious disruption of normal mental processes—either involving a dissociation of motor or sensory function (conversion) or a dissociation of awareness (dissociation). Further, in both cases, the patient's symptoms appeared to be motivated by the desire to achieve primary (symbolic) and/or secondary (external) gain.

In contrast, the *ICD-10* scheme, published in 1987, closely resembles the *DSM-IV* scheme except that—for similar reasons—it excludes conversion disorder from the somatoform disorders category and places it in the dissociative disorders category. While this approach has its merits, it overlooks the significant overlap between conversion disorder and the other somatoform disorders, especially somatization disorder (which includes conversion symptoms within its own diagnostic criteria). It therefore might be reasonable for future classification schemes to once again group all of the somatoform and dissociative disorders together within a single category.

Because of the association between dissociative symptoms and trauma, some clinicians have suggested that more severe dissociation doesn't occur in the absence of more severe trauma (especially repeated childhood trauma). In support of this theory, they note the high prevalence of recollections of childhood physical and sexual abuse among their dissociative disorder patients. However, it is not clear that childhood abuse *in itself* is either necessary or sufficient to cause lasting dissociation.

First, a large percentage of the population reports a history of childhood physical or sexual abuse (with 27% of women and 15% of men endorsed such a history in one telephone survey), but the overwhelming majority of them do not go on to develop dissociative disorders. *Second*, the majority of patients who develop post-traumatic stress disorder in the wake of a severe trauma are disabled not by *amnesia* but by an inability to *forget* the traumatic event. *Third*, childhood abuse places individuals at risk to develop *many* psychiatric disorders, including borderline and antisocial personality disorders, mood disorders, anxiety disorders, bulimia nervosa, and substance-related disorders. In the majority of these cases, dissociative phenomena do not occur.

Studies reporting a high frequency of childhood abuse in dissociative disorder patients typically do not distinguish between traumatic memories that were *always* remembered and those that were "retrieved" over the course of psychotherapy. Corroboration of the patients' reports of abuse typically hasn't been obtained from outside sources. This is an important consideration when studying a population of patients who by definition have unreliable memories.

Therefore, while is likely that childhood trauma is one important factor in the development of the dissociative disorders, one cannot generalize from this, as some therapists have done, to say that trauma is the "single cause" or "root cause" of dissociation, any more than it is the "cause" of the personality disorders, eating disorders, or anxiety disorders. Multiple intervening factors, including the influence of the psychotherapy itself, may contribute to the development of a dissociative disorder. Similarly, one cannot "work backward" from a dissociative disorder diagnosis to the inference that severe childhood trauma "must have occurred." Nor can one infer that if patients with a dissociative disorder cannot recall any childhood trauma, they must have "repressed the memory of the trauma."

Dissociation and Hypnosis

Are certain people more prone to engage in dissociation? What exactly is it that "occurs" during the process of dissociation? Some insight into dissociation can be gained by examining what transpires during *hypnosis* since this has been hypothesized to be a clinically induced dissociative state.

Contrary to popular belief, the hypnotist does not "gain control" over the subject, e.g., inducing the subject—for example, inducing the subject to act like a chicken against the subject's will. Nor does the induction of a hypnotic state require the subject to enter a "trance" or sleep-like state. Rather, subjects in a hypnotic state appear to be in a state of *relaxed wakefulness*. Similarly, EEG studies suggest that hypnotized subjects are fully awake and alert.

Even without entering a "hypnotic state," many subjects comply with requests by hypnotists due to the *contextual demands of the situa-*

tion, particularly when the hypnosis occurs in the medical setting with patients who present expecting to receive "hypnotherapy." The *authority of the therapist*, the *patient's urge to comply*, and the *strength of the therapeutic alliance* all contribute to patients complying with suggestions made by a therapist.

However, it does not appear that *all* of the benefits associated with hypnosis accrue from the contextual situation. For example, a subject who is not hypnotized may be able to *imagine* being regressed to 6 years of age, but likely won't *act the part*. Similarly, in the absence of hypnosis, a subject might be able to try to *ignore* pain during dental surgery but is unlikely to attain a state of *analgesia*. To achieve these latter effects, hypnosis appears to rely on an *alteration in the normal state of consciousness*. Researchers have described three main characteristics of this hypnotic state: absorption, dissociation, and suggestibility.

Absorption refers to the reduction of peripheral awareness while intensely focused on some central thought or object. Individuals who are intensely absorbed in some activity tend to *ignore* other perceptions, thoughts, memories, or motor activities. Similarly, during hypnotic age regression, subjects act as though they were younger by ignoring both their awareness of their actual age and their awareness of incongruity between their current behavior and their "normal," age-appropriate behavior. Their experience of acting like a 6-year-old is particularly vivid since they do not allow critical self-evaluations to intrude upon it. Similarly, patients in the midst of a hypnotically induced analgesic state remain *aware* of pain (e.g., when undergoing surgery or when placing a hand into a bucket of ice) but they *ignore* the pain by focusing their attention on other thoughts and experiences.

The phenomenon of **dissociation** mirrors that of absorption in that while one is intensely absorbed with some central object, other sensory perceptions, thoughts, or emotions are more easily dissociated (i.e., they remain outside the realm of conscious awareness). Dissociated information can still influence an individual, however. For example, a rape victim in the midst of dissociative amnesia still might experience intense anxiety when exposed to reminders of the rape despite her avowals of having no conscious recollection of the rape. In other words, the dissociated information is still "there" but is outside of conscious awareness due to an extreme form of selective attention.

Subjects in a hypnotic state also voluntarily relinquish the usual critical evaluative faculties and therefore enter into a state of heightened **suggestibility**. Instructions from the therapist may be accepted without question since the subject isn't paying attention to the irrationality of the requests. The subject also may have more difficulty distinguishing between outside suggestion and internally generated ideas or between outside suggestion and past memories. This places the subject in a particularly vulnerable position, one which can work either to the patient's benefit or detriment depending upon the patient's circumstances.

The extent to which individuals are "hypnotizable" is a *dimensional trait* that varies across the general population. It is not a pathologic sign of a particular illness, nor is it proof that some trauma has occurred. About three-quarters of the population is hypnotizable and about 10% of the population is highly hypnotizable. This capacity can be quantified using standardized assessment tools that assess the individual's responsiveness to suggestion. Hypnotizability is greatest during childhood and gradually declines into adulthood, but it remains relatively consistent over at least three decades of adulthood.

More highly hypnotizable individuals *tend to become more absorbed in their life experiences*. For example, individuals who become so absorbed in a film that they temporarily forget that they are in a movie theater are likely to be more hypnotizable. Similarly, more hypnotizable subjects also *tend to be more suggestible*, even when they are *not* in a trance state. Young children are especially prone to suggestion, and clinicians involved in cases involving allegations of child abuse need to interview children extremely carefully, making efforts to avoid asking leading questions (particularly when using anatomically correct dolls).

Studies of patients being treated for dissociative disorders reveal these individuals to have high degrees of hypnotizability. At this point it isn't clear whether this capacity has been present from birth or whether trauma has rendered them more susceptible to both hypnosis and spontaneous dissociation. Conceptually, however, dissociation can be thought of as a severe form of **selective attention** (discussed in the last chapter with reference to the somatoform disorders), in which individuals become highly absorbed in one aspect of their experience to the exclusion of one or more other aspects, most often in settings where they have been placed into a heightened state of suggestibility.

A large body of evidence has confirmed *that hypnotically enhanced recall is not more accurate than nonenhanced recall*. However, hypnosis does increase a subject's tendencies to: *(1)* report previously uncertain memories with strong feelings of conviction; *(2)* confabulate in those areas where the subject has little or no recollection; *(3)* distort memory such that it becomes more congruent with the subject's preexisting beliefs, hopes, and fantasies; and *(4)* incorporate cues from leading questions into "memories" that then are retained with strong conviction in their veracity. These same caveats apply to attempts to retrieve memories through so-called "drug-assisted" interviews utilizing amobarbital ("truth serum") or benzodiazepines. The assumption that memories retrieved with the assistance of hypnosis or with sedative medications are unadulterated and highly reliable is incorrect.

It goes without saying that child abuse occurs and that it occurs commonly. About 3 million cases of child abuse are reported in the United States each year, and one-third of these cases subsequently are substantiated. However, some patients, under the encouragement of their therapists, have broken off ties with family members or have pursued civil action against the alleged perpetrators of abuse. This can have disastrous consequences for all involved.

First, patients have been harmed in the process. Suing one's parents is not a simple matter and the court system was designed not to help patients heal but rather to determine the truth through a highly adversarial process. While some patients may achieve vindication, others may emerge from the process feeling revictimized and traumatized. Treatment providers who agree to testify on behalf of their patients in court in the expert witness role also are unlikely to achieve objectivity (particularly if they have not interviewed collateral informants such as family members) and—in moving from the role of treatment provider to expert—risk irreparably damaging the treatment relationship with the patient.

Second, some of these patients ultimately have gone on to "recant" their charges against the alleged perpetrators and to then successfully sue their therapists for malpractice. Accused family members also have successfully sued these therapists either for malpractice or for slander. Therapists who have been most vulnerable to these lawsuits have been those who have zealously attempted to "uncover" memories of abuse, who have repeatedly suggested to patients that abuse "must have occurred," or who have bolstered their suggestions through more unorthodox treatment techniques such as amobarbital interviews or hypnosis (usually by statements to the effect that any memories recovered through these techniques "must be accurate").

Asking patients about childhood abuse is an important and appropriate part of the psychiatric history. However, clinicians always should keep in mind the distinction between **narrative truth** (the "personal reality" of the stories that patients tell them, which might be distorted, exaggerated, inaccurately recalled, or completely false) and **historical truth** (the "external reality" of events from the patient's life as they actually occurred) Sitting in an office talking to the patient, the clinician may *never* know the historical truth about a patient's childhood. (If the patient is looking for this, she should hire a private investigator) Besides, the *goal* of psychotherapy has never been to help the patient uncover the historical "facts" of their lives. Rather, it is to help them come to terms with the "meaning" of their lives through techniques such as empathic listening, support, and interpretation.

Therefore, when patients report memories of sexual or physical abuse, clinicians should attempt to maintain an empathic, nonjudgmental, neutral stance toward the memories. As in the treatment of *all* patients, they then should perform a complete history and mental status evaluation, avoiding urges to prematurely focus on only one aspect of the patient's presentation to the exclusion of addressing treatable psychiatric conditions, and should attempt to avoid prejudging the causes of their patients' difficulties or the veracity of their reports.

Clinicians also should keep in mind that expressing strong convictions that sexual abuse or other factors "are" or "are not" the cause of their patients' problems sometimes interferes with the provision of effective care. For example, clinicians who prematurely express *disbelief* may even further alienate patients who *have* been abused but whose reports have not been believed by their families or friends. In contrast, clinicians who exert undue pressure on their patients—whether it is to believe in events that may not have occurred, to prematurely disrupt important personal relationships, or to make important life decisions based on clinical speculation—may also cause great harm, both to their patients and to their patients' families.

When a patient presents with *unclear* memories of possible abuse in the absence of readily available corroboration, the clinician might discuss with the patient the limitations of memory. He also might attempt to help the patient learn to live with uncertainty as opposed to offering premature, unfounded conclusions.

Phenomenology of Dissociative Amnesia Versus Amnestic Syndrome

As discussed in Chapter 4, there are two major forms of memory. **Declarative (explicit) memory** is memory that can be verbalized. It includes both *semantic memory* (memory for facts) and *episodic memory* (memory for events, whether public or autobiographical). **Nondeclarative (implicit) memory** is a memory for nonverbal procedures, such as how to type or how to drive a car.

These two types of memory are mediated by neuroanatomically distinct systems: declarative memory is mediated by a **medial temporal lobe circuit**, and nondeclarative memory is mediated by a **basal ganglia–frontal lobe circuit**. In advanced stages of *dementia*, all of these forms of memory are affected, while in the more limited *amnestic syndrome*, both aspects of declarative memory are typically impaired but procedural memory remains intact. In contrast, in *dissociative amnesia* and *dissociative fugue*, what is lost is solely episodic memory (without impairment in either semantic memory or implicit memory). Further, unlike the case with amnestic syndrome, here there is no anterograde component to the memory loss.

In other words, in dissociative amnesia what is lost is *retrograde memory,* either for a *circumscribed event* or for *several events that have a circumscribed theme.* Further, the forgotten event or events tend to specifically involve *traumatic or difficult-to-face subject matter*, and the memories sometimes are *restored following resolution of the amnesia or fugue state*. Obviously, the phenomenology of dissociative amnesia is much less consistent with a pathophysiologic disease process than with these memories still being "present" but being selectively "ignored," most likely at an unconscious level.

This deliberate, selective denial of specific aspects of cognition is especially apparent when dissociative amnesia or fugue is accompanied by the so-called **Ganser syndrome** (also called the "syndrome of approximate answers"). Individuals with this syndrome respond with answers that are so *obviously* wrong that even a person with severe brain injury would not have made such mistakes. The mistaken answers also are such "near misses" that it can be inferred that the individual must actually have had knowledge of the correct answer. For example, when asked, "How much is two plus two?" the patient might reply, "five." Similarly, when asked, "How many legs does a horse have?" the patient might reply, "three."

SPECIFIC DISSOCIATIVE DISORDERS

Depersonalization Disorder

Depersonalization, a feeling of detachment or estrangement from one's self, is a mental state transiently experienced by many people during periods of stress. The individual in the midst of a depersonalization state may feel like an "automaton" or as if he is "living in a dream or a movie." There may be a sensation of being an "outside observer" of one's mental processes or one's body. Various types of sensory anesthesia, affective detachment, and a sensation of lacking control of one's actions, including speech, often are present.

Transient depersonalization has been described by nearly one-third of individuals exposed to a life-threatening danger and by close to 40% of patients hospitalized for mental disorders. However, to be diagnosed with *depersonalization disorder* according to *DSM-IV* criteria, an individual should demonstrate evidence of *persistent or recurrent episodes of depersonalization*. The diagnosis of depersonalization disorder is made only when the symptoms are sufficiently severe to cause marked distress or to impair functioning.

Because depersonalization is a common associated feature of many other mental disorders, a separate diagnosis of depersonalization disorder is not assigned if feelings of depersonalization occur exclusively during the course of schizophrenia, panic disorder, acute stress disorder and PTSD, or another dissociative disorder. In addition, the disturbance should not be due to the physiological effects of an illicit drug intoxication or withdrawal, a medication, or a general medical condition.

Individuals with depersonalization disorder remain in contact with reality. For example, they are aware that this is only a *feeling*, that they are not *really* automatons. The duration of their episodes has been described as varying from seconds to years, although most often dissociative episodes are transient phenomena. Depersonalization following a life-threatening situation (e.g., military combat, a traumatic accident, or victimization in a violent crime) usually develops suddenly upon exposure to the trauma. More rarely, the course becomes chronic, with remissions and exacerbations. The latter may occur in association with actual or perceived new stressful events that resemble the original trauma.

Treatment involves first assessing for and treating any other diagnoses that might account for sensations of depersonalization. If none are found, treatment typically involves interventions such as education, cognitive therapy, and relaxation training.

Dissociative Amnesia and Dissociative Fugue

Dissociative amnesia (formerly called "psychogenic amnesia") is characterized by one or more episodes in which an individual becomes unable to recall important personal information. The information usually is autobiographically meaningful (typically involving a traumatic or stressful circumstance such as an assault or a rape) and is too extensive to be explained by ordinary forgetfulness. Because memory loss also can occur in association with other conditions with more extensive symptoms, including dissociative identity disorder, dissociative fugue, acute stress disorder, post-traumatic stress disorder, and somatization disorder, one wouldn't diagnose dissociative amnesia if symptoms of these other conditions are present. Also, like depersonalization disorder, dissociative amnesia shouldn't be diagnosed if the amnesia appears to reflect the effects of a substance (such as an alcoholic-related "blackout") or a neurological or other general medical condition (such as head trauma).

An even more extreme form of dissociation is *dissociative fugue* (formerly called "psychogenic fugue"). Here, a patient engages in sudden, unexpected, travel away from her home or customary place of daily activities and has an inability to recall some or all of her past. In contrast to dissociative amnesia, where the individual dissociates isolated *memories*, here the individual dissociates her entire *personal identity*. In rare cases, the individual even assumes a *new* identity (typically a more gregarious or uninhibited one). Travel can range from brief trips lasting hours or days to extensive travels across thousands of miles lasting for weeks or months.

Individuals in a dissociative fugue state generally don't attract attention since they appear to be acting quite normally. Ultimately, they may come to clinical attention as a result of complaints of amnesia or of a lack of awareness of their personal identity. Once having returned to their premorbid state, they may deny having any recollection of the events that transpired during the fugue state.

The prevalence of dissociative fugue is extremely low, likely a fraction of a percent of the population. The prevalence of dissociative amnesia also is likely extremely low, although again this has been called into question by reports of recovered memories of repeated episodes of abuse during childhood, each episode of which reportedly remained inaccessible to conscious awareness for years until "retrieved" at a later date in the setting of psychotherapy.

These two dissociative states often are self-limited, especially when they follow an isolated traumatic situation. Given this, therapy is typically supportive in nature. The use of hypnosis to treat more persistent cases also has been described.

Dissociative Identity Disorder (Formerly "Multiple Personality Disorder")

DID is the most severe form of dissociation, as it includes not only symptoms of amnesia but also the presence of different personality states that recurrently take control of the person's behavior. The *DSM-IV* diagnostic criteria for DID are listed in Table 14–1. This diagnosis is controversial and has evolved somewhat since it first appeared in *DSM-III* (1980) under the name multiple personality disorder (MPD). Significant questions remain about this condition's diagnostic reliability and validity, which reflect certain fundamental ambiguities about this disorder and about the nature of dissociation itself.

Ambiguity Over "Personality"

One key issue complicating discussion of DID is that different clinicians haven't agreed on what is meant by "personality." The *DSM-III* criteria for MPD required demonstration that within an individual there existed "two or more distinct personalities, each of which is dominant at a particular time," with "the personality that is dominant at any particular time determining the individual's behavior." Finally, the criteria required that each personality be "complex and integrated with its own unique behavior patterns and social relationships."

This definition had several problems. First, "personality" was never defined. Second, the in-

---

Table 14–1. *DSM-IV-TR* Criteria for Dissociative Identity Disorder

A. The presence of two or more distinct identities or personality states (each with its own relatively enduring pattern of perceiving, relating to, and thinking about the environment and self)

B. At least two of these identities or personality states recurrently take control of the person's behavior

C. Inability to recall important personal information that is too extensive to be explained by ordinary forgetfulness

D. The disturbance is not due to the direct physiological effects of a substance (e.g., blackouts or chaotic behavior during alcohol intoxication) or a general medical condition (e.g., complex partial seizures). Note: in children, the symptoms are not attributable to imaginary playmates or other fantasy play

Source: Reprinted with permission from the *Diagnostic and Statistical Manual of Mental Disorders, Fourth Edition, Text Revision*. Copyright 2000 American Psychiatric Association.

terrater reliability of these criteria had not been assessed. Finally, the criteria did not specify whether these symptoms had to have been evident *prior to* the onset of treatment, could have arisen *over the course of treatment*, or could be discerned even *only following major psychotherapeutic interventions*. For example, one clinician who has written extensively on DID, Richard Kluft, has stated that of his patients with MPD: 5% had "diagnosed themselves" but had been disbelieved by their previous psychiatrist; 15% had spontaneously dissociated either during the initial assessment or in the course of treatment; 40% had presented with "subtle signs" that could alert "a clinician with a high index of suspicion" to assess further for the presence of MPD; and 40% had been "highly disguised" cases that only were determined to have MPD following the use of a "special protocol." Would all of these cases equally qualify for the diagnosis of MPD, and do all of the cases represent the same condition?

Despite these ambiguities, clinicians who frequently treated DID argued in the early 1980s that the *DSM-III* criteria actually were overly strict since the "alters" seen in DID were rarely so well defined as the criteria suggested. Therefore, in *DSM-IIIR*, the criteria for multiple personality disorder were revised and now specified that the condition was characterized by "the existence within the person of two or more distinct personalities *or personality states* (each with its own relatively enduring pattern of perceiving, relating to, and thinking about the environment and self)." Thus, instead of discrete "personalities," the *DSM-IIIR* criteria required the existence of "personality states." Unfortunately, this didn't resolve the difficulties with reliability or validity, since different clinicians still didn't agree on what constituted a "personality state."

For example, Kluft has stated that personality states encountered in DID are "alternative ways of configuring aspects of the mental apparatus in relatively stable and enduring manners." In contrast, Frank Putnam, another authority on DID, has stated that personality states are "highly discrete states of consciousness organized around a prevailing affect, with a sense of self, with a limited repertoire of behaviors, and [with] a set of state-dependent memories." In further contrast, another authority, Colin Ross, has stated that per-

sonalities are "dissociated components of a single personality" and that "the most important thing to understand is that alter personalities are not people. . . . Alter personalities are highly stylized enactments of inner conflicts, drives, memories, and feelings. . . . They are fragmented parts of one person: there is only one person. The patient's conviction that there is more than one person in her is a dissociative delusion and should not be compounded by a folie a deux on the part of the therapist. . . . MPD is an elaborate pretending. The patient pretends that she is more than one person, in a very convincing manner. She actually believes it herself."

The *DSM-IV* did not clarify whether a "personality state" was an "alternative aspect of the mental apparatus," a "highly discrete state of consciousness," or merely "an elaborate pretending." Rather, it attempted to resolve the confusion by broadening the definition yet further, eliminating the word "personality" from the diagnostic label and substituting "identity." MPD became DID, which the criteria now defined as the existence of "two or more distinct *identities or personality states* (each with its own relatively enduring pattern of perceiving, relating to, and thinking about the environment and self)." Obviously, substituting "identity" for "personality" doesn't resolve the ambiguity over whether DID represents a true compartmentalization of consciousness or represents an "elaborate pretending."

In practice, this ambiguity sometimes translates into inconsistent behavior toward patients on the part of some therapists. For example, after having earlier explained to patients that alters are not separate "people" and only "aspects" or "fragments" of a single personality, some therapists later disregard this distinction by making comments such as, "I'd liked to speak with Billy now. Billy, you need to stop treating Robert this way." Such behavior might *reinforce* the patient's belief that various aspects of his personality actually are "separate people," thereby encouraging further fragmentation of identity and dissociative behavior.

Ambiguity Over Patients' Accountability for Their Behavior

Therapists also may be inconsistent in how they convey to patients whether or not they themselves should be held accountable for the behavior of their "alters." A therapist might inform the patient that all alters "will be held fully accountable" for everything that the other alters do, particularly if any of these alter engages in illegal behavior." However, he might also inform the patient that she has an illness that is causing her current symptoms, that having the illness is not her fault, and that the illness is out of her control.

The above therapist's inconsistent stance reflects an underlying ambiguity over whether patients who dissociate have an "illness" that is beyond their direct control (similar to schizophrenia or bipolar disorder), whether they are engaging in a behavior that is conscious but powerfully driven (similar to alcohol dependence), or whether they are engaging in behavior that is unconscious but still purposeful (similar to conversion disorder).

Clearly, DID appears closer to alcohol dependence or conversion disorder than to schizophrenia. For example, patients with DID frequently are able to conceal the existence of their condition from acquaintances. They also can "bring forth" alters at the request of the therapist. Both of these phenomena indicate *at least some degree of volitional control* over their dissociative behavior. Similarly, treatment for DID does not involve biological interventions such as might be employed for a disease such as schizophrenia; it involves "talk therapy" aimed at helping the patient to gain control over the alters and thereby achieve "fusion." This process more closely resembles strategies used to help alcoholics gain control of their drinking than strategies employed to treat diseases such as bipolar disorder or schizophrenia.

Ambiguity of Diagnostic Boundaries

The boundaries between DID and other psychiatric disorders (particularly the *somatoform disorders* and the *personality disorders*) are ambiguous as well. For example, some authorities on DID list a wide variety of nonspecific signs believed to be potentially indicative of an underlying DID, especially physical symptoms such as headache or gastrointestinal complaints. However, such symptoms also tend to also suggest the presence of somatization disorder. When patients meet the criteria for both disorders, some advocates of the DID diagnosis have stated that DID should be considered the "supraordinate diagnosis."

Similarly, some writers on this subject have suggested that when patients also are diagnosed with bipolar disorder, this too should be considered "secondary" to the DID since it is possible that only one alter has bipolar disorder and that with treatment of the DID, lithium therapy would not be required. Borderline personality disorder or bulimia nervosa also might be considered a "secondary" diagnosis. This conceptualization has led to the claim that the typical DID patient has received a "variety of incorrect diagnoses" by previous clinicians, such that it takes almost 7 years on average before the typical patient finally is "correctly" diagnosed with DID.

In contrast, critics of the DID diagnosis note that since so many DID patients also meet criteria for somatization disorder (20% of patients diagnosed with DID fulfill the diagnostic criteria for somatization disorder), somatization disorder should be considered the supraordinate diagnosis and DID might best be viewed as just one of the many bewildering symptoms might appear in this highly suggestible patient population.

Recall that somatization disorder is more common in women but appears to share a genetic linkage with antisocial personality disorder, which appears more commonly in male relatives. Similar findings have been noted in DID. For example, 90%–100% of patients in most samples series have been women, up to 70% of women with a diagnosis of DID also meet the diagnostic criteria for borderline personality disorder, and the most common associated personality disorder in men with DID has been antisocial personality disorder. Given this, it is notable that many symptoms commonly ascribed to DID also are seen in the majority of patients with borderline and antisocial personality disorders, including abrupt mood swings, identity disturbance, suicide attempts, impulsive behavior, depression, substance abuse, claims of amnesia, and histories of childhood physical and sexual abuse. Given this, while some advocates of the DID diagnosis have argued that many patients with DID have been "misdiagnosed" with borderline or antisocial personality disorder prior to their DID being finally "recognized," the converse also could be the case.

Since patients with borderline personality disorder, even in the *absence* of a diagnosis of dissociative disorder, tend to achieve higher scores on scales rating one's tendency to dissociate, the most parsimonious explanation for these findings is that is that there is an overlap between these conditions. The diagnoses of borderline and antisocial personality disorder describe *dimensional aspects* of one's temperament, while dissociative disorder describes particular *types of behavior* more likely to be engaged in by individuals with these dimensional features.

Ambiguity between "True" DID, "Iatrogenic" DID, and "Malingered" DID

Because the symptoms of DID are protean, even experts disagree on which symptoms are more suggestive of "true" DID, which are more suggestive of suggestion on the part of the therapist, and which are more suggestive of malingered (feigned) illness. For example, Putnam has noted that DID patients often refer to themselves as "we" rather than "I" or "me" and that when clinicians observe this phenomenon, it is a good sign of that the patient has "genuine" DID. In contrast, Ross has stated that it is rare for patients with "genuine" DID to refer to themselves in such an obvious manner and that when one sees this it should be a clue that the patient may be malingering DID.

Part of the problem here is that virtually any symptom can be ascribed to the disorder. For example, Ross (1989) has described the dissociative amnesia that can be seen in DID as follows:

> The blank spells may not be complete. Instead they may consist of "fuzzy" periods of partial recall. Such fuzzy periods should not be dismissed as due to drugs or alcohol, even when a patient abuses both. . . . The blank spells have usually occurred over an extended period of time, but there may be periods of years in the past when the alters were quiescent. A variation on this is the patient who reports a period of years during which she experienced frequent depersonalization but no amnesia. During this time the alters were copresent without amnesia. Or the MPD may simply have gone into remission. A general rule in MPD phenomenology is that all possibilities have happened to some patient somewhere. [pp. 104–105]

A further problem is that of iatrogenicity. It has been noted that the majority of patients diagnosed with DID are being treated by a relatively small minority of clinicians, and many clinicians report that they have never diagnosed a single case of DID. This suggests the possibility that "experts" on DID are overdiagnosing the disorder, even creating the disorder through their interactions with a highly suggestible patient population. Advocates of the DID diagnosis assert that this is not the case and say that other clinicians simply lack the specialized expertise to recognize DID. For example, they note that obsessive–compulsive disorder also was believed to be exceeding rare until quite recently, when epidemiologic studies that specifically screened for symptoms of the disorder revealed its prevalence in the United States to be about 2%.

How can one isolate "true" or "spontaneous" cases of DID from those "created" through undue influence by the treating clinician? One possibility would be for the examiner to remain totally nondirective in style, waiting to see if the patient spontaneously gives a history consistent with a DID diagnosis. However, DID advocates claim that clinicians who use this method often will miss the diagnosis, just as clinicians failed to diagnose obsessive–compulsive disorder since the symptoms of the latter also tend to go unreported by patients. Specialists in OCD recognize OCD more often than do typical clinicians because they engage in more *direct* inquiry into specific symptoms.

If an evaluator has used hypnosis to elicit the clinical phenomena of DID, this obviously creates further complications, since hypnotically refreshed recollections can be more unreliable. Note that even when these patients haven't submitted to *formal* hypnosis, many of them are highly hypnotizable and suggestible and therefore *spontaneously* enter states of heightened suggestibility in the course of psychotherapy. The emotional arousal and demand characteristics that are inherent in psychotherapy further encourage this process.

CONCLUSIONS

Overall, there is general agreement that the behavior of dissociation exists, but there is disagreement as to the relative contributions of genetic factors, early life trauma, the desire to adopt the sick role, and the influence of the therapist in the initiation and perpetuation of dissociative behavior. This is especially the case with dissociative identity disorder.

All parties agree that DID is diagnosed much more frequently now than it was two decades ago. The debate centers on whether this increased prevalence reflects greater awareness of a previously "hidden epidemic" (as has proven to be the case with obsessive–compulsive disorder) or whether DID is a socially constructed artifact generated in the course of the interaction between the patient and the therapist that is now being diagnosed with greater frequency because it is a "diagnostic fad."

As a result, there are two current schools of therapy. One school advocates *focusing on the dissociation*. Attempts are made to elicit the various alters, directly address them, encourage communication between them, and finally facilitate their integration into a single self. The other school advocates *drawing attention away from the dissociation* by removing patients from specialized "dissociative disorder units," refusing to reinforce the dissociative behavior, and directing the patient's attention to important issues of everyday living that he has been attempting to avoid through his dissociative behavior.

Recognition of dissociation as a behavior helps put this debate in better perspective in that the factors that *initiate* a pathologic behavior may not be the same factors that *perpetuate* the behavior. Even in cases where the therapist didn't "cause" the DID, it could be argued that therapists can play a major role in either *encouraging or discouraging the behavior* and in either *validating or invalidating the belief system* that comes to be associated with the behavior.

In theory, the question of how best to treat dissociation is an empirical one that might be resolved through clinical research. However, no studies to date have directly compared these two treatment techniques. By analogy, in the case of obsessive–compulsive disorder, while psychoanalytic psychotherapy was the treatment of choice for years, it now has fallen out of favor since it

has not proven itself to offer significant clinical efficacy, while behavioral therapy and serotonergic medication have done so. Similar comparative research needs to be conducted with regard to the dissociative disorders.

As is the case with all medical or psychiatric disorders, diagnostic reliability first must be established, followed by efforts to establish the validity of underlying theoretical constructs. While dissociation is far from a new phenomenon, it still is not reliably diagnosed in clinical practice, nor do we fully understand its underlying pathology.

However, recognizing dissociation as a behavior that follows principles similar to those that apply to other behavioral disorders may help clinicians to utilize a similar stepwise approach. First, the behavior needs to be recognized, and clinicians should attempt to help patients learn to control the behavior by helping them learn to recognize internal mood states and thoughts as well as external situations that act as triggers or reinforcers of the behavior.

Psychiatric comorbidity, especially mood disorders, anxiety disorders, somatoform disorders, substance-related disorders, and personality disorders, should be screened for and appropriately treated. These conditions should not simply be attributed to the dissociative disorder, since failure to recognize and treat such conditions sometimes leads to severe morbidity and even mortality. When patients are deteriorating (requiring multiple hospitalizations, engaging in an escalating cycle of self-injurious or parasuicidal behavior, declining in their ability to function in their daily life, etc.) one should "step back" and again consider one's diagnostic formulation and treatment plan. One should specifically examine whether one is failing to consider relevant state-related, trait-related, and behavior factors that might also be contributing to the patient's current clinical picture, including factors associated with the treatment relationship itself.

Chapter 15

Sexual and Gender Identity Disorders

Sexual behavior is ubiquitous and diverse. Beyond the sex act itself, sexuality permeates our culture and our daily lives. Therefore, as with all of the behavioral disorders, distinguishing "normal" from "abnormal" sexuality can be difficult. For example, there are no bright lines separating "low" sexual desire from "normal" sexual desire, or "premature" ejaculation from "normal" ejaculation. Whether a person even is bothered by a particular aspect of his or her sexuality is significantly influenced by personality, previous developmental experience, extent of education about sex, satisfaction with one's relationships in general, and surrounding cultural attitudes about sex.

Consider premature ejaculation. *DSM-IV* defines this as persistent or recurrent ejaculation with minimal sexual stimulation before, on, or shortly after penetration, and before the person wishes it. The definition is deliberately subjective, taking into account the quality of the individual's sexual relationship. Paradoxically, this subjective definition may be more reliable and valid than a definition based on the exact interval between penetration and ejaculation as measured by a stopwatch. Thus, while a man who ejaculates within a minute of vaginal entry might be considered by some people to be "premature," if he and his wife engage in a half-hour of very pleasurable foreplay, followed by mutual orgasms after a minute of pleasurable intercourse, he could not be considered to have a sexual "dysfunction." But a man who can engage in intercourse for 10 minutes prior to ejaculating might still be considered "premature" and to have a "dysfunction" if he only can do this by avoiding looking at his partner (finding this too stimulating), avoiding any foreplay, wearing several condoms, or attempting to distract himself mentally during the sex act.

Clearly, cultural expectations play an important role in the definition of "normal" and "abnormal" sexuality. In the 1940s, Kinsey found that three-quarters of men in the general population reached orgasm within 2 minutes. In contrast, in the 1970s, Hunt found that the mean duration of intercourse was 10–14 minutes. The major factor in this change appears to be that society now places a greater value on women achieving vaginal orgasm, so "the bar has been raised" for men. Currently, about 40% of men who present for treatment of a sexual disorder do so with a chief complaint of "premature ejaculation." This complaint is more common among men with a least a college education, suggesting that men with greater education are more concerned with their partner's satisfaction, as opposed to being predisposed to ejaculate more quickly than do men with lesser education.

As with other behavioral disorders, sexual disorders usually reflect the influence of multiple contributory factors. In some cases, biological factors play the primary role (e.g., diabetes causing impotence or fluoxetine causing anorgasmia), while in other cases, psychological factors play a greater role. However, as with other behavioral disorders, the factors that initiate a disturbance may not be the same factors that serve to perpetuate it later on.

For example, diabetic vasculopathy might account for a patient's initial *difficulty* achieving full erections, but the patient then may go on to develop "performance anxiety" that becomes an even greater source of disability in that it prevents him from obtaining any erections *at all* during intercourse. In other words, the physical disturbance (the vasculopathy) was the major initiating factor, while the psychological disturbance (the performance anxiety) was the major perpetuating factor.

DSM-IV divides sexual disorders into three major groups: sexual dysfunctions, paraphilias, and gender identity disorder.

- **Sexual dysfunctions** are characterized by a disturbance in some aspect of the sexual response cycle itself.
- **Paraphilias** are characterized by recurrent, intense sexual urges, fantasies, or behaviors that involve unusual objects, activities, or situations. The abnormality here is in the *type of sexual behavior* engaged in by the individual, rather than in the sexual response cycle itself (although a paraphilia might be accompanied by a sexual dysfunction).
- **Gender identity disorders** are characterized by strong and persistent cross-gender identification accompanied by persistent discomfort with one's assigned sex.

We will first discuss some general concepts of human sexuality and the normal sexual response cycle. Following this, we will discuss each class of disorder in turn.

HUMAN SEXUALITY

The term "human sexuality" describes a complex group of behaviors, but it also includes everything that *surrounds* these behaviors, from the individual's sense of sexual identity to the expectations of the surrounding culture. Sexual preferences, behaviors, and expectations vary within the population along a continuum. For example, sexual orientation can be heterosexual, homosexual, bisexual, or asexual (the last referring to absent or low desire for sexual partners). The major aspects of an individual's "sexuality" include his or her sexual identity, gender identity, gender role, sexual orientation, and sexual behavior.

Sexual identity refers to an individual's *biological sex*. It includes that individual's chromosomal *genotype* (XY for male, XX for female), *gonads* (testes or ovaries) *internal and external genitalia, hormone levels,* and *secondary sex characteristics.*

Sexual identity begins at conception but subsequently is influenced by a variety of factors. During the first few weeks of gestation, the gonads and genitalia aren't yet differentiated. If a Y chromosome is present, the gonads develop into testes and begin secreting testosterone. The testosterone in turn acts as an *androgen*, causing the genitalia to assume a male phenotype (i.e., epididymis, vas deferens, ejaculatory ducts, penis, and scrotum). In the absence of a Y chromosome, the gonads become ovaries, testosterone isn't secreted, and the genitalia assume a female phenotype (i.e., fallopian tubes, uterus, clitoris, and vagina).

Typically, there is no conflict between one's genotypic sexual identity and one's phenotypic sexual identity. Such cases do arise, however. When a genotypic female fetus (with ovaries) is exposed to androgen, either from an internal source (as in congenital adrenal hyperplasia) or from an external source (as is the case when exogenous androgens have been administered), she develops external male genitalia. Similarly, when a genotypic male fetus either has deficient androgen production by the testes or has defective androgen receptors in the periphery, he develops female genitalia.

Androgen receptors are contained not only within the nascent fetal genitalia but also within the fetal brain, and androgens exert a significant impact upon the development of brain structure and function. Gender-related differences (*sexual dimorphisms*) in the structure of the brain include the size of various brain nuclei, the number of neurons contained within these nuclei, the patterns of connections between neurons and between different brain regions, and axonal and dendritic branching patterns. Gender-related differences in the function of the brain include differences in the concentration of various neurotransmitters and differences in neuroregulation. In other contexts, we already have discussed sexual differences with regard to the presentation of most psychiatric disorders, including the mood and anxiety disorders, schizophrenia, and the eating disorders.

While sexual identity refers to one's biological sex, **gender identity** refers to one's *subjective self-awareness* of "maleness" or "femaleness." It can be influenced by a variety of prenatal and postnatal factors. The extent to which genetic factors or exposure of the fetal brain to androgen affects later sexual behavior remains uncertain. In other vertebrates, prenatal exposure to androgens irretrievably imprints the brain such that postnatal sexual behavior also is masculinized.

Research conducted during the 1950s and 1960s suggested that—in humans—gender identity remains highly malleable at birth. For example, children born with an XY phenotype but with highly ambiguous external genitalia (i.e., a "micropenis" resembling an enlarged clitoris) were treated surgically through castration, remodeling of the external genitalia to resemble female anatomy, and instructions to the parents to clearly and unambiguously treat their child as a female. When the child reached puberty, estrogen was prescribed.

While some contemporary reports suggested favorable outcomes—with these individuals continuing to view themselves as "female" and demonstrating good psychosocial adjustment to the female gender role—it later became apparent that at least some of these children rejected a female gender identification from a very young age and ultimately chose to receive testosterone therapy and to live as males. Given this, some clinicians now argue that infants with ambiguous genitalia should remain "uncorrected" until the child's gender identity becomes more apparent, in particular avoiding early surgical interventions that cannot be undone.

It may be that individuals with an XY chromosomal pattern who have more complete forms of *androgen insensitivity* are more likely to be successfully raised as females, since their brains, like their genitalia, have not been masculinized

in utero. Conversely, prenatal exposure of the fetal brain to testosterone may explain why some XY males with *5-α-reductase deficiency*, reared as females, voluntarily adopt a male sexual role at puberty. In this condition, an enzymatic defect prevents the conversion of testosterone to dihydrotestosterone, which is required for prenatal virilization of the genitalia. The individual therefore is born with female-appearing genitalia but experiences male sexual development (including phallic growth) at puberty in response to the developmental surge in testosterone.

In *gender identity disorder*, an individual's gender identity comes into conflict with his or her sexual identity. Individuals with this disorder have a strong desire to *be* of the other sex, even insisting that they actually *are* of the other sex despite external appearances. The relative roles of hormonal, neurobiological, and psychological influences in the etiology of this condition remain uncertain.

Gender role refers to the *behaviors* engaged in by an individual that serve to "identify" him or her as being "male" or "female." In other words, gender role reflects how "masculine" or "feminine" a person acts. This repertoire of behaviors is learned over the course of childhood development. For example, boys and girls observed on the playground act quite differently, with boys tending to be more physically and verbally aggressive than girls. Society is more forgiving of girls who engage in more masculine, rough-and-tumble play ("tomboys") than it is of more effeminate boys (who might be called "sissies" and be teased mercilessly by their peers). Over time, men and women also come to dress and behave differently in a variety of social settings.

Gender role and gender identity are not the same thing. While they closely correspond in most cases, they sometimes diverge. For example, men with *transvestic fetishism* have a male gender identity (i.e., they think of themselves as being "men") but nonetheless enjoy adopting the female gender role by dressing and acting like women. In contrast, individuals with gender identity disorder describe themselves as "feeling" like a member of the opposite biological sex and also adopt the gender role of the opposite sex.

Gender role also differs from **sexual orienta-**

tion. The latter refers merely to the *object* of one's sexual drives. For example, among men, there are heterosexuals who are more effeminate or more masculine and homosexuals who are more effeminate or more masculine.

As with all of the motivated behaviors, sexual orientation is a complex and multifaceted phenomenon. The term "**homosexuality**" is broad and subsumes four different behavioral dimensions: sexual fantasy, sexual activity, personal identity, and social role.

The most important dimension to examine in assessing homosexual orientation is **sexual fantasy** since erotic fantasy may be entirely private and may or may not motivate overt **sexual activity** with others. For example, an individual may be heterosexual or even celibate in terms of his sexual activity but homosexual in his sexual fantasy life (and therefore in his sexual orientation).

These different dimensions refer to different *aspects* of sexuality, and they sometimes come into conflict with each other. For example, the terms "gay" and "lesbian" usually refer to an individual's sense of belonging to a particular *social group*. In other words, they include elements of both **personal identity** and **social role**. Given this, one might be "homosexual" based upon the nature of one's *sexual fantasies* but still not consider oneself to be "gay" in terms of personal identity or social role. These latter dimensions can be at variance with each other, as well. For example, a "closeted" homosexual may have a homosexual personal identity while maintaining a heterosexual social role.

In *DSM-I* and *DSM-II*, homosexuality was considered a deviant behavior. However, in 1973 the American Psychiatric Association's Board of Trustees elected to remove homosexuality from the diagnostic manual, as organized psychiatry had shifted from seeing homosexuality as a pathological adaptation to seeing it as a normal variation. The decision was a controversial one, but was approved by the majority of the organization's membership. There do remain some psychiatrists who consider homosexuality to be a form of psychopathology but they are in the minority.

More recently, controversy has centered on whether certain biological markers or neuropathologic findings are more common among homosexual than among heterosexual individuals. Defining which subjects should be included in which group, since "sexual orientation" includes a spectrum of behaviors, is one difficulty that such studies face. For example, homoerotic play commonly occurs in both boys and girls as part of normal sexual development and is not predictive of adult homosexuality. In addition, men or women who are preferentially heterosexual still may engage in homosexual activity when placed in certain settings, such as single-sex boarding schools or prisons.

In 1948, Kinsey drew attention to the theory that homosexuality reflects variation along a *dimension of behavior* rather than being a *discrete attribute* of a person that is either "present" or "absent." He described occasional homosexual behavior as being more common than exclusive homosexuality. In his sample, 10% of men and 5% of women were exclusively homosexual but about 40% of people had engaged at some point in homosexual behavior. While more recent, larger studies have revised these figures downward, they have reached the same general conclusion. For example, a large 1994 survey of individuals between the ages of 18 and 59 found that while 2.8% of men and 1.4% of women described themselves as being homosexual in orientation, 9% of men and 5% of women reported having engaged in at least one homosexual experience since puberty.

A variety of factors have been postulated to contribute to homosexuality. Genetic influences likely play a role, since the concordance rate for homosexuality is greatest for monozygotic twins, followed by dizygotic twins, followed by adopted siblings. (The rates are about 50%, 20%, and 10%, respectively for men, and 50%, 15%, and 5% for women.) Environmental factors also must play a role, however, since the concordance rate for monozygotic twins is far from 100%. These also have been some case reports of concordance for homosexuality among monozygotic twins who were reared apart. While the absence of larger-scale studies limits the conclusions that one might draw from such case reports, given the low prevalence of homosexuality in the community they do suggest the possibility of a significant genetic contribution to homosexuality.

How such genetic factors might affect sexual orientation is less certain. A potential link between genotype and phenotype is the finding in one autopsy series involving a group of *interstitial nuclei in the anterior hypothalamus (INAH nuclei)*. These nuclei are **sexually dimorphic**—that is, different for males and females. While they are the same size in both sexes at birth, very soon after birth their size increases more in men than it does in women. This is especially the case for nucleus 3, which in men increases to a size that is twice that which is seen in women. The growth likely results from an immediate postnatal surge of testosterone in male but not female infants.

The function of the INAH nuclei is unclear, but in other mammals this area of the hypothalamus is known to be involved in the regulation of gonadotropin release and sexual behavior. In the autopsy series, INAH 3 was almost twice as large in heterosexual men as in gay men and in women. (Note that this finding is a statistical one, observed for each group in the *aggregate*. For example, one presumably homosexual man in this series had a large INAH 3 and one presumably heterosexual man had a small INAH 3, suggesting that hypothalamic size doesn't dictate sexual "destiny.")

Therefore, one possibility is that the genetic contribution to sexual orientation involves either postnatal testosterone release or the responsiveness of the hypothalamus to testosterone. However, even if this is the case, it doesn't explicate the *intermediate steps* in the development of homosexual behavior. In other words, genetic effects might be relatively *direct* (if these hypothalamic nuclei influence sexual fantasy and activity) or might be more *indirect* (if these nuclei influence gender-related behaviors or attachments, which then are either further reinforced or are extinguished during psychosexual development).

For example, while most women report having been tomboys to some degree as children, homosexual women are more likely than heterosexual women to report that they were "extreme" tomboys. In one study, 70% of homosexual women versus 16% of heterosexual women recalled having been "boylike" as children. Another study found that 71% of homosexual women versus 28% of heterosexual women greatly enjoyed sex-stereotyped boys' activities during childhood, such as baseball and football.

Similarly, 67% of homosexual men versus 3%

of heterosexual men recalled being "girl-like" as children (e.g., they had no male buddies, avoided boys' games, played predominantly with girls, and were teased and called "sissy" by other boys). In another study, 11% of homosexual men versus 70% of heterosexual men recalled having enjoyed sex-stereotyped boys' activities during childhood. Conversely, this study also found that only 11% of heterosexual men but 46% of homosexual men reported having enjoyed stereotypic girls' activities.

Overall, sexual orientation and sexual behavior appear to be multiply determined. It is unlikely that research will reveal a single biological "cause" for homosexuality, and "disease perspective" reasoning hasn't proven to be useful in understanding homosexuality. Sexual dimorphism, a biological measure that varies along a *biological dimension* and that likely has both genetic and neuroanatomic correlates, may play a role. However, the relationship between this biological correlate and expressed human sexual behavior may be indirect and may prove to be neither necessary nor sufficient in itself to account for variations in sexual orientation.

THE SEXUAL RESPONSE CYCLE

Regardless of one's gender identity, gender role, or sexual orientation, the sexual response cycle follows the same pattern. Based on research conducted by Masters and Johnson, this cycle has been divided into *four phases*: the desire phase, the excitement phase, the orgasm phase, and the resolution phase.

The **desire phase** involves the appetite, or craving, for sex. As we have seen in the case of other motivated behaviors, cravings can be influenced by a variety of internal and external factors. In this case, such factors include one's underlying degree of libido, the physical presence of a sexual partner or sexually suggestive materials, and whether the individual is currently fantasizing about sex.

The **excitement (arousal) phase** consists of a subjective sense of sexual arousal and also accompanying physiological changes. The major physiological changes in the male consist of penile tumescence and erection. The major changes in the female consist of vasocongestion in the pelvis, vaginal lubrication and expansion, and swelling of the external genitalia. Arousal requires *four systems to be working together*:

> *Psychological.* Feelings of arousal can be brought on either by fantasy, or by the presence of a sexual partner, or by more direct physical stimulation (e.g., the touching of either one's body in general or of more specific erogenous zones such as the genitalia or nipples). The resulting state of physiologic arousal further influences one's psychological state, and vice versa; a state of increased muscular tension and pelvic throbbing is accompanied by a feeling of spreading warmth and a changing sense of consciousness. In contrast, arousal can be adversely affected by psychological factors as well, including fatigue, anxiety, depression, anger, and distraction.

> *Neural.* Psychological arousal is associated with involuntary firing of the *parasympathetic* nervous system via the splanchnic nerves (S_2, S_3, S_4). This activity increases the amount of parasympathetic tone relative to sympathetic tone at the level of the smooth muscles of blood vessels leading to and from the penis or vagina.

> *Vascular.* In the male, in response to increased parasympathetic tone, the neurotransmitter *nitric oxide* is released in the corpus cavernosum of the penis. The nitric oxide in turn activates the enzyme *guanylate cyclase,* thereby resulting in increased levels of *cyclic guanosine monophosphate (cyclic GMP).* Cylic GMP in turn activates a specific protein kinase that phosphorylates various proteins and ion channels, resulting in the opening of potassium channels and closing of calcium channels, leading to hyperpolarization of smooth-muscle cell membranes. Penile arteries dilate while relaxation of the trabecular smooth muscle increases the compliance of the sinusoids, facilitating rapid filling and expansion of the sinusoidal system. Venous plexuses that allow for the outflow of blood in the flaccid state now become compressed between the trabeculae and the rigid tunica albuginea, resulting in almost total occlusion of venous outflow. Detumescence results either from of the cessation of neurotransmitter release, or from sympathetic discharge during ejaculation, or from cyclic GMP being hydrolyzed back to GMP by *phosphodiesterase type 5 (PDE5).* Contraction of the trabecular smooth muscle reopens the venous channels, thereby allowing for the drainage of the trapped blood.

> In the female, an analogous process takes place. Vasodilation of the circumvaginal blood vessels causes both clitoral erection and diffuse genital swelling and vaginal lubrication (the latter resulting from vascular transudation through the vaginal wall). In the female, an adequate level of estrogen must be present for this process to occur. Absent this, the vaginal mucosa becomes thin, dry, and atrophic, thereby making intercourse less comfortable or impossible.

> *Endocrine/Metabolic.* In both men and in women, testosterone facilitates arousal and orgasm. The mesolimbic dopamine system further facilitates these two processes. In contrast, serotonergic activity appears to play an inhibitory role.

The **orgasm** phase consists of a peaking of sexual pleasure, a release of sexual tension, and a slight clouding of consciousness, along with rhythmic contraction of the perineal muscles and reproductive organs. In the male, orgasm is associated with a sensation of ejaculatory inevitability, followed by the ejaculation of semen. In the female, orgasm is associated with contractions of the walls of the outer third of the vagina and sustained uterine contractions. In both genders, the anal sphincter rhythmically contracts. Centrally, *dopamine* appears to play a role in the pleasurable, rewarding sensations associated with orgasm via the mesolimbic pathway. Peripherally, *sympathetic* innervation from the hypogastric plexus is an important mediator of orgasm.

The **resolution phase** consists of a sense of muscular relaxation and general well-being. During this phase, males are physiologically refractory to further erection and orgasm for a period lasting from several minutes to several hours. In contrast, females may be able to respond to additional stimulation almost immediately.

All four factors (psychological, neural, vascular, and endocrine/metabolic) must be intact for normal sexual functioning to occur, and sexual functioning can be impaired by any illness or medication that disrupts one or more of these factors. The list of offending conditions includes *psychological insults* (stress, depression, or anxiety), *central or peripheral neurologic insults* (including multiple sclerosis, stroke, lumbar or sacral spinal stenosis, diabetic neuropathy, and nerve injury related to having undergone radical prostatectomy or other abdominal surgery), *vascular insults* (e.g., focal stenosis of the arteries leading to the penis due to extensive bicycle riding or due to diabetic or hypertensive vascu-lopathy), or *endocrine disorders* (e.g., hyperpro-lactinemia; hypothyroidism or hyperthyroidism; increased estrogen due to cirrhosis, diabetes, re-nal failure, or zinc deficiency). *Medications* can also interfere with sexual functioning at a sev-eral points.

> Medications with *anticholinergic activity* (e.g., an-tipsychotics, tricyclic antidepressants, and MAO inhibitors) can inhibit arousal, leading to impotence in men and impaired lubrication in women.
>
> *Antihypertensives* that decrease sympathetic nerv-ous system activity (e.g., clonidine, β-blockers) can impede one's ability to achieve orgasm, and β-adrenergic blockade also can impede arousal. In contrast, *trazodone* rarely has been associ-ated with excessive arousal and persistent erec-tion (*priapism*), perhaps due to its combination of powerful α-adrenergic blockade and minimal anticholinergic activity (which leads to a net in-crease in parasympathetic activity).
>
> *Antipsychotic* medications can impair arousal via several mechanisms, including dopamine blockade, anticholinergic effects, and increased prolactin release. Their α-adrenergic blocking effects likely account for their ability to cause anorgasmia.
>
> *SSRI medications* can inhibit arousal and orgasm through their serotonergic effects. Agents that antagonize the effects of serotonin on $5HT_2$ re-ceptors (nefazodone and mirtazapine) appear to carry a lower risk of causing antidepressant in-duced sexual dysfunction, while bupropion, which has no serotonergic effects and is *not* an SSRI, appears to carry the lowest risks (and sometimes even is used as an "antidote" to SSRI-induced sexual dysfunction).
>
> *Spironolactone, steroids, and estrogens* can de-crease sexual desire through their antiandro-genic effects.
>
> *Drugs of abuse such as alcohol, opiates, and co-caine* also can interfere with both arousal and orgasm, particularly in the setting of either sig-nificant intoxication or more chronic use.

SEXUAL DYSFUNCTION

Overview

Sexual dysfunction can occur *at any of the phases* of the sexual response cycle, and an in-dividual can have more than one dysfunction.

Sexual dysfunction can be either *lifelong*, (i.e., since the onset of sexual functioning) or *acquired* (having developed after a period of normal func-tioning). It can be *situational* (limited to certain types of situations or partners) or *generalized* (occurring in all situations). It can either be due to *psychological factors alone* or due to a *com-bination of psychological factors and a general medical condition or substance use*. If a general medical condition or substance use (including medication side effects) is sufficient in itself to account for the sexual dysfunction, one would make a diagnosis of sexual dysfunction due to a general medical condition or substance-induced sexual dysfunction. Sexual dysfunction includes several specific *DSM-IV* conditions, which are listed in Table 15–1.

Desire Disorders

Hypoactive Sexual Desire Disorder

In **hypoactive sexual desire disorder**, the pa-tient demonstrates a deficiency or absence of both sexual fantasies and the desire for sexual activity. The low sexual desire may be *global* (encompassing all forms of sexual expression) or may be *situational*—that is, limited to one part-ner or to a specific sexual activity (e.g., to inter-course but not to masturbation). The individual usually does not initiate sexual activity and may

Table 15–1. *DSM-IV-TR* Sexual Dysfunctions

DESIRE DISORDERS

Hypoactive sexual desire disorder
Sexual aversion disorder

SEXUAL AROUSAL DISORDERS

Female sexual arousal disorder
Male erectile disorder

ORGASMIC DISORDERS

Female orgasmic disorder
Male orgasmic disorder
Premature ejaculation

SEXUAL PAIN DISORDERS

Dyspareunia
Vaginismus

SEXUAL DYSFUNCTION DUE TO A GENERAL
MEDICAL CONDITION

SUBSTANCE-INDUCED SEXUAL DYSFUNCTION

only engage in it reluctantly when it is initiated by the partner. Although the frequency of intercourse with the partner is usually low, pressure from the partner or "nonsexual" needs (such as a desire for physical comfort or intimacy) may contribute to continued sexual activity.

Because of a lack of normative age-related or gender-related data on the frequency or degree of sexual desires, the diagnosis must rely on clinical judgment based on the individual's characteristics, the interpersonal determinants, the life context, and the cultural setting. While the frequency of intercourse often declines with marriage, it doesn't inevitably do so. In the 1994 University of Chicago survey, the greatest frequency of intercourse (twice a week or more) was reported by cohabiting single persons, but 41% of married couples reported the same frequency of activity. However, in various samples of happily married couples, up to a third of couples report that they engage in intercourse no more frequently than once every 1–2 months.

The clinician may need to assess both partners when discrepancies in sexual desire prompt the professional consultation. Apparent "low desire" in one partner may instead reflect an excessive desire for sex by the other partner. Alternatively, both partners may have levels of desire that fall within the normal range but at different ends of the continuum. Men may have relatively greater sex drive than their wives given that, in the 1994 University of Chicago survey, over half of men said they thought about sex every day or several times a day, while this was the case for only 20% of women. In addition, a quarter of the men masturbated at least once per week, versus 10% of the women.

Low sexual interest is frequently associated with other sexual dysfunctions, including difficulties achieving arousal and orgasm. The deficiency in sexual desire may be the *primary* dysfunction or may be *secondary* to emotional distress associated with these other dysfunctions. However, some individuals with low sexual desire retain the capacity for adequate sexual excitement and orgasm in response to sexual stimulation.

While some individuals describe a lifelong disorder (present since puberty), most individuals develop the condition in association with psychological distress, stressful life events, or interpersonal difficulties following a period of adequate sexual interest. The loss of sexual desire also may be *continuous* or *episodic*. An episodic pattern occurs in some individuals in association with problems with intimacy and commitment. Sometimes, the loss of desire reflects anger at one's partner. The pattern may become self-reinforcing, as prolonged sexual abstinence can lead to further suppression of libido.

Attention always should be paid to the possibility that the low sexual desire is secondary to either a *general medical condition* or to a *prescribed medication*. Further, the *psychological stress* associated with a medical condition (e.g., weakness, pain, problems with body image, concerns about survival) also can contribute to lower sexual desire. Depressive disorders often are associated with low libido, and hypoactive sexual desire disorder only should be diagnosed if the condition antedates the depression or becomes a separate focus of clinical attention.

Treatment of hypoactive sexual desire initially involves attending to any potential medical or pharmacologic causes of lowered libido. Testosterone therapy has been attempted and is useful in some cases. However, it typically has little beneficial effect on men if they present with normal baseline testosterone levels, and benefits are variable in patients who present with low testosterone levels. It also can cause virilization in women.

Typically, treatment consists of either individual or couples therapy combining cognitive–behavioral and psychodynamic principles. Most often, the couple itself is considered to be "the patient," and participation by both partners is a requirement of the therapy. In many cases, lack of education about normal sexuality contributes to anxieties or guilt about sex. Sometimes, simply offering sexual education to both partners leads to significant improvement.

Cognitive–behavioral approaches involve exercises that are given to the couple and practiced in the privacy of the home. Results of these exercises then are discussed at the subsequent session. Typically, homework assignments involve attempts to combat performance anxiety, increase intimacy, improve communication, and allow each person to gain a better understanding of what gives their partner pleasure. Sexual intercourse may even be proscribed at first, both to decrease performance anxiety and to interrupt problematic behavior patterns that have arisen in relation to the couple's current sexual practices. Emphasis instead is placed on reestablishing intimacy and mutual pleasure.

One commonly prescribed course of behavioral exercises involves *sensate focus*. Initial assignments involve mutual light touching and caressing (avoiding the breast or genital areas). Each partner attends to both the positive and negative feelings that accompany these activities. The exercises ultimately come to include oral or manual genital exploration without penetration, and later by penetration.

While the results of cognitive–behavioral therapy are gratifying for some couples, interpersonal problems may arise that quickly confound this approach. When this occurs, the therapist must step back and shift the focus of therapy, employing a more *psychodynamic or interpersonal approach* to these relationship problems. The interpersonal difficulties may underlie the couple's sexual difficulties or may simply have arisen because of them.

Hypoactive sexual desire can be the most difficult to treat of the sexual dysfunctions. While sensate focus exercises can be very effective for arousal and orgasmic disorders (since they help diffuse the performance anxiety that accompanies these conditions), many patients with hypoactive sexual desire don't *desire* intimacy with their partner and may even be "turned off" by the partner. Pressuring such patients to engage in sensate focus exercises may even be countertherapeutic. These patients sometimes benefit from being encouraged to stimulate their libido and bypass anxieties through erotic fantasy, through fantasy accompanied by masturbation, and through fantasy during intercourse. "Courtship" assignments also may be given, either to help discern sources of interpersonal conflict or to help interrupt the couple's usual pattern of interaction.

Sexual Aversion Disorder

As with patients with hypoactive sexual desire disorder, patients with **sexual aversion disorder** typically present with a complaint of decreased frequency of intercourse. However, in this case, the individual expresses an *active aversion* to genital sexual contact with the sexual partner, leading to this decreased activity. While in hypoactive sexual desire disorder, the individual primarily experiences a *lack of libido*, here the individual experiences negative emotions such as *anxiety, fear, or disgust* when the opportunity for sex arises.

This aversion to genital contact might focus on a *particular* aspect of sexual experience (e.g., genital secretions, vaginal penetration), but some individuals experience a more *generalized* revulsion to *all* sexual stimuli, even kissing and touching. The intensity of the reaction may range from moderate anxiety and lack of pleasure to extreme psychological distress, even panic attacks.

In practice, it can be difficult to distinguish between this disorder and hypoactive sexual desire disorder, and both conditions can coexist. While the aversion sometimes is the result of interpersonal problems within the relationship, it also can be a reflection of aversive behavioral conditioning. For example, the patient may have developed an aversion to sexual activity secondary to another, preexisting sexual dysfunction such as premature ejaculation or dyspareunia. In such cases, both diagnoses should be assigned.

A 34-year-old woman with two young children presents for evaluation out of concern that her marriage may be in jeopardy, as she has been refusing to have intercourse with her husband. She hasn't asked her husband to accompany her to the evaluation, since talking about intercourse in front of him "would be too difficult." She describes herself as always having been "sexually inhibited." Her husband has been her only sexual partner. Since the earliest days of their relationship, she only has engaged in intercourse with him when she has wanted to conceive. She never undresses in front of him, and she typically goes to bed later than her husband as one means of avoiding proposals of sexual contact. Intercourse has never been pleasurable for her, and even thinking about having intercourse engenders tremendous anxiety. She reports that she loves her husband, and she feels that they are compatible in all other areas of their relationship except for sexuality. On further questioning, she reports that she is not comfortable with looking at her own nude body, and she has never masturbated.

In contrast to the treatment of hypoactive sexual desire disorder, treatment of sexual aversion disorder is similar to that for a phobic disorder, including graded in vivo desensitization. This must progress at a slow and careful pace. Sometimes augmenting the exercises with an anxiolytic agent (such as a benzodiazepine) is useful. Helen Singer Kaplan (1995) has described this process:

During in vivo desensitization assignments, phobic patients are instructed to attempt to remain physically in the presence of a small manageable piece of the feared and previously avoided sexual situation (e g., kissing, body caressing, genital touching, looking at the partner's nude body, holding hands) until their negative feelings have abated. After they become entirely comfortable with that level of exposure, they advance to the next step. For example, patients who are phobic and aversive to vaginal penetration are typically too frightened to look at their genitalia. As an initial assignment, a female patient might be encouraged to view her genitalia in a mirror. Although at first such assignments typically make patients quite anxious, after a few repetitions of the assignment, most become accustomed to the sight. The next assignment is for the patient to place the tip of her index finger at her vaginal introitus, perhaps for 2 minutes each day. After the patient's anxiety has abated sufficiently so she can do this easily, she proceeds to the next step, which might entail inserting her finger more deeply into her vagina and for longer periods of time. After that, I usually begin the stretching aspect of treatment by having the patient work with progressively larger vaginal dilators until she can comfortably accommodate an object the size of her partner's erect penis. Thereafter, most couples progress rapidly to comfortable intercourse.

Sexual Arousal Disorders

Female Sexual Arousal Disorder

In **female sexual arousal disorder**, there is a persistent or recurrent inability to attain, or to maintain until completion of sexual activity, an adequate lubrication–swelling response during the sexual excitement phase. This disorder rarely occurs in isolation; more often, it occurs in combination with hypoactive sexual desire disorder, with female orgasmic disorder, or with both of these conditions.

To fulfill the diagnostic criteria for this disorder, the patient's difficulty shouldn't be due solely to a general medical condition or the side effects of a medication. Most commonly, women with these symptoms either are *postmenopausal with low estrogen levels* or are *taking a medication with anticholinergic side effects*. Reduced

vaginal lubrication also can occur with *atrophic vaginitis, diabetes mellitus*, and *during lactation*. The condition often can be treated with a combination of estrogen replacement therapy and a topical lubricant.

Male Erectile Disorder

Male erectile disorder (also known as erectile dysfunction or impotence) is defined as a persistent or recurrent inability to attain, or to maintain until completion of sexual activity, an adequate penile erection. As with female sexual arousal disorder, in making this diagnosis the clinician must take into account the patient's age, relevant psychosocial factors, and the circumstances of the patient's life. There is no standardized measure of the adequacy or duration of erection that an individual must fall below in order to be considered to have erectile "failure," nor is there a specific number of episodes of such failure that must occur before one would be considered to have an erectile "disorder." Rather, the diagnoses is a mixture of objective and subjective assessment such that the clinician assigns the diagnosis this disorder if the patient's erection is not "adequate" and if the condition causes the patient to experience "marked distress or interpersonal difficulty."

Male erectile disorder is the most common presenting complaint to sex therapy clinics and is present in 50% of new patients. The reported prevalence of this disorder in the general population has varied in different studies, which is likely a reflection of varying definitions and ascertainment methods, but it has been estimated to be present in about 10% of males. The prevalence increases with age: the percentage of men who are totally impotent ranges from 7% of men who are 20–30 years old to about 50% of men who are 40–70 years old. The increased prevalence in older men may be due more to injury or specific diseases associated with aging than to aging per se.

Male erectile disorder has been found to occur even more commonly among patients who present to the primary care setting, likely because the erectile response is so vulnerable to a wide variety of pathologies and medications. For example, at one outpatient clinic, over a third of male patients were found to have erectile dysfunction. Fifty percent of males with diabetes ultimately develop erectile dysfunction. Unfortunately, only about 10% of men with erectile dysfunction ever seek treatment, and many physicians don't routinely inquire into erectile functioning during their clinical examination.

A wide variety of *psychological, neurologic, vascular*, and *endocrine* insults can contribute to impotence. Impotence also can occur as a side effect of a variety of commonly prescribed *medications* (including β-adrenergic blockers, thiazides, cimetidine, antidepressants,and antipsychotics) and as a result of *alcohol or drug abuse*. Several decades ago, it was believed that up to 90% of cases of erectile dysfunction were "psychogenic" in nature, with the remaining 10% being caused by a physical illness. However, it now appears that the opposite is the case: subtle or occult medical conditions are found to be present in about 90% of cases.

The most important of these factors are *aging*, *diabetes* (which affects the responsiveness of penile tissue, causes vascular disease, and causes peripheral neuropathy), and *vascular disease* (present in about 70% of cases of erectile dysfunction). Other risk factors for vascular disease, such as *hypercholesterolemia* and *cigarette smoking,* also appear to exert independent effects on erectile tissue. Erectile dysfunction also occurs as a consequence of mood and anxiety disorders.

Regardless of precipitating factors, erectile dysfunction can become self-perpetuating due to the development of superimposed "performance anxiety" and "spectatoring" (i.e., excessive monitoring of one's sexual performance during intercourse). Since anxiety in itself can impede one's ability to achieve an erection, fears of erectile failure become "self-fulfilling prophecies." Preexisting psychological or relationship difficulties also can become heightened due to sexual dysfunction, which in turn further exacerbates both anxiety during intercourse and erectile dysfunction

The *sexual history* should inquire into the circumstances of the onset of the problem (e.g., age at onset, sudden versus gradual onset), the degree of erectile failure, its relationship to other sexual dysfunctions, its relation to alcohol or other medication use, and whether the patient is able to achieve erections in nonperformance situations (e.g., upon awakening in the morning, or in response to masturbation). If the patient can achieve erections in such nonperformance situations, it is unlikely that significant organic impairment is present. It also is important to explore both the patient's and his partner's *reactions* to the sexual dysfunction and their openness to various somatic or conjoint behavioral treatment strategies. The *physical examination* should include attention to secondary sexual characteristics, palpation of the penis, sensory testing of the perineum, and evaluation of lower-extremity vascular function.

> A 60-year-old man with no medical problems presents with a chief complaint of progressively worsening erectile difficulties. He and his wife are interviewed separately. His initial fear is that his difficulty might be a symptom of a physical problem such as prostate cancer. However, his internist has performed a prostate examination and has checked his prostate-specific antigen (PSA) and both of these were unremarkable. His blood pressure also is normal. He therefore has attributed the situation to "life stress" and has tried not to pay too much attention to the problem. He hasn't discussed it with his wife, hoping that his erectile function would improve over time. It hasn't done so, however, and he has become increasing anxious during intercourse. He can achieve a partial erection, but then loses the erection prior to penetration. He also occasionally experiences premature ejaculation. He is becoming more emotionally withdrawn from his wife. His wife reports that she herself has just gone through menopause and has worried that perhaps her husband no longer finds her attractive. She also has been concerned that her husband might be having an extramarital affair. However, she hasn't discussed his sexual performance difficulties or these other concerns with him, out of fear of "what he might tell me." Following the assessment, the clinician meets with the patient and his wife together. Open discussion of the patient's erectile problems and the provision of education about how the problem is common and potentially treatable brings dramatic relief to both partners, even prior to the initiation of any specific treatment intervention.

Commonly performed ancillary studies include *blood glucose testing* (to assess for diabetes), *liver and thyroid function studies*, and *hormonal studies* (including testosterone, prolactin, and follicle-stimulating hormone). More specific studies, performed when indicated, include: *noc-*

turnal penile tumescence testing (which utilizes a spring gauge on the penis during sleep to determine the degree of erectile function during REM sleep), doppler flow studies (to assess blood flow in the internal pudendal artery, which then might be supplemented by penile blood pressure testing, selective pudendal angiogram, or dynamic cavernosography), and dorsal nerve somatosensory evoked potentials (to assess the integrity of nerve innnervation).

When contributory medical conditions are present, these should be appropriately managed. Given the older age of many patients, these conditions often are present although their relationship to the erectile difficulties may remain unclear. When hypogonadism is present, secondary erectile dysfunction may respond to testosterone administration, either by intramuscular injection at 2 week intervals or through a transdermal cream. Hyperprolactinemia may respond to the administration of bromocriptine.

Psychological treatment can be helpful even when "organic" conditions play a major etiologic role. The therapy typically includes couples therapy and education. The goal is to help the couple deal with relationship difficulties, frustrations, and anxieties that may have arisen secondary to the erectile dysfunction, as well as providing behavioral therapy. The latter usually includes sensate focus exercises, which place the emphasis on sexual pleasure rather than on "performance," and—when erectile function sufficient for penetration remains present but is psychologically inhibited—in vivo desensitization exercises ultimately leading to vaginal entry.

Nonpharmacologic somatic interventions include external vacuum devices and penile prosthetic implants. Vacuum devices employ a plastic cylinder that is placed over the flaccid penis. Pumping the air out of the cylinder creates negative pressure around the penis, which in turn draws blood into the corpora cavernosa, leading to erection. An elastic band then is slid off of the cylinder and around the base of penis, preventing venous outflow. This produces an erection sufficient for penetration lasting for up to 30 minutes. The most common complaints with this treatment include discomfort, difficulty ejaculating, and lack of sexual spontaneity. Overall, however, these devices are accepted by about 80% of men. Penile prostheses (either an inflat-

able implant or a bendable rod) can be relatively effective, but preoperative counseling is essential, since many couples expect that with such a device there will be a full return to premorbid functioning. Despite improved rigidity, the implant won't relieve premature ejaculation or other coexisting sexual dysfunctions, and the implant sometimes contributes to a decreased intensity of orgasm.

Fortunately, a growing number of pharmacologic agents have become available. These are effective not only in many cases of erectile dysfunction associated with diabetes and vascular disease but also in many cases that appear to be primarily "psychogenic" in origin. They also may be more acceptable to a couple than is an intensive behavioral program.

The first such treatments were intracavernosal injections of agents that led to relaxation of arterial and cavernosal smooth muscle, such as **papaverine** (a smooth-muscle relaxant), **phenoxybenzamine** (an α-adnrenergic blocker), and **prostaglandin E$_1$**, in the form of **alprostadil (Caverject)** The patient must receive appropriate training before beginning home injections. The goal is to achieve an erection that is adequate for sexual intercourse but does not last for more than 1 hour. The two major side effects of intracavernous injection are priapism and fibrosis. Although the response rate is high, up to 80% of patients ultimately discontinue the injections due to complaints of pain, fear of injections, lack of spontaneity, or cost.

Alprostadil also is available in a more convenient urethral suppository form (Muse). While this form of therapy is not associated with fibrosis or priapism, some patients complain of penile pain (32%) or urethral irritation (12%). Further, the response rate for the suppository form of alprostadil is lower than for the injectable form (40% versus 70%, respectively).

Oral agents rapidly have become the preferred form of therapy since 1998, with the introduction of the only agent currently on the market, **sildenafil (Viagra)**. Oral agents not only are more convenient, but they allow the majority of cases to be managed by primary care physicians without the need for referral to a urologist or psychotherapist. Being able to initiate an empiric course of therapy with sildenafil also obviates the need to first obtain extensive ancillary tests such as nocturnal penile tumescence studies or vascular flow studies. (Of course, it remains essential for clinicians to assess for underlying general medical or pharmacologic causes of erectile dysfunction and to address these before initiating empiric therapy.)

After sildenafil was introduced, physicians found themselves deluged with requests for prescriptions, indicating the vast number of patients with erectile dysfunction who had suffered in silence until then. It is effective in about half of cases of erectile dysfunction due to radical prostate surgery or long-standing diabetes. However, it doesn't improve libido and doesn't increase erectile performance beyond what might be expected for age.

Sildenafil doesn't exert direct effects on the smooth muscles in the penis. Rather, it inhibits the activity of the enzyme phosphodiesterase 5 (PDE5), thereby decreasing the breakdown of cyclic GMP. It therefore indirectly amplifies the effects of nitric oxide on penile blood flow in response to sexual stimulation. Sildenafil has no effect on the penis in the absence of sexual stimulation, when the concentrations of nitric oxide and cyclic GMP are low.

Sildenafil can produce erections in men with severe organic impotence caused by diabetes (60%), spinal cord injuries (80%), and radical prostatectomy (40%) and in men taking various medications (including antidepressants, antipsychotics, antihypertensives, and diuretics). It also produces erections in 80% of men felt to primarily have psychogenic impotence. (In contrast, response rates associated with placebo are about 10%–15% for impotence from organic causes and 25% in men with psychogenic impotence.)

Side effects of sildenafil are mild and include headache (16%), flushing (10%), and dyspepsia (7%). Visual changes, such as mild and temporary changes in blue/green color perception and increased sensitivity to light can also occur. Because sildenafil potentiates the hypotensive effects of nitrates, resulting in severe hypotension, it should not be administered to patients taking these agents (including cardiac patients who don't take standing doses of nitrates but who might develop angina during intercourse that might require treatment with sublingual nitroglycerin). In addition, sildenafil should not be prescribed to patients with more advanced cardiac or cerebrovascular disease, for whom strenuous physical exertion (including sexual intercourse) would be inadvisable. It may be appropriate to obtain cardiac stress testing to better assess a patient's risk of cardiac ischemia during intercourse.

Sildenafil is well absorbed. Plasma concentrations reach their maximal level within 30 to 120 minutes (60 minutes on average). It is eliminated predominantly by hepatic metabolism and has a half-life of about 4 hours. The recommended starting dose is 50 mg taken 1 hour before sexual activity. The maximal recommended frequency is once per day. Depending upon its effectiveness and side effects, the dose may be increased to 100 mg or decreased to 25 mg. Half-dosages should be prescribed for older patients or for those with renal or hepatic disease. Patients who do not respond to oral therapy may still respond to intracavernous or transurethral therapy or to nonpharmacologic somatic interventions.

Orgasmic Disorders

Female Orgasmic Disorder

Female orgasmic disorder (formerly called inhibited female orgasm) is defined as a persistent or recurrent delay in, or absence of, orgasm following a normal excitement phase. The prevalence of this condition is variable. Delayed or absent orgasm only is considered to be a sexual dysfunction when a woman is *troubled* by it, since *satisfaction* with orgasm is related not only to a woman's consistency of achieving organism but also to her overall satisfaction with the sexual relationship. For example, one survey that examined a group of almost 2500 women visiting a gynecological clinic found that 25% of women experienced "infrequent" orgasm (defined as orgasm occurring less than 30% of the times that they engaged in intercourse) but that only 25% of these women were distressed about it.

The ease with which women can achieve orgasm may fall along a bell-shaped curve. Some women can achieve orgasm *without any genital stimulation* (via fantasy, kissing, or breast stimulation). Some can achieve orgasm (or multiple orgasms) via *coitus alone*. Some can achieve orgasm *only via direct clitoral stimulation* (either alone or during intercourse). Some can achieve orgasm *only via masturbation*. Finally, some women are *unable to achieve orgasm by any means*. The majority of women do not regularly have "vaginal" orgasms but still can experience orgasm following clitoral stimulation; again, they are not considered to have a sexual dysfunction unless this situation causes "marked distress or interpersonal difficulty."

As with hypoactive sexual desire disorder and female sexual arousal disorder, clinicians should direct their attention while taking a medical history to any current general medical conditions or medications that might impede orgasm. **Primary anorgasmia** (i.e., where a woman has never achieved orgasm) has a prevalence of about 5%–10% in the general population. The prognosis is good: most women are ultimately able to achieve orgasm after having received education about genital anatomy, the sexual response cycle, and how to achieve orgasm through masturbation. Following this, couples therapy could be added. Couples may be offered education about the variety of ways that women might achieve orgasm beyond or in addition to coitus, homework assignments aimed at fostering improved communication about sexual matters, and sensate focus exercises.

Secondary anorgasmia (i.e., where a woman only is anorgasmic in certain situations) occurs in up to a third of women. The response rate to treatment is lower in secondary anorgasmia than in primary anorgasmia (about 50%). This group is more heterogeneous, and the response to treatment typically depends on other issues in the couple's relationship, the couple's motivation to engage in treatment, and whether the patient's partner is willing to become involved in the therapy.

Male Orgasmic Disorder

Male orgasmic disorder (also called inhibited male orgasm) is characterized by a persistent or recurrent delay in, or absence of, orgasm following a normal sexual excitement phase. In judging whether orgasm is "delayed," the clinician should take into account the man's age and whether sexual stimulation has been adequate in focus, intensity, and duration. Most men who present for treatment complain of absence of orgasm rather than of a delay in achieving orgasm. Most commonly, the difficulty is *situational* rather than *global*. For example, the man might

be unable to reach orgasm intravaginally although he can ejaculate following manual or oral stimulation by his partner or following masturbation. Some individuals with male orgasmic disorder can reach coital orgasm but only after prolonged and intense noncoital stimulation.

In some cases, the patient is an older man who has been engaging in frequent sexual activity. These patients may respond to education about how the latency period prior to orgasm can become prolonged with age and with increased frequency of sexual contact. While many patients have decided that they need not achieve orgasm on every occasion, others report significant disruption of their marital or sexual relationships. For example, if a man has hidden his lack of coital orgasms from his wife, the couple may present with infertility of unknown cause. Further, while anorgasmia may be the presenting complaint, additional history may reveal that the more significant problem actually is an associated hypoactive sexual desire disorder or paraphilia.

Male orgasmic disorder is the least frequent male complaint in sex clinics. It has been estimated to be present in well under 10% of men. One therefore should be careful in such cases to rule out anorgasmia due to either a general medical condition or substance use, especially when the condition isn't accompanied by hypoactive sexual desire disorder. The sympathetic pathways supplying the penis appear to be more sensitive to various insults than are the parasympathetic pathways that mediate erection, so anorgasmia may be the earliest sign of subtle nerve injury or side effects from pharmacologic agents such as antihypertensives, benzodiazepines, alcohol, and antidepressants.

Treatment might include *behavioral interventions* to minimize performance anxiety (sensate focus, increased stimulation prior to coitus via oral or manual fondling) and/or pharmacologic interventions (e.g., cyproheptadine, a serotonin antagonist, or yohimbine, an α-2 presynaptic antagonist, each taken 1–2 hours prior to intercourse). In more severe cases of anorgasmia due to nerve injury, *anal stimulation* (via an inserted anal probe) may be the most effective intervention.

Premature Ejaculation

Premature ejaculation describes the persistent or recurrent onset of orgasm and ejaculation with minimal sexual stimulation before, upon, or shortly after penetration, and before the person wishes it. The clinician must take into account the presence of various factors that can affect the duration of the excitement phase of the sexual response cycle. These include *age* (latency time increases naturally with aging, and men also may gain greater control with increased sexual experience), *novelty* of the sexual partner or situation, and the current *frequency of sexual activity* (since latency time increases along with increased frequency of intercourse).

The majority of males with this condition can delay orgasm during masturbation for a considerably longer time than during coitus. The man's estimate of the duration of time that typically lapses from the beginning of sexual activity until ejaculation may vary significantly from the report of his partner. The same may be the case with the man's and his partners opinion as to whether the premature ejaculation is a "problem."

Lifelong premature ejaculation is more commonly seen in younger men, while *acquired* premature ejaculation is more often seen in older men in association with male erectile disorder, along with "performance anxiety" and fears of losing the erection during intercourse. The former is the more common presentation, with premature ejaculation occurring in up to 40% of all men. Patients typically present for treatment in their 20s or 30s.

The cause of premature ejaculation is unknown. *Psychological theories* have suggested that the man's feelings toward the sexual partner may play an important role. *Behavioral theories* have suggested that the rapid ejaculatory response may have been "learned" by some individuals during adolescent masturbation (with fears of being discovered by one's parents leading to attempts to reach orgasm rapidly) and also that some men may lack the ability to accurately perceive increasing levels of arousal and to modulate their response to this. However, none of these theories has been proven, and comparison with control groups of men without premature ejaculation has failed to reveal differences in any of these aspects of sexuality.

The most successful treatment strategy has been *behavioral therapy*, which is effective in 80%–97% of cases. The two major behavioral techniques are the *"stop–start" (or "pause")* *procedure* and the *"squeeze" procedure*. Since the male typically finds vaginal intercourse excessively arousing, therapy begins either with masturbation or with manual or oral stimulation by the partner. As the male senses that he is nearing the point of inevitable orgasm, his partner either *pauses* in providing any sexual stimulation until the man's arousal diminishes or else firmly *squeezes* the penis at the coronal ridge (i.e., where the glans joins the shaft) using the thumb and first two fingers. In both cases, the man experiences decreased arousal.

The couple then continues with this pattern of stimulation–interruption several times, ultimately progressing to the point of ejaculation. Over several such sessions, the individual generally gains greater control over arousal and ejaculation such that the periods of stimulation can be increased in duration. At this point, vaginal intercourse can be introduced, using the same technique. Initially, there should be little stimulation or thrusting following penetration, followed by progressive increases over time in the duration of stimulation.

Partners may have difficulty complying with this regimen. The female partner may have become frustrated over the preceding years by her needs not having been met by the patient, and the therapist is now encouraging even *more* attention on her part to her husband's pleasure. Therefore, the couple should be encouraged to include opportunities for the patient to bring his partner to orgasm. The patient might bring his partner to orgasm by providing manual, oral, or vibrator stimulation before engaging in the premature ejaculation exercises. Alternatively, the couple might alternate these "exercise" sessions with other sessions where they focus exclusively on the partner's pleasure.

A potentially more convenient approach is through *pharmacologic interventions*. *Clomipramine*, a serotonergic antidepressant, has been used, given that some patients who have taken this medication to treat obsessive–compulisve disorder have reported increased ejaculatory latency. However, its use has been limited by significant side effects. More recently, clomipramine has been supplanted by the SSRIs. The latter have been prescribed either as a standing daily dose or as a single dose that is taken several hours before intercourse. These agents generally are tolerated well, but sexual side effects can occur, including decreased libido, decreased intensity of orgasm, and erectile dysfunction. These side effects sometimes respond to dosage reduction.

Sexual Pain Disorders

Dyspareunia

Dyspareunia is characterized by genital pain that occurs in association with sexual intercourse. Although it most commonly is experienced during coitus, it also can occur before or after intercourse. The intensity of the symptoms may range from mild discomfort to sharp pain. While the disorder can occur in both males and females, it is much more common in females and typically presents to mental health clinicians only after a previous evaluation by a gynecologist. It may be accompanied by **vaginismus** (discussed below), and it can be difficult to determine whether the vaginismus is occurring secondary to pain, or vice versa.

Dyspareunia due to a general medical condition can accompany *infections* (of the vagina, urinary tract, cervix, or fallopian tubes), *endometriosis*, *surgical scar tissue from an episiotomy*, and *ovarian cysts and tumors*. In postmenopausal and lactating women, *estrogen deficiency* can contribute to decreased vaginal lubrication. *Radiation therapy* for pelvic malignancy is associated with vaginal atrophy and with an increased propensity for traumatic injury and pain. *Vulvar vestibulitis* is a syndrome characterized by pain in the vaginal introitus associated with multiple tiny erythematous sores in the vulvar vestibule. It has been associated with subclinical infection with human papillomavirus, chronic recurrent candidiasis, chronic recurrent bacterial vaginitis, and with the use of certain chemical agents.

Even when dyspareunia has been *initiated* by some medical condition, over the course of time the pain and discomfort can become closely associated with the experience of intercourse, and as a result *phobic avoidance* may be present.

Treatment typically involves treatment of underlying medical problems that are amenable to intervention, education, relaxation exercises, exploratory masturbation, and the use of a lubricant when significant vaginal dryness is present. Sometimes, the use of progressively larger vaginal dilators prior to attempts at intercourse with the partner proves to be useful.

Vaginismus

In **vaginismus**, the patient experiences recurrent or persistent involuntary contraction of the perineal muscles surrounding the outer third of the vagina when vaginal penetration (with penis, a finger, a speculum, sometimes even a tampon) is attempted. In some females, even the *anticipation* of vaginal penetration results in muscle spasm. The degree of muscular contraction may range from mild (inducing a sensation a sensation of moderate tightness and discomfort) to severe (preventing any penetration).

Other aspects of the sexual response cycle (desire, pleasure, orgasmic capacity) may not be impaired unless penetration is attempted or anticipated. The patient may even have an active sex life through manual or oral stimulation. However, the physical obstruction due to muscle contraction usually prevents coitus. For this reason, the condition can limit the development of new sexual relationships and can disrupt existing relationships. Some patients present for treatment due to unconsummated marriage or infertility. Patients and their partners may be quite distressed, especially those who wish to conceive.

Psychological factors often play an important contributory role in vaginismus. Many women with vaginismus developed it as a complication of dyspareunia, with the vaginismus having persisted following treatment for the underlying medical cause of the dyspareunia. Other women present with a history of having been sexually abused or having been indoctrinated during childhood with the notion that sex is "dirty," or "sinful." Some cases are idiopathic.

Treatment involves relaxation training, followed by graded exposure. The approach is similar to that employed to treat sexual aversion disorder. The patient first is taught to gradually explore her own genitalia, followed by attempts to insert her smallest finger or a dilator in the vagina with the assistance of a lubricant. The patient later attempts to insert a larger finger or dilator. When this can be successfully done, the partner can be involved in the therapy through sensate focus exercises ultimately leading to attempts at penetration.

PARAPHILIAS

Phenomenology

In contrast to sexual dysfunction, the **paraphilias** don't involve difficulties in the sexual response cycle. Rather, in the paraphilias, patients' sexual attractions or behaviors are directed at inappropriate *objects*. Paraphilias are characterized by persistent (over a period of at least 6 months), recurrent, intense, sexually arousing fantasies, urges, or behaviors that generally involve either *nonhuman objects, the suffering or humiliation of oneself or one's partner*, or *children or other nonconsenting persons*.

Paraphilias included in the *DSM-IV* include **exhibitionism** (exposing one's genitals), **fetishism** (using nonliving objects), **frotteurism** (touching and rubbing against nonconsenting persons), **pedophilia** (focusing on prepubescent children), **sexual masochism** (receiving humiliation or suffering), **sexual sadism** (inflicting humiliation or suffering), **transvestic fetishism** (cross-dressing), and **voyeurism** (observing sexual activity). A residual category, **paraphilia not otherwise specified**, includes other, less frequently encountered paraphilias. These include **telephone scatologia** (making obscene phone calls), **necrophilia** (being attracted to corpses), **partialism** (exclusively focusing on part of the body), **zoophilia** (being attracted to animals), **coprophilia** (focusing on feces), **klismaphilia** (focusing on enemas), **urophilia** (focusing on urine), and **hypoxyphilia** (focusing on self-asphyxiation during sexual arousal).

Paraphilias are *socially defined constructs*. If a man is greatly aroused by women who wear lingerie or high heels or enjoys "role playing" during intercourse, and if his partner is not bothered by these preferences or even enjoys them herself, his pattern of sexual arousal is not considered to be "deviant." However, should his fantasies, urges, or behaviors be disturbing or dangerous to himself or to those around him, he could be diagnosed as having a paraphilia.

It also should be noted that an individual can engage in *inappropriate* and even *illegal* sexual conduct and still not have a paraphilia, provided that the individual does not experience *recurrent, deviant sexual urges*. For example, a college student who becomes intoxicated at a football game and "moons" the crowd but who otherwise does not experience recurrent urges to expose himself to strangers would not be considered to have exhibitionism despite having committed the crime of "indecent exposure."

With rare exceptions (primarily involving sadomasochistic practices), virtually all individuals with paraphilia are male. For some of these individuals, the paraphilia is *exclusive*—that is, paraphiliac fantasies or stimuli are obligatory for them to experience erotic arousal and their sexual preferences are always included in sexual activity. In other cases, the paraphilia is *nonexclusive*—that is, the individual can experiences both conventional and paraphiliac sexual desires, although the paraphiliac activities often are preferred.

Paraphiliac urges or behaviors may occur only *episodically*, particularly during periods of increased stress. While early studies suggested that individuals with paraphilia typically only have a single paraphiliac interest and rarely "cross over" into other paraphiliac behaviors, more recent research suggests that individuals with one paraphilia actually are quite likely to have one or more others. Therefore, a detailed and directive history exploring all aspects of sexual arousal is essential in evaluating paraphilia.

As we have seen in the case of other disorders of motivated behavior such as the substance-related disorders and the eating disorders, there are some individuals who are distressed by their cravings and unsuccessfully attempt to resist them such that their cravings are considered to be "ego dystonic." In other cases, however, the individual believes that the cravings are acceptable or even desirable, such that the cravings are considered "ego syntonic." This is also the case with paraphilias.

Not surprisingly, treatment interventions are generally much less effective when sexual cravings are ego syntonic. Patients who lack the *desire* to stop engaging in aberrant behaviors are unlikely to do so as a result of individual or group therapy. Rather, they usually persist in rationalizing, minimizing, or denying the significance of their behaviors and its impact on others.

Further, many individuals with paraphilias have been referred for treatment by a court order. Those who have not yet gone to trial and who are averring innocence of all criminal charges generally have little incentive to cooperate with the evaluation or to admit to any wrongdoing. Even in cases where the evaluee already has been convicted of a sexual offense and where treatment is an obligatory aspect of his sentence, he may be more interested in demonstrating to the court his cooperation with therapy and his ultimate "cure" than with truly changing his behavior. In general, treatment is more likely to be effective both when the evaluation takes place after a criminal defendant has been found guilty of an offense and when the duration of the sentence hasn't been made contingent on the outcome of treatment.

However, it is likely that many individuals residing in the community have paraphilias and are genuinely disturbed by their sexual cravings or behaviors. The population encountered by most clinicians almost certainly is not representative, given that individuals referred by the court have been *arrested* for their behavior while most deviant sexual behavior in the community goes undetected. Unfortunately, embarrassment about deviant sexual urges and behaviors makes it unlikely that most individuals will present for treatment of their own initiative. In addition, it is unlikely that individuals with pedophilia will present for treatment voluntarily given that physicians are ethically and legally bound to report patients known to be engaging in child abuse. Ironically, providing treatment to individuals with pedophilia is likely the most effective way to protect children from them.

It is likely that paraphilias are extremely common in the community. Many individuals with socially unacceptable sexual cravings probably either resist their urges or integrate them into "acceptable" sexual practices. Examples of the latter include engaging in private fantasy during intercourse or engaging in role playing with a willing partner or a hired prostitute. Individuals who instead engage in illegal paraphiliac activity often have an additional clinical condition that contributes to behavioral disinhibition or exploitation of others such as a personality disorder, or a substance-related disorder or a mood disorder.

As with all behavioral conditions, paraphiliac behavior likely occurs in the general population along a spectrum of severity, with those individuals who present for treatment likely representing the most severe cases—the "tip of the iceberg." For example, one survey asked 94 males in the community to describe their fantasies during masturbation or intercourse. Sixty-two percent reported fantasies of initiating a young girl into sexuality, 33% described fantasies of raping adult females, 11% had masochistic fantasies, 5% had fantasies of having sex with an animal, and 3% had fantasies of initiating a young boy into sexuality.

Another survey asked 60 male undergraduates about their participation in and/or fantasies involving sexual behavior. Sixty-five percent actually had engaged in some paraphiliac activity: 42% had participated in voyeurism, 35% in frottage, 8% obscene phone calls, 5% coercive sexual activity, 3% sexual contact with girls under 12 years of age, and 2% exhibitionism. Further, 54% desired to be involved in some voyeuristic activity, 7% desired participation in exhibitionistic behavior, and 5% reported a desire for sexual activity with girls under the age of 12.

Individuals with paraphilias are rarely self-referred and usually come to the attention of mental health professionals only when their behavior has brought them into conflict with sexual partners or society. Often, the individual denies having any inappropriate urges. Physiologic testing can be a useful adjunct to the clinical evaluation in some of these cases. For example, *penile plethysmography* assesses for evidence of penile erection as the subject is presented with a variety of paraphiliac stimuli. A positive test can be used to help persuade the patient to admit to a deviant pattern of arousal. Similarly, in the setting of *group therapy* specifically targeted at convicted sexual offenders, individuals who initially deny ever having experienced deviant sexual urges ultimately might admit to having had them following confrontation by other members of the group.

However, there is no specific test that allows the clinician to reliably determine whether an individual truly experiences recurrent, powerful, deviant sexual urges in the face of that individual adamantly denying having such urges. Even the penile plethysmograph is not a "lie detector," since some individuals can successfully suppress their sexual responses. Nor is there a "personality profile" that allows one to say with any certainty that an individual does or does not have a paraphilia. There likely are many individuals with paraphiliac disorders who lead otherwise-"normal" lives.

Sometimes the individual's lifestyle can present clues from which the presence of a paraphilia can be *inferred*. For example, a person with pedophilia may be noted to be friends with many children in the neighborhood, or he may have entered a profession that involves frequent contact with children. If the individual is discovered to have a collection of pornography, the type of pornography may reflect his preferred erotic stimulus (children, high-heeled shoes, crossdressing, etc.). Sexual dysfunction in the individual's current sexual relationship may be present due to the individual attempting to engage in sexual intercourse in the absence of the preferred erotic stimulus.

Paraphilia represents a major public health problem. Twenty percent of adult women have been the victim of individuals with either exhibitionism or voyeurism. Exhibitionists engage in their behavior a median of 50 times before they ultimately are arrested. Similarly, almost 30% of women and 15% of men report having been sexually abused prior to age 18, in many cases by individuals with pedophilia. Studies of nonincarcerated individuals with pedophilia reveal them to have engaged in an extremely large number of paraphiliac acts prior to having entered treatment, ranging from 23 to 282 acts. Therefore, while society clearly needs to protect children, the best way to protect the greatest number of children would be to provide intensive, proactive treatment to individuals with pedophilia.

Unfortunately, treatment is not readily available to most individuals with paraphilia either in the correctional setting or in the community. Most psychiatrists, and certainly most physicians, receive little training in the treatment of these disorders. The primary intervention has been incarceration. Over 10% of the prison population in the United States consists of sex offenders. While it is appropriate for individuals to be held accountable for their behavior, there is little evidence that incarceration in itself is an effective treatment strategy. For example, an individual may continue to masturbate to deviant fantasies throughout his period of incarceration, the paraphiliac arousal pattern thereby being preferentially reinforced given the unavailability of more appropriate sexual activity.

Etiology

Clearly, biological factors play a role in shaping sexual preference and sexual drives. However, no specific biological factor has been isolated that accounts for paraphiliac behavior. Further, most studies of various biomarkers in paraphilia have involved men who have engaged in sexually aggressive acts, so the findings may not be applicable to all paraphilias.

In some violent and/or sexually violent men, testosterone levels are abnormally high. However, this has not been a consistent finding. In two studies, aggressive pedophiles and age-matched control subjects were injected with gonadotropin-releasing hormone (which stimulates release of luteinizing hormone, which in turn stimulates testosterone release). The pedophiles tended to oversecrete luteinizing hormone, suggesting hyperactivity at the level of the hypothalamic–pituitary axis. This difference was noted even after controlling for the presence of alcohol or drug abuse, violence, and comorbid mental illness.

There may be a higher-than-expected prevalence of learning disorders and neurologic soft signs in the sex offender population, and some neuroimaging studies have suggested the possibility of smaller left temporal parietal regions in this group as well. However, other studies have found no differences between subjects with paraphilia and control subjects in either neuroimaging tests or neuropsychological tests.

Taken together, these findings suggest that some individuals with paraphilias may be predisposed to engage in their behavior by subtle neuropsychological deficits or hormonal abnormalities. However, whether these findings relate to the paraphiliac behaviors themselves or to distinct comorbid contributory factors (such as learning disorder or personality disorder) remains uncertain.

One *ethnological theory* suggests that paraphilia appears selectively in men because male sexual appetites are different from female sexual appetites. In early societies, the man who had sex with 50 women could sire over 50 children; in contrast, the woman who had sex with 50 men would have no more descendants than the woman who slept with one man. Therefore, from an evolutionary perspective, men seeking to maximize their reproductive advantage should seek *quantity* in sexual partners, while women should seek *quality*—that is, secure resources and good genes. Men also appear to be drawn preferentially to younger and more nubile-appearing women, perhaps to further their reproductive advantage. Given that men are less selective in general, perhaps the fact that some men are drawn to preadolescent girls or even preadolescent boys may represent excessive variation along a biologically driven dimension of behavior.

Potential examples of this ethnologic theory can be seen on modern college campuses. When asked how many sexual partners they would like to have in the next 2 years, most college-age males reply, "Eight." In contrast, most college-age women reply, "One." Similarly, one group of researchers hired attractive assistants to approach college students of the opposite sex and sexually proposition them, out of the blue. Seventy-five percent of the males that the female assistants approached accepted the proposition (with many of the remaining 25% asking for a "rain check"), but 0% of the women accepted the proposition.

Many individuals with paraphilia begin to show a pattern of deviant sexual behavior during early adolescence. In pedophilia, the deviant pattern of arousal occurs before age 19 in half of all cases, often before the age of 15. Almost all paraphilias are well established by age 25. Ideally, clinical intervention would be aimed at these adolescents, with the goal being to remedy maladaptive thoughts and behaviors before they become more firmly established.

Parents might rationalize deviant sexual behavior engaged in by their adolescent child as simply being "sexual exploration." Certainly, one must be cautious about labeling *any* sexual contact between children or adolescents of different ages as reflecting pedophilia. However, in one study of adolescent males with paraphilia, the age of onset of nondeviant sexual behavior tended to predate the age of onset of deviant sexual behavior. This finding is consistent with the hypothesis that deviant sexual behavior isn't sim-

ply early exploration. Rather, deviant sexual behavior appears later but then is *preferentially reinforced*. Similarly, in one study of convicted adult rapists and child molesters, many subjects recalled a gradual progression from nonviolent sex crimes during adolescence to more serious sexual assaults during early adulthood.

It is likely that several factors contribute to this initiation of deviant sexual behavior during adolescence. These include having been sexually or physically abused. For example, a child who has been strangled may develop a predilection for autoerotic asphyxiation, while a child whose parents gave him frequent enemas might develop klismaphilia. Portrayals of violent or deviant sexuality in the media also may play an important contributory role.

The process of coming to ultimately prefer one particular paraphiliac object may be a result of early happenstance or of trial and error. For example, an individual may have spied on his sister and become sexually aroused, or may have found his mother's underwear and become aroused, leading to voyeurism or transvestic fetishism, respectively. Similarly, the precociously sexual adolescent may have experimented sexually with a preadolescent child due to the child's availability and found that there were no negative consequences. After this, the individual may have begun masturbating to fantasies involving sexual activity with preadolescents; as a result, his fetish became increasingly associated with orgasm, a powerful reinforcer. Ultimately, pedophilia therefore may have become his *preferred* sexual outlet.

However, the general belief that pedophilia is "caused" by childhood molestation is unfounded. The prevalence of childhood sexual abuse among imprisoned pedophiles has been found to be less than the prevalence among inmates who are not pedophiles. Clearly, childhood molestation is an important *risk factor* for pedophilia, with 24% of people who molest girls and 40% of people who molest boys reporting that they themselves were molested as children. However, this means that the *majority* of individuals with pedophilia were *not* abused as children. Further, 10% of all men in the general population report that they were sexually abused as children, but the overwhelming majority of them do not become pedophiles. Similarly, while 20% of women report having been sexually abused as children, pedophilia is essentially nonexistent among women.

Overall, while the origins of paraphilia remain uncertain, it is likely that—as in other behavioral disorders—some individuals carry a greater risk of developing the disorder due to biological vulnerability, while factors arising during childhood and adolescence likely help to initiate and then shape the behavior. However, paraphiliac behavior ultimately becomes *self-reinforcing*, even in the absence of the original initiating factors. Treatment therefore must attempt to address the ongoing behavior itself.

Treatment

As with other behavioral disorders, it is important to confront the individual early on about the need to stop engaging in problematic behavior. Many individuals present for treatment as a result of legal coercion (usually a probation agreement), and their continued freedom from incarceration depends upon their continuing to abstain from paraphiliac behavior. In other cases, fear of rearrest can play an important motivational role.

Some individuals also are motivated to address their paraphilia by an appreciation of the negative consequences of their behavior for others. However, other individuals rely excessively on cognitive distortions such as extensive rationalization and projection. For example, the individual with pedophilia may state that a 6-year-old boy was old enough to make a "rational choice" about engaging in intercourse with him and may even state that the child "initiated" the sexual activity and that he was helpless to resist the sexual pressures that this boy placed on him. Similarly, the exhibitionist may interpret a woman's surprise when he exposed himself as her having been impressed and aroused by the sight of his penis. Sexual offenders also may repeatedly insist that "nobody was harmed" by their illegal actions.

While psychodynamic therapy may be helpful in allowing some individuals to understand themselves better, it has not proven to be very effective in interrupting ingrained behavioral patterns and reducing criminal recidivism. Cognitive–behavioral therapy, using a *relapse-prevention approach* similar to that used to treat substance abuse, is the most common type of therapy offered by sex-offender treatment programs.

Typically, an individual's patterns of arousal are explored with him, sometimes with the assistance of penile plethysmography testing. The goal is to help the individual identify high-risk situations and how to manage them better or avoid them. Group therapy can be helpful in encouraging the patient to confront cognitive distortions, to avoid reinforcing stimuli (e.g., pornography related to his paraphilia), and to engage in other life activities. The patient also may be encouraged to engage in empathy training exercises through discussion and written exercises centering on the effects of childhood molestation on victims' later lives.

Psychotherapy may be augmented by *pharmacologic agents* aimed at decreasing sexual cravings. **Antiandrogen agents** decrease sex drive overall and therefore also can decrease paraphiliac cravings. Following the administration of these agents, an individual ideally still can engage in nonparaphiliac sexual activities but will gain a greater ability to resist deviant sexual urges. Individuals treated with these agents sometimes feel very relieved, as their paraphiliac fantasies have been intense, repetitive, and distracting.

Cyproterone acetate acts directly to block central and peripheral androgen receptors. It has been used abroad but is not available in the United States. **Medroxyprogesterone acetate (Provera)**, available in sustained release form as Depo-Provera, is the antiandrogen employed most commonly in the United States. In contrast to cyproterone, it decreases testosterone levels indirectly. A synthetic progestogenic hormone, it exerts negative feedback effects, leading to decreased release of both luteinizing hormone (LH) and follicle-stimulating hormone (FSH), which in turn leads to reduced androgen output by the testicles. It also appears to increase the clearance of serum testosterone through increased hepatic metabolism. **Leuprolide acetate (Lupron)** is a synthetic analogue of gonadotropin-releasing hormone. Like medroxyprogesterone, it is available in a long-acting injectable form. While it initially triggers an increase in testosterone release, chronic administration suppresses serum testosterone release due to depletion of LH. The circulating testosterone levels achieved with use of leuprolide are lower than those achieved with medroxyprogesterone. Whether this allows for greater efficacy is unclear since the testosterone levels achieved with both agents are below prepubertal levels.

Neither antiandrogen medication nor surgical castration is a "cure" for paraphilia. Individuals still can commit sex offenses while taking these medications, even after surgical castration. Further, antiandrogen medications can cause significant side effects, including weight gain. hypertension, impaired glucose tolerance, and gallbladder disease. Given this, most clinicians who treat sex offenders consider it unethical to force these medications on patients.

Serotonin reuptake inhibitors (SSRIs) also appear to be useful in treating some individuals with paraphilia. Like antiandrogen agents, they appear to reduce intrusive sexual fantasies and urges and to improve control over sexual impulses. It remains uncertain at this point whether they are more or less effective than antiandrogen medications. It also isn't certain whether their benefits arise from antiobsessional effects, anti-impulsiveness effects, or libido-suppressive effects.

GENDER IDENTITY DISORDERS (TRANSSEXUALISM)

Individuals with **gender identity disorder** exhibit a strong, persistent cross-gender identification. They have a strong desire to *be* of the other sex, or they insist that they actually *are* of the other sex despite their external appearance. This cross-gender identification should not simply reflect a desire to achieve perceived *cultural advantages* that accrue to individuals of other sex Rather, there should be evidence of persistent discomfort about one's assigned sex or a sense of inappropriateness of the gender role associated with that sex.

This disorder is rare. While there are no epidemiological studies to provide data on its prevalence, data from smaller countries in Europe with access to total population statistics and referrals suggest that roughly 1 in 30,000 adult males and 1 in 100,000 adult females seek sex-reassignment surgery.

The cross-gender identification typically begins between the ages of 2 and 4. Boys may cross-dress and pretend to be women. They typically enjoy engaging in feminine activities such as playing house (acting the part of female figures such as the mother), drawing pictures of beautiful girls and princesses, watching television or videos of their favorite female characters, and playing with Barbie dolls. They avoid rough-and-tumble play and competitive sports, and they demonstrate little interest in cars, trucks, or other stereotypical "boy's" toys. They may express a wish to be a girl or assert that they will grow up to be a woman. They may insist on sitting to urinate and may pretend not to have a penis by pushing it between their legs.

Girls with the disorder may prefer boy's clothing and short hair and often are misidentified by strangers as being boys. They may ask to be called by a boy's name. Their fantasy heroes are most often powerful male figures, such as Batman or Superman. They prefer boys as playmates and prefer to engage in contact sports, rough-and-tumble play, and traditional boyhood games. They usually show little interest in dolls or any form of feminine dress-up or role-play activity. They might refuse to urinate in a sitting position. They may claim that they have or will soon "grow" a penis, that they don't want to grow breasts or menstruate, and that they will grow up to be a man.

Children tend to be referred for evaluation around the time of school entry due to parental concern that what initially appeared to be a "phase" does not seem to be passing. Only a fraction of children with gender identity disorder continue to have symptoms that fulfill the criteria for gender identity disorder into later adolescence or adulthood. Over time, most of them display less overt cross-gender behaviors, especially in the face of ongoing negative responses from parents and peers. By late adolescence or adulthood, about three-quarters of boys with childhood gender identity disorder report that they have a homosexual or bisexual orientation but do not experience strong cross-gender identification. Most of the remainder report having a heterosexual orientation, but again without cross-gender identification. The corresponding percentages for sexual orientation in girls are not known. However, some adolescents continue to demonstrate strong cross-gender identification and may present requesting sex-reassignment surgery.

Individuals who continue to demonstrate gender identity disorder into adulthood remain preoccupied with their wish to live as a member of the other sex and voice discomfort at being viewed by other members of society as a member of their assigned sex. In private, they may spend a great deal of time cross-dressed, and many ultimately attempt to pass in public as the other sex. With cross-dressing and hormonal treatment (and for males, electrolysis), many individuals with this disorder are convincingly able to do so. They may express an intense desire to acquire the physical appearance of the other sex through hormonal or surgical manipulation. Their sexual activity with same-sex partners is generally constrained by their preference that their partners neither see nor touch their genitals, and for some males, sexual activity with a woman is accompanied by the fantasy that they are lesbian lovers or that his partner is a man and he is a woman.

When patients present requesting sex-reassignment surgery or hormonal treatment, careful assessment is necessary. To begin with, not all of these individuals have gender identity disorder. Some individuals with *severe personality disorders*, especially borderline personality disorder, exhibit a disturbance in their sense of identity in general (not simply their gender identity), and some of them come to believe that all of these problems will magically resolve following a sex change operation. *Effeminate homosexuals* may present with a desire to change sex in order for their behavior to be more socially acceptable. Individuals with *transvestic fetishism* sometimes develop gender dysphoria at a later stage, again perhaps seeing this as a way of making their transvestic impulses more acceptable. In each of these latter cases, careful questioning (and sometimes the use of collateral informants) reveals that the individual's gender identity actually is consistent with his or her biologic sex. Given this, the appropriate treatment is psychotherapy aimed at helping the individual learn to deal with chronic identity disturbance and the superimposed life crises that may have precipitated the desire to seek surgical intervention.

Obviously, sex-reassignment surgery is permanent. While the outcome can be favorable in selected cases, it isn't a panacea. Clinical outcomes appear to be best for those individuals who are psychologically stable, who have lived successfully in their desired gender role for at least a year prior to the surgery (with the assistance of hormonal therapy), and who have engaged in psychotherapy prior to and following the surgery. The goals of psychotherapy are to confirm that the diagnosis is correct and also to make certain that patients have realistic expectations of the surgery and have fully considered other options.

SUMMARY

"Sexuality" refers to a complex group of behaviors mediated not only by neurologic, vascular, and endocrine systems but also by societal and personal attitudes. The major aspects of an individual's "sexuality" include sexual identity, gender identity, gender role, sexual orientation, and sexual behavior. The sexual response cycle is sensitive to a variety of insults, including aging, medical and psychiatric illness, and stress. In addition, since sexual coupling requires contact with others, one cannot think about the individual with a sexual disorder in isolation.

In this chapter, we have discussed the sexual dysfunctions (characterized by a disturbance in some aspect of the sexual response cycle), the paraphilias (characterized by a disturbance not in one's sexual drive or sexual performance but in the *object* of one's sexual drives), and gender identity disorder (characterized by strong and persistent cross-gender identification).

Treatment of these conditions in the primary care setting begins with taking a complete history (including a detailed sexual history, social history, medical history, and psychiatric history) and conducting a physical examination. Following this, patients usually are provided with basic education (which may in itself be an effective treatment intervention), followed by behavioral and psychotherapeutic interventions (often involving the patient and his or her partner). Urologic or psychiatric referral is indicated in some cases.

Chapter 16

Suicide

Every physician at some point must deal with patients who either previously have attempted suicide or who will commit suicide while under the
physician's care. Suicide is the ninth leading cause
of death in the United States, accounting for
30,000 deaths each year. It is especially important
for primary care physicians to have some understanding of how to assess for suicidality since
most individuals who attempt or complete suicide
seek medical treatment shortly before doing so,
most often from their primary care physician.

People encountered in the primary care setting
are at higher risk for committing suicide than are
other members of the general population. This
likely reflects the higher rate of suicide among
people with medical illnesses and also the fact
that persons with mental illnesses that predispose
to suicide (such as major depressive disorder or
panic disorder) also are more likely to require
general medical care.

Retrospective studies involving individuals
who have successfully committed suicide reveal
them to have visited their primary care practitioners more often during the 4-month period before the suicide than during the previous 4
months. About 80% of those who commit suicide visit their physician within 6 months of the
suicide, 50% within 1 month of the suicide, and
40% within 1 week of the suicide. However, despite this potential opportunity for intervention,
doctors frequently do not detect suicidal ideation
in their patients.

While suicide occurs more frequently *in the
setting* of particular psychiatric diseases such as
major depressive disorder, schizophrenia, and
substance dependence, suicide *itself* is not a diagnosis. Rather, suicide is a *behavior*. While individuals with particular diseases engage in this
behavior with greater frequency than do other individuals, suicidal behavior cuts across a wide
variety of diagnoses.

Similarly, being "suicidal" is not an enduring
personality trait. Given this, one shouldn't waste
one's time attempting to determine whether an
individual is or is not a "suicidal person." No single suicidal personality has been identified, just
as no particular "alcoholic personality" or
"anorexic personality" has been identified.
Whether a person is "suicidal" may even change
from one day to the next, which is hardly consistent with "suicidal" being a personality trait.

Like other behaviors, suicidal thoughts and behaviors occur commonly among members of the
the general population and fall along a spectrum
of severity. Suicidal *ideation* is common, occurring at some point in up to a third of the population. Far fewer people actually have attempted
suicide. Among this group are individuals who
actually have engaged in suicidal *gestures*—that
is, deliberately nonlethal attempts designed more

to elicit "rescue" by friends or family than to cause their own death. Also among this group are individuals who truly desired to die at the time of their attempt but who shortly after the attempt expressed regret over the attempt as well as relief at having survived. Finally, this group also includes individuals who strongly desire to end their lives and ultimately succeed in doing so.

Retrospective analyses reveal that 90% of individuals who have successfully committed suicide had some psychiatric illness at the time of the suicide, most commonly major depressive disorder, alcohol dependence, or schizophrenia. However, no single disorder is "synonymous" with suicide. For example, while up to 15% of people hospitalized with more severe major depressive disorder ultimately die by suicide, this means that over 85% of these individuals do *not* commit suicide. Suicidal behavior therefore appears to be multidetermined, even in the case of individuals with severe mental illness.

Suicidal patients reach clinical attention in several ways. Some present to their physician or to an emergency room explicitly requesting help for their suicidal thoughts. Others present for treatment of physical complaints but upon further questioning reveal that they are having suicidal thoughts. Yet others present to the emergency room for medical attention following a failed suicide attempt. In all of these scenarios, several questions immediately present themselves: Is the patient still "suicidal"? Is a particular course of treatment indicated? Can the patient be released or should he be admitted to a psychiatric inpatient unit? Can he be admitted to the hospital on a voluntary basis, or does he require involuntary civil commitment to the hospital?

A psychiatrist is called to assess a 40-year-old white male auto mechanic following an "overdose" with 10 acetaminophen tablets. The patient began to feel nauseated shortly after this ingestion and presented to the emergency room for treatment. Only after further questioning did he ultimately admit to having taken the overdose, leading to the consultation. The patient states that he has been going through a difficult separation from his wife over the past several months, during which time he has been living in an efficiency apartment with few possessions or furniture. While he previously drank alcohol only on weekends, since the separation he has been drinking during the week as well. A few hours before the overdose, he learned that his wife was dating a male friend of his. He took the pills impulsively, after about 5 minutes of thought. He had not been drinking at the time. He did not speak to anybody prior to taking the pills. Asked why he had not done so, he replies that he doesn't have many close friends.

When asked how he picked the number of tablets to take, the patient replies that this was the number of tablets left in the bottle. He describes having experienced a lower mood over the past few weeks, with difficulty sleeping, anhedonia, loss of appetite, and difficulty concentrating at work. His past psychiatric history is notable for having taken a similar overdose 3 years earlier, following an argument with his wife during which she had threatened to leave him. He reports past periods of lower mood lasting up to several weeks for which he has never received psychiatric evaluation or treatment. He reports a family history of depression in his mother, treated years ago with electroconvulsive therapy, and also notes that his maternal uncle committed suicide but that he doesn't know any of the details about this. His past medical history is notable for peptic ulcer disease and hypertension.

The patient reports that he is still having suicidal thoughts. However, he feels that he'll "be all right" and he refuses voluntary psychiatric hospitalization. He states that he'll lose his job if he doesn't show up the next day because he has been tardy on several occasions over the past few weeks. The psychiatrist decides to pursue involuntary civil commitment. He diagnoses major depressive disorder, alcohol abuse, and possible dependent personality disorder. On the inpatient unit, the patient is initially observed by the nursing staff every 15 minutes as a "suicide precaution." Upon admission, he is asked to sign a "suicide contract" in which he formally agrees to let the staff know if he is feeling like hurting himself, and he reluctantly does so. He also agrees to take an antidepressant medication.

Over the next 2 days, the patient is noted to be superficially social with peers but reluctant to discuss any personal issues with the nursing staff, with the attending psychiatrist, and in therapy groups. He reports that his mood is improving, however, and after his second day on the inpatient unit he consistently denies experiencing any suicidal thoughts. He attends an Alcoholics Anonymous meeting and reports afterward that he found this to be helpful.

On his third inpatient day, the patient's 15-minute-check status is discontinued and he is allowed to leave the unit with staff accompaniment.

On his fourth hospital day, he attempts to telephone his wife but she refuses to speak with him.

Following this incident, he discusses with his nurse his feelings of frustration, grief, and jealousy. The nurse sees this as having been a "good session" since the patient for the first time has been able to talk about his feelings. At the end of the session, the patient has a brighter affect and tells the nurse that the session was very helpful and helped him "put things in better perspective." He tells the nurse that he is looking forward to addressing these issues further in psychotherapy following his hospital discharge. One hour later, he sneaks off the unit as the meal trays are being wheeled in, jumps from the roof of the hospital parking garage, and dies.

This case raises several important questions. First, *can clinicians accurately predict who is or isn't going to commit suicide?* Involuntary civil commitment—that is, detaining a person in a psychiatric facility against his or her will—is predicated in most states on the clinician asserting to legal authorities following a clinical evaluation that it is his opinion that "the patient is a danger to himself or others." If clinicians cannot accurately predict who will or will not ultimately go on to commit suicide, should the legal system be allowed to detain *any* individuals?

Second, *when is psychiatric hospitalization indicated?* Placing a person in the hospital, whether voluntarily or involuntarily, isn't always beneficial. For example, the patient in the above example was concerned about the possibility of losing his job if he were hospitalized. If this had happened, perhaps it would have increased rather than decreased his risk of suicide following hospital discharge. Third, *are some clinical variables more predictive of suicide than others?* Finally, even if higher-risk patients *can* be identified based on the clinical evaluation, *what steps should be taken* to reduce this risk?

WHY CLINICIANS CAN'T "PREDICT" SUICIDE

In answer to the first question, several large studies have reached the same conclusion: clinicians are not able to accurately predict which particular patients ultimately will or will not commit suicide. Why is this the case?

First, while epidemiologic studies have identified relevant *risk factors* for suicide that are statistically valid when applied to *groups* of patients, these risk factors are too numerous and too nonspecific to be useful when applied to an *individual* patient. Second, suicide occurs *so rarely* in the general population that even excellent clinicians cannot avoid overpredicting suicide in their clinical practice. Third, other factors that are outside of the clinician's control commonly are present that impede reliable prediction of suicide, particularly prediction over the longer term. These include the potential unreliability of the information provided by patients (who might either minimize their suicide potential or exaggerate it) and also the potential for the patient to encounter intervening variables subsequent to the clinical evaluation that alter his risk of committing suicide but that were unforeseeable at the time of the evaluation.

Relevance of Risk Factors in Specific Cases

The two most significant studies concerning the effort to predict suicide, involving thousands of patients, were conducted by Pokorny in 1983 and by Goldstein and associates in 1991. The Pokorney study prospectively followed 4800 consecutive psychiatric inpatients for 5 years following their hospital discharge in an attempt to determine whether particular variables predicted which patients ultimately went on to commit suicide. Data were collected using several instruments and included demographic information as well as rating scales for depression, anxiety, and psychotic symptoms. In all, 21 different items were used to identify a group of 803 patients who were considered to be at a higher risk of suicide.

Of the original group of 4800 patients, 67 patients committed suicide over the next 5 years. Only 30 (less than half of this group) had been in the high-risk group. In addition, while 30 of the 803 high-risk patients (3.7%) did go on to commit suicide, 773 of these patients (96.3%) did *not* go on to commit suicide.

Goldstein and associates modified Pokorney's statistical model. They prospectively followed 1906 patients who had been admitted to the hospital for treatment of a mood disorder. Again, while statistically significant risk factors could be identified for the *entire* group, the model wasn't sensitive or specific enough to prospectively identify which *particular* patients later went on to commit suicide.

The Base-Rate Problem

While suicide occurs commonly enough to constitute a major cause of mortality, it occurs rarely enough that most patients being assessed for suicide will not go on to commit suicide, even when the patient has multiple high-risk factors. Given this, if a clinician predicts that a given patient will go on to commit suicide, he will be wrong much more often than he is right. This doesn't reflect poor interviewing skills or clinical acumen. It simply reflects the nature of low baserate phenomena.

For example, we know that in the general population, 10–12 out of 100,000 people in the general population (0.01%) commit suicide. Let us therefore assume that the frequency of suicide among the patients encountered by the psychiatrists in one particular emergency room is 10 times this number, or 1 out of every 1000 patients. (Note that I am only postulating this figure and that it is not based on actual patient samples.) Let us also assume that the psychiatrists in this emergency room are brilliant clinicians and can predict which patients ultimately will go on to commit suicide with 95% accuracy.

Therefore, of 100,000 patients evaluated, 100 patients (1 in 1000) ultimately will commit suicide, while the remaining 99,900 ultimately won't commit suicide. Since these psychiatrists are 95% accurate in their predictions, of the 100 patients who do go on to commit suicide, 95 patients will be correctly predicted. However, of the 99,900 patients who do *not* go on to commit suicide, 5% (i.e., 4995 people) will be wrongly predicted to commit suicide. In other words, because suicide is a behavior with a very low base rate, even a highly sensitive and specific test will produce many false positives.

This base-rate problem isn't unique to psychiatry. Any time that a diagnostic test for a particular condition is used to screen a large population (rather than to screen members of a specific high-risk group), the base rate of the condition will be lower and the number of false positives will be commensurately higher.

Inability to Trust
Patient Disavowals

In making a diagnosis, clinicians typically rely upon the history and mental status examination, which in turn depend on the patient's ability and willingness to introspect and then accurately describe internal mental experiences to the clinician. In routine clinical practice, this is not a major issue because most patients who present voluntarily for medical care have little incentive to lie.

However, patients who seriously wish to commit suicide and do not wish to be prevented from doing so are more likely to lie to evaluating clinicians. Most patients view treatment providers as resources and allies, but suicidal patients sometimes view them as obstacles. Given this, the clinician needs to consider the *entire* clinical scenario and not simply a patient's avowals or disavowals of suicidal thoughts or intent. Clinicians who in the past have been "burned" by a patient who alleged not to have any suicidal intent but who then went on commit suicide understandably may become more "conservative" in their management approach, preferring to err on the side of protection even when this requires involuntarily hospitalizing the patient.

"Parasuicide" and Malingering

The opposite also can be true. There are a large number of individuals who engage in self-harm *without* the expectation of dying. Some of these individuals are **malingering**—feigning mental illness or suicidal thinking in order to gain admission to a psychiatric unit and avoid situations such as incarceration or homelessness.

Other individuals engage in self-injurious behavior in order to get attention from significant others rather than in order to die. Their "suicide attempts" are usually of lower lethality and involve a greater expectation of rescue. For example, they might superficially cut their wrists or take a small number of pills and then immediately telephone a friend or their therapist to inform them that they have done so.

Such behavior has been termed "**parasuicide**." Parasuicidal patients are more likely to be younger (under age 35), female, and to have an adjustment disorder or cluster B personality disorder as their primary diagnosis. In contrast, suicide "completers" are more likely to be male, over age 60, and to have major depressive disorder, a psychotic disorder, and/or a substance-related disorder (especially alcohol dependence) as their primary diagnosis.

However, clinicians must take all suicide attempts seriously, even when they suspect parasuicide or malingering. For example, 10% of patients evaluated for what appears to be parasuicide ultimately go on to successfully commit suicide. In some cases, the later suicide is unintentional. For example, the patient may not realize that overdosing on an over-the-counter medication such as acetaminophen can be lethal or that in cutting one's wrist "superficially" one also might accidentally lacerate a major blood vessel. In other cases, a patient who has been parasuicidal earlier in life becomes genuinely suicidal at a later point.

Even when the clinician strongly suspects malingering—for example, when the individual has "attempted suicide" on the same day that he has been arrested and admitted to jail, the clinician also must avoid relying on overly simplistic rules of thumb (e.g., "jail equals malingering"). For example, suicide is the major cause of death in jails, and the majority of jailhouse suicides occur on the day of admission.

Intervening Variables Impede Long-Term Prediction

Predicting the likelihood that a patient will engage in suicidal or violent behavior is like predicting the weather: one's predictions are more likely to be accurate in the short term (e.g., over the next 24–48 hours) than over the long term (e.g., over the next 5 years). The intrusion of unforeseeable, intervening variables diminishes any clinician's ability to make longer-term predictions of behavior.

Such variables might include *life events* (such as losing one's job or being hired for a new one, meeting a new lover or being rejected by a current one, or experiencing a death in the family), the *waxing or waning of one's psychiatric condition*, or *chance factors*. Chance factors could include finding oneself with more ready access to lethal means during a period in which one is feeling suicidal (e.g., being at a friend's house and discovering pills in a medicine cabinet).

While short-term clinical predictions of suicidality likely are more accurate than longer-term predictions, research into the accuracy of any predictions is impeded by obvious ethical considerations. For example, one can't simply follow patients predicted to be at high acute risk for suicide over time without offering clinical intervention. In fact, those patients judged to be at the highest risk for suicide usually end up receiving the most intensive clinical intervention. Given this, if a research study finds that many patients initially judged to be at high risk of committing suicide ultimately did not do so, it may not be able to determine whether this finding reflects inaccurate prediction or accurate prediction followed by subsequent clinical interventions that altered the patient's previous trajectory.

DANGEROUSNESS AND RISK ASSESSMENT

Dangerousness: A Social Rather Than Clinical Term

When clinicians are asked at civil commitment hearings whether particular patients constitute a "danger" to themselves or to other people, what are they being asked? In other words, what is dangerousness? It isn't a clinical diagnosis. It isn't even a clinical symptom. Rather, it is a *legal term of art*.

The general public typically thinks of "dangerousness" as a single *trait* that an individual either does or does not possess. Clinicians therefore might find themselves being asked to determine whether a given evaluee either is or is not a "dangerous person." Further, the clinician's determination might be considered in retrospect to have been either "right" or "wrong," depending upon how the evaluee subsequently behaved weeks, months, even years after the assessment.

However, clinicians aren't trained to assess "dangerousness." They are trained to assess for particular *clinical symptoms* and to assign particular *clinical diagnoses*. Some of these diagnoses are associated with a greater *risk* that the affected individual will engage in particular *behaviors*. Therefore, clinicians speak in terms of the *statistical likelihood* that an evaluee will engage in some particular behavior in the future (such as suicide or homicide) based upon her diagnosis, current symptoms, and other relevant factors.

When we consider whether or not a person is dangerous, we are referring to two particular aspects of the person's potential behavior. The first aspect is the *magnitude* of the behavior, and the other is the *likelihood* that the person will engage in the behavior.

For example, a patient with borderline personality disorder might be followed as an outpatient over a period of several years, during which time she might superficially cut herself 50 times. On each of these occasions, despite the high *likelihood* that she will again engage in this behavior at some point in the future, her therapist does not pursue involuntary hospitalization because the *magnitude* of her behavior has been relatively low.

In contrast, another patient might be seen in the emergency room after having shot himself with a rifle. During the evaluation, he expresses extreme regret for his actions, calling his suicide attempt a "colossal mistake." The clinician might estimate that the *likelihood* that this patient will make another attempt in the near future is quite low, perhaps under 10%. Despite this, she elects to pursue involuntary civil commitment because the *magnitude* of the suicide attempt was so great that it remains cause for concern.

Clinicians often have difficulty deciding whether to pursue hospitalization, especially when the patient declines voluntarily admission. They often end up debating their decisions with the patient (or the patient's family members), with colleagues, or with attorneys. They get into these debates not because their clinical judgment is wrong but because whether an individual should be placed in the hospital against her will isn't simply a clinical decision. It is a social decision. In other words, whether a patient's risk of self-harm is *so* great that it outweighs his or her constitutionally guaranteed liberty interests is a question that cannot be answered solely on clinical grounds.

For example, let us assume that the clinician estimates that a particular patient's risk of suicide is about 20%. Is this enough to justify forcing her into the hospital? The patient (or her attorney) may argue at the civil commitment hearing that since there is an 80% chance that she will not engage in any self-harm, and since she has committed no crime, the doctors should not be allowed to detain her in a hospital against her will. If the clinician *doesn't* pursue commitment, however, and the patient then goes home and takes her life, her survivors may sue the clinician, arguing that it was malpractice to release a patient from the hospital who was known to have a 20% likelihood of committing suicide if released.

In both scenarios, the "clinical facts" are the same. This suggests the great degree to which the decision as to which of various competing interests (the paternalistic desire to protect mentally ill patients from their illnesses, the libertarian desire to respect patients' autonomy) is a *social* rather than a clinical one. (Obviously, however, it is a decision that should be clinically *informed*.)

Doctors and lawyers are trained differently with regard to how to answer such questions. Doctors are trained to believe, paternalistically, that above all they should "do no harm." This has led to the clinical maxim, "When in doubt, admit," since a relatively brief loss of personal liberty is seen as being outweighed by the patient's potential for inflicting serious harm on himself or on those around him.

In contrast, lawyers are trained to believe that liberty is our society's highest value. Thus, the standard of proof in *criminal* cases, where a defendant's personal liberty is at stake, is extremely rigorous—that is, "beyond a reasonable doubt." The standard is deliberately stricter than that used in civil cases ("more likely than not"), since in the latter case what is at stake is money rather than individual liberty. This has led to the legal maxim, "Better that ten guilty men should go free than one innocent man be deprived of liberty," or more succinctly, "When in doubt, acquit."

Risk Assessment Rather Than Prediction

Despite these inherent limitations on the value of predictions, clinicians frequently are called upon to use their diagnostic skills to determine who "is" potentially suicidal or violent and who "is not." Legal decisions that demand such clinical input include not only civil commitment but also sentencing in criminal trials, transfers from the Department of Corrections to the hospital and back again, and various release decisions (e.g., release from the hospital or release from the correctional system). The court system also might request clinical input in determining the treatment needs of a variety of individuals, including spouse abusers, individuals on parole or probation, insanity acquittees, and sexual offenders.

Given clinicians' limited ability to predict future human behavior and given that legal determinations involving patients' rights are based as much on a weighing of social issues as on clinical judgment, clinicians should attempt to *restrict the scope of their opinions to the clinical issues* and also should *avoid making "predictions" of "future dangerousness."*

Rather, clinicians should perform a *risk assessment*—that is, they should attempt to determine whether patients appear to be at a *greater or lesser risk* of engaging in specific behaviors such as suicide or severe violence. Even if they can't predict with certainty whether particular patients are going to commit suicide, they can be much more certain about whether or not such patients fall into a group that is at *high risk* for committing suicide. Clinicians also should *avoid making absolute statements* such as, "I predict that if this patient isn't committed, he will commit suicide." Rather, the clinician should speak in terms of the *relative probability* of the patient committing suicide.

Clinicians also should distinguish the *determination of risk* (a clinical task) from the ultimate *societal weighing of whether this level of risk justifies involuntary confinement* (a legal task). When a clinician feels that the patient requires hospitalization, he should attempt to persuade the patient of this. The patient has a legal right to refuse hospital admission, but this right can be overruled by a judge under particular circumstances. Should this become necessary, the clinician's task is to explain the clinical situation to the judge, who will then use this information, along with any other relevant information (e.g., the testimony of the patient, of family members, of other witnesses to the patient's behavior, or of potential victims of violence) to determine whether the *legal criteria* for civil commitment have been met.

Once the clinician has identified the patient as posing a particular level of risk of engaging in suicidal or violent behavior, she needs to formulate a treatment plan. The goal of this plan is not to eliminate *all risk* of suicide or violence. This goal either could never be achieved or could be achieved only at unacceptable costs (e.g., continuous physical restraint or indefinite hospitalization). Rather, the goal is to ascertain which risk factors for suicide or violence are amenable to clinical intervention, and then to initiate interventions that address these specific risk factors.

Such a risk assessment should be performed and documented *whenever major clinical decisions are made.* For example, the patient's level of risk should be assessed when one is deciding whether or not to admit the patient to the hospital, when deciding whether to continue or discontinue "15-minute checks," when deciding whether or not to expand off-unit "privileges," when deciding whether or not the patient should be allowed to leave the unit on an extended pass, and when deciding whether to discharge the patient from the hospital.

When deciding whether or not to utilize various clinical interventions, a *risk–benefit analysis* should be performed. For example, discontinuing "15-minute checks" does increase a patient's ability to commit suicide, but at some point the benefits of taking this step (e.g., it allows the patient greater autonomy and it also allows the staff to better assess the patient's ability to handle increased responsibility prior to hospital discharge) will outweigh the increased level of risk.

Similar arguments could be made for giving the patient an out-of-hospital pass in the company of a family member shortly before hospital discharge. Here, while the risk of suicide clearly is greater, it may be outweighed by the need to assess whether the patient is capable of handling the transition to the outpatient setting. For example, if the patient—during a 5-hour home visit—begins to feel more suicidal, it might indicate that he is not yet ready for discharge from the hospital. Further, the elements of the visit that contributed to the increased suicidal thoughts now can be explored.

In summary, if clinicians can't accurately predict which patients will or will not commit suicide, why assess for suicidality at all? The reply to this question is that the goal of the assessment is not to predict suicide. The goal is to determine a particular patient's *degree of risk* for suicide along a continuum of risk, to identify relevant suicide *risk factors* that are present or absent in the particular case, and to offer more informed *treatment interventions.* The goal is not to prevent all suicides but to *balance* safety concerns with other clinical, ethical, and legal considerations, including respecting the patient's dignity and civil rights and maintaining a therapeutic working relationship.

Risk Factors: Static and Dynamic

In performing a risk assessment for suicide, there are two major types of risk factors that a clini-

Table 16–1. Static and Dynamic Risk Factors Associated with Suicide

STATIC RISK FACTORS

Demographic variables (older, male, Caucasian more common)
Psychiatric diagnosis (depression, schizophrenia, alcohol and substance abuse)
Prior suicide attempts
Medical illness
Trait vulnerabilities (personality disorder)

DYNAMIC RISK FACTORS

Clinical variables (current depressive symptoms, anxiety symptoms, hallucinations, delusions, alcohol or drug use, therapeutic alliance, impulsive aggression)
Situational variables (social supports, interpersonal conflict, occupational status, access to lethal means such as a gun)

cian should consider: static factors and dynamic factors. The most relevant factors are listed in Table 16–1. **Static factors** are risk factors that are not subject to change with clinical intervention. Examples include: demographic variables (age, race, sex), the presence of a psychiatric diagnosis, a history of previous suicide attempts, the presence of comorbid medical illnesses, and enduring traits such as mental retardation or personality disorder.

Dynamic factors are risk factors that are potentially amenable to clinical intervention. Some of these dynamic factors will be **clinical variables**, such as current symptoms of mental illness (depressive symptoms, command hallucinations, ongoing alcohol use) and also the presence (or absence) of a therapeutic alliance. Other dynamic factors will be **situational variables**, such as limited social support, a current interpersonal conflict, unemployment, or access to a gun. We will discuss each of these risk factors in turn. Following this, we will discuss how to design a treatment plan aimed at addressing these risk factors in an attempt to lower the patient's risk of engaging in suicidal behavior.

STATIC RISK FACTORS

Demographic Variables

As noted above, the suicide rate in the United States is about 10–12 per 100,000, and this statistic has not changed over the past several decades despite advances in the treatment of depression. However, the rate of suicide is not evenly distributed across all segments of the population.

For example, while females attempt suicide three to four times more frequently than do males, males are successful two to three times more frequently than females, largely because they tend to employ more lethal means. (Males more often utilize hanging, shooting, or jumping while females more often utilize overdosing or drowning.)

While race does appear to play a contributory role, it often is outweighed by other factors. In general, Caucasians are at highest risk for suicide, followed by Native Americans, African Americans, Hispanic Americans, and Asian Americans. Seventy-three percent of all suicides in the United States are committed by white males. However, rates among minorities may be much higher for particular subgroups, including inner-city youths, and recent immigrants.

Patients who live with others or who are married are at lower risk of committing suicide than are patients who live alone or who are separated, divorced, or widowed. Patients who are unemployed also have a greater suicide risk than those who are employed, likely because they experience greater psychological, social, and economic stress.

The rate of suicide increases with age. While younger patients are the most likely to *attempt* suicide, older patients are more likely to *succeed*. For example, among men aged 65 and older the rate of suicide is 40 per 100,000, which is four times the rate in the general population. The majority of these suicides are committed using a firearm.

Several factors likely contribute to this increased degree of risk. One is untreated depression. While the prevalence of depression isn't higher among older versus younger patients, depression presents differently in older patients (more often with complaints of anxiety, somatic complaints, or cognitive complaints than with complaints of "sadness") and depression therefore is less likely to be recognized and appropriately treated. Other predisposing factors in older individuals include alcohol abuse or dependence, social isolation, spousal loss, medical problems, and anxiety due to financial instability. Individuals with the greatest level of risk tend to have multiple demographic risk factors (e.g , an older, white male who is recently widowed, has comorbid medical problems, and is depressed and/or is abusing alcohol).

However, suicide does occur in younger patients as well, and it is the third leading cause of death in persons 15–34 years of age. As in the elderly, depression is a major risk factor. In adolescents, depression leading to suicide often is accompanied by substance abuse, conduct problems, and family discord.

While demographic variables are helpful in guiding a clinical assessment, they aren't sensitive or specific enough in themselves to allow for prediction in individual cases. Single males with no children who are in a higher-risk age group account for over 5 million individuals in the United States: most of these men will never attempt suicide. Viewed another way, in one study of 134 consecutive cases of suicide, only 16% of the cases were in a higher-risk demographic group. Therefore, demographic considerations might help the clinician formulate a treatment plan, but should not dictate it.

Psychiatric Diagnosis

Ninety percent of people who commit suicide have been found to have some Axis I psychiatric disorder at the time of death, most commonly a major depressive episode (50%–70% of suicides), schizophrenia (10%–15%), or alcohol and substance abuse (15%–25%). It likely that some of these suicides might have been potentially preventable through clinical intervention. Again, though, while suicide is a known complication of these disorders, the majority of individuals with these disorders never attempt suicide. For example, while clinical depression is the disorder with the greatest associate suicide risk, in any given year over 99% of depressed individuals do *not* commit suicide.

In about 10% of suicides, no underlying psychiatric disorder is noted. A small percentage of these suicides occur in response to recent life stressors, especially some sort of loss (interpersonal, financial, or occupational), while up to 5% of suicides are engaged in by individuals in response to a severe illness such as cancer, spinal cord injury, multiple sclerosis, and HIV disease.

Depression

The most common psychiatric diagnosis associated with suicide is depression. A major depressive episode (whether in the context of major depressive disorder or bipolar disorder) is present in between 50% and 70% of completed suicides. About 25% of all depressed patients attempt suicide at some point, and up to 15% of depressed patients discharged from an inpatient hospitalization ultimately die by suicide. Since depression is encountered so commonly in the primary care setting, and since up to half of patients who commit suicide see their doctor in the preceding month, the first step in lowering the risk of suicide is to recognize and treat depression.

The second step is to determine whether a *particular* depressed patient appears to be at greater risk of committing suicide. Such an assessment requires the clinician to recognize the complex interactions that can occur between depression and other static and dynamic risk factors. For example, studies comparing depressed patients who have attempted suicide with depressed patients who have not done so find that those who attempted suicide more often were male, were socially isolated (single, separated, divorced, widowed, or recently bereaved), were middle aged or elderly, reported more subjective depression and hopelessness, reported more severe suicidal ideation, and perceived fewer reasons for living (despite having the same objective severity of illness and a similar number of adverse life events as the depressed patients who have not attempted suicide). They also are more likely to demonstrate aggressive or impulsive personality traits in other aspects of their lives (e.g., relationships, jobs) and are more likely to have engaged in previous suicide attempts.

About 10% of depressed patients have a *family history of suicide*, and this subset of patients appears to be at higher risk for committing suicide themselves, particularly violent suicide. This suggests the possibility that they have inherited two genetic diatheses, one toward depression and the other toward impulsive aggression and/or suicide.

Particular depressive symptoms may be more associated with suicide. The NIMH Collaborative Program on the Psychobiology of Depression followed 954 depressed patients longitudinally. During the first 8 years of the study, 32

(3%) of the patients committed suicide. (This rate is lower than the rate among depressed individuals in the general population and may reflect the fact that these patients were receiving treatment.) Forty percent of the suicides took place during the first year of follow-up and were thus considered "short-term" suicides, while 60% took place at some point after a year and were considered "long-term" suicides. Nine clinical symptoms were found to be prospectively associated with suicide. Six of the nine symptoms— *panic attacks, anxiety, decreased concentration, insomnia, alcohol abuse, and anhedonia*—were associated with short-term suicide. Three of the nine symptoms—*hopelessness, suicidal ideation, and a past history of attempts*—were associated with long-term suicide.

It again should be noted that these are statistical associations. While they can help guide clinical decision making, they aren't sensitive or specific enough to allow for prediction in individual cases. For example, a subjective sense of *hopelessness* is one of the strongest "predictors" of suicide. This experience can be measured by the Beck Hopelessness Scale, and a recent study using this scale showed the instrument capable, over a 10-year period, of identifying 16 of 17 suicides among 1958 consecutive outpatients. Therefore, while the *sensitivity* of this scale is 94%, the *specificity* is only 41%, with over 1145 patients being labeled as high risk who did *not* commit suicide. Viewed another way, while almost every person who commits suicide does so in the face of severe feelings of hopelessness, only 1 or 2 out of every 100 people with severe hopelessness commit suicide. Clearly one cannot involuntarily hospitalize every depressed patient who reports feeling severely hopeless.

Suicide may be more common at *certain stages of treatment for depression*. It is more likely to occur at the onset of or at the end of a depressive episode. The first months after discharge from a psychiatric hospitalization are a period of especially high risk. One commonly held clinical maxim is that one must be especially vigilant in assessing for suicidal ideation during the first few weeks of antidepressant therapy. The idea is that patients may remain hopeless at this point but may also have gained enough energy and drive as a result of treatment to carry out a suicide plan. However, empirical evidence in support of this maxim is lacking.

Similarly, suggestions that some antidepressants may actually increase suicide risk due either to their direct lethality in an overdose or to medication side effects (such as agitation, restlessness, or insomnia) are not well substantiated. Nevertheless, clinicians should closely monitor for suicidality in patients at the start of treatment, particularly when initiating treatment with medications that might be associated with adverse side effects that might increase a patient's level of distress. They also should attempt to avoid prescribing lethal quantities of medication to potentially suicidal patients.

Alcoholism

About 20% of those who commit suicide have a primary diagnosis of alcoholism, and the rate of suicide among individuals with alcoholism is about 3%. As with depression, the suicide rate is a bit higher for those individuals who have received inpatient treatment than for those who only have received outpatient treatment (3.4% versus 2.2% respectively). Up to 40% of the former group commit suicide within a year of the last hospitalization.

Again, there are interactions between alcoholism and other risk factors that might help the clinician better determine *which* alcoholic patients are at the highest risk of suicide. Suicide completers with alcoholism tend to be male (80% of the time), white, middle-aged, divorced or separated, socially isolated, and actively drinking. Typically, the alcoholism has been present for years. Up to 40% of these individuals have made a previous suicide attempt. Alcoholism itself is more common in men than in women, and there also is a greater tendency for men to be socially isolated (since women are more likely to have children in the home). These two facts may largely account for the more general finding that suicide is more common in men than in women. In one recent study, when the two factors of alcoholism and children in the home were controlled for, no gender difference was noted in the rate of suicide.

Many alcoholic patients hospitalized for suicidal ideation who ultimately commit suicide are noted to be depressed during their inpatient stays. In many cases, it isn't clear whether the depression is secondary to the alcohol abuse, is secondary to medical concomitants of alcoholism such as head injury or malnutrition or constitutes an independent condition.

Depression in alcoholic patients often is exacerbated by the social isolation that results from the patient having "burned his bridges" with family and friends. Up to 50% of alcoholics who commit suicide have lost a close relationship during the previous year. In many cases, the depression hasn't been treated with antidepressants, while in other cases the patient has been noncompliant with antidepressant therapy. Further, since alcohol intoxication can be associated both with a depressed mood and with a loss of normal inhibitions, it isn't surprising that many of these individuals commit suicide while intoxicated.

Finally, since many alcohol-dependent individuals utilize alcohol's sedative, anxiolytic, and rewarding properties as a way of coping with internal or interpersonal difficulties, some individuals may be at greater risk for suicide following "successful" detoxification, particularly in the absence of adequate social supports. Bolstering existing support systems (family, friends, religious affiliations) or enlisting new supports (AA, rehab programs, support groups, psychotherapy) can be essential in such cases.

Substance Abuse

While a primary diagnosis of alcoholism is strongly associated with suicide, polysubstance abuse is even more strongly associated. In the San Diego Suicide Study, polysubstance abuse was noted in almost 70% of completed suicides in youths and young adults and in nearly half of suicides in adults of age 30 and older. Most commonly, these individuals have a history of drug overdoses and comorbid depression, the latter being diagnosed either as a separate condition or secondary to the substance use. As noted in Chapter 12, depression occurring during a cocaine withdrawal "crash" makes this a particular period of higher risk for suicide. As with alcohol, despite histories of substance abuse going back years, these suicides tend to be precipitated by some recent event, often occurring within several weeks of some interpersonal loss.

Schizophrenia

About 30% of individuals with schizophrenia attempt suicide and 10% ultimately die by suicide. Most (75%) are men in their 20s or 30s who have a chronic illness characterized by multiple hospital admissions. About 50% have made previous suicide attempts.

In contrast to depressed patients, most patients with schizophrenia who commit suicide do so during the first years of the illness. They tend to be unmarried, to be socially isolated, and to express feelings of inadequacy and hopelessness. However, greater severity of negative symptoms does not correlate with a higher risk of suicide. Rather, it is the patients with later onset of illness, better premorbid functioning, a greater capacity for abstract thinking, and greater insight (i.e., the patients who might be expected to have a *better* prognosis) who also have a greater risk of suicide. While negative symptoms (such as loss of drive, decreased affective range, and indifference toward the future) contribute to greater *disability*, they may actually mitigate the painful self-awareness that causes some patients with schizophrenia to turn to suicide.

In further contrast to what might be expected, it is much less common for patients to commit suicide due to their positive symptoms—for example, in response to command hallucinations or in order to escape from delusions of persecution. Rather, suicide occurs in most cases during *a postpsychotic depressive episode*. About a third of patients with schizophrenia who commit suicide were hospitalized several weeks to months before the suicide, and another third commit suicide while still inpatients. Other higher-risk situations include periods when the patient must go through a significant *loss* (e.g., the end of a relationship or marriage, the loss of a job, a change of therapist, or being asked to leave the home) and periods when the patient is gaining greater *insight into having a chronic illness* (perhaps in response to the institution of a new antipsychotic medication).

Despite the above caveat about the relative rarity of suicide in response to command hallucinations or persecutory delusions, clinicians still should inquire into these. Some authors have speculated that the reason suicides are rarely noted in response to hallucinations demanding that the patient to kill himself is that clinicians have such a low threshold for hospitalizing the patient and aggressively treating such symptoms, thereby possibility averting suicide. In contrast, clinicians are less likely to aggressively recognize and treat postpsychotic depression. Therefore, *both* risk factors should be explored and taken very seriously.

Prior Suicide Attempts

The rate of completed suicide among those who have made previous suicide attempts is over 100 times greater than the rate in the general population, and the risk is highest during the year following a previous suicide attempt.

A history of previous suicide attempts is an important risk factor for another suicide attempt, since between 10% and 40% of people who successfully commit suicide have made a prior attempt. However, between 60% and 90% of persons who commit suicide have *not* previously attempted suicide. In other words, if every person who had attempted suicide in the past were somehow prevented from doing so in the future, most suicides still would occur.

Clinicians frequently are asked to assess an individual shortly after a suicide attempt in order to determine if the individual is at imminent risk for another attempt. Only about 10% of these individuals will be hospitalized. The majority of suicide attempts are impulsive: two-thirds of those who attempt suicide have first thought about doing so less than an hour before the attempt. Suicide attempters who go on to become suicide completers are more likely to have the demographic and clinical characteristics noted above.

Weisman and Worden have emphasized that when one attempts to assess the significance of a suicide attempt, one should consider not only the *risk* associated with the attempt (i.e., potential lethality) but also the *relationship* between this *risk* and the *likelihood of rescue*. Both previous attempts and current attempts are subject to such a "risk–rescue" analysis. One should assess how dangerous the suicide method was, whether the patient actually believed she would die, whether she was surprised to have survived, and whether the attempt was impulsive or highly planned. One also should assess whether the patient took steps to either decrease or increase the likelihood of being rescued (such as choosing a remote location as opposed to overdosing in front of a family member). Table 16–2 outlines four common clinical scenarios:

Table 16–2. Weisman and Worden's Risk–Rescue Rating System

Rescue	Risk	
	High	Low
High	A	B
Low	C	D

Source: Adapted from a theoretical model presented in Weisman AD, Worden JW: "Risk–Rescue Rating in Suicide Assessment." *Arch Gen Psychiatry* 26:553–560, 1972.

Scenario A: high-risk, high-rescue. For example, in front of his wife, a patient points a gun at his head and threatens to shoot himself, but his wife "somehow" is able to wrest the gun away from him. While this can be considered a "suicide gesture," the level of lethality should increase the clinician's level of concern, particularly when the patient's behavior is impulsive, highly aggressive, or escalating in severity.

Scenario B: low-risk, high-rescue. For example, a patient takes a small number of sleeping pills and immediately goes into the next room to tell her mother, who takes her to the emergency room. These are the patients most likely to be labeled as having made a "suicide gesture."

Scenario C: high-risk, low-rescue. For example, a patient attempts to hang himself in an isolated hotel, having put his financial affairs in order, and only fails in his attempt due to his having been fortuitously interrupted by the hotel maid. Clearly, this is the most ominous scenario.

Scenario D: low-risk, low-rescue. For example, a patient superficially cuts her forearm while alone and does not tell anybody that she has done so. While such patients might be considered to have made a "suicide gesture," they often deny actual suicidal intent and therefore might better be categorized as having engaged in "self-injurious behavior."

Medical Illness

Retrospective studies reveal some medical illness to have been present in between 25% and 75% of suicide completers. However, many of these medical conditions are commonly associated with either clinical depression (e.g., cancer, epilepsy, multiple sclerosis, head injury, cardiac disease, Huntington's disease, dementia, AIDS) or with alcoholism (e.g., peptic ulcer disease, cirrhosis). Some of these conditions also can be associated with feelings of hopelessness independent of a major depressive episode. The presence of comorbid medical illness may be overlooked when performing a risk assessment on a "psychiatric patient." For example, the patient in the case example presented at the beginning of this chapter had a history of peptic ulcer disease and hypertension.

Medical illness and age are not independent risk factors since medical illness becomes an important risk factor only later in life. In adolescents and young adult suicide victims, the primary contributory life stressors appear to be interpersonal conflicts, separations, and rejections. In contrast, in the 40–60-year-old suicide victims, economic problems appear to have been the most important stressor. For suicide victims over the age of 60, medical illness plays a more prominent contributory role, and for victims over age 80 it appears to be the most significant risk factor.

A detailed examination of the ethics of **physician-assisted suicide** for patients who have a severe medical illness is beyond the scope of this text. However, one should keep in mind that physician-assisted suicide is still suicide and that the same risk assessment principles therefore should apply. Whenever a patient requests a physician's assistance in dying, the physician should carefully assess the patient for dynamic, potentially reversible risk factors and should be especially attentive to the possible presence of a treatable psychiatric condition such as major depressive disorder.

In 1997, the U.S. Supreme Court ruled that state laws that prohibit physician-assisted suicide do not violate patients' constitutional rights to due process or to equal protection under the law. The patients who petitioned the court were not asking that the "right to die" be extended to *all* people who wished to commit suicide, only to terminally ill patients who would otherwise die protracted and very painful deaths.

The underlying assumption of the plaintiff's case was that medicine had little to offer many terminally ill patients beyond assistance in committing suicide. While this may be true on rare occasions, it is not true in the overwhelming majority of cases. While pain control may be underutilized in current general medical practice, most terminally ill patients' pain can be controlled throughout the dying process without an

excessive risk of sedation, anesthesia, or respiratory depression.

In fact, in actual clinical practice the demand for euthanasia does not come principally from patients seeking relief from physical pain. A study reviewing such euthanasia requests in Washington State found that neither severe pain nor dyspnea was a common patient concern. Other studies have found that patients who are experiencing severe pain are not more inclined to request euthanasia than other patients.

Why, then, do some patients request physician-assisted suicide? Most of them do so out of a concern that—at some point in the future—their pain will become intolerable, they will suffer a severe loss of dignity, they will become excessively dependent upon others, or they will become an excessive burden on their families. Clinicians often can address these concerns by providing assurances that they will remain committed to providing adequate pain control and by assisting the patient to confront their underlying fears of pain and excessive dependency. Clinicians who work with terminally ill patients have noted that in many cases, once patients have been assisted in confronting these fears, their initial desire for death passes and they achieve a greater sense of meaning in their final days.

As is the case with all suicidal patients, *clinical depression* commonly is found to be present in those terminally ill patients who are expressing suicidal ideation. In one study of 44 terminally ill cancer patients, all but one of the 11 clinically depressed patients expressed some wish to die, while none of the remaining 33 expressed such a wish. The failure to recognize alternative presentations of major depressive disorder in elderly patients represents a similar obstacle to treatment in the terminally ill patient population to that found in the general patient population.

Even in an ideal system of medical care—one that recognizes and appropriately treats pain, fears of dying, and depression—there likely will remain a small number of patients for whom medicine has little to offer. Assuming that these patients, with the assistance of their physician, can competently make an informed decision about the issue, assisted suicide might be considered appropriate. However, a key question is whether physicians can be relied upon to limit euthanasia to this small fraction of patients. Case studies from the United States and the Netherlands suggest that a physician's *willingness* to assist in suicide in itself can powerfully influence their patient's decision with regard to euthanasia. Therefore, physicians cannot objectively assess the impact of their own attitudes on the patient's final decision.

Trait Vulnerabilities and Personality Disorder

Personality disorder has been retrospectively diagnosed in up to 25% of suicide completers and in about half of suicide attempters. The most common personality disorder diagnosis is borderline personality disorder, which includes suicide attempts in its diagnostic criteria. The lifetime mortality from suicide in borderline personality disorder is about 10%, and the lifetime mortality in antisocial personality disorder is about 5%.

A postmortem study in Finland examined 229 randomly selected individuals who had committed suicide over a 12 month period. Through the use of collateral informants, personality disorder diagnoses could be assigned to 67 individuals (29%). Only one subject had a cluster A diagnosis, while 43 subjects (19%) had a cluster B disorder (usually borderline personality disorder), and 23 subjects (10%) had a cluster C diagnosis. The most important finding was that all suicide victims with a personality disorder also were found to have an Axis I diagnosis. In 95% of the cases, it was major depressive disorder, a substance-related disorder, or both. While the clinical variables for the subjects with a cluster C personality disorder were not significantly different from those of the subjects without personality disorder, subjects with cluster B disorders were more likely to have a history of substance abuse and previous suicide attempts and were less likely to have a comorbid medical condition.

DYNAMIC RISK FACTORS

Clinical Variables

While the *presence* of a psychiatric disorder such as major depressive disorder, schizophrenia, or a substance-related disorder constitutes a static risk factor (i.e., a factor that cannot be changed), the current *severity* of a patient's clinical symptoms constitutes a dynamic factor. Depressive symptoms, anxiety symptoms, hallucinations, delusions, and current alcohol or drug use all may be amenable to clinical intervention, thereby lowering the risk of suicide associated with these psychiatric conditions.

Another factor that also should be assessed is the *presence or absence of a therapeutic alliance*. For example, in the clinical vignette presented at the beginning of the chapter, the patient had multiple demographic and clinical risk factors for suicide, including being an older, white male with concurrent medical problems, depression, alcoholism, and a history of a previous suicide attempt. Dynamic factors included current symptoms of depression, active drinking, and social isolation. It also was noteworthy that, once on the inpatient unit, the patient remained quiet in groups, only "superficially social," and only spoke about his personal problems "reluctantly." Despite this, the staff discontinued his 15-minute-check status after he denied feeling suicidal. Should the patient have been believed? Perhaps his limited engagement in the treatment process should have alerted the treatment team to investigate his suicide risk further, especially after he became even more upset following his wife's refusal to speak with him.

Also, note that the patient in the clinical vignette signed a *"no self-harm contract."* Is this significant? Keep in mind that such agreements certainly aren't binding in any way and that they carry no legal protection for the clinician if the patient ultimately commits suicide in violation of the contract. However, such contracts can be useful for two reasons.

First, a contract can solidify the therapeutic alliance between the patient and the clinician and can encourage the patient to commit to working with the clinician to get well. (Of course, the degree to which this is the case depends upon the preexistence of such a therapeutic alliance. An agreement on the part of a patient to notify a clinician of worsening suicidal thoughts likely is more meaningful when the patients and the clinician have been working together for months than when the patient is asked to contract with an emergency room physician that he has known for less than an hour.)

Second, asking a patient if he can "contract for

safety" provides a useful means of gauging the patient's reaction to such a request. It is true that some patients who strongly desire to commit suicide might readily agree to make such a contract only to violate it later on. (This may have been the case in the above example, in which case the patient's willingness to sign a contract may have given the staff a false sense of security.) However, when a patient either hesitates to contract for safety or states that he simply can't trust himself to abide by such a contract, this certainly raises the clinician's level of concern by an additional notch.

Unfortunately, some clinicians assign far too much weight to no-harm contracts. An agreement on the part of the patient to "contract for safety" is never a substitute for a more comprehensive assessment of overall suicide risk.

Impulsive Aggression as a Clinical Variable

A patient's personality or temperament can constitute either a source of protection from suicide or a vulnerability that increases one's risk. In general, one's personality does not change over time, such that personality disorder constitutes a static risk factor. However, particular *aspects* of temperament may be amenable to pharmacologic or psychotherapeutic intervention, thereby making them dynamic variables. For example, a consistent research finding has been the association of low serotonin activity with impaired impulse control. Such impairments can contribute to aggression that is either "directed outward" at others or "turned inward" in the form of self-injurious behavior or suicide.

Research highlighting the role of neurotransmitters in temperament and behavior began in the 1960s with the postmortem study of individuals who had died by violent suicide. Compared to individuals who had died in accidents, the suicide victims had lower cerebrospinal fluid levels of 5-HIAA, the principal metabolite of serotonin. More recent studies with still-living patients have found that depressed subjects who previously have attempted suicide, as compared to nonsuicidal depressed subjects, also have lower cerebrospinal fluid levels of 5-HIAA. Indirect methods also indicate an increased number of 5-HT_{2A} receptors in suicide victims, consistent with receptor upregulation in the face of a serotonin deficiency.

Studies in individuals diagnosed with more severe personality disorders also reveal lower levels of 5-HIAA specifically in those subjects with lifetime histories of aggression and suicidal behavior. Of note, studies of violent criminal offenders have found that 5HIAA levels are lower in some of these individuals, but only those who have a history of *impulsive violence*, as opposed to nonimpulsive (i.e., premeditated) violence. This is consistent with the notion that lower CNS serotonin activity corresponds to a general tendency toward *impaired impulse control* rather than to a tendency toward violent or sociopathic behavior.

In lower mammals, administrating pharmacologic agents that decrease the animal's CNS serotonin levels causes the animal to demonstrate an increase in aggressive behaviors. In contrast, interventions that increase the animal's serotonin levels cause a reduction in aggressive behaviors. Recent studies in research subjects with personality disorders or with histories of impulsive-aggressive and irritable behaviors have demonstrated that treating the subjects with SSRIs is associated with a decrease in impulsive and aggressive behavior. (Of note, subjects with a history of major depressive disorder were deliberately excluded from these studies.)

However, it is likely that serotonin isn't the only neurotransmitter involved with impulse control. Indirect evidence suggests that while *serotonin plays an inhibitory role* in aggression, *norepinephrine and dopamine play facilitating roles*. For example, while some patients with borderline personality disorder and comorbid depression who are treated with amitriptyline demonstrate a decrease in depressive symptoms, two-thirds of the patients in one study who received amitriptyline also demonstrated a worsening of hostility and paranoia. In this same study, among the subjects who were nonresponders to either amitriptyline or placebo, the amitriptyline nonresponders developed more paranoid ideation, impulsiveness, assaultiveness, and suicidal threats by the sixth week of therapy, an effect that wasn't observed in subjects who received placebo. This suggests that these symptoms weren't simply due to the borderline personality disorder itself.

Since tricyclic antidepressants raise the levels of both norepinephrine and serotonin, what may be important here is the balance between the two.

Similarly, antipsychotic agents sometimes prove to be useful in decreasing impulsivity and aggression, likely because of their dopaminergic antagonism. The newer atypical antipsychotic agents may have further antiaggressive effects because, in addition to the dopamine-receptor-blocking effects, they add serotonin-receptor-blocking effects, which in might combat the serotonin receptor upregulation that occurs in response to lower synaptic serotonin levels.

Situational Variables

In attempting to tailor a risk assessment to a particular patient, attention should be paid to the patient's current circumstances—that is, to the presence or absence of social supports, interpersonal conflicts, and financial, occupational, and residential stability.

One situational variable that can play a key role is the availability of lethal means to commit suicide. For example, detoxification of the domestic gas supplied to homes in England and Japan led to a reduction in the rate of successful suicides in both countries. In the United States, the risk of suicide strongly correlates with the presence of a firearm in the home, particularly for adolescents. This is the case even when the firearm has been locked away and the ammunition has been stored separately. Individuals who purchase a handgun are 57 times more likely than the general population to commit suicide in the week after the purchase, and they continue to have a higher risk of suicide even after 6 years. Removing firearms from the home of a suicidal person would likely decrease the risk of that person committing suicide because even though the person could still obtain a gun elsewhere, it would be that much more difficult.

Decreasing a person's ready access to lethal means is also the rationale for attempting to "suicide proof" inpatient psychiatric units. In actuality, no psychiatric unit is completely suicide proof. For example, if all psychiatric inpatients were kept nude and restrained to their beds for their entire hospital stay, their risk of suicide clearly would be reduced, but obviously no meaningful therapy could occur and many patients would even be psychologically harmed. Obviously, this is an extreme example, but what about strip searching all patients upon their arrival to the unit in order to decrease the likeli-

hood that they might smuggle in a razor blade or other contraband? What about taking away their belts and shoelaces to lessen the risk of them hanging themselves? What about searching patients' handbags? Most units attempt to strike a balance between protecting patients from self-harm and respecting their autonomy and dignity when devising such policies.

For example, using shower curtain rods that break away when any weight is placed on them, in order to prevent hanging, is a relatively innocuous measure. Searching patients' belongings upon their arrival to the unit, taking away their shoelaces, and not allowing them to keep razor blades or lighters are more intrusive but commonly utilized interventions. More extreme measures, however, such as strip searches or random searches of patients' rooms are rarely employed except for particular higher-risk situations (e.g., when admitting a patient known to have smuggled a razor blade onto the unit during a previous admission).

The mental status examination should always include not only questions related to the presence of **suicidal ideation** but also ones related to whether the patient has active **suicidal intent** and has formulated a specific **suicide plan**. If the patient does have such a plan, one next should attempt to attempt to ascertain if the patient has **taken steps toward carrying out the plan**.

For example, if the plan is to overdose, has the patient hoarded medications? If the plan is to die by gunshot wound, does the patient have access to a gun or has the patient made plans to buy one? In addition to using these questions to gauge the severity of the suicidal ideation, the clinician can use this information to help formulate a treatment plan aimed at decreasing ready access to lethal means. This strategy is especially important in the case of patients who may be tempted to act impulsively. For example, family members can be enlisted to remove firearms or pills from the home prior to the patient being discharged from the hospital.

One particular life circumstance that also has been associated with suicide is involvement with the legal system, either through incarceration or a pending court appearance. The suicide rate is nine times higher in the correctional setting than in the general population. About 40% of these suicides occur within the first 30 days of incarceration, and about half occur within a few days of a court appearance. Almost all suicides in the correctional setting are by hanging, and almost all of these inmates have been housed alone. Most of them are found in retrospect to have had a treatable psychiatric illness. These findings argue for the need for psychiatric screening of all newly incarcerated inmates for the presence of either a psychiatric history or suicidal ideation. Correctional staff should receive education about suicide, and potentially suicidal inmates should not be housed alone in a cell.

AFTER THE RISK ASSESSMENT

After the risk assessment has been completed, the clinician's goal is to formulate a treatment plan designed to decrease the risk of suicide. The clinician should identify relevant dynamic risk factors that are amenable to clinical intervention and should consider the risks and benefits of specific interventions.

The clinician then should document this thought process. The best protection against a future lawsuit for negligent care is sound clinical practice. In the event of a lawsuit, courts tend to be less concerned with whether the physician ultimately was able to prevent a suicide than with whether the clinician's performed a reasonable risk assessment and initiated a reasonable treatment plan.

One maxim clinicians frequently hear from attorneys is: "If something is not documented in the chart, it didn't occur." Unfortunately, some clinicians believe (mistakenly) that if they make no reference to a patient's suicidal statements, then no liability can be assigned since one could infer that the patient never mentioned suicide to the clinician. In fact, failure to document an inquiry into suicidal ideation may expose the clinician to greater liability since it might be inferred that the clinician never took the care to inquire into suicide or to formulate a treatment plan designed to minimize the risk of suicide. In short, a clinician is less likely to be held liable for honest errors of judgment than for errors of omission.

Therefore, the clinician should write some sentences in the chart documenting that she has considered certain risk factors to be the most relevant ones and that she has considered the risks

Table 16–3. Example of a Treatment Plan to Address Dynamic Risk Factors

Risk Factors	Steps to Address Them
1. Alcohol dependence	1. Patient to attend AA meetings while inpatient; addictions consultation for placement in outpatient rehab; random drug and alcohol screens; discuss naltrexone and disulfiram with him
2. Low mood, vegetative symptoms, hopelessness	2. Antidepressant medication (will use SSRI; avoid TCA due to overdose risk and possible increased impulsivity); supportive psychotherapy
3. Command hallucinations	3. Initiate antipsychotic medication; discuss using Haldol Decanoate due to poor past compliance
4. Gun in home	4. Brother to remove gun from home
5. Lives alone; little social support	5. Family meeting by social work; can patient temporarily stay with brother after discharge? Arrange outpatient psychotherapy

and benefits of various steps that might be taken to address these risks. One simple technique in documenting a risk assessment is to list all relevant dynamic risk factors in one column and then list the steps being taken to address each risk factor in an adjoining column, as illustrated in Table 16–3. Even if one doesn't use this format, one can use the same conceptual approach when formulating one's opinion.

When patients are discharged from the emergency room following a suicidal gesture or attempt rather than admitted to an inpatient psychiatric unit, the most important question is this: "What will be different now than it was prior to the attempt?" Even though only a brief period of time may have elapsed since the attempt, the situation might in fact be quite different. For example, the major interpersonal stressor may no longer be present (if she and her boyfriend now have resolved the argument that preceded the attempt), or the patient may now be agreeing to attend outpatient psychotherapy, or the patient may never have realized until now the effect that her suicide attempt would have on her family. Patients should not be sent home from the emergency room without either timely follow-up or information about who to call in case of an emergency.

Formulating a *contingency plan for suicide*

can aid the clinician in assessing the patient's ability to "think things through" should she again feel suicidal in the future. It also can help the patient avert a future crisis. Who will the patient call if she feels suicidal again? Who will she call if *that* person isn't home? The ultimate "safety net" in any such plan usually is for the patient to call 911 or return to the emergency room to seek inpatient admission.

When formulating a treatment plan, the clinician must have realistic expectations. Is the patient *really* going to stop drinking as he says he is? Is he *really* likely to appear for his outpatient follow-up appointment? Are his avowals of having "learned a lot about myself and how much I have to live for" *credible*? If not, voluntary or involuntary inpatient admission should be pursued.

When a less restrictive intervention is taken— for example, sending the patient home from the emergency room rather than seeking involuntary commitment, a *risk–benefit analysis should be documented*. This can be brief but should document the clinician's thought process in weighing the various pros and cons of hospitalization. For example, the clinician might note:

> The patient regrets the overdose attempt, immediately sought help after having taken a small number of pills, denies any current suicidal ideation, contracts for safety, plans to stay with his brother for now, and has an appointment with his therapist tomorrow afternoon. Short-term hospitalization likely would have little effect in decreasing his longer-term suicide risk. Hospitalization might even be detrimental in that the patient fears that

he will lose his job if he doesn't appear for work tomorrow and he would also have to explain his absence to his coworkers. He is agreeable to outpatient follow-up, and I worry that seeking involuntarily commitment might alienate him from the mental health system in general and jeopardize the longer-term treatment plan. I have contacted his outpatient therapist to discuss the case, and she agrees with this plan.

CONCLUSION

Suicide is a behavior. When it occurs, it most commonly is associated with an underlying psychiatric disorder, but no single disorder is synonymous with suicide, and the overwhelming majority of people with any given psychiatric disorder do not commit suicide. However, in treating patients with psychiatric disorders, it is essential to assess for the presence of suicidality, and in talking with patients who voice suicidal ideation it is important to assess for the presence of treatable psychiatric disorders.

However, the presence of a psychiatric illness is only one risk factor for suicide. While suicide cannot be reliably predicted in individual cases, clinicians still can attempt to gauge a patient's level of risk by conducting a comprehensive risk assessment. They should delineate static and dynamic risk factors and identify which factors are potentially amenable to clinical intervention. Since all clinical interventions carry potential risks as well as potential benefits, one must weigh these competing considerations in attempting to tailor a treatment plan to the specific needs of the patient.

Chapter 17

Violence

Virtually all clinicians at some point must deal with violence in the course of working with patients. Clinicians may have to manage acutely violent patients in the medical setting. They also may be called upon to determine whether particular patients are at higher risk of engaging in violence. For example, a clinical determination that a patient, as a result of a mental illness, is "dangerous" to himself or others is a prerequisite for involuntary psychiatric hospitalization (civil commitment). In addition, under some circumstances clinicians may find it necessary to take appropriate steps to protect "third parties"—that is, other members of society who might be harmed by the patient. In such situations, the clinician's societal obligations may come into conflict with ethical obligations to the patient (i.e., respecting the patient's autonomy and safeguarding the confidentiality of the patient's disclosures).

Like suicidality, dangerousness is not a clinical diagnosis. Unlike suicidality, it does not even describe a specific behavior. Rather, it is a legal term of art that refers to an individual's general propensity to engage in one or more types of aggressive acts. In addition, a patient's propensity toward "dangerous" behavior must rise to a particular level of *severity* before being considered "dangerous enough" to justify involuntary containment. The latter is a social rather than a clinical determination. In other words, even if two observers agree on an individuals absolute level of risk, they still might disagree as to whether that level of risk outweighs a patient's civil liberty rights and justifies involuntary detention.

While clinicians are not able to *predict* whether a given individual will engage in future acts of violence with a high degree of accuracy, they *are* capable of assessing whether that individual is at high, medium, or low *risk* for engaging in future violence. Obviously, clinicians can't exert total control over how a patient will behave in the future. Given this, whether it ultimately turns out that the clinician was "right" about the patient's risk of violence once released from an emergency room or an inpatient unit is less important than whether the clinician "asked the right questions" and responded appropriately by attempting to address those risk factors for violence that might be amenable to clinical intervention.

In this chapter, we first will discuss violence as a behavior. After this, we will discuss two common social contexts for violence: domestic violence and workplace violence. One example of the latter is violence in the health-care setting. The latter should be of particular concern to clinicians because they themselves have become the victims of assault by patients on occasion.

Aggression is multifactorial in origin, with

genetic, neurobiological, developmental, and cultural factors all playing important contributory roles. Clinicians who are aware of these elements can weave an assessment of relevant risk factors into their history and mental status examination such that risk assessment for violence becomes an integral part of their routine clinical practice.

VIOLENCE AS A BEHAVIOR

Four aspects of violent behavior can be delineated. The first of these is the *magnitude* of violent behavior. This spans a continuum, with verbal outbursts at one end, followed by pushing, slapping or hitting, followed by violence that is severe enough for the victim to require medical attention, and ultimately followed by homicide.

The second aspect is the *likelihood* of violence, which always is considered along with the magnitude of violence. For example, a patient who drinks on a daily basis and gets into at least one bar fight per week might be assessed in the emergency room as having a high likelihood of engaging in violence over the next several days. However, he still might be released given the relatively low magnitude of the violence. In contrast, a patient with no history of violent behavior who states during a psychotherapy sessions that he gets so angry at his employer that "I could just shoot him," but who readily disavows that he ever "would actually do such a thing," also might be released. While the magnitude of the possible behavior is great, the likelihood appears to be quite low. Many people seen in the emergency room fall somewhere in between these two extremes. For example, when a patient with schizophrenia states that he hears voices telling him to kill his daughter because she is possessed by demons, the potential magnitude of violence is high, so that the clinical risk assessment would focus on attempting to determine how likely it is that he would do what the voices were telling him to do.

The third aspect is the *imminence* of potential violence. Some patients present with long histories of severe violence, and it can be presumed that *at some point* in the future they will engage in another severe act of violence. However, unless there is evidence that such violent behavior is "imminent" the clinician might not be justified in detaining a patient. The word "imminent" is included in some state's civil commitment statutes, but not in others. Some states include the term but deliberately avoid defining it, while others may offer definitions (e.g., within 48–72 hours). Because of the wealth of potential intervening variables, clinicians are more accurate in predicting imminent violence than in predicting longer-term violence, much as a meteorologist is more accurate in making shorter-term predictions about the weather.

The fourth aspect is the *frequency* of violence. Some patients frequently engage in violence, as in the above example of the alcoholic patient who frequently got into fights at bars. Other violent acts may be of greater cause for concern even if they occur infrequently. For example, if a clinician believes that the patient is engaging in child abuse, even infrequently, this would be enough to trigger the legal obligation to notify the Department of Social Services.

As was the case with suicide, aggressiveness occurs along a spectrum of severity, cuts across psychiatric diagnoses, and even can occur in the absence of any psychiatric diagnosis. Many individuals in society are "aggressive," but not all of them are *violent*. For example, a physician who insults his patients and yells at the hospital nursing staff might be reprimanded but would not be arrested, since his aggression has been expressed verbally and not physically. As discussed in the last chapter, the trait of "impulsive aggression" has been associated with lowered lower levels of serotonin activity (and possibly higher levels of norepinephrine and dopamine activity) in populations of individuals who either have committed suicide by violent means or have engaged in severe violence against other people.

In itself, however, impulsive aggression doesn't necessarily constitute a liability. In some settings—such as in the business, sports, and military arenas—aggressiveness might be an enviable trait, an asset. Both the likelihood that an aggressive individual will become violent and the extent of the violence likely are influenced by many factors, including cultural factors, prior life experience, personality vulnerabilities, and clinical variables (including the presence of alcohol or drug abuse and the presence of particular symptoms of mental illness such as anger, depression, anxiety, and psychotic symptoms).

VIOLENCE AS A PUBLIC HEALTH PROBLEM

One cannot glance at movie marquees or prime-time television without quickly reaching the conclusion that violence permeates modern American culture. Violence constitutes a major public health problem. According to the Department of Justice, there were 6.6 million violent victimizations in 1992. These included 141,000 rapes, 1.2 million robberies, and 5.3 million assaults. In 1992, 5% of all households had a member victimized by violence. A 12-year-old American has an 80% chance of being the victim of a serious crime at some point in his or her life, greater than his or her chance of being injured in a motor vehicle accident.

Homicide was the 14th leading cause of death in the United States in 1996. Each year, about 10 out of every 100,000 people are murdered. Over the past decade, the homicide rate in the United States has been declining, but it remains dramatically higher than the homicide rate in Europe. For example, according to the Centers for Disease Control and Prevention (CDC), in England and Wales the homicide rate for 1994 was only 0.5 per 100,000, 20 times less than the rate in the United States. In Switzerland, the homicide rate is about 1.3 per 100,000, and in Germany it 1.2 per 100,000. There are more violent countries than the United States, including Russia (about 20 per 100,000), Botswana (13 per 100,000), Panama (14 per 100,000), and Grenada (8 per 100,000). However, among Western industrialized nations, the United States clearly stands head and shoulders above the rest. More troubling, the number of homicides committed by children doubled in the decade after 1985, a trend that has not occurred in other countries.

Domestic Violence

Clinicians have become increasingly aware of the need to recognize the clinical concomitants of *domestic violence* because such violence often isn't reported to legal authorities. Battering of females affects at least 4.4 million women in the United States each year; 8% of this country's women are abused each year, 3% severely. One-quarter to one-half of married women are violently assaulted by their male partner at some point in the marriage, and similar rates of assault have been described in nonmarital relationships. About one-third of emergency room visits by women are the result of domestic violence.

The most severe form of domestic violence is homicide. While 22% of homicides are committed by a stranger (half of these during the commission of a felony), 44% are committed by an acquaintance and 20% by a family member. A homicide victim is the wife or girlfriend of the murderer in 11% of all homicides, and about half of all women who are murdered in the United States are killed by a current or former male partner.

Battered women experience high rates of depression, substance abuse, and PTSD. In addition, children who live in households where the female partner is being abused are at increased risk of being physically abused themselves. Usually the abuse is by the male partner, but sometimes it is by the female partner. Given this, clinicians who uncover one form of domestic violence should continue to explore for other forms.

When spousal abuse occurs in a household where there are children present, even when the child hasn't been physically injured he or she typically has witnessed the spousal abuse. This can lead to emotional consequences for the child, including low self-esteem, anxiety, the development of a personality disorder, and being at increased risk for engaging in violence themselves later in life. In addition to their early exposure to domestic violence, children who grow up in violent households typically are exposed to related factors that place them at higher risk for engaging in violence themselves. These include exposure to psychiatric illness or substance abuse in one or both parents, household disarray (such as frequent arguments, relocations, and involvement with the court system), and socioeconomic factors (including poverty, unemployment, lower education, and cultural factors).

Violence and Children

The perpetrators and the victims of violence often are children. When the CDC compared 26 countries, it found that 73% of homicides occurred in the United States, and the homicide rate for children was five times higher in the United States than for the other 25 countries combined. (In the same survey, 54% of suicides also occurred in the United States, and the suicide rate here was two times higher than the combined rates for the other 25 countries.)

One cause of these dramatically higher homicide and suicide rates appears to be the more ready availability of firearms in the United States. A 1993 survey revealed that guns are present in 40%–50% of American households, and 50% are handguns. Keeping a firearm in the home increases the probability that a household member will be killed by a factor of 2.7. When the CDC examined the rates of firearm-related death among children under age 15 for the 26 industrialized countries in 1997, they found that 86% of firearm-related deaths occurred in the United States (50% were homicides, 20% suicides, 22% unintentional, and 3% "intention undetermined"). The overall firearm related death rate for children in the United States was almost 12 times higher than for children in the other 25 countries combined.

This is not to say that the availability of firearms is the *only* factor that accounts for the high death rate among U.S. children. For example, while there is a high density of firearms in some rural, ethnically homogeneous areas, the homicide rate in these areas is far below that seen in some urban areas with a lower density of firearms. Epidemiologic research also has revealed associations between rates of childhood death and other social factors, including low funding for social programs, economic stress related to participation of women in the workforce, divorce, ethnic heterogeneity, and increased social acceptance of violence.

Workplace Violence

Workplace violence has become a source of increasing concern over the past decade. It is a major cause of lost work time and productivity, occupational injury, and even death. Workplace violence is generally defined as verbal or physical assault or any violence that occurs in the workplace even if its source is unrelated to the work environment (e.g., a self-directed assault such as suicide, or an act of violence by a spouse who assaults his partner at her work setting).

The most common attacker in the workplace is a customer (44%), followed by a stranger (24%), coworker (20%), or boss (7%), with former employees only accounting for 3% of incidents despite this last group tending to receive the most publicity. The three most common motivators of workplace violence are revenge, jealousy, and financial gain.

The rate of workplace homicide appears to have dramatically increased over the past two decades. Overall, in the United States it is the third most common cause of occupational death overall (following motor vehicle and machinery accidents), and for women it is the number 1 cause of occupational death. In 1993 there were 1004 homicides in the workplace, an average of four every working day. Most of these murders were robbery-related crimes., which occurred in either the retail sector (particularly jewelry, grocery, and liquor stores) or in the service sector (e.g., gas stations, convenience stores, taxicabs).

Nonfatal assault is 16 times more common in the health-care sector than in the private sector. Almost 20% of teaching hospitals report that threats involving the display of a weapon occur at their facility at least once a month. Half of all of these institutions confiscate weapons at least once a month, and almost half report one or more physical attacks on members of the medical staff each month. About half of all health-care workers are physically assaulted at some point in their careers. In 1995, the Washington State Department of Labor identified the health-care professional as the person most likely to be injured on the job (ranking just above police officers and taxicab drivers).

According to the Occupational Safety and Health Administration (OSHA), the reasons for the high prevalence of assaults in health-care facilities include: 24-hour "open-door" policies, an increased prevalence of patients with active symptoms of mental illness and substance abuse, the availability of drugs and money in the hospital setting, staff downsizing within the health-care industry (with staff members who are working the night shift often having to do so alone), and factors related to the overall hospital milieu (distraught family members, trauma patients, gang members, crowded waiting rooms, intoxicated patients, etc.). Another important factor is the high prevalence of patients who carry weapons. For example, between 4% and 8% of patients bring weapons with them to the psychiatric emergency room, and the only way that these patients have been distinguished from patients who aren't carrying weapons has been through routine screening of all patients.

Job stress and employee "burnout" are problems that both contribute to workplace violence and result from workplace violence. In the wake of an episode of violence, both the victim and his or her coworkers may experience pervasive fear, stress, or depression. Some of them fulfill the diagnostic criteria for major depressive disorder, panic disorder, PTSD, or alcohol or substance abuse. They may express anger at their employers or managers for having failed to sufficiently protect them. Preventive programs aimed at improving interpersonal relations, reducing workplace stress and harassment, and recognizing situations that ultimately might escalate to the point of violence may help to lower the prevalence of workplace violence. Mental health clinicians are increasingly being called upon to consult to private industry in the design and implementation of such programs.

Violence on Inpatient Psychiatric Units

Violence on psychiatric units occurs so commonly that staff members tend to become inured to it. For example, researchers at one site found that five times as many assaults on staff occurred on the unit than were documented by incident reports. A 5-year review by one state facility determined that an average of three to four assaults occurred per day despite the facility having experienced a 33% decrease in the census during the 5 year period.

The prevalence of violent assaults on inpatient psychiatric units may be increasing for a variety of reasons: deinstitutionalization policies have led to those patients who are less violent having been discharged into the community while laws granting patients greater latitude to refuse treatment with antipsychotic medications has increased the proportion of patients on inpatient units who have an untreated psychotic illness. In addition, fears of lawsuits probably have led emergency room clinicians to admit more evaluees who have severe character disorders and histories of violence despite many these individuals having no treatable psychiatric illnesses.

However, most psychiatric inpatients are not violent. A small core group of about 10% of inpatients accounts for most of these violent inci-

dents. The most common psychiatric diagnoses associated with inpatient assault varies depending on the inpatient setting being examined. For example, it shouldn't be particularly surprising that on psychiatric units that primarily treat patients with chronic schizophrenia, schizophrenia is the most common diagnosis associated with assault. The same applies to the finding that on geriatric units it is patients with dementia who are the most likely to assault a staff member. Overall, though, the diagnoses most commonly associated with assaultive behavior on inpatient units are schizophrenia, mania, personality disorder, alcoholism, delirium, and dementia.

Of note, patients who only have made *threats* of violence prior to admission, even threats not directed toward treatment staff, are as likely to engage in violent behavior once on the inpatient unit as are patients who actually have engaged in a violent act prior to hospital admission. In one study, about 30% of patients with schizophrenia and mania who had made violent threats prior to hospital admission engaged in assaultive behavior in the hospital.

Manic patients are more likely to engage in assaultive behavior in the absence of prior threats than are patients with schizophrenia. Violence by manic patients most often is the result of general behavioral disinhibition and irritability. In contrast, patients with schizophrenia of the paranoid subtype and patients with delusional disorder of the persecutory type are more likely to engage in premeditated violence in the community, often in response to paranoid delusions. These patients, in comparison with patients with schizophrenia of the disorganized subtype, are better able to carry out organized, planned behaviors such as buying a firearm, traveling to another city, locating victims, etc. In contrast, patients with schizophrenia of the disorganized subtype are more likely to engage in violence on longer-term inpatient units. The patients are more likely to engage in unplanned (and therefore unforeseen) acts of aggression, such as suddenly punching a nurse in the face as she is handing out medication.

Not surprisingly, violent behavior is more prevalent on acute admissions wards and locked units because such units deliberately select for more "unstable" patients. In addition, violence may occur more frequently on more overcrowded units. Inpatients who engage in violence typically due so early on their hospital stay before the prescribed treatment has begun to take effect. (Of course, whether patients remain in the hospital often depends on whether they continue to pose an ongoing risk of violence, such that the longer-stay patient population also becomes fortified with the most violent individuals.)

Assaults may be most common on visiting days, perhaps due to the increased activity or the anxiety, anger, or ambivalence commonly associated with family visits. Assaults also may occur more commonly during periods of the day when there are fewer structured activities, although they also can occur when a period of relative inactivity is followed by increased demands being placed on the patient. Inconsistent limit setting also plays a role in some cases. Some staff members may unconsciously or subtly provoke violence by displacing their personal aggression onto the patient. Staff members described as "rigid," "intolerant," "adversarial," or "authoritarian" may be at greater risk of being assaulted.

Most assaults in the inpatient setting are related to the use of seclusion or restraint. In other words, the patient already has demonstrated the potential for violence or losing control, and a staff member then becomes injured while attempting to restrain the patient. This argues for the importance of training staff in the proper techniques of placing patients in seclusion and restraint and also for the importance of having a sufficient number of personnel present during the restraint procedure to ensure personal safety.

Risk assessment for violence potential should be a routine part of the psychiatric hospital admissions process because hospital staff should be forewarned and interventions in higher-risk cases should occur early in the hospital stay. Even outside of the psychiatric arena, all health-care professionals should have an understanding of the risk factors for potential violence in the health-care setting in order to better protect not only the medical staff but also other patients.

RISK ASSESSMENT FOR VIOLENCE

A 32-year-old man with a history of schizophrenia and cocaine abuse presents to the emergency room with persecutory delusions involving his father,

who he feels is conspiring to kill him by poisoning his medications. He is admitted to the inpatient psychiatric unit and treated with haloperidol. Over the next few days, the delusions remit, and he appears much more organized. His attending psychiatrist wonders if he is ready for discharge. How should he assess for this, and what relevant risk factors should he address?

The caveats related to risk assessment for suicide discussed in the previous chapter also apply to risk assessment for violence. First, clinicians should avoid making *predictions* of future behavior; rather, they should assess whether the patient is at higher or lower *risk* of engaging in particular behaviors. Second, *absolute*, categorical statements should be avoided; rather, clinicians should speak in terms of relative *probabilities*. Even highly astute clinicians are unable to make predictions with a high degree of certainty due to factors beyond their control such as low base rates of violence and potential intervening variables. Third, the determination of risk is to be distinguished from the ultimate societal weighing of whether a given level of risk justifies or does not justify civil commitment.

Fourth, the goal of the treatment plan is not to eliminate *all* risk of violence but to determine the risk factors that might be modifiable and to address these to a feasible extent. Given the multidetermined nature of violence and the interdependent nature of violence risk factors, no single intervention is likely to prevent future violence. Multiple targets for intervention will exist in many cases but will differ from person to person. However, this also means that effective intervention need not *eliminate* all or even most of a person's risk factors. It may be sufficient for intervention simply to reduce the total, combined effect of all of these risk factors to a level that is below the threshold for overt violence.

Fifth, a risk assessment should be performed and documented at major decision points throughout the treatment. Levels of risk change over the course of treatment, and it is appropriate to modify one's risk assessment accordingly. In this regard, clinicians' determinations of the risk of violence resemble meteorologists' assessments of the risk of inclement weather, which they modify on a daily basis. The public has grown accustomed to meteorologists defining the risk of inclement weather in probabilistic language (e.g., stating that there is a "40% chance of precipitation today"), although when the magnitude of the risk is particularly great, they also are accustomed to taking significant steps to minimize the probability of harm even when the likelihood of harm is low (e.g., they may evacuate their homes in response to a "tornado warning" even though they recognize that there is a significant chance that the tornado never may materialize). By analogy, a patient might initially be committed in response to a "violence" warning, but it might be quite appropriate to release the patient a few days later following further assessment and possibly by the initiation of treatment.

Sixth, a *risk–benefit analysis* also should be a part of clinical decision making at each of these stages. As discussed in the previous chapter, every treatment option offers potential short-term and longer-term costs as well as potential benefits. Clinicians must weigh these against each other throughout the course of treatment. When the risk of imminent violence appears to be very high, involuntary hospitalization may be quite justified, despite the expense, the potential stigma, and the potential risk of alienating the patient. However, as the patient's level of risk declines over the course of the hospital stay, further inpatient hospitalization at some point will no longer be justified. Patients typically are not retained in the hospital until their level of risk has declined to zero—only until the benefits of hospitalization no longer outweigh the disadvantages of hospitalization.

As discussed in the last chapter, in the context of risk assessment for suicide, risk factors for violence can be divided into those that are static (i.e., not subject to change) and those that are dynamic (i.e., amenable to clinical intervention). These factors are listed in Table 17–1. **Static risk factors** include the presence or absence of particular *demographic variables* (age, race, sex whether raised in a violent family), the presence or absence of a *psychiatric diagnosis*, enduring *trait vulnerabilities* such as mental retardation or psychopathy, and a *prior history of violence*. **Dynamic risk factors** include both **clinical variables** (e.g., *psychotic symptoms, alcohol or drug use*, presence or absence of a *therapeutic alliance*, presence or absence of *impulsive aggression*) and **situational variables** (e.g., *social sup-*

Table 17–1. Static and Dynamic Risk Factors Associated with Violence

STATIC RISK FACTORS

Psychiatric diagnosis (depression, schizophrenia, alcohol and drug abuse, dementia or brain injury)
Demographic variables (younger, male, raised in violent or unstable family)
Trait vulnerabilities (mental retardation, psychopathy)
Prior violent acts

DYNAMIC RISK FACTORS

Clinical variables (psychotic symptoms, alcohol or drug use, impulsive aggression, therapeutic alliance)
Situational variables (social supports, interpersonal conflict, occupational status, availability of weapons, availability of potential victims)

ports, interpersonal conflict, occupational status, access to a weapon such as a gun, and the *availability of potential victims*).

In general, one first should estimate a patient's *actuarial* risk of violence by considering demographic groups into which the patient falls and known base rates for violence by members of such groups. Just as local meteorologists use actuarial information from the National Weather Service as a starting point for their local forecast but then revise this data upward or downward to adjust for particular local idiosyncrasies, clinicians should *adjust their estimation* of a specific patient's violence risk based upon the patient's particular clinical and situational variables (each of which may serve to either increase or decrease the risk of violence).

Clinicians who rely solely on patients' current clinical symptoms and ignore actuarial data may significantly underestimate or overestimate a patient's risk of violence. One never can be sure that one's "clinical judgment" is particularly accurate because clinicians don't routinely track down former patients to determine how accurate their forecasts turned out to be. Clinicians tend to develop "rules of thumb" over the years about the relationship between particular symptoms (e.g., "command" hallucinations or paranoid delusions) and future outcomes. These heuristic "rules of thumb" may be of limited utility, may distract the clinician from attending to more predictive variables, and sometimes turn out to be just plain wrong. For example, one study found that mental health clinicians asked to predict violence risk based solely upon mental status examination data were less accurate in their predictions than were nonclinicians who were provided with information about the patients' histories of previous violence.

Further, recent research suggests that some of the best predictors of future violence relate not to particular psychotic or mood symptoms but to particular *dimensional personality features* that clinicians don't routinely or explicitly assess for during briefer examinations. These factors tend to become more apparent if clinicians perform a detailed *social history*, particularly if they fortify their history with a few additional questions related specifically to the theme of past violent behavior attitudes known to be associated with a greater propensity for violence.

While most physicians don't routinely perform such detailed social histories, it becomes more important for them to do so in specific cases where they have reason to be concerned that a patient may be at higher risk for violence (e.g., the patient has a significant history of violent behavior or was admitted to the hospital due to having made violent threats). Examples of dimensional factors that one should assess for in conducting a more detailed social history include "core" antisocial personality traits (emotional detachment with a lack of empathy or remorse), an antisocial behavior style (a tendency to act in ways that violate societal norms or the rights of others), a tendency toward impulsiveness, a tendency to anger easily, and the presence of violent fantasies (particularly escalating fantasies).

STATIC RISK FACTORS

Psychiatric Diagnosis

Are psychiatric patients more prone to engage in violent behavior than are other members of the general population? The general public tends to assume that this is case based primarily upon extensive media coverage whenever a mentally ill individual engages in an act of severe violence. This assumption is a primary cause of stigma attaching to the mentally ill. In other words, many people support treating the mentally ill in the community setting provided that it isn't in *their* community, often due to concerns about the potential for such patients to behave violently.

Is there any objective basis for such concerns? Swanson and associates attempted to address this question using data from the Epidemiologic Catchment Area survey of over 10,000 individuals living in the community. While this study wasn't originally designed to address the relationship between mental illness and violence, it did assign *DSM-III* psychiatric diagnoses and also did include five "yes/no" questions related to more severe violent behavior over the previous year:

1. Did you ever hit or throw things at your spouse/husband/partner?
2. Have you ever spanked or hit a child (yours or anyone else's) hard enough so that he or she had bruises or had to stay in bed or see a doctor?
3. Since age 18, have you been in more than one fight that came to swapping blows, other than fights with your spouse/husband/partner?
4. Have you ever used a weapon like a stick, knife, or gun in a fight since you were 18?
5. Have you ever gotten into physical fights while drinking?

The researchers found that the base rate of violence among individuals with no mental disorder diagnosis was 2%. In contrast, the base rate of violence for individuals with almost any of the major Axis I diagnoses (obsessive–compulsive disorder, panic disorder, major depressive disorder, bipolar disorder, and schizophrenia) was about 12%—that is, six times higher than the rate for the general population. However, this rate of violence still pales in comparison to the rate that they found for individuals with substance-related disorders, whether due to cannabis (a base rate of 19%), alcohol (25%), or other drugs (35%).

Many psychiatric patients carry more than one diagnosis. In such patients, these psychiatric diagnoses can interact in a synergistic way to further increase their risk of violence. For example, when one considers patients with histories of an anxiety disorder, mood disorder, or schizophrenia who do *not* also have a history of a substance-related disorder, the rates of violence are much lower (2%, 3%, and 8%, respectively). In contrast, when one considers patients who *only* have a substance-related disorder, the rate of violence is considerably higher (21%). The highest rates, however, occur in those patients who have *both* an anxiety disorder and a substance-related disorder (20%), a mood disorder and substance-related disorder (29%), or schizophrenia and a substance-related disorder (30%).

In this study, gender and age also played important contributory roles. Violence was twice as prevalent among males as among females and seven times as prevalent among younger individuals as among older individuals.

Several other community surveys have confirmed the conclusion that psychiatric patients residing in the community demonstrate more violent behavior than do members of the population without a history of mental illness. However, one must keep firmly in mind that this is a *statistical* association, revealing an increased *relative risk* for violence among individuals with mental illness. In contrast, the *absolute risk* of violence by individuals with mental illness, particularly more severe violence, remains very small. Only a small proportion of the violence that occurs in our society is attributable to individuals with a mental illness. Further, substance abuse is a much more significant risk factor for violence than other Axis I conditions such as anxiety disorders, mood disorders, or psychotic disorders.

Neuropsychiatric disorders including dementia, delirium, traumatic brain injury, and epilepsy also have been associated with increased rates of aggression. Researchers have examined the relationship between brain injury and violence in two ways: populations selected on the basis of known brain injury have been examined for evidence of violent behavior, and violent populations (particularly prison inmates) have been examined with neuropsychological and neurologic examinations to assess for evidence of subtle brain injury.

Among the very old, *dementia* is the most common cause of violent behavior. Surprisingly, statistics gathered by a nursing union have documented that working in a nursing home is more dangerous than working in mines, construction, or private industry. When individuals with dementia engage in violent behavior, it often occurs in the context of "catastrophic reactions," during attempts to redirect them or assist them with bathing, toileting, or dressing. Their violence also tends to occur more commonly in the evening, consistent with aggressiveness being exacerbated by the "sundowning" phenomenon.

Patients with *closed head injuries* often demonstrate a combination of neuropsychological abnormalities; nonspecific, subtle neurologic abnormalities (neurologic "soft signs"); EEG abnormalities; and personality changes. The last typically include a combination of apathy, impulsiveness, irritability, and—on occasion—violent outbursts.

Rarely, patients with a *seizure disorder* become violent during the ictal state or while postictally confused. This aggression typically is disorganized and is not goal-directed. While some individuals with seizure disorders demonstrate violent outbursts that are out of proportion to any external provocation, it isn't clear that these outbursts caused by seizure activity. Rather, such individuals may have underlying neuropsychological impairments, lower I.Q., or a comorbid psychiatric illness.

How does brain injury contribute to an increased propensity for violence? Animal research and case reports involving humans with regional brain injuries suggest that aggression can be associated with injury to *specific neuroanatomic locations*. In animals, stimulation of some brain regions leads to increased aggressive behavior, while stimulation of other areas leads to behavioral inhibition. For example, stimulation of one area of the amygdala leads to a rage response, while stimulation of another areas of the amygdala only 3 millimeters away inhibits the expression of anger.

As discussed in Chapter 4, specific brain regions are involved in the modulation of emotion. These regions in turn connect to other brain regions, thereby forming *circuits* that allow the brain to integrate perceptions of the external environment, internal physiologic states, memories of past experiences, moods, biological drives, and behaviors into a coherent whole. The regions that appear to be the most important with regard to violence all relate to the *limbic system* and include the hypothalamus, various temporal lobe structures (especially the amygdala), and the frontal lobes.

The *hypothalamus* appears to play a key role in integrating the somatic, visceral, and affective components of emotional responses. In animals, hypothalamic lesions lead to *sham rage reactions*—that is, intense anger and undirected aggression with little or no external provocation, accompanied by sympathetic hyperarousal. The behavior is stereotyped, independent of both past experience and current environmental cues, and isn't modified by learning.

Structures within the *temporal lobes*, particularly the *amygdala*, appear to play a role in associating past experience with related emotions and behaviors. The amygdala receives input from each sensory modality and also from the prefrontal cortex. Its output projects to the extrapyramidal system and hypothalamus. In general, *stimulating* the amygdala and surrounding regions of the temporal lobe (the "extended amygdala") leads to an *increase* in emotional reactivity to external stimuli and aggression. In contrast, *lesions* to this area lead to *decreased* emotional reactivity to external stimuli. In monkeys, this takes the form of **Klüver-Bucy syndrome**: a loss of aggressive responses, accompanied by hyperorality and hypersexuality. The latter two symptoms can be explained by the monkeys having lost *selectivity* in their behavioral drives—having lost their past associations to foods and sexual partners, they attempt to eat anything and have sex with anybody. Therefore, in contrast to hypothalamic lesions, where aggression becomes autonomous, with amygdala lesions the behavior is closely tied to environmental stimuli but isn't appropriately *modulated*. Patients with histories of violent behavior sometimes demonstrate temporal lobe EEG abnormalities, although this is a nonspecific finding.

The *frontal lobes* are involved in regulating "executive function"—that is, synthesizing external stimuli, internal mood states, and memory; setting goals; and organizing behaviors in such a way as to achieve these goals. Frontal lobe injury is associated with impaired planning and cognitive flexibility. Personality changes also can be seen. Lesions of the orbitofrontal region (which has reciprocal connections to the amygdala) have been associated with irritability or violent behavior. Histories of severe violence in various clinical populations also have been associated with decreased frontal lobe metabolism in several functional neuroimaging studies, and violent patients sometimes demonstrate slowing of EEG activity in the frontal region.

The above research involves studying brain–behavior relationships by making brain disease the independent variable and violence the dependent variable. Another area of research has taken the opposite tack, looking for evidence of brain disease in particularly violent individuals. A high rate of subtle neuropsychological and neurological deficits has been noted among individuals incarcerated for violent offenses. The direction of causality remains unclear, however. For example, while neuropsychological deficits might contribute to psychopathy or to impulsive aggression, the opposite also could be true: the latter two traits might contribute to an individual leading a higher-risk lifestyle that includes multiple subacute head injuries (e.g., fights leading to blows to the head, car accidents, falling off of roofs, chronic substance use, or car accidents).

Even when a violent individual demonstrates a subtle neurophysiologic abnormality, it may be impossible to determine with any degree of certainty whether the violence is causally related to the abnormality. The diagnosis of **intermittent explosive disorder** has been applied to individuals who experience discrete episodes of aggression that result in serious assaults or destruction of property: the degree of aggressiveness expressed during an episode is grossly out of proportion to any provocation or precipitating psychosocial stressor.

However, the diagnosis of intermittent explosive disorder is poorly validated and controversial. Many individuals who receive this diagnosis also have been diagnosed with a cluster B personality disorder (such as borderline, narcissistic, or antisocial personality disorder), which themselves are characterized by impulsive aggression. Others have also had other Axis I disorders including bipolar disorder, conduct disorder, attention-deficit hyperactivity disorder, a substance-related disorder, dementia, or traumatic brain injury. Given this, the *DSM-IV* has retained the diagnosis but has relegated it to being a *diagnosis of exclusion*. One should only diagnose intermittent explosive disorder in those rare cases when none of these other diagnoses is present.

While there is a higher rate of EEG abnormalities among impulsive and aggressive individuals, these are nonspecific findings and in any given individual might be purely incidental. Epileptiform activity has been noted in 1%–10% of the nonepileptic general population and also is occasionally seen in nonepileptic patients who are taking antidepressant or antipsychotic medications or who are withdrawing from sedative–hypnotic medications. When EEG testing is performed on all patients admitted to a psychiatric unit, abnormalities are found in up to 20% of cases; only rarely do they lead to any change in the clinical diagnosis, however. Further, while anticonvulsant drugs sometimes are useful in attenuating impulsive aggression in cases where EEG abnormalities have been detected, they also have been useful when no such abnormalities have been detected since they appear to exert nonspecific, antiaggressive effects in addition to their anticonvulsant effects.

To reiterate a key tenet of the behavioral perspective, it is unlikely that abnormal activity in a particular brain region is enough *in itself* to explain violent behavior in most cases. Rather, localized brain dysfunction is but one factor that—in combination with other psychiatric symptoms, personality vulnerabilities, lower intelligence, substance abuse, previous life experience, and/or current life circumstances—may *contribute* to the ultimate behavioral outcome.

Demographic Variables

In the general population *age* is an important risk factor. Younger age is associated with a higher risk of violence, with a window of particularly high risk stretching from the late teens through the early 20s. Psychopathy also appears to decline with age in some (but certainly not all) individuals with antisocial personality disorder. An increase in the rate of violence occurs in individuals over age 70, associated with an increasing prevalence of dementia in this group. *Sex* also is an important risk factor, since men are three times more likely to engage in violence than are women.

However, while these relationships hold true for the general population, other factors may greatly outweigh them in specific cases. For example, while age may be an important factor when assessing an individual with a personality disorder, it may be less important in the context of an individual with a severe mental illness associated with persecutory delusional beliefs. The same reasoning applies to male versus female sex

One prospective study that asked emergency room psychiatrists to predict whether patients that they were evaluating would become violent

during the following 6 months found that the psychiatrists were more accurate in their predictions for male patients than for female patients. To determine why this might be the case, the researchers asked the clinicians to estimate base rates of violence for the men and women who presented to their emergency room. The clinicians estimated that the base rate among men was 45%, which was very close to the actual base rate, which was 42%. In contrast, they estimated that the base rate for women was 22%, when the actual base rate turned out to be 49%. In other words, while women are much less likely to become violent than men in general, this is not the case for women suffering symptoms of acute psychiatric illness. In the face of the latter, gender differences disappear, such that the rates of violence for male and female become the same.

The nature of the aggressive behaviors exhibited by men and women differs. The targets of aggressive or violent acts by women are more likely to be family members, while the targets of such acts by men are more likely to be either acquaintances or strangers rather than family members. Similarly, violent behavior by women is more likely to take place at home, whereas violence by men is more likely to take place outdoors on the streets. Violence by men is more likely to be associated with alcohol or substance intoxication, and it is more likely to result in serious injury to the target, resulting in the need for medical attention. Perhaps as a result, violent behavior by men is more likely to result in arrest.

Dimensional Vulnerabilities

Many individuals who engage in impulsive aggression do so as a result of low frustration tolerance and difficulty controlling anger. Dimensional vulnerabilities such as personality disorder and lower intelligence increase these propensities. In previous chapters, we have discussed how some *personality disorders* (particularly *borderline and antisocial personality disorders*) include affective instability, impulsiveness, and aggressive behavior in their diagnostic criteria. These disorders also have been associated with evidence of subtle neurophysiologic dysfunction, including neuropsychological abnormalities, decreased cortical arousal and excessive temporal lobe activity on EEG studies, and neurotransmitter abnormalities (most notably, evidence of lower serotonergic activity).

Individuals with *lower intelligence* (even those whose I.Q. doesn't fall within the mental retardation range) also are at greater risk for engaging in violent behavior. This likely reflects the fact that, in the face of a frustrating or upsetting situation, they have greater difficulty devising appropriate alternatives to violence that better serve their longer-term best interests.

Individuals with a history of a childhood *learning disorder* and/or *attention-deficit hyperactivity disorder* also may be at increased risk for becoming violent, both due to the impairments in impulse control associated with these conditions and because of their association with the later development of conduct disorder (and subsequently, in some cases, antisocial personality disorder). One theory proposes that individuals with attention and learning difficulties receive little reward from academics, become disruptive, and ultimately drop out of school. Enjoying little support from either their family or the school system, their impulsiveness is more likely to become linked to socially disruptive behaviors.

Both personality disorders and mental retardation—when considered as global constructs—are enduring dispositions. They therefore are considered to be "static" risk factors even though some aspects of temperament (especially impulsivity and irritability) might be considered "dynamic" in that they may respond to medication or to psychotherapy (such as supportive therapy or anger management training). In other words, an individual with antisocial personality disorder who is prescribed an SSRI such as fluoxetine, while still exhibiting antisocial attitudes, may still experience a reduction in impulsive aggression.

In taking the social history, one should focus on *childhood developmental factors* that have been associated with an increased likelihood of later violence, including separation from parents (particularly from one's father) during childhood or early adolescence, childhood physical abuse, and a parental history of substance abuse or violence. Childhood abuse and neglect might result in future violent behavior due to modeling of violent behavior and/or from lack of self-control developing in children who have not been received adequate supervision during early childhood (when one's "moral sense" develops).

One also should focus on past incidents that indicate a predisposition toward impulsive behavior, poor response to criticism, low frustration tolerance, or reckless behavior. For example, patients may indicate having worked multiple jobs, but none for very long. They might report having impulsively quit these jobs, either out of anger over some minor incident or simply out of boredom. They may describe a history of arrests for driving offenses, public intoxication, fights, shoplifting, or writing bad checks. They also may report a history of attitudes and behaviors typically seen in association with conduct disorder and antisocial personality disorder, such as childhood fire-setting or cruelty to animals, school truancy and suspensions, fights, drug use, sexual promiscuity, coercive sexual activity, destruction of property, substance use, deceitfulness, and lack of remorse.

Prior Violent Behavior

The best predictor of future behavior is past behavior, and a *previous history of violent behavior* is the single best predictor of future violent behavior. Virtually all violent crime committed by released psychiatric inpatients is committed by those individuals who already had extensive criminal records prior to the hospitalization. In addition, the risk of future violence increases with number of past violent acts: the probability of being arrested again for a person with four prior arrests is about 80%; the probability with five prior arrests is virtually 100%.

One way of quickly eliciting a history of violence is to *directly ask the patient*: "What's the most violent thing that you've ever done?" Surprisingly (given the social unacceptability of violent behavior), many patients are very willing to answer this question in extensive detail. Two other useful screening questions are: "Have you ever seriously injured another person?" and "Do you ever now think about harming someone else?" When available, *collateral informants* can be very important sources of information about past violent behavior. Informants might include family members, records from past hospitalizations, and the potential victim of any current violent threats.

When the patient endorses past episodes of violence, one can explore these in more detail. The goal of this questioning is to discern any *patterns of violence* and to determine how the patient's current situation resembles or differs from these past situations. One also is looking for points in these past situations where intervention might have been feasible. For example, who said what first? How soon was it before the patient acted violently that he decided to do so? What was he thinking at the time? Did he use a weapon? Were these isolated incidents or repetitive or escalating patterns of behavior? In listening to the patient's description of past incidents, one also should be assessing the degree to which the patient appears to demonstrate *remorse* for these violent acts or *empathy* for the victims of the violence.

Was the patient *intoxicated* at the time of the assaultive behavior? (If so, substance rehabilitation might be the major intervention employed to minimize the risk of future violence.) Was the patient compliant with prescribed medications at the time of the violent incident? (If not, this suggests that one will particularly need to address the issue of treatment compliance if one hopes to reduce the risk of future incidents.)

Where has past violence taken place? In considering this question, one should ask questions about *domestic violence* involving the patient's spouse and children. The most common victims of violence by psychiatric patients are family members, and this violence more commonly occurs in chaotic or crowded homes. Has the patient engaged in assaultive behavior even in highly structured settings such as in an inpatient psychiatric unit or in jail?

Patients might describe two types of violence. **Reactive aggression** (also called "affective" or "impulsive" aggression) describes aggressive behavior that is unplanned and that occurs in response to acute provocation. This type of violence might be amenable to psychotherapy using an "anger management" or "relapse prevention" model. The goal of this type of therapy is to help the patient identify the typical situations that tend to provoke his anger to devise more effective and appropriate coping strategies. This type of aggression also is more likely to be amenable to pharmacotherapy.

In contrast, **instrumental aggression** (also called "predatory" aggression) refers to aggressive behavior that is premeditated and goal-directed. This latter pattern of violence is seen in antisocial individuals and obviously much more difficult to modify. Patients who demonstrate isolated episodes of reactive aggression may express remorse for their behavior once they have calmed down. They therefore may be open to trying to change their behavior. In contrast, patients who engage in instrumental aggression usually don't regret their behavior (although they may be upset about their behavior's negative *consequences*, such as incarceration). Note that while reactive aggression can occur in isolation, most individuals who demonstrate a consistent pattern of instrumental aggression also tend to experience superimposed episodes of reactive aggression.

Some patients come across as having "overcontrolled" aggression. In other words, they might deny having virtually *any* violent urges, despite obvious objective evidence to contrary. For example, an individual arrested for having stalked and shot his wife following a separation might insist that he was "not upset at all" after he discovered his wife's infidelity toward him and when she left him to be with the other man. When asked how he came to kill his wife he might answer, "I can't really explain it." Such patients appear to have a very limited ability to recognize and appropriately channel their angry impulses so that they can suppress their anger. At some point, they fly into an acute rage that might come as a surprise even to themselves.

One should assess any *current threats* of violence using similar questions. Is the threat of violence impulsive or is it well planned? Has the patient been "escalating" in his recent behavior? Detailed questioning about the potential *outcome* of any threatened acts of violence can serve two purposes. First, it can provide information about the nature of the threat (e.g., whether it is reactive or instrumental) and how serious the patient is about carrying out the threat. Second, in some cases this questioning might prove to be therapeutic for reactive individuals who haven't really "thought the whole thing through." Consider the following two examples:

A 27-year-old man states that he is furious at his wife for cheating on him, and that he plans to kill her. When asked by the psychiatrist what he plans to do *after* having killed her, the patient appears surprised and asks, "What do you mean?" The psychiatrist again asks what the patient thinks will happen *after* he kills his wife. The patient pauses and replies, "You know, I never really thought about that. I guess I would be arrested." When asked what likely would happen after this, the patient replies, "Well, I guess they'd lock me up for a long time, maybe even for life." The psychiatrist asks how the patient feels about that, and the patient replies, "I don't like it. It's not worth throwing my whole life away just for her. She's not worth it. Maybe I won't kill her, but, God, I'm really mad at her." The patient agrees to a voluntary hospital admission with the goal of "helping him to learn to handle his anger."

A 27-year-old man states that he is furious at his wife for cheating on him, and that he plans to kill her. When asked by the psychiatrist what he plans to do *after* killing her, the patient appears surprised and asks, "What do you mean?" The psychiatrist again asks what he thinks will happen *after* he kills his wife. The patient pauses and replies, "Well, there's no way I'm going to jail for the rest of my life. My plan is to shoot her in the head and then shoot myself in the head, too."

The second example also illustrates another important clinical maxim. When patients make homicidal threats, one also should inquire into *suicidal ideation*. The risk of violence is of even greater concern from patients who plan to commit suicide afterward because they are not likely to be deterred by the threat of future punishment for their actions. In addition, one should inquire into past suicide attempts and the nature of these: patients with histories of violent suicide attempts also are more likely to engage in violence against others.

But when a depressed patient reports suicidal ideation, one also should inquire about homicidal thoughts. Male and female patients may differ in this regard. A male patient who plans to kill himself might decide to kill his entire family first out of *jealous* concerns about that his wife will marry another man after his death and that his children will think of this man as their father. A female patient who plans to kill herself might decide to kill her children first out of more *altruistic* concerns about her children otherwise being left alone in the world without a mother.

Finally, one should assess the *potential availability of the victim of the threatened violence.* Clearly it is of greater cause for concern if the victim is readily available, as would be the case when the potential victim is an employer, supervisor, or spouse.

DYNAMIC RISK FACTORS

Clinical Variables

Delusions

While individuals with mental illness have a higher risk of engaging in violence relative to individuals without mental illness, these findings do not tell the "whole story." They don't explain *why* individuals with mental illness are more likely to engage in violence, and they also don't explain why *one* individual with a given mental illness might engage in violence and another individual with the same mental illness might not. Given that most patients with any given mental disorder do *not* become violent, it is likely that particular symptoms associated with those disorders account for the increased risk.

For example, some large community studies have suggested that specifc types of *paranoid delusions* (i.e., delusions in which patients believe that people are seeking to harm them or that outside forces are controlling their minds, both of which have been called *"threat/control override" delusions*) account almost entirely for the higher rate of violence among individuals with mental illness. These researchers found that when they controlled for these specific delusions, the rates of violence among mentally ill individuals and among nonill individuals were the same. (Again, this is not to say that these symptoms *predicted* violence in individual cases. Most individuals who expressed these symptoms didn't engage in violence, just as most young males don't commit violence, despite this being a statistically significant risk factor.)

However, a more recent study, the MacArthur Study of Mental Disorder and Violence, did not find a relationship between delusions and violence. This study prospectively examined over 1000 patients recruited from inpatient psychiatric units. They assessed these patients for 134 risk factors while the patients were still in the hospital, and they then followed through serial interviews every 10 weeks over a 1 year period from the date of hospital discharge.

At baseline, 29% of the patient sample manifested delusions. When delusions were present, they were assessed with regard to the degree of conviction to which the patient held them, associated negative affects, the patient's history of having acted on their beliefs, the patient's degree of preoccupation with their beliefs, and the pervasiveness of the beliefs. Remarkably, the researchers found a weak *negative* relationship between delusions and violence. In other words, delusional patients were *less* likely to become violent than were nondelusional patients. This conclusion held even when the type of delusions, their content (including violent content), and patient's histories of having acted on their delusions were taken into account. It may be that the findings from earlier researchers resulted from their having used self-report inventories (thereby including some individuals whose comments that there were others who "wished to do them harm" weren't in fact delusional) and also from having—through these particular questions—selected a group of individuals who were more angry and suspicious in general, both of which are risk factors in themselves for violence.

These researchers were quick to point out that these findings must be interpreted appropriately. They should not be taken as evidence that delusions never cause violence. Clinical experience confirms that severe acts of violence by psychiatric patients do occur and sometimes are motivated by their delusional beliefs. However, such acts fortunately appear to be relatively rare.

From the *public policy* perspective, it is important to recognize that, as a group, delusional persons do not appear to be more violent than persons with other mental illnesses or even than their nonill neighbors. Perhaps this reflects that fact that delusions tend to occur in the context of chronic psychotic conditions and that these conditions also are associated with social withdrawal and with the development of smaller social networks. Chronically ill, delusional individuals therefore may have less desire and fewer opportunities than other individuals to engage in the kind of interpersonal interactions that might lead to acts of instrumental violence.

From the *clinical* perspective, however, it remains very important to assess carefully for evidence from one's examination of past violent incidents and of recent events for any discernable relationship between the patient's delusions and violent behavior. It remains possible that a person who has acted violently in the past on the basis of his delusions may well do so again. Nor do they provide support for neglecting the potential threat of an acutely destabilized, delusional person in an emergency setting, in which the person's past history of violence and community supports are unknown. However, the persistence of delusions in a person who has been hospitalized and treated, and who otherwise is ready for release, should not—in itself—preclude the formulation of an appropriate discharge plan.

Another useful approach to assessing persecutory delusions is to ask the patient to speculate as to how he might act in the future should his worst fears actually come to pass. For example, if the patient believes that people on the street are "all looking at him" and "trying to insert thoughts into his head," one might ask him what he would do if there were a knock at the door and the people who have been spying at him for so long were standing right there. If the patient replies that he would "try to run away," one might be less concerned than if he states that he keeps a loaded gun next to the front door and that if anybody does knock on his door he will "shoot first and ask questions later."

Some less common types of delusions might be encountered in specific patient populations. For example, some investigators have noted that when *delusional disorder of the erotomanic type* leads to violence, the aggression initially is aimed at individuals who stand in the way of the patient and the object of his or her affection (e.g., loved person's spouse). However, should the loved person finally succeed in frustrating the patient's romantic ambitions, the patient ultimately may decide to engage in violence directed against the loved person.

Elderly patients with *dementia* sometimes become violent in response to delusions. For example, a patient may believe that family members are stealing personal belongings that she actually has misplaced, or she may come to believe that family members have been replaced by imposters (**Capgras's syndrome**).

In the case of patients who are taking antipsychotic medication, one should consider the possibility that the patient's agitation actually is a manifestation of *akathisia*. In such cases, one should consider lowering the medication dose, adding a β-adrenergic antagonist such as propranolol, or switching to an atypical antipsychotic medication.

Hallucinations

Empirical research has produced very similar results with regard to the role of *"command" hallucinations* in violence, having failed to reveal a clear relationship between assaultive behavior and hallucinated "commands." Up to two-thirds of patients with schizophrenia and about one-fifth of patients with bipolar disorder experience hallucinations. Patients experiencing hallucinations rarely have them in isolation; while some studies have indicated that the presence of hallucinations at the time of hospital admission corresponds to assaultiveness, these patients typically were experiencing multiple other kinds of psychotic symptoms as well.

In one series, about one-third of auditory hallucinations involved "commands," the most common being commands to commit suicide (51%), but also including homicide (5%), non-lethal injury to the patient or others (12%), benign actions (14%), and "unspecified" (17%). Patients with hallucinations were more likely to require seclusion (suggesting increased aggression) but there was no difference between those with "command" hallucinations or hallucinations of other types.

Similarly, in the MacArthur study, neither having hallucinations nor having "command" hallucinations in general was significantly related to acts of violence during the year following hospitalization. Violence also wasn't related to the duration that the patient had been experiencing hallucinations, the patient's belief that the voices had to be obeyed, a history of having obeyed the voices in the past, or the patient's belief that he or she would obey the voices in the future. However, when patients specifically reported "command" hallucinations that involved commands to commit *acts of violence* against other people, they were significantly more likely to be violent during the year following hospitalization. (Forty-five percent of these patients engaged in violence versus 24% of patients who

did not report command hallucinations involving interpersonal violence.) This was the case whether or not these patients had a history of having obeyed the voices commanding violence in the past.

While the relationship between hallucinations and violence remains a weak one and likely is outweighed in many cases by other factors, most clinicians have encountered patients who *have* acted in response to "command" hallucinations. Given this, and given the clinical maxim that the best predictor of future behavior is past behavior, one still should assess not only for whether the patient is experiencing "command" hallucinations but also for what the commands are telling the patient to do and for whether the patient has responded to such commands in the past.

Why do some patients act on command hallucinations while others do not? One small series found that those patients who acted on their hallucinations were more likely to either be experiencing an associated delusional belief and/or to be experiencing hallucinations of a recognizable and trusted person. For example, a patient who heard a voice telling him to assault his psychiatrist might be more likely to act on this if he *also* believed that the psychiatrist was part of a conspiracy to poison him with "fake medications" and if the hallucination involved the voice of trusted figure, such as his wife.

Alcohol and Drug Use

Two-thirds of violent offenders were drinking *alcohol* shortly before having committed their crime. This rate is about double that seen with nonviolent crimes. The risk of engaging in violence also has been associated with greater *chronicity* of drinking: chronic drinkers are at greater risk for engaging in a violent offense even when they are not intoxicated at the time of their offense.

Similarly, some *illicit drugs* appear to be especially likely to cause behavioral disinhibition and aggression. These include the psychostimulants, cocaine, PCP, and anabolic steroids. As noted above, alcohol or drug use also can be associated with other Axis I conditions, including schizophrenia and mood disorder, leading to much higher rates of violence than for individuals who have these latter disorders in the absence of substance abuse. In the MacArthur study, 54% of patients who engaged in a violent act during the year following hospital discharge reported having been drinking just before the incident, while 23% reported having used illegal drugs just before the incident.

Impulsive Aggression

Impulsive aggression has been discussed above in the context of static risk factors. However, it is listed here so that clinicians will keep in mind that in some cases it also is a dynamic risk factor that may be amenable to clinical interventions.

Therapeutic Alliance

Does the patient have a therapeutic alliance with a treatment provider? In assessing for this, one should assess not only whether the patient is currently "in treatment" but also whether she is *compliant with visits and with all treatment recommendations*. Does the patient have insight into being ill and needing treatment? Is the patient attending treatment only due to a court order or pressure from her family, or is she actually *invested* in treatment?

In addition, has the patient engaged in acts of violence *despite* being in regular treatment? For example, has the patient engaged in violence on a Wednesday despite having psychotherapy visits every Monday and Friday? If so, it might argue in favor of initiating more intensive or restrictive treatment interventions, such as inpatient hospitalization.

Situational Variables

What type of situation will the patient be discharged into after release from the emergency room or from the hospital? Will this situation be any less stressful than the situation that existed at the time when the patient initially presented? Will it be more stressful?

Does the patient have close *social supports*? Even if he does have many friends, are they the type of friends who are likely to *encourage* substance use and violence rather than discourage it? What is the patient's current *home situation*? Is it supportive or is it a source of distress? Does the patient have a job? If so, is it a stabilizing influence or is it one more source of distress to him?

Does the patient own a potentially *lethal weapon* (especially a gun)? How available are such weapons? If they are readily available, can they be removed by a family member prior to hospital discharge?

Finally, how accessible is *the victim* of the threatened violence? Is the victim in any way provoking a violent response from the patient?

AFTER THE RISK ASSESSMENT

Formulating a Treatment Plan

After the risk assessment has been completed, the clinician's next step is to formulate a treatment plan designed to minimize the risk of future violence. In doing so, one should attempt to identify relevant dynamic risk factors that are amenable to clinical intervention and consider the risks and benefits of specific interventions.

The clinician should document this thought process. As discussed in the last chapter, the best defense against future assertions that the care that one offered was negligent is to engage in sound clinical practice. In the event of a lawsuit, courts tend to be less concerned with whether the physician was able to prevent violence than if the clinician performed a reasonable risk assessment and initiated reasonable clinical interventions. The technique of listing the relevant dynamic risk factors and then listing the steps taken to address each of these (illustrated for a risk assessment for suicide in Table 16–3 in the previous chapter) can be a useful in more complex cases.

As discussed with regard to assessing the risk of suicide, when relying upon less restrictive interventions (e.g., discharging the patient home from the emergency room rather than seeking hospitalization) the *rationale* for the decision based upon a risk–benefit analysis should be documented. Again, this can be brief but should include discussion of the key clinical concerns. For example, the clinician might note:

> The patient threatened to kill his wife during an argument tonight, but both he and his wife confirm the absence of any previous history of violence toward her, only verbal outbursts. I see no evidence at this point of depression or psychotic symptoms that would necessitate initial inpatient treatment, and he is not interested in voluntary admission. He appears to have features of narcissistic personality

disorder with angry outbursts. While he is at high risk for continuing to engage in such behavior, he appears to be at low risk for physically harming his wife. He and his wife have agreed to begin couples therapy, and they can be seen for an intake visit next week. His wife states that she is not afraid of him at this point, but I gave her information on how to call for help or seek admission to a shelter if her husband's behavior does escalate further.

Treatment of dynamic risk factors may include primary pharmacologic intervention not only for depressive, anxious, manic, or psychotic symptoms but also for impulsive aggression, whether this occurs concomitantly with a mood disorder or psychotic disorder or as part of an underlying personality disorder. However, the research supporting their efficacy in this setting has consisted of small case series rather than controlled studies or head-to-head comparisons.

Large-scale pharmaceutical trials usually are conducted with the ultimate goal of obtaining Food and Drug Administration approval for an additional prescribing indication. However, the FDA has been reluctant to offer approval for treatment of "aggression" given that aggression isn't a clinical diagnosis and that there isn't even a universally accepted definition of aggression as a symptom.

Clinicians therefore should rely on their clinical judgment, and sometimes on trial and error, when choosing an appropriate agent. A general rule of thumb is that one first should attempt to select a medication that is appropriate for a patient's *primary* psychiatric disorder but that also possesses antiaggressive properties. When one is prescribing an agent primarily to treat *aggression itself*, one should include the fact that this is an "off-label" (i.e., "unapproved") indication in one's discussions with the patient and obtain appropriate informed consent.

For example, an *antipsychotic medication* would be the first choice in a patient with either schizophrenia or delusional disorder, as well as in the patient with dementia who is engaging in violence in response to delusions or hallucinations. One should strongly consider using an atypical agent, both because akathisia can contribute to aggression and because several studies have documented that atypical agents may have greater antiaggressive effects in patients with schizophrenia than do traditional agents, independent of their antipsychotic and sedative effects. This might relate to their serotonin antagonist effects.

An *SSRI* would be an appropriate choice in a patient with major depressive disorder, dysthymic disorder, or a persistent, dysphoric mood in the context of a personality disorder. Again, research suggests that SSRIs may have antiaggressive properties independent of their antidepressant effects—for example, in patients with personality disorders who do not have a mood disorder.

Mood stabilizers (such as lithium, valproate, and carbamazepine) also have been demonstrated to have antiaggressive properties in a variety of populations, including in patients with bipolar disorder, schizophrenia (even in the absence of affective symptoms), mental retardation, dementia, head injury, borderline personality disorder, and conduct disorder. One might consider using an anticonvulsant agent first in those patients noted to demonstrate paroxysmal activity on an EEG.

Beta-adrenergic antagonists (most commonly propranolol) have been shown to have antiaggressive effects in patients with more severe mental retardation and with traumatic brain injury. *Trazodone* and *buspirone* also have also been shown to be efficacious in these populations, as well as in patients with agitation associated with dementia.

The Duty to Protect Potential Victims of Violence

In general society, people have no legal duty to protect other people from injury caused by a third party. For example, if one sees a blind person about to be hit by a car, one has no legal obligation to protect the blind person from the driver of the car. This is not to say that one wouldn't have an *ethical* obligation to protect the blind person. However, one couldn't be found *legally liable* to the blind person for the failure to have taken steps to protect him. The traditional exception to this rule has been those situations where an individual does have some degree of control over the third party due to a "special relationship." For example, if the car's driver were a minor and I am the minor's parent, I myself could be held liable since I am expected to have some degree of *control* over my child.

Similarly, clinicians have traditionally owed obligations only to their patients. If a clinician provides negligent care that leads to the *patient* being harmed, the patient has the right to sue the clinician. However, if the patient has harmed some third party, *that* person hasn't had the right to sue the clinician because the clinician has no obligation to that third party. In other words, if the patient were going to hit a blind person with a car, the therapist would not be obligated to protect the blind person, since patients have been considered to be autonomous agents rather than children, over whom clinicians do not have control.

This changed in 1974, after a patient in the midst of receiving therapy sessions at the student health clinic at the University of California made threats to kill a woman he knew named Tarasoff. He ultimately did so, and her family later sued the patient's treatment providers on her behalf, arguing that they should have warned her about the patient's homicidal ideation.

The trial court dismissed the case on the grounds that therapists had no obligations toward third parties and third parties therefore had no basis to bring a lawsuit. However, the family appealed and the case ultimately reached the California Supreme Court, which in turn ruled that therapists *do* have obligations to third parties who might be harmed by their patients. The court stated that this obligation stems from the fact that therapists have access to key information due to their relationship with the patient, and that this therefore constituted a "special relationship." In other words, they made a connection between a therapist's having particular *information* to their having some degree of *control* over the patient. The court stated that when a therapist determines or "should have determined" that the patient posed a risk of harming another person, the therapist must *warn* the potential victim.

Several organizations, including the American Psychiatric Association, strongly disagreed with this decision. The APA had six major concerns. First, the court's decision didn't address the baserate problem. Since most patients don't go on to commit serious violence, clinicians would be forced to make many unnecessary warnings, violating confidentiality in each of these cases. Second, there is no objective standard to use when deciding whether a clinician "should have

known" that the patient posed a danger to the victim.

Third, this problem can be exacerbated by "hindsight bias" by a plaintiff's expert, since it is always easier for a somebody *retrospectively* reviewing a patient's chart (i.e., after the patient has killed or serious injured another person) to recognize how "obvious it should have been" that a particular patient was dangerous. In actuality, things aren't as clear *prospectively*.

Fourth, the decision was seen as a serious intrusion on doctor–patient confidentiality. For therapy itself to be ethically permissible, clinicians essentially would have to issue "Miranda" warnings at the outset of therapy, warning their patients that anything that they said that raised concerns about potential harm to another person might lead to the clinician to issuing a warning. This might exert a "chilling effect" on psychotherapy such that patients no longer would be able to openly discuss any aggressive feelings.

Fifth, by requiring that clinicians issue warnings to potential victims in all cases, the decision didn't take into account other potentially available options that might be more appropriate. For example, a clinician might decide to commit the patient to the hospital. This could protect a potential victim without violating doctor–patient confidentiality.

Sixth, the court didn't consider the effects of warning a potential victim on the course of therapy and the patient's future behavior, or whether *warning* potential victims always is the most effective way to *protect* them. For example, what if a patient becomes so upset after a warning has been issued about the violation of his confidentiality that he drops out of treatment? Ultimately, patients such as this could become *more* of a risk to others.

In response to these concerns, the California Supreme Court agreed to reconsider the case, and they issued a new ruling in 1976. This time, they ruled that the therapist didn't have a duty to *warn* potential victims of patients but did have a duty to take steps to *protect* these potential victims. The duty could be carried out by a variety of means, of which issuing a warning was but one.

The court's ruling received a mixed reception. On the one hand, therapists in California now weren't obligated to immediately violate confidentiality in all cases. On the other hand, a well-defined duty (picking up the telephone) had been replaced by a much vaguer standard. Now, plaintiffs' attorneys easily might argue (again, with the benefit of hindsight) that a therapist "should have done even more than he did" to protect the victim and that the therapist obviously *hadn't* done enough, based on the fact that the patient ultimately had attacked the victim.

In the decades following this original decision, almost every state has addressed the so-called "Tarasoff issue" through either court decisions or legislation. Clinicians should familiarize themselves with their state's legal standard. For example, some states have found that clinicians owe *no* obligations to protect third parties, while other states have *expanded* these obligations— for example, to include *any* potential victims and not simply potential victims that the patient has explicitly identified in the course of a treatment session.

Regardless of what the law says, clinicians always should "think clinically" before "thinking legally." What is the patient's diagnosis? What is the patient's level of risk for harming others? How can the risk to others best be minimized? What is best for the patient? Is there a way to protect other members of society while *also* looking out for the patient's best interest? Is there a way to discharge one's "Tarasoff obligations" in a way that moves therapy *forward* rather than *sabotages* it?

Again, clinicians should keep in mind that the obligation to potential victims is to *take appropriate precautions to protect them, not simply to warn them*. Therefore, when a patient has a history of violent behavior, or when the patient expresses current desires to harm others, the clinician is not automatically obligated to begin warning every person with whom the patient might have any contact. Rather, the clinician should *perform a risk assessment for violence*, as detailed in this chapter. Warning the victim should be thought of as *one option for helping to minimize the risk of harm*. Other potential options include the following: increasing the *frequency of sessions*; *adjusting medications* to decrease psychotic symptoms; involving the *patient's family* in therapy; involving the *potential victim* in therapy (although the goals in such cases needs to be carefully weighed against the risks); increasing the extent of *social supports*

(e.g., the Department of Social Services, a substance rehabilitation program, Alcoholics Anonymous, outreach mental health programs for noncompliant patients, etc.); *voluntary hospitalization*; and *involuntary hospitalization*

Notification of the police or of a potential victim ultimately still may prove to be necessary. This is most likely to be the case when a significant risk to the potential victim is likely to remain despite any of the above interventions. However, this still ideally should be turned into a *doctor–patient therapy issue* rather than simply the fulfilling of a doctor's ethical and legal obligations. After all, issuing a warning may actually be in the patient's best interest if it helps the patient avoid committing an impulsive act that he later would regret.

For example, the patient might be encouraged to issue the warning *himself*. This strategy not only encourages the patient to assume responsibility for his impulses but also addressees any concerns about potential breach of confidentiality. In addition, the patient's attitudes and behaviors during such an intervention can provide further valuable clinical data to include in one's ongoing risk assessment

Even when a patient declines to take such an active role in issuing a warning, clinical experience suggests that the outcome of therapy is better when any such warnings have been discussed with the patient in advance of issuing them. Even in cases where the patient disagrees with the clinician's plan to warn the victim, if the plan has been discussed with her and she has been allowed to have some "voice" in the process, she often will state that she "can understand why the doctor did it—he was just doing his job." The patient therefore may be less likely to feel angry and betrayed and to drop out of treatment. In contrast, consider the patient who comes to work one day and abruptly is informed by her boss: "Your therapist called me yesterday and says that you feel like killing me." Would it be any surprise if this patient becomes even angrier?

The clinician's responsibility to a potential victim does not end with having issued a warning. The clinician also should attempt to answer any questions that the potential victim might have. Depending on the urgency and nature of the situation, a direct interview usually is preferable to a phone call (which in turn is preferable to a letter or telegram). In some situations, a follow-up contact with the potential victim to ensure that no harm has occurred might be clinically appropriate. In cases where intervention with the patient has little chance of benefit, intervention could potentially *primarily* involve the victim—for example, encouraging a battered spouse to move out of the home and into a shelter.

SUMMARY

Aggression and violence are complex, multidetermined behaviors rather than a discrete psychiatric diagnoses. A variety of psychiatric illness can increase the risk of aggressive or violent behavior, but most individuals with these psychiatric disorders do not engage in severe acts of violence, while many individuals who do engage in severe acts of violence do not have a psychiatric diagnosis.

While clinicians cannot accurately *predict* future violence (particularly over the longer term), they are able to perform an appropriate *clinical evaluation* and then attempt to gauge a patient's *level of risk* based upon consideration of relevant risk factors. The predictive nature of risk assessment under conditions of uncertainty forces clinicians and legal decision makers to expect and to tolerate a certain degree of error in their judgments. Unconscious bias, lack of access to relevant data (unavailable records or informants), and misrepresentation of historical data or clinical symptoms by the patient all may inflate this error.

In performing a risk assessment, one should conduct one's routine evaluation but should supplement each element of the history and mental status examination with questions designed to assess particular static and dynamic risk factors for violence. *Static risk factors* include a patient's psychiatric diagnosis, demographic variables, trait vulnerabilities, and violence history. *Dynamic risk factors* include both *clinical variables* (including psychotic symptoms, ongoing substance use, impulsive aggression, and whether there is a therapeutic alliance) and *situational variables* (degree of social supports, interpersonal conflict, occupational status, availability of weapons, and the availability of potential victims).

Particularly when higher-magnitude violence is at issue, clinicians (and society) tend to be more concerned with achieving higher sensitivity than with achieving higher specificity. In other words, they are willing to tolerate "false negatives" (i.e., to "err on the safe side" by involuntarily confining an individual in the hospital due to a greater risk of violence, even if the patient ultimately might *not* have engaged in violence). By analogy, it is not "wrong" for an individual to respond to a tornado warning even when she knows that there is a good chance that no tornado ultimately will materialize. However, some individuals will refuse to leave their homes. Such individuals, despite agreeing on the statistical likelihood that a tornado will appear, have different priorities and are willing to tolerate a greater degree of risk.

Degrees of risk vary along a continuum of severity; *all* persons present *some* level of risk for engaging in violent behavior, but the level ranges from very low to very high. However, clinical and legal decisions (e.g., issuing a warning, involuntarily committing a patient to the hospital, medicating a patient over his objections) usually are dichotomous (i.e., "all or none") in nature. Two clinicians may honestly disagree over whether a patient's degree of risk is "high enough" to cross a particular threshold, depending upon where they "draw the line." Where they draw the line will be influenced by clinicians' personal biases and by the degree of risk that they are willing to tolerate. Similarly, legal decision makers bring their own biases and priorities to the table, and these may differ from those of a patient's treating clinician. Lawyers and judges often place a higher premium on a patient's liberty interests than on his medical interests.

One source of clinicians' discomfort when they are asked to assess for and address violence is the uncertainty inherent in making such decisions, the high stakes that often are involved, and the implications of being wrong. The other source of distress relates to the differences between the disease perspective and the behavior perspective. Clinicians are most comfortable with the disease perspective, which hinges on discovering the underlying cause of a patient's symptoms and—following this—on prescribing the appropriate treatment. In the ideal case (e.g., pneumococcal pneumonia), one discovers a single underlying cause and can prescribe a single treatment, a "magic bullet" (such as penicillin) that selectively targets the underlying disease entity.

In contrast, the behavior perspective hinges on the proposition that complex social behaviors cannot be traced back to single, underlying causes. Given this, there also are no single solutions, no magic bullets. Clinicians are unable to prescribe a cure for violence just as they are unable to prescribe "cures" for eating disorders or substance-related disorders (two other conditions that engender anxiety and frustration in clinicians). However, clinicians' anxieties may be lessened somewhat when working with behavioral disorders if they focus their energies on helping patients learn to manage their behaviors rather than on working toward a "cure." In the case of violent behavior, clinical intervention involves working with patients, their families, and the surrounding community in an attempt to help individuals who are at higher risk of engaging in violence gain a greater degree of control of their impulses through appropriate, targeted interventions.

Chapter 18

Psychotherapy

In Chapter 3, the important features of the life-story perspective were discussed. To recap briefly, this perspective seeks to understand the patient as an individual with a unique story. There are as many stories as there are lives and many stories within each life. Stories are not data, but are *narrative*—that is, a series of interpretive connections made between pieces of data in an attempt to "make sense" of the data. Stories also are not facts. They are "true" only to the extent that they are accepted by and prove useful to the therapist and the patient. Of the many stories that a therapist and a patient might potentially construct, the one that they ultimately will choose will be one that sufficiently illuminates the clinical issue at hand. Thus, the "truth" of the story is not validated in the same manner as a scientific theory might be. Its truth is "narrative truth" rather than "historical truth."

We use the logic of the life-story perspective every day in our personal lives. Without the life-story perspective, we would have no sense of our lives having meaning. Our lives would appear to be a random series of events, without any subjective sense of personal identity, relationships to family and coworkers, opinions about the past, or predictions about the future.

In using the life-story perspective, we do not examine a person's "external" reality but rather the person's inner *representation* of that reality.

By analogy, we might consider this inner reality a "map" of the outside world, similar to a paper map used to find one's way around an unfamiliar city. If a paper map exactly paralleled every detail of the city it represented, it would be unusable; the purpose of a map is to simplify reality by highlighting important elements and leaving out nonessential elements.

One's internal map is constructed during childhood development and modified to a greater or lesser degree throughout one's entire life. The accuracy of the map is influenced by one's underlying genetic endowments, including intelligence, temperament, and personality. Thus, the most significant distortions occur as a result of brain injury, mental retardation, personality disorder, or mental illness. Once an individual has constructed a biased or more inaccurate map due to maladaptive childhood experiences, he or she may only modify it with some difficulty. For example, the map of a child who has experienced early abuse or neglect may include the rules, "You cannot trust other people," and "I am an ineffective person and must rely on others to get by." Individuals may retain these attitudes into adulthood even in the face of evidence to the contrary. The attitudes also may contribute to social maladjustment such that they become self-fulfilling prophecies.

In psychodynamic theory, this internal map is

called one's **object relations**. The map is considered to be an internal representation of oneself, of the significant others in one's life (i.e., "objects"), and of one's relationship to them. In cognitive therapy, this internal map is called a **cognitive schema**. Some examples of adaptive and maladaptive cognitive schemas are listed in Chapter 7, Table 7–13.

The extent to which this map is encoded in the brain's neural "hardware" versus its biochemical or psychological "software" is uncertain. Given that—even in adults—there remains room for changes in the "hardware" in response to life experience (**synaptic plasticity**), the "hardware–software" dichotomy is overly simplistic and has led to overly dogmatic distinctions between psychiatric syndromes ("endogenous" versus "reactive" depression, "psychotic" versus "neurotic" depression, and so on). It also has led to artificial distinctions between "biological" and "psychological" approaches to the treatment of mental disorders. Obviously, medications don't change people lives, but sometimes they greatly assist people to do so. Similarly, talking to patients likely causes changes in the brain structure and function.

This brings us to psychotherapy. *All* physicians likely practice psychotherapy to some extent. However, some physicians probably use it to greater effect than do others. Like medications, psychotherapy can provide powerful benefits but also can cause significant adverse effects. Given this, physicians need have a basic understanding of psychotherapy and its putative mechanisms of action. In this chapter, we will define psychotherapy, delineate its most important components, and examine how psychotherapeutic techniques can be used to advantage even in routine physician–patient interactions.

DEFINING PSYCHOTHERAPY

Psychotherapy is a form of treatment in which an individual who is suffering from some distress comes to a socially sanctioned healer, who in turn attempts to relieve this distress by using personal influence to mobilize change in the sufferer. "Formal" psychotherapy is practiced by physicians, psychologists, nurses, social workers, and a variety of counselors. Some of these practitioners receive specialized, supervised

training leading official certification, while others do not.

However, this broad definition also includes other, "informal" variants of psychological healing not typically thought of as falling under the umbrella of "psychotherapy." These include the counseling offered to individuals by nonpsychiatric physicians, chiropractors, naturopaths, and other "alternative" healers. Members of the clergy obviously provide psychotherapy, grounded in their religious as well as their secular authority. This definition also encompasses the activities of faith or religious healers. Nowadays, counseling sometimes is provided by telephone or by electronic mail, either by certified therapists or by a variety of "alternative" counselors (including "psychics"). While these latter interactions are typically brief (with services sometimes being billed by the minute), they contain the "active ingredients" of psychotherapy described in more detail below.

While most psychotherapy involves a dyadic sufferer–healer relationship, some psychological treatment takes place in a group setting. In "formal" **group psychotherapy**, a group leader provides authority and structure, organizing the experience in such a way that members of the group support each other but also challenge each other to change established patterns of thinking, feeling, and behaving. In peer-run **self-help groups** such as Alcoholics Anonymous (AA), the authority and structure might be provided by a book written by the group's founder. (Members of AA refer to this as the "Big Book" or "our bible.") The book assumes the role played by the therapist in individual psychotherapy, providing an explanation for the suffering of the people who present for treatment and prescribing a series of steps that the sufferer must take in order to become well.

EFFICACY OF PSYCHOTHERAPY

Research suggests that psychotherapy is successful in about 70%–80% of cases in alleviating patient suffering in a variety of contexts. Psychotherapy also is cost effective. Psychiatric consultation and psychotherapy can decrease medical costs (including primary care physician visits, X-rays, blood work, prescriptions, and length of stay during inpatient hospital admissions) by about a third. This cost-offset effect likely relates to the fact that psychological factors that accompany medical illnesses can worsen the symptoms associated with the illness and can worsen functional disability in general. For example, the total medical costs of patients with major depressive disorder are double the costs of nondepressed patients, while the costs of patients with somatization disorder are nine times the costs of other patients. Patients who are receiving psychotherapy therefore tend to require fewer laboratory tests and hospital admissions and sometimes can be discharged from the hospital a bit sooner.

Similarly, patients with psychiatric disorders who receive psychotherapy are less likely to require hospitalization for suicidal ideation and are more likely to respond to pharmacologic treatments. Among patients with borderline personality disorder, intensive (twice weekly) psychotherapy over the course of a year can lead to an average savings of about $10,000 per patient due to a decreased frequency of self-mutilating behaviors, suicide attempts, and hospitalization when compared to patients receiving a more typical course of psychotherapy (an average of 20 visits per year). Similarly, when family therapy and education is added to medication management for patients with schizophrenia, relapse and hospitalization rates are lower, especially when the patient's family interactions are characterized by a high degree of "expressed emotion."

Some of the studies demonstrating the cost-effectiveness of psychotherapy date back to the 1970s and early 1980s. Since that time, there has been a greater emphasis on cost containment in medical care in general, and managed care organizations have placed greater restrictions on the use of expensive diagnostic tests and hospitalization. This may offset some of the economic savings previously realized from psychotherapy. However, even assuming that the margin of economic benefit to the medical system afforded by psychotherapy now is smaller, psychotherapy still can be justified. After all, the cost-effectiveness of any treatment should include more than cost offset; it also should include whether the treatment has "value." For example, psychotherapy often improves a patient's quality of life, ability to parent, and ability to return to work, all of which provide social and economic benefits for the patient and for society as a whole.

For example, patients who experience a major depressive disorder following a myocardial infarction have five times the mortality of patients matched for cardiac status who are not depressed. Even if psychotherapy turned out to add to the cost of caring for these patients, it likely would be money well spent.

Patient surveys indicate that most patients who have received psychotherapy believe that they benefited from it and are glad that they received it. *Consumer Reports* conducted the largest such survey in 1995. Of 4000 readers who had received care from a mental health professional, 43% stated that their emotional state at the time of seeking therapy was either very poor ("I barely managed to deal with things") or fairly poor ("Life was usually pretty tough"). Of the "very poor" group, 90% felt that therapy had been helpful, with 50% saying that it had "helped a lot." A similar pattern was seen in the "fairly poor" group, although the people who started out "very poor" may have demonstrated a more dramatic response to treatment. Of those respondents who were no longer in treatment at the time of the survey, two-thirds said they had left treatment because their problems had been resolved or were now easier to deal with.

For those respondents who received treatment from family physicians, the results were less impressive. The duration of treatment was shorter, there was a greater emphasis on medications, and patient satisfaction with the outcome was lower. Even when patients hadn't responded well to treatment by the family physician, referral to an outside therapist occurred in only one out of four cases.

The major response to psychotherapy typically occurs quite rapidly, within the first few weeks. While a therapist might assume that patients who "drop out" of treatment early on are demonstrating "resistance" to change, studies where such patients were actually tracked down and interviewed have found that many of them dropped out because they were feeling better. Figure 18–1 summarizes a large number of studies involving different types of patients seen in a variety of treatment settings. It superimposes a "dose–response" curve for psychotherapy over average patient attendance.

The top curve represents symptomatic improvement as measured by an independent rater's

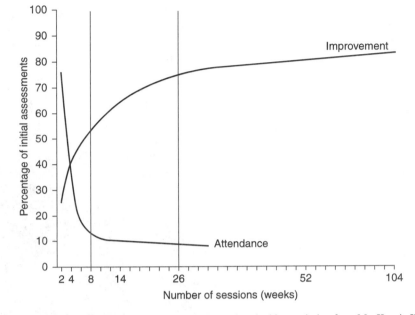

Figure 18–1. Psychotherapy dose–response curve. Reproduced with permission from MacKenzie KR: "The Time-Limited Psychotherapies: An Overview." *American Psychiatric Press Review of Psychiatry, Vol. 15.* Edited by Dickstein LJ, Riba MB, Oldham JM. Washington, DC, American Psychiatric Press, 1996.

objective assessment. (Given that patient's or therapist's ratings usually are more positive than those of independent raters, this is a relatively conservative measure.) Fifty percent of patients demonstrate rapid improvement over the first 2 months of psychotherapy, and another 25% of patients demonstrate strong improvement over the following 4 months. The curve rises much more slowly after this for up to 2 years, and the final response rate is about 85%. Even patients who remain in treatment 1 or 2 years later have reported that they experienced their greatest symptomatic response early on. This outcome curve reflects a highly significant improvement over that which is observed in patients who did not receive psychotherapy.

In studies assessing the efficacy of new pharmaceutical agents, the effective dosage of a medication is usually defined as the dosage that offers at least a 50% reduction in clinical symptoms. If this standard were to be applied to psychotherapy, six to eight sessions over a 12-week period could be considered the average "effective dosage," although these figures obviously may not be applicable for every patient presenting with every particular problem. This curve appears to be consistent across many different serv-

ice systems. While the point where the sharp bend in the attendance curve occurs varies a bit in different systems, the rapid initial falloff is universal.

Even in sites that specialize in the provision of long-term psychotherapy, over 80% of patients receive fewer than eight therapy sessions, and fewer than 15% of patients remain in treatment after 6 months. Patients who do remain in treatment after 6 months have a higher likelihood of remaining in treatment over many subsequent months.

COMMON FACTORS IN PSYCHOTHERAPY

Throughout this text, we have discussed various theoretical "schools" of psychotherapy. For example, we have discussed psychodynamic and cognitive therapy in the treatment of the mood and the anxiety disorders and behavior therapy in the treatment of phobias and obsessive–compulsive symptoms. We have discussed how behavior therapy can be combined with cognitive, psychodynamic, and marital therapy in the treatment of sexual dysfunction. Finally, we have discussed how group therapy can play an important role in the treatment of behavioral disorders such as eating disorders, substance-related disorders, and paraphilias.

These are only the most common schools of psychotherapy since—by some counts—there are over 400 different ones. However, while there is little argument that psychotherapy *in general* is effective, no particular form of therapy has proven to be significantly more effective than any other form of therapy for most conditions (with only a few noteworthy exceptions, such as the use of behavioral therapy to treat phobias and compulsions).

Proponents of one form of therapy (who typically have received extensive training in that modality) often emphasize those research findings suggesting that their form of therapy offers mild benefits with regard to some symptoms for some patients, but such differences tend to be quite minor. Some third-party payers therefore have sought to refer all patients to less expensive (and less experienced) therapists on the assumption that "it's all the same." Similarly, many insurance companies limit patients' access to psychotherapy, seeing it as unnecessary and costly. However, these conclusions are inappropriate for several reasons.

First, while research has not revealed any single form of psychotherapy to be dramatically more effective than other forms of therapy for large *groups* of patients, this is not the same as saying that one approach might not be more effective for *particular* patients. Second, the training and experience of the therapist—regardless of the therapist's school of therapy—clearly makes a difference in the management of more complex cases. For example, in some studies, sympathetic college professors asked to provide supportive psychotherapy to students did quite well, but they soon "ran out of things to talk about." More experienced clinicians rarely encounter this difficulty.

Third—and most importantly—to say that two schools of psychotherapy are equally effective is not the same as saying that neither is effective. Jerome Frank, a psychiatrist at Johns Hopkins University, first noted this in the late 1950s. He emphasized that all psychotherapies have shared elements and was chagrined that theorists from different schools emphasized the differences between different types of therapy rather than these similarities. He theorized that these shared elements might account not only for *different types of therapy being equally effective for the same condition* but also for each school of psychotherapy being nonspecifically effective in treating a *variety of conditions*, including psychotic illnesses, nonpsychotic depression and anxiety, and personality disorders.

By analogy, consider acetylsalicylic acid (aspirin). It is available in a variety of forms, under different trade names, with different appearances. It can come as a liquid or as a pill. In the latter case, the pill might be larger or smaller and it can come in different colors. Different manufacturers of aspirin-containing remedies often tout their products as being "uniquely effective." If one were to analyze two very different-appearing "cold remedy" pills, each of which contained aspirin along with a variety of other ingredients (both active and inert), and found that these remedies were equally efficacious, one would not conclude that both pills contained only inert substances or that patients shouldn't bother to take either medication. Rather, one would try to figure out which ingredients were the active ones and which are the inert ones. Similarly, aspirin-containing products are effective for a wide variety of conditions, including headache, inflammatory arthritis, heart disease, and fever or pain regardless of the underlying pathology. However, to say that aspirin offers a wide variety of nonspecific benefits is not to say that aspirin is ineffective.

A similar argument can be made for psychotherapy. While different forms of psychotherapy may contain unique "active ingredients," these differences may be overwhelmed by even more powerful shared elements, just as a pill that contains aspirin, acetaminophen, and ibuprofen may demonstrate only mild benefit over a pill that contains aspirin alone despite each of these three ingredient being "active." Several commentators have proposed conceptual schemes that delineate the shared elements of all psychotherapies. Frank's scheme remains one of the clearest and is elaborated here.

Frank calls a patient's internal map or schema his **assumptive world** since each individual evaluates internal and external stimuli in the light of underlying *assumptions* about what is dangerous, safe, important, unimportant, and so on.

These assumptions become organized into *attitudes*, which are sets of highly structured, interacting values, expectations, and images of oneself and of those around us. These attitudes have *cognitive, affective, and behavioral components*.

Not all patients with mood swings, delusions, or sexual difficulties present to clinicians requesting help. What patients who do present for treatment tend to have in common, regardless of their underlying specific symptoms, is that they are in a state where their assumptive world is in conflict with their current situation. As a result, they are experiencing various degrees of helplessness, hopelessness, confusion, and subjective incompetence. Frank calls this state of mind **demoralization**.

All psychotherapies first attempt to combat this general state of demoralization and to heighten the patient's hopes of relief regardless of the underlying pathology that has contributed to the development of the demoralized state. All forms of psychotherapy do this implicitly regardless of their explicit aims. Next, they attempt to help the patient feel better and function better by encouraging appropriate modifications in the patient's assumptive world, thereby transforming the meanings of the patient's experiences to ones that are more favorable.

Because major assumptive systems, especially unhealthy ones, are resistant to change, the changes produced directly by psychotherapy are usually minor. Fortunately, they often suffice. Small improvements in one assumptive system may initiate changes in several others. While different schools of psychotherapy focus primarily on one or another aspect of a patient's attitudes (emotions, cognition, or behavior), since all three components are interrelated, the particular component that a given school of therapy chooses to emphasize may be relatively inconsequential.

For example, even purely "behavioral" therapy begins with an intake evaluation. During this evaluation, the therapist, through detailed questioning, expresses an interest in the patient's health, attempts to put the patient's problems in perspective, and proposes a course of treatment. In doing so, the therapist addresses the patient's feelings of alienation and isolation and inspires hope that recovery is possible. While the emphasis in behavioral therapy obviously is on modifying the patient's behavior, patients who

do so may in turn achieve improvements in their dysfunctional cognitions (i.e., they achieve greater "insight") and in their feelings of depression or anxiety.

In contrast, psychodynamic therapy emphasizes the achievement of "insight." However, patients who achieve insight are unlikely to significantly benefit until they can translate this insight into emotional and behavioral change. Fortunately, insight typically serves a catalytic function. Armed with a better understanding of *why* she behaves a certain way, and feeling a strong desire to demonstrate to the therapist and to herself that the therapy is "working," the patient feels powerfully compelled to change her behavior.

Therefore, both psychodynamic and behavioral therapy ultimately demand that therapists attempt to help patients address all aspects of their assumptive worlds—cognitive, emotional, and behavioral. Patients who are successful in doing so are able to replace the state of demoralization with a new state—one of *mastery*. This improvement can occur quite rapidly, as noted above. Clinicians may be able to maximize the likelihood that their patients will be able to achieve a state of mastery by emphasizing the most important shared elements of psychotherapy. What are these elements? Frank proposes that there are four major ones: a *therapeutic alliance*, a *healing setting*, a *rationale (or "myth")*, and a *healing ritual*. These elements, listed in Table 18–1, each will be considered in turn.

The Therapeutic Alliance

Perhaps the most essential ingredient of successful psychotherapy is the relationship be-

Table 18–1. Common Elements of All Psychotherapies

1. An emotionally charged, confiding relationship with a helping person (often with the participation of a group)
2. A healing setting
3. A rationale, conceptual scheme, or myth that provides a plausible explanation for the patient's symptoms and prescribes a ritual or procedure for resolving them
4. A ritual or procedure that requires the active participation of both patient and therapist and that is believed by both to be the means of restoring the patient's health

Source: Adapted from Frank JD, Frank JB: *Persuasion and Healing: A Comparative Study of Psychotherapy*, 3rd edition. Baltimore, Johns Hopkins University Press, 1991.

tween the patient and therapist. Research suggests that, regardless of the form of therapy being studied, the presence of a strong therapeutic alliance is one of the best predictors of a positive outcome. Patients present to clinicians with certain expectations. The societal role of the clinician (whether the clinician is a physician, a psychologist, a nurse, or a social worker) is that of a person with healing skills acquired through specialized training who has been socially sanctioned to listen to the patient's complaints and offer solutions.

Nonindustrialized societies grant such special status to the shaman. In Western cultures, the attitude toward healers, especially psychotherapists, is more ambivalent. We might tell jokes about psychotherapy (often involving the phrase, "And how did you feel about that?"). Our ambivalence also is reflected in representations of psychiatrists in Hollywood films, which generally depict them as either wise sages or dimwitted clowns.

The strength of the therapeutic alliance depends on features of the therapist, on features of the patient, and on whether there is a good "fit" between both parties. The initial phase of individual psychotherapy consists of a patient presenting for help after alternative methods of relief (e.g., distraction, problem solving, talking to friends) have failed. The initial interview represents a pre-alliance negotiation or "courtship" phase. Based on the patient's initial impressions of the therapist's professional skills and personal qualities and on the therapist's perceptions of whether the patient is someone he can help, a collaboration is proposed.

Clearly, there is an initial power imbalance. The patient must be willing to trust and depend upon the therapist; this is easier to do if the therapist doesn't appear overly threatening or judgmental and if his approach is "in synch" with the patient's expectations. Initially, the therapist's authority derives from the healing setting itself (discussed below) as well as from his formal training, the latter being reflected in the questions that he asks and perhaps in the initial interpretations or patient education that he provides. Over time, the personal qualities of the therapist come to assume more importance.

Qualities of the patient matter, as well, however. Patients who have difficulty relinquishing control or trusting other people are less able to form an alliance, at least at the outset. Further, patients who are presenting for treatment solely due to coercion by family members or employers or the court system will be less likely to allow themselves to trust or to depend upon the therapist.

The equivalent of the therapeutic alliance in group therapy is *group cohesion*. As in individual psychotherapy, group psychotherapy also includes an initial courtship phase. During this phase, members of the group tentatively reveal aspects of their personal histories. Not uncommonly, new group members present in a demoralized state, feeling that their problems are unique or that they prove that they are "losing their minds" or are "out of control." Empathic, accepting comments by other members of the group allow the new group member to gain a sense of acceptance and also help him to recognize that some aspects of his problems are universal. Members of the group typically do not begin to challenge each other until after sufficient group cohesion has been established.

A Healing Setting

Most psychotherapy takes place in a setting that reinforces the authority and healing powers of the therapist: either in a clinic located within a prestigious university or in a private office. Most such offices prominently display evidence of specialized training, such as diplomas, licenses, and textbooks. The healer's office is the secular equivalent of the churches, temples, and sacred groves where religious healing historically has taken place. The healing setting not only highlights the authority and power of the therapist but also helps inspire a sense of safety in the patient. The therapist's office is thought of by many patients as being separate from "the outside world," a place where personal disclosures will be accepted and kept confidential.

A Rationale or Myth and Healing Rituals

While every school of therapy agrees on the importance of the therapeutic alliance, each school has its own theory of human behavior. Based on this theory, each school prescribes a different type of procedure, be it cognitive restructuring, exploration of childhood trauma, hypnosis, behavior modification, or exploration of existential fears of death. The therapeutic rationale and the procedures that relate to this rational serve several functions.

First, the rationale and procedures combat the patient's sense of alienation and strengthen the therapeutic relationship. The therapist's adherence to the rationale helps her to accept the patient, even when the patient describes socially objectionable thoughts or behaviors. Similarly, the patient comes to feel accepted and understood because of the theoretical explanations offered by the therapist. The ritual also gives the therapist and patient something to do together and sustains their mutual interest, even during periods where it appears that little progress is being made.

Second, they inspire and maintain the patient's expectations of help. As discussed in Chapter 14 with regard to hypnosis, a patient enters treatment with certain expectations. Having been provided with a coherent theory that is acceptable to her, that appears to explain her symptoms, and is linked to a procedure that is expected to help her get well, she often experiences rapid and powerful relief. Several studies have shown that a preliminary "role-induction interview" at the time of the first session increases the likelihood of achieving positive outcomes. Such an interview explains to the patient what the psychotherapy procedure involves, the respective roles of the therapist and the patient, and the potential benefits of psychotherapy. The major goal this procedure is to teach the patient the "rules of the game," thereby bringing the patient's expectations in line with what will occur in therapy and maximizing the patient's anticipation of improvement.

Third, they provide new learning experiences, accompanied by emotional arousal. All schools of therapy agree that insight unaccompanied by more substantive attitudinal and behavior changes (so-called "empty" insight) is of little benefit. Patients are more likely to alter deeply ingrained beliefs and behaviors if they can engage in active learning while in an emotionally "charged" state. For example, in psychodynamic therapy, examination of painful past experiences and examination of current transference feelings toward the therapist offer opportunities for active learning experience as well as emotional arousal. In cognitive therapy, examination of cognitive distortions, homework exercises, and role playing offer similar benefits. In group therapy, fellow group members are enlisted to both support and confront the patient, again providing for experiential learning in an emotionally charged setting.

Fourth, the rationale and ritual enhance the patient's sense of mastery and personal effectiveness. The conceptual scheme provided by the therapist provides an explanation for the patient's suffering, thereby offering some measure of relief even when the patient's symptoms persist. Patients often have worries that they have ruminated about but have never voiced. Simply doing so can be cathartic and can help the patient feel more in control of her life circumstances. This has been called the "Rumpelstiltskin effect" (after the dwarf in the fairy tale who loses his power over the queen after she speaks his name aloud). The ritual also provides opportunities for the patient to experience some degree of success and personal control—for example, after achieving a new insight or fighting a phobia.

Finally, they encourage the patient to practice and implement what he has learned in therapy in the setting of the "outside world" so that insights gained in therapy might "generalize" to apply to other interpersonal relationships. This is generally the final stage of therapy, following the establishment of a trusting relationship and the practicing of new attitudes and behaviors within the therapy sessions themselves. This final implementation phase of psychotherapy may continue even after the completion of the psychotherapy itself. For example, patients frequently describe having imaginary conversations with their therapist or having an awareness of "what my therapist would have told me about this situation if she were here." In other words, the patient ultimately *internalizes* the rationale of the therapy.

EXPRESSIVE AND SUPPORTIVE PSYCHOTHERAPY

Psychoanalytic theorists have described two major types of psychotherapy, although we can apply these same distinctions to the enterprise of psychotherapy as a whole. **Expressive psychotherapy** (also called **insight-oriented psychotherapy**) involves helping the patient *ex-*

amine unconscious desires, conflicts, and defense mechanisms. The assumption in expressive psychotherapy is that patients' mental health might improve once they gain insight into various aspects of their selves, resolve unconscious conflicts, and give up pathological defenses. However, some patients are not able to tolerate psychotherapy that is so emotionally arousing and evocative. Examples include patients with psychotic illnesses, brain injury, or severe personality disorders. Such patients might regress, "act out" their conflicts through problematic behavior (such as self-injury or aggression), or experience an exacerbation of psychotic symptoms.

In contrast, **supportive psychotherapy** attempts to relieve suffering by emphasizing the *support of an authority figure (the therapist) and a bolstering of the patient's more mature defenses.* Through empathy and validation of the patient's experiences, it places greater emphasis on "here and now" issues of daily living and on *conscious* thoughts and conflicts.

While the distinction between expressive and supportive psychotherapy is useful, this traditional dichotomous conceptualization is artificial and overly simplistic. The conventional assumption has been that expressive psychotherapy is the clearly preferred mode of therapy, particularly for those patients who have the ability to tolerate it and who have the resources to afford it, while supportive psychotherapy can be helpful, if "more superficial," for the remainder of patients. However, as might be expected from the previous discussion, there is no evidence that patients benefit any less from supportive psychotherapy than from expressive therapy. In fact, detailed analyses of 42 patients treated in the Menninger Foundation Psychotherapy Research Project revealed that *all* forms of psychotherapy contain a *mixture of expressive and supportive elements* and that a variety of interventions fall along a *continuum*, ranging from the purely expressive to the purely supportive.

The researchers therefore coined the term "expressive–supportive psychotherapy" to describe this therapy process. Throughout the psychotherapy process, the therapist needs to continually assess *how and when* to either "step forward" and make an interpretation or "step back" and be more unconditionally supportive, depending on the needs of the patient at that given point in time. Psychiatrist Glen Gabbard has described the various elements of the expressive–supportive continuum that is illustrated in Figure 18–2. These elements include interpretation, confrontation, encouragement to elaborate, empathic validation, and advice or praise.

Interpretation is the most "expressive" of these interventions. Interpretations often hinge upon the suggestion by the therapist that a conscious behavior might reflect an unconscious motivation. For example, the therapist might say: "While you say you aren't angry at your father's behavior toward you as a child, you have described several comments he made to you that would have made most people pretty angry. You also say that you have trouble expressing anger toward anybody. Maybe you were angry at your father but weren't able to express it because you feared he would hurt you, and still feel that way about expressing anger toward anybody else." Interpretations also might involve comments about possible transference feelings or resistances that the patient might be developing in the setting of the evolving relationship between patient and the therapist.

Since interpretations are meaningful connections, the most important thing about an interpretation is that it weaves the events in the patient's life into a coherent *story*. Therefore, interpretations don't have to be "psychoanalytic." For example, the therapist might note: "It seems like every situation that you have described where you have felt anxious has involved a fear of being rejected or laughed at by other

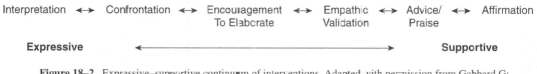

Interpretation ⟷ Confrontation ⟷ Encouragement ⟷ Empathic ⟷ Advice/ ⟷ Affirmation
To Elaborate   Validation   Praise

Expressive ⟵————————————————————⟶ **Supportive**

Figure 18–2. Expressive–supportive continuum of interventions. Adapted with permission from Gabbard G: *Psychodynamic Psychiatry in Clinical Practice: The DSM-IV Edition.* Washington, DC, American Psychiatric Press, 1994.

people. It also seems that one of the most important things to you is that you be liked and accepted by others."

Sometimes, therapists present these interpretations prematurely, before the patient is ready to accept them. For example, for the patient to do so might require her to admit to harboring "unacceptable" feelings or attitudes. The therapeutic alliance also might not yet be strong enough to sustain such interpretations. What might appear to be "obvious" to the therapist by the end of them first session might become apparent to the patient only after several more sessions (or even longer). Sometimes a therapist makes suggestions that go seemingly unacknowledged by the patient, followed by the patient "spontaneously" reaching similar conclusions later in the course of therapy.

It is noteworthy that the *expectations of the therapist* help to shape this process. Even when these expectations are unspoken, or when the therapist is convinced that she has remained "neutral," subtle forms of unconscious influence still can occur. For example, simply asking more questions about one area of discussion than another can convey to a patient that the therapist is more interested in exploring the former areas. Such effects are enhanced both by the degree of status or prestige associated with the therapist and by the patient's degree of motivation to "find answers" and to "get better."

The role of very subtle demand characteristics was demonstrated in a classic experiment by Rosenthal (1969). He recruited two groups of individuals. One group acted as "experimenters" and the other acted as "research subjects." The experimenters were instructed to show a series of pictures of faces to the subjects and to then ask the subjects to rate the degree of "success" or "failure" expressed in the faces, using a rating scale ranging from -10 (extreme failure) to $+10$ (extreme success). In actuality, the faces had been deliberately chosen to be *neutral*, such that the average score given by the subjects should have been zero.

All of the experimenters were provided with the same instructions with regard to how to administer the test, with one exception. Half of the them were told that the *purpose* of the experiment was to reproduce previous studies that had shown that research subjects tend to rate such faces more toward failure; the other half were told that previous studies had shown that research subjects tend to rate such faces more toward success. However, all experimenters were explicitly instructed *not to convey this information to the subjects*; rather, they were simply to read the instructions and adhere strictly to the protocol.

Despite this instruction, the researchers repeatedly found that the ratings given to the faces by the "subjects" were biased in the direction of the information that had previously been given to the "experimenters." This bias occurred rapidly: it often was seen in the very first answers given by the subjects. Therefore, the expectations of the experimenters must somehow have been transmitted to the subjects through subtle visual or auditory cues while greeting the subject or while reading the instructions. The perceived power or status of the "experimenter" also played a significant role in biasing the outcomes. For example, when the "subjects" were college students, the biasing effect was almost four times greater when the "experimenters" had a higher status than when they also were college students.

Confrontation is the next most expressive intervention. Confrontation is typically gentle and involves helping patients to address areas that they would like to minimize or avoid. For example, the therapist might comment: "You say that when your husband hits you it's probably your own fault, but you also say that you would never say such a thing about a friend of yours in the same situation. Why is it that you would never say such a thing about a friend but always seem to say it about yourself?"

Clarification involves pulling together several comments made by patients in order to help put into words something that they have been attempting to understand or to convey. For example, the therapist might say: "It sounds as if you get the most angry not when your boss puts you down but when he does so without even listening first to what you were trying to tell him." Clarification differs from confrontation in that it involves material that the patient isn't necessarily minimizing or denying. Typically, patients respond by saying, "That's exactly right."

Encouragement to elaborate is extensively used in most forms of psychotherapy. It falls somewhere at the center of the continuum between expressive and supportive interventions.

Here, the therapist asks the patient for more details about either an event or a relationship or about his feelings or attitudes. The therapist might ask, "Can you tell me more about that?" or might ask, "How did you feel about that?"

Empathic validation falls more toward the supportive end of the continuum. However, it also is an essential part of expressive psychotherapy since a therapist's interpretations will fail to carry any weight with the patient at all unless he also can convey that he has some appreciation of the patient's subjective experience. An example of an empathic comment would be: "It sounds like you were really devastated by that experience. I can see why you couldn't stop thinking about it."

Advice and praise are actually two interventions that both share the common features of prescribing and reinforcing certain activities. These clearly represent a departure from the "therapeutic neutrality" that characterizes more expressive forms of psychotherapy. An example of advice would be: "If I am going to help you, you also need to attend an alcohol rehabilitation program. You also need to try to tell me about when you're feeling stressed rather than acting it out by cutting on yourself and then calling me on the phone to tell me what you've just done." An example of praise would be: "I think it's great that you've gone 2 months without either having taken a drink of alcohol or cutting yourself. I know it hasn't been easy, but I think we're making progress."

Affirmation is engaged in throughout the course of psychotherapy. It conveys both that the therapist is listening to what the patient is saying and that the therapist understands what the patient is trying to convey. Simple acts such as nodding or saying, "Uh-huh," or, "I see what you mean," can be powerful supportive interventions. This is especially the case when a patient is describing previously unspoken, embarrassing thoughts or feelings. By expressing tacit acceptance (rather than shouting, "That's ridiculous," or, "I'm disgusted—get out of my office") the therapist helps to provide a "corrective emotional experience" to the patients' sense of guilt or shame.

For example, a woman who is a new mother might hesitantly tell her therapist, "I'm a horrible mother. I'm so embarrassed to say this, but last week I got so upset when my baby wouldn't stop crying in the middle of the night that I finally just felt like throwing him against the wall." The therapist might reply, "Sure, but the fact is that you didn't throw him against the wall. It seems to me that most parents, including myself, at some point have been in the same boat as you. I know that I've had those feelings, and I've felt guilty, too."

Note that in addition to having provided the patient with affirmation, the therapist in this example also has engaged in **self-disclosure**. The disclosure is a limited one, is brief, and is used for a particular strategic purpose. In such cases, self-disclosure potentially helps to strengthen the therapeutic alliance and also helps combat demoralization by providing an example of another individual having learned to live with "unacceptable" emotions. However, *indiscriminate or excessive* self-disclosure may greatly interfere with successful psychotherapy. For example, it may remove the pressure on the patient to explore how *she* feels about a matter (as opposed to how the therapist feels about it). It may also lead to the therapy becoming "more about the therapist than about the patient."

More expressive strategies are typically employed in treating patients who have a strong motivation to understand themselves and who also can tolerate powerful emotions in the course of the therapy without becoming overwhelmed, regressed, or suicidal. More supportive strategies are indicated for patients who are psychotic, who have severe major depressive disorder or bipolar disorder, who demonstrate poor impulse control, who have a more severe personality disorder (such as antisocial personality disorder, paranoid personality disorder, or severe borderline personality disorder), or who are of lower intelligence or are brain-injured.

BRIEF AND LONG-TERM PSYCHOTHERAPY

Over the past several decades, psychotherapy has increasingly come to emphasize "briefer" forms of treatment, usually consisting of somewhere between 8 and 26 weekly sessions (i.e., a total course of therapy lasting from 2 to 6 months). By default, given the patient dropout rates noted in Figure 18–1, *most* psychotherapy is "brief."

However, several models have been proposed that deliberately impose a *fixed number of sessions* or a *prearranged date of termination*. The goal in imposing these limits is to increase the pace of psychotherapeutic progress by using the fact that the termination date always remains in sight. The potential constraints of brief therapy are discussed explicitly with the patient at the outset of therapy.

Brief psychotherapy tends to be more structured than longer-term, "open-ended" psychotherapy. In brief psychotherapy, a few key issues are delineated following the intake interview, and the therapist attempts to keep the focus of the therapy on these particular issues. However, many patients also demonstrate improvement in other areas, even following the completion of the course of psychotherapy. Patients with particular vulnerabilities sometimes return for another course of psychotherapy at a later date, usually in the context of some new life crisis. (In this regard, prescribing a short course of psychotherapy resembles prescribing short courses of antibiotics for recurrent episodes of bronchitis.) Therefore, although a termination date is imposed at the outset, the "door is always left open" following "termination" of therapy.

Brief psychotherapy requires that clinicians select patients carefully since this form of therapy isn't appropriate for everyone. The relative contraindications listed above for more expressive forms of psychotherapy also apply to brief psychotherapy, since both types of therapy tend to be more evocative and can exacerbate symptoms or cause regression in patients with schizophrenia, more severe mood disorders, mental retardation, brain injury, or more severe personality disorders.

Figure 18–1 has two demarcations—the first at 8 weeks and the second at about 26 weeks. These correspond to two common forms of brief psychotherapy. **Crisis intervention** typically lasts for up to about eight visits, although some patients benefit even from a single psychiatric evaluation in the emergency room or outpatient clinic. The goal of crisis intervention is to help the patient achieve rapid mastery and a return to functioning by focusing on the specific crisis that has led the patient to seek help. The therapy emphasizes supportive, directive techniques. Crisis intervention is the most common form of therapy applied to most patients. It also is the form of therapy most likely to be employed by primary care physicians. **Time-limited psychotherapy**, which typically lasts for up to about 26 visits, sets more ambitious (albeit still limited) goals, and it places a greater emphasis on expressive techniques.

Longer-term psychotherapy lasts for over 6 months, sometimes even for several years. For many patients, symptomatic improvement continues over the duration of therapy, although after the first few months the gains tend to be much milder. However, many patients remain in longer-term therapy not to achieve new gains but to *maintain* their current degree of functioning. In this regard, "maintenance psychotherapy" resembles maintenance pharmacotherapy with an antidepressant or antipsychotic agent. The goals in such cases might include prevention of illness exacerbations, job loss, or psychiatric hospitalization. As all of these compensations contribute to illness morbidity as well as to societal costs, longer-term psychotherapy often remains cost-effective. In many cases, longer-term psychotherapy can utilize group therapy, which may allow for more efficient delivery of services to larger patient populations.

PSYCHOTHERAPY IN MEDICAL PRACTICE AND THE PLACEBO EFFECT

In Chapter 13, we discussed how many patients present to the primary care setting with somatic complaints believed to be related to psychological factors. In the current chapter, we have noted that the common elements of all forms of psychotherapy are an authoritative healer, a visit to a healing setting, an explanation for the patient's suffering, and a course of treatment prescribed by the healer. The other essential component is hope—that is, the expectation on the part of both the healer and the patient that the proposed course of treatment will be of benefit. Finally, we have discussed how many patients demonstrate a rapid response to psychotherapeutic intervention, even after a single visit.

All of the above suggests that when patients present to their primary care physicians, at least some of the benefit that they achieve from the visit derives from the *doctor–patient interac-*

tion—that is, from nonspecific, psychotherapeutic aspects of the visit—and not simply from the *specific treatments* that the physician prescribes during the visit. This will be the case regardless of the patient's presenting complaint.

Given that all medical treatment contains a mixture of nonspecific and specific effects, is there some way to "dissect out" the percentage of benefit that derives from the arousal of hope and the expectation of improvement? One way to accomplish this is to provide patients with an inactive placebo in place of the prescribed medication while keeping all other aspects of the physician visit the same. In these cases, any benefits that the patient obtains following the visit with either reflect the natural course of disease or psychotherapeutic aspects of the visit.

These nonspecific benefits of treatment have been termed "placebo effects." However, viewed another way, placebo effects are in reality "psychotherapy effects." While many physicians tend to think of placebos merely as a means of satisfying demanding patients through the use of deception (in fact, the word "placebo" literally means "I shall please"), in actuality, placebo treatment offers real benefits to the patient A second implication of viewing placebo effects in this light is that physicians commonly discount the effectiveness of a drug when it performs only marginally better than placebo when they should instead be asking which particular aspects of the pharmaceutical trial led to the placebo group having demonstrated such significant improvement.

Physicians always should keep in mind that the placebo/psychotherapy effect is a component of every encounter between a physician and a patient, even when the physician has a limited interaction with the patient or when potent pharmaceutical agents are being prescribed. They also should keep in mind that until this century, almost *all* of the benefits that patients obtained through the interventions of physicians were predominantly the result of placebo effects.

Even in the twentieth century, patients who received invasive surgical procedures in actuality benefited primarily from placebo effects. For example, many patients with cardiovascular disease were treated with *mammary artery ligation*, the goal of which was to divert a greater supply of blood to the heart. The benefits of this intervention were suggested by research demonstrating

that about 40% of patients who received the procedure experienced dramatic improvement in their angina and also were able to exercise at a greater intensity before ischemic changes became apparent in their cardiograms. However, in the late 1950s (before informed consent became an integral part of biomedical research), Cobb and associates performed a remarkable study. They performed mammary artery ligation on every other patient, alternating this with a "mock" operation during which the patient received only anesthesia and a chest incision. Both groups achieved equal benefits, suggesting that the surgical intervention was in actuality a placebo treatment (albeit a powerful one).

Raising the expectation of cure is such a powerful effect that it can even overcome the effects of active pharmaceutical treatments. For example, in one study a pregnant patient with hyperemesis gravidarum (excessive vomiting) was administered the drug ipecac (which *induces* vomiting rather than relieves it) while her stomach motility was monitored. As would be expected, she experienced a cessation of normal motility, followed by a worsening of her nausea and vomiting. However, when the same patient was administered ipecac through a nasogastric tube (so that she wouldn't recognize it by taste) and was told that it was a powerful *antiemetic* drug that would *cure* her vomiting, she rapidly experienced a resolution of her nausea and resumption of normal gastric motility.

Certain factors appear to enhance the placebo effect. *Physicians who have an upbeat, confident, hopeful manner and who communicate well with patients* tend to achieve higher treatment response rates, lower rates of patient noncompliance, and fewer malpractice claims against them. The *placebo pill itself* can affect patient expectations of success. Multiple pills, larger pills, capsules, and colored pills tend to be associated with stronger placebo effects.

Patient and physician expectations also play a role; this factor can confounding supposedly "double-blind" drug studies, especially when the investigators and subjects aren't surveyed about their presumptions about whether a given subject actually received active medication. For example, both the investigator and the subject might surmise that the subject is receiving active medication rather than placebo when typical side effects occur (e.g., a dry mouth or constipation in a depression study involving the tricyclic agent imipramine). Some pharmaceutical studies have attempted to control for this effect by employing *pharmacologically active placebos*, which mimic potential side effects of the actual drug being studied but lack any known therapeutic effects. For example, atropine, a drug with anticholinergic but no antidepressant effects, might be used as the placebo in a study testing the efficacy of imipramine.

Studies employing such pharmacologically active placebos tend to find that placebo effects are amplified over those seen with pharmacologically inert placebos. Not surprisingly, the incremental benefit of the medication being studied over placebo tends to diminish. In other words, placebos with adverse side effects paradoxically offer *greater* therapeutic benefits, presumably because side effects enhance expectations on the part of the patient that he has been fortunate enough to be assigned to the "active treatment" group and therefore is more likely to respond to treatment.

The general clinician should come away with several important points from this discussion. First, as Francis Peabody noted in a classic 1927 article, "The secret of care of the patient is in caring for the patient." A strong doctor–patient relationship *itself* constitutes a potent medicine. The goal when sitting down with a patient is not simply to make an accurate diagnosis but to maximize the psychotherapeutic or "placebo" benefits to the patient that the encounter might confer. Unfortunately, changes in the administration and financing of medicine have forced physicians to spend less time with each patient. They are more likely to feel that they are "performing a job" than "answering a calling." In addition, as medical technology has evolved, more ancillary tests have become available and the "laying on of hands" has become less frequent and less extensive.

However, unless physicians continue to strive to form a trusting doctor–patient relationship with patients (the "medical" equivalent of the therapeutic alliance), patients may derive less benefit overall from their medical care. Given this, here are several simple suggestions aimed at fostering such relationships and maximizing nonspecific psychotherapy effects within the constraints of current medical practice.

First, you should *strive to be a professional*, since psychotherapeutic benefits accrue from the clinician's authority as a healer. However, it also is important to *be yourself*, since psychotherapeutic benefit *doesn't* accrue in the absence of a therapeutic alliance. One can have authority without being an authoritarian. The best way to achieve this goal is to be open and personable in speaking with your patients. They likely will appreciate your honesty and will respond in kind.

Respect the patient. This is especially the case when patients come from a lower-class background. Keep in mind that such patients often have questions but are less likely to ask them. Regardless of social class, many patients benefit simply from an authority figure having listened attentively and respectfully and having validated their concerns.

Initially, emphasize supportive interview techniques (such as affirmation, advice and praise, empathic validation, and encouragement to elaborate). *Only later utilize expressive techniques, if indicated* (such as clarification, confrontation, and interpretation).

Support the patient by emphasizing her strengths. However, you must do this with honesty. Emphasizing a patient's strengths is not the same as offering insincere praise or naïve optimism. Patients typically readily see through the latter and also end up feeling that the clinician hasn't really appreciated the gravity of their difficulties. One can recognize that the patient's life is hard while also reminding the patient how far she has come during the course of treatment and emphasizing how the patient deserves some of the credit for this improvement.

SUMMARY

Psychotherapy approaches patients from the perspective of their unique life story. Even when a physician admits a patient with diabetes to the hospital for the primary purpose of gaining better control over the patient's blood sugar, the patient typically views the diabetes, the impact of the diabetes (and its treatment) on her life, and her discussions with the physician as elements in an evolving narrative. Patients usually present their histories in this narrative form, with themselves as the protagonist. In contrast, clinicians then reformulate this narrative in their hospital admission note, using the language of the disease perspective, such that the protagonist of the story becomes the illness rather than the patient. Therefore, when providing psychotherapy, the clinician may have to deliberately shift from one employing one perspective to using another.

Psychotherapy, loosely defined, refers to any form of treatment in which an individual who is suffering from some distress comes to a socially sanctioned healer who attempts to relieve the individual's distress by using personal influence to mobilize change in the sufferer. There are over 400 different "schools" of psychotherapy, and therapists with a wide variety of training backgrounds practice psychotherapy. While some forms of psychotherapy may be more effective for some categories of patients (for example, cognitive–behavioral therapy may be the most effective psychotherapy for phobic and obsessive–compulsive disorders), the "active ingredients" of these therapies include several nonspecific elements. These include therapeutic alliance, a healing setting, a therapeutic rationale (or myth), and a prescribed healing ritual (talking, attending support groups, taking herbs or medications, undergoing surgery, etc.).

Psychotherapy is effective in the majority of cases, and in most cases these effects occur within weeks. A significant percentage of the benefit observed over the course of short-term psychiatric hospitalizations, medical hospitalizations, and pharmaceutical research trials relates to such psychotherapy effects. When patients benefit from these effects despite having been administered pharmacologically inert substances, these effects are called "placebo effects." *Research trials* attempt to *minimize* placebo effects in order to better elucidate the more specific effect of the clinical treatment being studied. However, in the *clinical care* setting, clinicians who achieve the best clinical outcomes frequently do so by *maximizing* the contribution of placebo effects to the more specific treatments that they offer the patient.

Psychotherapy employs a combination of supportive and expressive (interpretive) techniques, depending upon the patient, the condition being treated, the intended duration of treatment, and the ultimate treatment goals that are sought. Such techniques are not unique to formal psychotherapy, and they can be integrated into general medical practice regardless of the practitioner's specialty.

Chapter 19

Childhood Disorders

Evaluating children is inherently more difficult than evaluating adults since children often cannot fully examine their feelings and therefore are more prone to "demonstrate" psychiatric disturbances through problematic behavior. In assessing children, clinicians often must "work backwards," inferring the presence of a clinical disorder on the basis of these behaviors. Often, clinicians must assemble data from multiple sources, supplementing history provided by the child with descriptions of the child's behavior in other settings provided by parents and teachers. Ancillary studies such as intelligence testing, educational testing, and projective testing often play more important roles in child psychiatry than in adult psychiatry. Sometimes children only express how they are feeling indirectly, through their drawings or their free play. Clinicians therefore have to be able and willing to engage children by using language and behavior that is appropriate for their particular developmental level.

Most of the adult psychiatric disorders can present during childhood, including the mood disorders, anxiety disorders, and schizophrenia. However, their phenomenology may differ in children since children aren't simply "little adults." For example, until recently, clinicians believed that neither major depressive disorder nor bipolar disorder presented before adolescence. However, a variety of case series and prospective studies has demonstrated that these disorders do in fact occur during childhood and that they often respond to the same treatments employed in adults. In contrast, there are other disorders that almost exclusively first present during infancy, childhood, or adolescence. These disorders include mental retardation, learning disorders, attention-deficit hyperactivity disorder, conduct disorder, and autism.

Two factors further complicate matters. First, children with one disorder frequently are found to also have several *comorbid disorders*. For example, attention-deficit hyperactivity disorder (ADHD) commonly occurs along with learning disorder (LD), and individuals who have both disorders are at greater risk of developing conduct disorder. Conduct problems may represent a pure "response" to the first two disorders, but more likely genetic factors and environmental influences also influence whether a child also develops conduct disorder.

Second, most of the childhood disorders involve behaviors that aren't considered to be pathological for children who are at one stage of development but *are* considered to be abnormal when they *persist beyond that point* or *return* at a point when they would not be considered to be age appropriate. For example, one wouldn't diagnose oppositional defiant disorder in a 2-year-old who is having tantrums and refusing to cooperate with adults. (In fact, it might be of greater concern if a 2-year-old child *wasn't* behaving in an oppositional manner.) However, one would be quite concerned to see an 8-year-old child behaving this way. Therefore, clinicians working with children must possess an understanding of *normal* childhood development.

The appearance of childhood psychiatric disorders at the same time that normal developmental changes are taking place obviously makes the task of diagnosis more difficult. One doesn't want to "pathologize" a child who is engaging in developmentally appropriate coping behaviors in the face of life stressors, but one also doesn't want to make the reverse mistake—that is, "explaining away" the symptoms of serious mental illness by suggesting that a child "is just going through a stage." For example, an adult who insists that he is Superman and assaults people would readily be diagnosed with mania (associated with severe, mood-congruent, grandiose delusions). In contrast, a 13-year-old who makes the same statements and is equally assaultive might be misdiagnosed as having an "overactive fantasy life" rather than diagnosed with early-onset mania. Due to space constraints, normal childhood development isn't fully explored in this chapter, but it will be referenced at various points in order to help distinguish when problematic behaviors should be considered symptoms of a psychiatric disorder.

As with adult disorders, any given patient's overall presentation can be viewed from each of the four perspectives; in addition, each of the specific disorders can be approached from more than one perspective. For example, ADHD is here considered primarily from the disease perspective. However, deficits in attention also can be considered from the dimensional or behavior perspectives, and ADHD often is associated with low self-esteem and underachievement that are best appreciated from the life-story perspective. Similarly, separation anxiety disorder is described here primarily from the disease perspective (given its possible links to mood disorders and anxiety disorders), but it also has a prominent behavioral component and frequently responds to behavioral interventions.

THE DISEASE PERSPECTIVE

All of the major adult diseases can first present during childhood. We initially will consider the mood disorders, the anxiety disorders, and schizophrenia. We then will discuss some conditions that almost always first present during infancy, childhood, or early adolescence. These include separation anxiety disorder, reactive attachment disorder of infancy or early childhood, the pervasive developmental disorders, and attention-deficit hyperactivity disorder.

Mood Disorders

In assessing for the presence of a major depressive episode in children and adolescents, the clinician must attempt to determine whether the child's depressed mood reflects an attempt to deal with conflicts arising out of a developmental stage or is an early symptom of either **major depressive disorder** or **bipolar disorder**. This can be especially difficult when examining preadolescents, since the "classic" symptoms of these disorders may not be present. Further, youths diagnosed with mood disorder may be experiencing their first episode of illness, and so one cannot rely upon a history of past episodes to help validate the diagnosis.

Most patients with bipolar disorder cycle through several episodes of depression before ultimately having their first manic episode. Given that bipolar disorder tends to have an earlier age of onset than major depressive disorder, one always should consider the possibility that a depressed child actually may have bipolar disorder. The "switch" rate from unipolar depressive illness to bipolar illness in adults is generally under 10%; in contrast, 20%–30% of depressed children are rediagnosed as having bipolar disorder by the time that they have reached their teens or early 20s. One must be especially vigilant for this possibility when treating depressed children with antidepressant medications since these might precipitate manic or mixed episodes.

In contrast to depressed adolescents and adults, preadolescent children with major depressive disorder are less likely to demonstrate hypersomnia, weight loss, or delusions. They are more likely to present with prominent somatic complaints, irritability, and social withdrawal. In the case of bipolar disorder, children or adolescents who become manic seldom present with a "euphoric" mood; rather, they most commonly are extremely irritable and might exhibit severe temper outbursts ("affective storms"). While "atypical" forms of mania (mixed or dysphoric mania, or rapid cycling between mania and depression) are the *exception* in adults (about 20% of cases), they are the *rule* in children (about 80% of cases). Further, while the course of bipolar disorder in adults is characterized most often by acute, episodic exacerbations, the course in children and adolescents more often is continuous.

Children or adolescents with bipolar disorder most often present for treatment having already been diagnosed by other clinicians with conduct disorder and/or with "very severe" ADHD, and they typically have received unsuccessful trials of stimulant medication. (One longitudinal study has revealed that 20% of children initially diagnosed with ADHD go on to develop bipolar disorder.) In addition, they often have been diagnosed as having a severe depression rather than a severe mania, given that depression in youths also can present with prominent irritability. However, compared to children with major depressive disorder, conduct disorder, or ADHD, children with bipolar disorder tend to display irritability that is more severe, more persistent, and often reaches the point of violence (sometimes necessitating hospitalization).

When attempting to treat patients who present with a likely manic episode but who might have ADHD and/or an agitated depression, clinicians usually will first attempt to manage the manic symptoms by using a mood stabilizer. *Lithium* is the best-studied mood stabilizer in children, although *carbamazepine* and *valproate* also are used in clinical practice, especially with patients who are lithium nonresponders. Since mood stabilizers aren't effective for comorbid ADHD and usually are only mildly effective for depression, *stimulant* and/or *antidepressant medications* sometimes are cautiously added later if necessary. Obviously, one needs to weigh such options against both the risk of worsening the mania and the goal of minimizing the use of polypharmacy in children.

As in adults, major depressive disorder commonly co-occurs with other psychiatric conditions in children. Comorbid conditions are present in 80%–95% of depressed youths, and when one takes into account factors that distinguish children from adults, the patterns of comorbidity are remarkably similar. In both children and adults, comorbid *dysthymic disorder* occurs in about 30% of cases. (The only difference in the diagnostic criteria for dysthymic disorder in children is that they need only demonstrate depressive symptoms for 1 year, as opposed to 2 years in adults, since this duration still represents a significant period of time relative to the child's age.) Comorbid *anxiety disorders* also commonly co-occur. In adults, the most common of these is generalized anxiety disorder, while in children it is separation anxiety disorder. (Of note, children with separation anxiety disorder frequently go on to meet the criteria for generalized anxiety disorder as adults.) *Substance-related disorders*, another common comorbidity in depressed adults, are difficult to diagnosis in young children given the stringent diagnostic criteria, but 15% of depressed children have a comorbid *conduct disorder*, which might be the closest "childhood equivalent."

It is essential to assess for suicidal thoughts in depressed youths. A 1999 national survey of 10,0000 high school students found that during the preceding 12 month period, 19% had seriously considered attempting suicide, nearly 15% had made a "serious" suicide plan, 8% had attempted suicide, and 2.6% had made a suicide attempt that required medical attention. These results reflect the suicide risk in the *general* adolescent population. Studies of children and adolescents with major depressive disorder indicate that the risk in this population is even higher: 25% eventually attempt suicide, 2.5% of depressed children kill themselves by late adolescence, and 7.7% of such adolescents kill themselves by early adulthood.

The average length of a depressive episode in children and adolescents is about 9 months. Given that this is the same length as the school year, the morbidity associated with a depressive episode can be significant. About half of depressed youths go on to experience another episode in the future, most often within the first 3 years after the child was diagnosed with the first episode.

Treatment for depression can involve individual and family psychotherapy, but sometimes antidepressant medication is required. Cognitive therapy, supportive therapy, and family therapy all have been demonstrated to be effective in relieving depression, reducing suicidality, and improving overall functioning, although cognitive therapy appears to be most effective in the short term. Cognitive therapy has not been studied in small children. It may not be feasible for most young children since it requires the patient to think abstractly about the relationship between one's automatic thoughts (e.g., overgeneralizations, arbitrary inferences, catastrophic thoughts) and one's emotions and to then try to correct these irrational thoughts. Any adult who has attempted to correct a 5-year-old's irrational thoughts will immediately recognize the limitations of cognitive therapy in young children.

Case reports and clinical experience suggest that depression in children does respond to pharmacotherapy. However until recently almost all placebo-controlled trials have failed to reveal significant benefits of medication therapy over placebo treatment. This has particularly been the case for the tricyclic antidepressants (TCAs). Fortunately, recent studies using fluoxetine and paroxetine suggest that these selective serotonin reuptake inhibitors (SSRIs) are at least modestly more effective than placebo. Despite the relative dearth of evidence for the clinical efficacy of antidepressants in children, their use has become widespread due to the significant morbidity and mortality associated with childhood depression.

The unforeseeable risks associated with exposing children to newer pharmaceutical agents, whether in clinical practice or in research trials, obviously are a concern for both parents and physicians and account for the limited number of pharmaceutical trials involving children. While the largest amount of data is available for the TCAs, these medications have been supplanted by newer antidepressants because of their toxicity in overdose and their association with cardiac arrhythmia even at therapeutic doses (with desipramine in rare cases having been associated with sudden death in children).

When prescribing a TCA, it is essential to obtain a detailed personal and family cardiac history, to perform a physical examination, and to obtain an ECG prior to prescribing a TCA. One

also should consider monitoring serum drug levels over the course of therapy and obtaining serial electrocardiograms to assess for conduction delay when one is prescribing doses that are greater than 3 mg/kg/day.

In contrast to the TCAs, the SSRIs have fewer side effects, aren't associated with adverse cardiac effects, and are much safer in an overdose. They have been demonstrated to be useful in treating childhood obsessive–compulsive disorder and appear to be modestly efficacious in childhood major depressive disorder. The onset of response to treatment may be delayed, with little response being observed over the first few weeks; thus, clinicians should wait at least 10 weeks before switching to an alternative agent.

Various theories have been offered to explain the weaker response pattern to pharmacotherapy among depressed youths. Perhaps their neurotransmitter systems or the balance between competing neurotransmitter systems is different than in adults (particularly given the widespread neuronal "pruning" that occurs during adolescence). For example, perhaps their noradrenergic systems have not matured to the same extent as their serotonergic systems. (This might help account for why SSRIs appear to be more effective than TCAs.) Perhaps illness heterogeneity accounts for the lower response rate since admixed with cases of major depressive disorder are cases of what later will be rediagnosed as bipolar disorder; depressive episodes associated with the latter condition tend to be less responsive to antidepressant medication. Finally, perhaps childhood depression is a distinct form of depression that is more treatment refractory. Consistent with this hypothesis, some research suggests that adults with medication-refractory depression are more likely than adults with medication responsive depression to have experienced the onset of their illness in childhood.

Anxiety Disorders

As discussed in Chapter 9, anxiety is a physiologic reaction that occurs in multiple settings. These include: a *normal reaction* that everybody experiences in response to stressful life circumstances; a reflection of *personality vulnerabilities* (particularly cluster C traits); a reflection of *underlying biologic vulnerabilities* that predispose an individual to develop generalized anxiety or panic attacks; and *conditioned associations* between specific environmental stimuli and the anxiety response (as occurs with phobias, obsessive–compulsive phenomena, and post-traumatic anxiety).

All of these conditions also occur in children. For example, **obsessive–compulsive disorder (OCD)** first occurs during childhood in between a third and a half of all cases. It presents similarly in children as in adults, although children more commonly describe difficulties with repetitive rituals than with obsessional thoughts. Treatment includes behavior therapy, clomipramine, and/or the SSRIs.

Panic disorder with or without agoraphobia also can occur in children, although they are less likely to report fears of dying, going crazy, or doing something uncontrolled during an attack than are adults. Treatment typically consists of psychotherapy, sometimes augmented with benzodiazepines, TCAs, or SSRIs.

Post-traumatic stress disorder (PTSD) also can occur in children. It most commonly presents with separation anxiety, fears of death, and social withdrawal. Reexperiencing of the event may occur through nightmares, daydreams, or repetitive reenactments of the trauma through symbolic play or drawings rather than through intrusive flashbacks. Affected children may regress (engaging in behavior from earlier developmental stages) and often experience somatic symptoms (especially headaches and stomachaches). Treatment typically consists of individual and family psychotherapy, sometimes including systematic desensitization. Pharmacological interventions have received less study in children than in adults, although there have been anecdotal reports of using SSRIs and TCAs for core symptoms of depression, arousal, and reexperiencing. Propranolol and clonidine have been reported to be useful in some cases to treat autonomic arousal.

Generalized anxiety disorder (GAD) also can have a childhood onset and is present in about 3% of school-age children. Before *DSM-IV*, these children would have been diagnosed with "overanxious disorder of childhood." However, since over half of adult patients with GAD report onset of their symptoms during childhood, and since the symptoms of GAD and overanxious disorder were essentially the same, *DSM-IV* merged these two diagnoses. Children with GAD appear shy and self-deprecating and typically report multiple somatic symptoms. They may engage in stereotyped nervous habits, such as nail biting, hair pulling, or thumb sucking. Treatment typically includes behavioral therapy in younger children and cognitive therapy in older children, with the emphasis being on assertiveness training. These children often have parents who are highly anxious as well, and family therapy therefore can be useful. While antihistamines frequently have been prescribed for anxiety in children, data for their efficacy are lacking, and they are not recommended for first-line therapy. The use of benzodiazepines also has been described for short-term therapy, but the risk of behavioral disinhibition may be greater in younger patients. Buspirone may be useful in some younger patients and does not appear to be associated with behavioral disinhibition. SSRIs have not received significant study in childhood GAD but have largely supplanted other agents as first-line therapy for adult GAD. Given this, many practitioners prescribe SSRIs for children with GAD, especially when anxious symptoms occur admixed with depressive symptoms.

Phobias occur in children as well. **Social phobia** can have childhood onset (where it was formerly called "avoidant disorder of childhood") and occurs in 1% of school-age children. Children with social phobia are extremely shy and withdrawn in unfamiliar situations. They may cry, freeze, have tantrums, cling to parents, and refuse to engage in normal social activities or group play. Some children engage in selective mutism, a refusal to speak in specific social situations. (This condition is described below.) School-age children usually exhibit poor classroom performance and avoid age-appropriate social activities or dating. They sometimes refuse to attend school at all.

Social phobia is the most stable of the childhood anxiety disorders. Because it interferes with academic performance and normal psychosocial development, it sets up the individual for problems throughout later life. There have been no placebo-controlled pharmacologic studies in children for this condition, and clinicians have tended to attempt therapy with agents that have been successful with adults (SSRIs and benzodiazepines) in combination with behavior and family therapy.

Schizophrenia

The term "childhood-onset schizophrenia" historically has referred to what is now recognized as a mixed group of conditions, including neurologic conditions, mood or dissociative disorders, mental retardation, and (most commonly) autism and pervasive developmental disorder (discussed below). While true schizophrenia does occur prior to age 15, it only does so rarely, occurring in 0.014% of children. While schizophrenia has been described in children as young as age 5, the onset of symptoms in almost all childhood cases occurs after puberty. The diagnostic criteria for schizophrenia are the same in children and adults.

As discussed in Chapter 8, schizophrenia likely is a condition in which genetic and environmental factors combine to cause neurodevelopmental brain injury. Cases with very early onset therefore may constitute a more homogeneous group, with biological factors playing a greater contributory role, such that the individual develops symptoms at a younger age. Such factors might include a stronger genetic or perinatal component or perhaps more prominent associated hormonal abnormalities. Consistent with this hypothesis, 80% of children diagnosed with schizophrenia also experienced severe language deficits and motor developmental problems prior to age 6, and 40% experienced symptoms of pervasive developmental disorder prior to the onset of the symptoms of schizophrenia.

Adolescents with schizophrenia are primarily male (as might be expected given the earlier age of onset of schizophrenia in men than in women) and demonstrate both positive and negative symptoms, including flat or inappropriate affect, deterioration of social and academic skills, avolition, alogia, and prominent hallucinations and delusions. The onset of illness is typically insidious, with a prodrome characterized by deterioration in school performance, social withdrawal, disorganized behavior, and decreased ability to perform basic activities of daily living such as personal hygiene. Their response to medications and their overall outcome tend to be poor.

Separation Anxiety Disorder

While **separation anxiety disorder** is listed in the *DSM-IV* as a childhood disorder, it likely is related to the adult anxiety disorders. The cognitive, behavioral, and somatic manifestations of the disorder overlap with those of generalized anxiety disorder and social phobia, although they also represent an exaggeration of *normal* separation anxiety. The latter is a developmental milestone that first appears by about 7 months of age and peaks at between 13 and 18 months of age before gradually subsiding.

In separation anxiety disorder, the child's anxiety is much greater than what would be considered developmentally appropriate. Table 19–1 lists the diagnostic criteria for this condition. These children experience severe anxiety upon separation from home or major attachment figures. Upon separation, they often need to know these attachment figures' whereabouts, need to stay in touch with them (by telephone, for example), and become extremely homesick and preoccupied with reunion fantasies. Even when they are *with* the attachment figures, they often continue to experience pervasive fears that an accident or illness will lead to permanent separation.

They usually are extremely shy, demonstrating the personality trait of *behavioral inhibition* (discussed in Chapter 9). The disorder becomes more apparent at about age 7 or 8, when children typically begin to spend more time away from home. They may refuse to go to school, to friend's houses for sleepovers, or to camp. They may "shadow" or "cling" to their parents. While bedtime sometimes is anxiety-provoking for all children (depending on their current stage of development), children with separation anxiety disorder may refuse to go to sleep alone and have nightmares that articulate their worst fears (such as separation from the family through murder, fire, or some other catastrophe). They often complain of somatic complaints (stomachaches, headaches, nausea, and vomiting in younger children, and palpitations and lightheadedness in older children). In contrast to generalized anxiety disorder, where somatic complaints are more "free-floating," in separation anxiety disorder they are associated either with actual separations or with anticipation of impending separation.

Patients with separation anxiety disorder also often meet the diagnostic criteria for other mood and anxiety disorders, including social phobia, generalized anxiety disorder (in which case they also are more nonspecifically anxious), panic disorder, major depressive disorder, dysthymic

Table 19–1. *DSM-IV-TR* Criteria for Separation Anxiety Disorder

A. Developmentally inappropriate and excessive anxiety concerning separation from home or from those to whom the individual is attached, as evidenced by three (or more) of the following:
  1. Recurrent excessive distress when separation from home or major attachment figures occurs or is anticipated
  2. Persistent and excessive worry about losing, or about possible harm befalling, major attachment figures
  3. Persistent and excessive worry that an untoward event will lead to separation from a major attachment figure (e.g., getting lost or being kidnapped)
  4. Persistent reluctance or refusal to go to school or elsewhere because of fear of separation
  5. Persistently and excessively fearful or reluctant to be alone or without major attachment figures at home or without significant adults in other settings
  6. Persistent reluctance or refusal to go to sleep without being near a major attachment figure or to sleep away from home
  7. Repeated nightmares involving the theme of separation
  8. Repeated complaints of physical symptoms (such as headaches, stomachaches, nausea, or vomiting) when separation from major attachment figures occurs or is anticipated
B. The duration of the disturbance is at least 4 weeks
C. The onset is before age 18 years
D. The disturbance causes clinically significant distress or impairment in social, academic (occupational), or other important areas of functioning
E. The disturbance does not occur exclusively during the course of a pervasive developmental disorder, schizophrenia, or other psychotic disorder and, in adolescents and adults, is not better accounted for by panic disorder with agoraphobia

SPECIFY IF

Early Onset

If onset occurs before age 6 years

Source: Reprinted with permission from the *Diagnostic and Statistical Manual of Mental Disorders, Fourth Edition, Text Revision.* Copyright 2000 American Psychiatric Association.

disorder, and cluster C personality disorders. Even when they don't complain of being depressed, children with this disorder are as likely to demonstrate nonsuppression on the Dexamethasone Suppression Test as are children who present with major depressive disorder. This finding is consistent with a possible shared biologic diathesis.

These children often have a prominent family history of anxiety, including higher familial rates of panic disorder. Their mothers often are described as having "insecure attachments" themselves. For example, the child's mother might herself become anxious upon separation from the child, might be overly preoccupied with the child's somatic complaints, and might herself feel ambivalent about sending her child off to school. Therefore, it is likely that the disorder reflects the contributions of both a genetic predisposition toward introverted personality traits and physiologic hyperarousal and superimposed phobic avoidance behavior modeled or reinforced by significant attachment figures.

Like social phobia, the course of separation anxiety disorder tends to be chronic. Even after

these children have been coaxed to attend school, they often remain underachievers. When they have grown to adulthood, they might have difficulty in workplace settings, exhibiting absenteeism and failure to perform to their potential. Similarly, they often have difficulty handling major life changes such as moving or getting married and can become overly concerned about the safety of their spouses and children. Many ultimately develop other anxiety disorders. For example, retrospective studies of adult patients with panic disorder reveal that those who had a childhood history of separation anxiety disorder had an earlier onset of panic attacks and more severe symptoms.

While these children may first present for pediatric or psychiatric evaluation following their having refused to attend school, separation anxiety disorder is not synonymous with "school refusal" (also called "school phobia" or "absenteeism"). School refusal refers to a specific *behavior*, which can have several causes: separation anxiety disorder is just one of them. For example, 75% of adults recall having failed to go to school at some point. In some inner-city schools, absenteeism is as high as 90%. Social forces ("peer pressure") explain some cases. Other cases are associated with a more extensive pattern of problematic behaviors associated with conduct disorder.

In evaluating the child who presents with "school refusal," special attention should be paid to the possibility of an underlying anxiety or mood disorder (particularly separation anxiety disorder, generalized anxiety disorder, panic disorder with agoraphobia, social phobia, major depressive disorder, or dysthymia). In addition, the refusal to attend school could reflect the presence of an underlying learning or communication disorder, and the child is refusing to go to school out of frustration and embarrassment. These conditions might only be recognized through formal testing.

Treatment of separation anxiety disorder requires that the clinician recognize that the disorder is more than a simple behavioral disturbance. To treat the component of "school refusal," behavioral strategies involving the patient, family, and school often are helpful, particularly progressively increased exposure to the school setting. One might even give the child a coin with which to telephone or page a parent if necessary. The child typically only has to telephone the parent once or twice; however, the coin itself ultimately becomes a "transition object," a substitute for the attachment figure that the child can keep nearby to help ease anxiety.

One should remember, though, that addressing school refusal alone typically is insufficient since most children's anxiety is more pervasive. Many other treatment approaches have been employed, including individual psychotherapy and family therapy. Parents need to be educated about the need to be supportive while attempting to avoid being overly indulgent or reinforcing their child's fears. Sometimes parents must be treated (or referred for treatment) for their own anxiety disorder.

More severe cases of separation anxiety disorder may require pharmacotherapy. A mainstay of treatment for years was TCAs, although—once again—SSRIs have become the first-line drugs due to their greater margin of safety. Buspirone is an alternative treatment. "As needed" dosages of a benzodiazepine or β-adrenergic blocking agent may be useful in treating episodes of anxiety related to exposure to feared situations.

Following treatment, most children no longer meet the diagnostic criteria for separation anxiety disorder by the following next year. However, many of these children continue to be fearful and avoidant and they remain at risk for developing other anxiety and mood disorders. Comprehensive care includes trying to help the child acquire a greater sense of confidence and autonomy.

Selective Mutism

From about ages 3 to 5, most children become mute when around strangers. However, for children with **selective mutism**, this behavior *persists* beyond this developmental stage and *increases* in severity. Selective mutism is characterized by the consistent failure to speak in specific social situations despite having the ability to speak in other situations. Typically, the child's speech is normal when he or she is at home or alone with family. However, the child won't speak around other children, teachers, or strangers. It is this selectivity that distinguishes selective mutism from more pervasive conditions that can include disturbances of spoken language, such as language disorder, autistic disorder, and mental retardation.

This rare condition (occurring in 0.03%–0.08% of children), most commonly is diagnosed in children between 5 and 8 years of age. Almost all of these children are behaviorally inhibited and almost all of them also meet the diagnostic criteria for *social phobia*. In other words, they demonstrate significant anxiety-related social impairments *beyond* those that are attributable to their failure to speak. Although most children with selective mutism have normal language capabilities, about a third of them also do have a language disorder and about half of them have a history of delayed speech development. These preexisting language vulnerabilities, combined with an underlying anxious temperament, combined with behavioral reinforcement by anxious family members (with the family dynamic often resembling that observed for children with separation anxiety disorder), may shape the presentation of children with social phobia so that it includes symptoms of selective mutism.

Like social phobia and separation anxiety disorder, treatment typically involves individual and family therapy, both emphasizing assertiveness training. Psychotherapy often is augmented by pharmacotherapy, most commonly with an an SSRI (although the use of MAO inhibitors also has been reported).

Behavioral therapy may be helpful in teaching parents how to selectively reinforce more appropriate behaviors. However, as with separation anxiety disorder, the treatment goals include not only management of the aberrant behavior itself but also promotion of greater personal effectiveness and autonomy. The symptom of mutism may respond to treatment within several weeks but in some cases it continues for several years. Even when the child is teased by peers and experiences comorbid depression or anxiety, mutism can become a source of significant secondary gain. The prognosis appears to be poorer in cases where mutism persists beyond the age of 10, likely because by that point the disturbance has become a significant part of the child's social identity.

Reactive Attachment Disorder of Infancy or Early Childhood

This disorder first appeared in *DSM-III* in 1980. This was an attempt to include a syndrome well known to pediatricians under various names, including "failure to thrive," "hospitalism," "psychosocial dwarfism," "maternal deprivation syndrome," and "anaclitic depression." *DSM-III* described this disorder as one that occurs in infants who clearly have experienced grossly inappropriate care. Symptoms reflect a loss of normal social responsiveness, including: a weak cry, excessive sleep, lack of interest in the environment, hypomobility, poor muscle tone, and weak rooting and grasping upon feeding attempts.

While infants clearly exist who display this syndrome, there were some problems with this definition. First, as discussed in Chapter 7, attachment is a complex phenomenon and can be disturbed for other reasons beyond "grossly inappropriate care." For example, some children repeatedly are admitted to the hospital due to a chronic medical illness; others are raised in serial foster care settings following the death of parents; others are shuttled between parents in the midst of a divorce. Although there may be no gross "neglect" or "abuse," in such cases, children may be left without a consistent, nurturing attachment figure.

In addition, while older children who find themselves in such circumstances may not display the life-threatening "failure to thrive" that is observed in infants, they still can demonstrate significant abnormalities in their social behavior. In some cases, they become excessively inhibited and anxious; in other cases, their attachments exhibit no selectivity, so they are overly familiar and sociable even with relative strangers.

These concerns led researchers and clinicians to broaden the definition of reactive attachment disorder in *DSM-IIIR* and again in *DSM-IV*. The latter criteria are listed in Table 19–2. The current definition continues to emphasize the etiologic role of "pathogenic care" (giving reactive attachment disorder the distinction of being the only childhood disorder to require that a specific precipitating factor be present, a distinction shared in the adult disorders only by PTSD). However, the criteria for both the *type of abuse or neglect* and the *type of symptoms* have been broadened and now include more generalized *impairments in forming attachments* rather than simply a "failure to thrive."

Treatment obviously depends upon the specific social situation. The immediate goal of treatment is to *ensure the safety of the child*. This might require removing the child from the current home setting if it is determined that child abuse or neglect is occurring there. Similarly, *medical complications* such as malnutrition, dehydration, fractures, and infection must be treated. In some cases, this may require inpatient hospitalization. When the situation is not emergent, a concerted effort is made (sometimes involving the Department of Social Services and the legal system) to *improve the quality of the patient's attachments*, through family education, psychotherapy, and increased social supports.

Pervasive Developmental Disorders

Pervasive developmental disorders are characterized by severe and pervasive impairment across multiple areas of development. The manifestations of these disorders can vary greatly depending on the affected individual's developmental level and chronological age, but three primary types of deficits may be present: deficits in *reciprocal social interaction*, deficits in *communication*, and deficits exemplified by the *pres-*

Table 19–2. *DSM-IV-TR* Criteria for Reactive Attachment Disorder of Infancy or Early Childhood

A. Markedly disturbed and developmentally inappropriate social relatedness in most contexts, beginning before age 5 years, as evidenced by either 1 or 2:
   1. Persistent failure to initiate or respond in a developmentally appropriate fashion to most social interactions, as manifested by excessively inhibited, hypervigilant, or highly ambivalent and contradictory responses (e.g., the child may respond to caregivers with a mixture of approach, avoidance, and resistance to comforting, or may exhibit frozen watchfulness)
   2. Diffuse attachments as manifested by indiscriminate sociability with marked inability to exhibit appropriate selective attachments (e.g., excessive familiarity with relative strangers or lack of selectivity in choice of attachment figures)
B. The disturbance in criterion A is not accounted for solely by developmental delay (as in mental retardation) and does not meet criteria for a pervasive developmental disorder
C. Pathogenic care as evidenced by at least one of the following:
   1. Persistent disregard of the child's basic emotional needs for comfort, stimulation, and affection
   2. Persistent disregard of the child's basic physical needs
   3. Repeated changes of primary caregiver that prevent formation of stable attachments (e.g , frequent changes in foster care)
D. There is a presumption that the care in criterion C is responsible for the disturbed behavior in criterion A (e.g., the disturbances in criterion A began following the pathogenic care in criterion C)

SPECIFY TYPE

Inhibited Type

If criterion A1 predominates in the clinical presentation

Disinhibited Type

If criterion A2 predominates in the clinical presentation

Source: Reprinted with permission from the *Diagnostic and Statistical Manual of Mental Disorders, Fourth Edition, Text Revision.* Copyright 2000 American Psychiatric Association.

ence of stereotyped behavior, interests, and activities. Until recently, these disorders were labeled "childhood psychosis" or "childhood schizophrenia." However, while the rare child with a pervasive developmental disorder ultimately does go on to also develop schizophrenia, these two syndromes appear to represent distinct diagnostic entities.

Autistic Disorder

The prototypical pervasive developmental disorder is **autistic disorder**, which occurs in about 0.05% of children. (When other "autistic spectrum conditions" are included, the prevalence is as high as 0.1%.) In autistic disorder, all three of the above features are present, as detailed in Table 19–3. Children with autistic disorder typically are brought in by their parents for evaluation prior to the age of 3 due to concerns that the child isn't demonstrating normal reciprocal interactions or "relatedness" with the parents. Despite early theories that posited that distant or aloof parenting is responsible for this condition, no differences have been found in the parenting styles of the parents of autistic children, and these

parents usually are very concerned about their child's behavior.

For example, very young children with autistic disorder don't make eye contact, cuddle, lift their arms to be picked up, or smile in response to stimulation. While they may begin to interact more as they grow older, they typically remain aloof from other children and exhibit deficits in "getting" normal social interactions that other children pick up naturally, such as responding appropriately to various facial expressions or tones of voice or engaging in reciprocal play.

While other children are beginning to babble and ultimately to speak, up to half of all autistic children remain silent. Autistic children who do learn to speak frequently have difficulty with *semantics* (e.g., they may say "you," instead of "I") and may engage in *echolalia* (e.g., repeating jingles or phrases from television in situations where they have no relevance). Their speech also typically lacks *normal prosody* (inflection) and may have a monotone or "singsong" quality. They also demonstrate *impaired nonverbal communication* (e.g., failing to wave hello or goodbye or to communicate their anger or happiness

Table 19–3. *DSM-IV-TR* Criteria for Autistic Disorder

A. A total of six (or more) items from 1, 2, and 3, with at least two from 1, and one each from 2 and 3:
  1. Qualitative impairment in social interaction, as manifested by at least two of the following:
    a. Marked impairment in the use of multiple nonverbal behaviors such as eye-to-eye gaze, facial expression, body postures, and gestures to regulate social interaction
    b. Failure to develop peer relationships appropriate to developmental level
    c. A lack of spontaneous seeking to share enjoyment, interests, or achievements with other people (e.g., by a lack of showing, bringing, or pointing out objects of interest)
    d. Lack of social or emotional reciprocity
  2. Qualitative impairments in communication as manifested by at least one of the following:
    a. Delay in, or total lack of, the development of spoken language (not accompanied by an attempt to compensate through alternative modes of communication such as gesture or mime)
    b. In individuals with adequate speech, marked impairment in the ability to initiate or sustain a conversation with others
    c. Stereotyped and repetitive use of language or idiosyncratic language
    d. Lack of varied, spontaneous make-believe play or social imitative play appropriate to developmental level
  3. Restricted repetitive and stereotyped patterns of behavior, interests, and activities, as manifested by at least one of the following:
    a. Encompassing preoccupation with one or more stereotyped and restricted patterns of interest that is abnormal either in intensity or focus
    b. Apparently inflexible adherence to specific, nonfunctional routines or rituals
    c. Stereotyped and repetitive motor mannerisms (e.g., hand or finger flapping or twisting, or complex whole-body movements)
    d. Persistent preoccupation with parts of objects
B. Delays or abnormal functioning in at least one of the following areas, with onset prior to age 3 years: (1) social interaction, (2) language as used in social communication, or (3) symbolic or imaginative play
C. The disturbance is not better accounted for by Rett's disorder or childhood disintegrative disorder

Source: Reprinted with permission from the *Diagnostic and Statistical Manual of Mental Disorders, Fourth Edition, Text Revision.* Copyright 2000 American Psychiatric Association.

through facial expression or body language). Similarly, their play tends to be *stereotyped and noncreative* (e.g., lining up an exact number of blocks over and over, rather than building anything *with* the blocks).

Children with autistic disorder may insist on sameness and show resistance to or distress over trivial changes. For example, a younger child may exhibit a "catastrophic reaction" following even a minor change in the environment such as a new set of curtains or a change in place at the dinner table. Similarly, they may insist on always following the same *rituals or routines*, such as taking exactly the same route to school every day. (Note that—unlike the preoccupations seen in OCD—these rituals don't seem to the child to be unreasonable or distressing, and aren't resisted by the child.) Autistic children also may exhibit *stereotyped body movements* involving the hands (clapping, finger flicking) or the whole body (rocking, dipping, and swaying), or *abnormalities of posture* (e.g., walking on tiptoe, or odd hand movements and body postures).

Autistic children may show a persistent pre-

occupation with *parts* of objects (especially moving parts) rather than with the object itself. For example, they may repetitively spin the tires of a toy truck rather pretending to *drive* the truck, or they may play with the buttons on a doll's dress rather than with the doll itself. The child also might develop a strong attachment to some inanimate object, such as a particular piece of string or rubber band.

Associated features can include *impaired attention and hyperactivity, impulsiveness, aggressiveness*, and *temper tantrums*. Some children also exhibit *self-injurious behaviors*, such as head banging or hand biting. They may be overly sensitive to benign stimuli and yet display an inappropriate lack of fear in dangerous situations. Some repeated behaviors may resemble obsessive–compulsive phenomena, such as only eating certain foods or repeating the same activities in the same, stereotyped way.

While autistic disorder sometimes is confused with schizophrenia, children with autistic disorder do not experience hallucinations, delusions, or loose associations. They also are more likely to demonstrate evidence of a prenatal insult, including seizures (in up to one-third of cases) and mental retardation (in up to 70% of cases). Further, the age of onset in autism is younger than even the earliest reported cases of childhood schizophrenia.

Autistic disorder is associated with *mental retardation*, but unlike typical cases of mental retardation, where cognitive deficits tends to be consistently lower across various types of tasks, in autistic disorder the distribution of cognitive deficits is typically uneven. The patient can have "islands" of intact functioning or even of very high functioning. (However, "autistic savants"—individuals who can memorize long lists of numbers or play complex pieces of music perfectly after a single hearing—are extremely rare.)

The differential diagnosis for autistic disorder also includes congenital deafness. Deaf children, however, despite their inability to hear, still develop *reciprocal interactions* using mouth and body language. The same is true for children with congenital blindness.

Autistic disorder is three to five times more common in males than in females. However, when it occurs in females the symptoms often are more severe and there is more likely to be a family history of cognitive impairment. The etiology of autistic disorder remains unknown. The disorder occurs in all racial, ethnic, and social groups. Some medical conditions that also can be associated with Mental Retardation and seizures have been associated with autistic disorder, including *congenital rubella, phenylketonuria*, and *tuberous scerlosis*. However, in most cases of autistic disorder, no comorbid medical condition is discovered.

At one time, autism was thought to be related to childhood vaccination, specifically the measles–mumps–rubella (MMR) vaccine. However, reviews of the evidence by several panels of experts have concluded that current evidence does not support this theory. Given this, the CDC, the American Academy of Pediatrics, and the American Academy of Family Physicians all have recommended that physicians continue to counsel parents to follow the current recommended childhood immunization schedule.

Genetic factors appear to play an important etiologic role. If a family has one child with autistic disorder, there is a 5%–10% chance that they will have another child with autistic disorder (as opposed to a 0.1%–0.2% if the family does not already have a child with autistic disorder). There also is a much higher concordance for autistic disorder in monozygotic than in dizygotic twins. Finally, research involving family members also has demonstrated that "unaffected" family members sometimes exhibit subtle language disturbances.

The medical workup should include a *physical examination* that includes measurement of head circumference, inspection for minor physical anomalies (which are more common in autism) and for the skin changes that might suggest the presence of tuberous sclerosis ("ash leaf patches," adenoma sebaceum, or "shagreen patches"), along with a neurologic exam. The child's *visual acuity and hearing* should be tested. *Neuropsychological testing* can help to delineate the extent of cognitive and communication impairments. While *MRI and EEG* testing also usually are performed, in autistic disorder the results tend to be abnormal but nonspecific. *Serologic workup* includes testing for lead toxicity, inborn errors of metabolism, and chromosomal studies (including a screen for fragile X syndrome).

Expert committees reviewing the extensive literature on autistic disorder have concluded that there is insufficient evidence to support the use of various other laboratory tests that have been propounded. These include hair analysis for trace elements, celiac antibodies, allergy testing (particularly for food allergies to gluten, casein, candida, and other molds), testing for immunologic or neurochemical abnormalities and micronutrient or vitamin levels, intestinal permeability studies, stool analysis, urinary peptides, testing for mitochondrial disorders (including lactate and pyruvate), thyroid function tests and erythrocyte glutathione peroxidase studies.

The course of autistic disorder is variable. Individuals can achieve some gradual improvement if the condition is identified early and appropriate interventions are initiated. These interventions are multimodal in nature, including educational interventions, behavior management, speech therapy, social skills training, vocational training, and family counseling. (Obviously, the availability of such resources in one's community is an important concern.)

Improvement usually isn't uniform across the spectrum of symptoms and may occur in fits and starts. In milder cases of autistic disorder, the individual may ultimately be able to live in adult society, although often there will be continued evidence of an impaired ability to interact socially and an inability to perform creative work. Individuals with more severe forms of the condition may still be able to learn some adaptive skills.

Treatment also should include treatment for comorbid mood disorders, anxiety disorders (especially panic and obsessive–compulsive disorders), and attention-deficit hyperactivity disorder. Behavior therapy may be helpful in controlling self-injurious or other problematic behaviors, but sometimes pharmacotherapy is required.

Virtually every available class of psychotropic agent has been studied in this regard. Initial positive open-label reports frequently have been followed by disappointing results in controlled trial. For example, the most recently such agent has been *secretin*, a gastrointestinal polypeptide hormone. A series of three patients given open-label secretin as part of a diagnostic evaluation for gastrointestinal problems were described as having demonstrated dramatic improvement in their language and social relatedness. Following extensive media coverage touting a "possible new cure" for autism, subsequent placebo-controlled studies did not find secretin to be efficacious.

Several studies conducted during the 1960s and 1970s demonstrated that *lower-potency traditional antipsychotic agents* reduced motor hyperactivity and aggression in children with autistic disorder. However, since these agents also are sedating and can exacerbate cognitive deficits due to their anticholinergic effects, clinicians most often turned to the higher-potency typical agent, *haloperidol*. Haloperidol has received the largest amount of empiric study to date of the various pharmacologic alternatives. While it does appear to reduce hyperactivity, irritability, aggression, and repetitive behaviors in many cases, it also causes tardive dyskinesia in a significant percentage of these.

The *atypical antipsychotic agents* appear to be promising alternatives; some small, open-label studies suggest that they also can reduce these target symptoms and that they may prove to be less likely to cause tardive dyskinesia. Weight gain has been a limiting side effect for some individuals. The *SSRIs* and *buspirone* also appear to be useful in addressing these symptoms. Larger, controlled trials of the atypical antipsychotics, the SSRIs, and buspirone have not been conducted, however.

Naltrexone and *clonidine* both have been employed, but while they may be modestly useful in treating hyperactivity and aggression, their effects usually are modest and transient. *Psychostimulants* such as methylphenidate also are useful in some cases, but they can exacerbate irritability, insomnia, and aggression in other cases. While β-adrenergic blockers, lithium, and various anticonvulsant drugs (including carbemazepine, valproate, and lamotrigine) also have been reported to be of some utility in small patient samples, their clinical utility also remains to be determined.

Other Pervasive Developmental Disorders

Other pervasive developmental disorders are even more rare than autistic disorder. **Childhood disintegrative disorder** has similar symptoms, but presents at about age 3 or 4—following a period of at least 2 years of normal development—with marked deterioration that progresses over a period of several months. While the condition stabilizes after several months, most individuals remain impaired into adulthood and require institutionalization. This condition appears to be about four times more common in men than in women. Its etiology remains unknown. Clinical management is similar to that employed for autistic disorder, but even more intensive behavioral support usually is required.

Rett's disorder is a progressive neurodegenerative illness of unknown etiology that occurs only in girls. In this condition, a period of normal development over the first 5–48 months of life is followed by the development of autistic symptoms, deceleration of head growth, loss of motor skills in the hands (along with characteristic hand stereotypies, including hand wringing and wetting the hands with saliva), and a disturbance of gait. No specific treatment is available beyond supportive care, behavioral management, and targeted pharmacotherapy for specific behavioral problems when indicated.

Asperger's disorder resembles autistic disorder in that affected individuals also exhibit severe and sustained impairments in their social interactions and demonstrate restricted and repetitive patterns of behavior, interests, and activities. However, in contrast to individuals with autistic disorder, those with Asperger's disorder *don't demonstrate significant language dysfunction or significant delays in cognitive development.* They demonstrate normal curiosity about their environment and are able to acquire age-appropriate learning skills and adaptive behaviors in all areas *except* for the realm of interpersonal functioning.

Younger children with Asperger's disorder may display little or no interest in establishing friendships. As they age, while they may develop an interest in having friendships, they continue to lack the ability to grasp normal social conventions. For example, they lack normal "emotional reciprocity," and even when they involve others in their play activities, they typically "use" the child as just another object. While social deficits also occur in autistic disorder, individual's with Asperger's disorder demonstrate an *eccentric and one-sided* social approach (e.g., pursuing a particular conversational topic regardless of other people's reactions) rather than the *complete social and emotional indifference* exhibited by individuals with autistic disorder.

Similarly, while *language* functioning is essentially preserved in Asperger's disorder, an affected individual's communication isn't completely "normal" due to the intrusion of idiosyncratic preoccupations with certain topics, excessive verbosity, and an inability to follow normal conversational conventions (e.g., recognizing nonverbal cues, engaging in conversational reciprocity, and monitoring the flow of conversation).

Because these children develop language and motor skills at developmentally appropriate ages, their parents (despite perhaps having taken note of some subtle interpersonal difficulties) may only first become more concerned when their child is exposed to other children of the same age (e.g., in preschool). At that point, their child's interpersonal deficits begin to become more apparent and the child begins to experience difficulty "fitting in."

In further contrast to individuals with autistic disorder, those with Asperger's disorder usually don't have mental retardation (although occasional cases associated with mild mental retardation have been described). However, as with autism, subtle and nonspecific neurologic difficulties may be present, such as mild "clumsiness," inattention, and hyperactivity. (Not surprisingly, many affected individuals already have been treated for ADHD prior to having been diagnosed with Asperger's disorder.) Later in childhood, some of these individuals develop depressive symptoms, although the symptoms frequently reflect the teasing and social rejection that the children encounter from peers.

As with autistic disorder, the etiology of Asperger's disorder is unknown. Its prevalence has been estimated at about 0.05% of the population. The condition has received attention from clinicians and researchers and therefore is now being diagnosed more frequently. (Whether it is being overdiagnosed remains uncertain.) As with autistic disorder, the condition is about five times more prevalent in males than in females. It also appears to run in families and may occur more frequently when there is a family history of autistic disorder. It is possible that this condition represents a higher-functioning variant of autistic disorder or variation along an autistic spectrum.

The relationship between Asperger's disorder and *schizoid personality disorder* is unclear. In general, though, the social difficulties in Asperger's disorder are more severe and of earlier onset. Obviously, Asperger's disorder also must be distinguished from *"normal" social awkwardness.* Asperger's disorder only should be diagnosed if a child's social deficits are severe and if the preoccupations are all-encompassing and interfere with the acquisition of basic skills.

Attention-Deficit Hyperactivity Disorder

While **attention-deficit hyperactivity disorder** (**ADHD**) has traditionally been considered a "behavioral" disorder, it is more appropriately considered a chronic neurodevelopmental disorder with both genetic and environmental influences.

The simplest way to assess for ADHD is to ask the patient (and family members) screening questions based on the *DSM-IV* diagnostic criteria for ADHD, listed in Table 19–4. Children

Table 19–4. *DSM-IV-TR* Criteria for Attention-Deficit Hyperactivity Disorder

A. Either 1 or 2:
  1. **Inattention:** six (or more) of the following symptoms of inattention have persisted for at least 6 months to a degree that is maladaptive and inconsistent with developmental level:
     a. Often fails to give close attention to details or makes careless mistakes in schoolwork, work, or other activities
     b. Often has difficulty sustaining attention in tasks or play activities
     c. Often does not seem to listen when spoken to directly
     d. Often does not follow through on instructions and fails to finish schoolwork, chores, or duties in the workplace (not due to oppositional behavior or failure to understand instructions)
     e. Often has difficulty organizing tasks and activities
     f. Often avoids, dislikes, or is reluctant to engage in tasks that require sustained mental effort (such as schoolwork or homework)
     g. Often loses things necessary for tasks or activities (e.g., toys, school assignments, pencils, books, or tools)
     h. Is often easily distracted by extraneous stimuli
     i. Is often forgetful in daily activities
  2. **Hyperactivity–impulsivity:** six (or more) of the following symptoms of hyperactivity–impulsivity have persisted for at least 6 months to a degree that is maladaptive and inconsistent with developmental level:

     HYPERACTIVITY

     a. Often fidgets with hands or feet or squirms in seat
     b. Often leaves seat in classroom or in other situations in which remaining seated is expected
     c. Often runs about or climbs excessively in situations in which it is inappropriate (in adolescents or adults, may be limited to subjective feelings of restlessness)
     d. Often has difficulty playing or engaging in leisure activities quietly
     e. Is often "on the go" or often acts as if "driven by a motor"
     f. Often talks excessively

     IMPULSIVITY

     g. Often blurts out answers before questions have been completed
     h. Often has difficulty awaiting turn
     i. Often interrupts or intrudes on others (e.g., butts into conversations or games)
B. Some hyperactive–impulsive or inattentive symptoms that caused impairment were present before age 7 years
C. Some impairment from the symptoms is present in two or more settings (e.g., at school [or work] and at home)
D. There must be clear evidence of clinically significant impairment in social, academic, or occupational functioning
E. The symptoms do not occur exclusively during the course of a pervasive developmental disorder, schizophrenia, or other psychotic disorder and are not better accounted for by another mental disorder (e.g., mood disorder, anxiety disorder, dissociative disorder, or a personality disorder)

CODE BASED ON TYPE

Attention-Deficit/Hyperactivity Disorder, Combined Type
If both criteria A1 and A2 are met for the past 6 months

Attention-Deficit Hyperactivity Disorder, Predominantly Inattentive Type
If criterion A1 is met but criterion A2 is not met for the past 6 months

Attention-Deficit Hyperactivity Disorder, Predominantly Hyperactive-Impulsive Type
If criterion A2 is met but criterion A1 is not met for the past 6 months

Source: Reprinted with permission from the *Diagnostic and Statistical Manual of Mental Disorders, Fourth Edition, Text Revision.* Copyright 2000 American Psychiatric Association.

with ADHD typically demonstrate *inattentiveness, hyperactivity,* and *impulsivity.* The severity of their symptoms is excessive and inappropriate for their current developmental stage. Associated symptoms include low frustration tolerance, frequent shifting of activities, difficulty getting organized, and excessive daydreaming.

Since antiquity, this cognitive–behavioral syndrome has been recognized under a variety of names, including "disorder of moral control," "minimal brain damage," and "hyperkinetic impulse control disorder." Among most clinicians, the existence of ADHD and the importance of treating it are not a subject of controversy. In the

United States, ADHD has been recognized by the Department of Education, the National Institutes of Health, the surgeon general, the courts, and all of the major medical, psychiatric, psychological, and educational associations.

Despite this, public controversy has centered on two primary issues. The first issue relates to the *prevalence and diagnostic reliability* of ADHD. Some critics express concern that ADHD either does not exist at all or is tremendously overdiagnosed. They accuse physicians (perhaps under excessive influence from pharmaceutical firms that manufacture stimulant medications and sponsor medical conferences) of inappropriately applying a stigmatizing "medical" label to large numbers of children, when in fact the true causes of these children's problems are dysfunctional homes and overcrowded classrooms. They also charge that the diagnosis of "residual" ADHD in adults, by "medicalizing" various prob-lematic behaviors, relieves individuals of having to take personal responsibility for their actions. The second, related issue involves the *widespread practice of prescribing stimulant medications to children diagnosed with ADHD*, even to preschool-age children. Every few months, another newspaper headline asks a variation of the same question: "Are We Overmedicating Our Children?"

Therefore, as we have done throughout this text, we will begin with the issues of reliability and validity. As is the case with virtually *all* psychiatric disorders, there is no single ancillary test that can confirm or refute that an individual has ADHD. The diagnosis is assigned to an individual based upon clinical phenomenology. However, large studies utilizing structured interviews demonstrate that the diagnosis of ADHD can be made with a high degree of diagnostic reliability. This having been said, it is apparent that some busy clinicians don't conduct detailed diagnostic evaluations and don't carefully apply the current diagnostic criteria. Given this, ADHD may be overdiagnosed by some clinicians. However, ADHD also may *underdiagnosed* by other clinicians, depending upon the direction of their diagnostic bias.

In attempting to achieve greater diagnostic reliability, several key points should be kept in mind. Regardless of whether ADHD is diagnosed in a child or in an adult, the symptoms should have *first* appeared during early childhood (before age 7). The symptoms also should be present in *more than just one particular setting* (e.g., they shouldn't occur only at school), should should express themselves through *multiple behaviors*, and should be so severe that they can be considered a source of *significant functional impairment*.

Two primary symptom domains have been identified in ADHD: *inattention* and *hyperactivity–impulsivity*. ADHD is diagnosed when six or more symptoms are present from either of these domains. Collateral information from parents and teachers (in the case of children) or from spouses and coworkers (in the case of adults) can be invaluable. Even when evaluating adults for ADHD, a patients' parents may be able to offer important recollections about the patient's childhood behavior. Although not "diagnostic," symptom-rating scales, checklists completed by parents and teachers, and neuropsychological tests are other useful sources of information.

The hyperactivity is the most noticeable symptom in children, although clinicians obviously must attempt to distinguish "hyperactivity" from "normal" motor activity in young children. With aging, the hyperactivity becomes less prominent but impulsivity tends to remain. For example, older adolescents and adults with ADHD may continue to blurt out answers to questions or interrupt others in conversation and frequently complain of feeling "restless" or "bored." These difficulties may be less noticeable in adults with ADHD who have deliberately chosen vocations where they wouldn't be forced to remain seated for extended periods (in contrast to children, who are required to sit at a classroom desk for much of the day).

Note that being able to diagnose a condition with a high degree of *reliability* does not assure that the condition is a *valid diagnostic entity*. High reliability simply guarantees that two clinicians are likely to agree on which children should or should not be assigned a particular diagnostic label. Also, note that since stimulant medications improve concentration and quiet impulsive behaviors even in children and adults who do *not* have a diagnosis of ADHD, a positive clinical response to a trial of stimulant medication is not diagnostic of ADHD in a particular case and does not prove the existence of the diagnosis in general.

Given all of this, is ADHD an actual biological condition? A significant amount of research suggests that it is. First, ADHD appears to have a very strong *genetic component*. Siblings of a child with ADHD are twice as likely to have ADHD as are children in the general population. In addition, the concordance rate for ADHD in monozygotic twins is much higher than it is in dizygotic twins (92% versus 33%). Finally, the biological parents of adopted-away children with ADHD are more likely to have ADHD themselves than are the child's adoptive parents, suggesting an important role for genetic transmission. Overall, research suggests that ADHD has a heritability approaching 80%.

Second, *neurobiologic research* has demonstrated evidence of specific, regional neurophysiologic disturbances in individuals diagnosed with ADHD compared to control subjects without ADHD. ADHD may result from dysfunction within specific *frontal or frontal–striatal neuronal networks*. For example, studies involving functional neuroimaging (PET, SPECT, and functional MRI) in children, adolescents, and adults have demonstrated that individuals with ADHD—when compared to controls—have decreased striatal metabolism at rest and decreased prefrontal and striatal activity during tasks requiring inhibition of planned motor responses.

The *dopamine system* appears to play an important role in mediating this regional dysfunction. Stimulant drugs, which increase dopaminergic activity, are the most effective available treatment for ADHD. Further, the complaint of motor restlessness described by individuals with ADHD phenomenologically resembles the *akathisia* described by individuals treated with antipsychotic (dopamine-receptor antagonist) agents. Consistent with this, one functional MRI study has found adults with ADHD to have twice the dopamine transporter binding potential of control subjects. Molecular genetics research is currently exploring a possible etiologic role for the genes that code for dopamine D_2 and D_4 receptors and for the dopamine transporter protein.

Norepinephrine and serotonin also may play important mediating roles, although their relative contributions to ADHD remain uncertain. Animal research suggests that *dopamine* regulates novelty seeking and the ability to focus attention on a particular stimulus, that *norepinephrine* reg-

ulates general arousal and responsiveness to reinforcement, and that *serotonin* regulates the inhibition of drives and impulses. Variations in the degree of involvement of these neurotransmitter systems in different individuals might explain why some patients predominantly demonstrate inattention (20%–30% of cases), others predominantly demonstrate impaired impulse control (under 15% of cases), and others demonstrate both symptom clusters (50%–75% of cases). Such variations also might explain why so many individuals with ADHD go on to subsequently develop other psychiatric illnesses, such as mood and anxiety disorders and substance-related disorders. Unfortunately, while researchers may only be able to delineate the relative contributions of different neurotransmitter systems if they study specific subtypes of ADHD individually, the validity of various subtyping schemes currently remains uncertain.

If ADHD does represent a developmental disorder involving frontal and basal ganglia circuits, it might help explain the observed overlap between ADHD and other conditions that also are characterized by a failure to inhibit various behaviors and that also have been linked to these particular regions. For example, children with *obsessive–compulsive disorder* have difficulty inhibiting their repetitive compulsive behaviors, and children with *Tourette's disorder* (and other related tic disorders) have difficulty inhibiting their motor and vocal tics. About half of children with Tourette's disorder also fulfill the diagnostic criteria for ADHD, and two-thirds of them also fulfill the diagnostic criteria for obsessive–compulsive disorder. It also is noteworthy that their motor and vocal tics are suppressed by dopamine-receptor antagonists (i.e., antipsychotic medications) and are exacerbated by dopaminergic agents (i.e., stimulant medications), again suggesting that dopamine plays a contributory role in the etiology of all of these disorders.

Unfortunately, behavioral disinhibition, inattention, irritability, and hyperactivity are relatively nonspecific psychiatric symptoms that also occur, for example, in childhood major depressive disorder, childhood bipolar disorder, learning disorders, and even as part of the prodromal syndrome that precedes psychotic illness ("schizotaxia"). For example, 20%–30% of depressed youth and 50%–90% of bipolar youth also fulfill the diagnostic criteria for ADHD. Do all of these children really have both conditions? It therefore is likely that a subgroup of children diagnosed as having ADHD actually have early or more nonspecific manifestations of other psychiatric disorders, although—given that all of these other conditions also are increasingly being recognized as being lifelong neurodevelopmental disorders—it may be quite reasonable to diagnosis *both* ADHD and the other, comorbid, condition. Often, these other psychiatric disorders ultimately will "declare themselves" at some later point when more specific symptoms finally appear (depressive symptoms, manic symptoms, panic attacks, etc.). Given this, clinicians must *continually reassess* children who they are treating for presumed ADHD at regular intervals. As noted earlier, such diagnostic ambiguity comes with the territory when working with children.

Is ADHD overdiagnosed in children and adults? If anything, epidemiologic research actually suggests that—overall—ADHD is *underdiagnosed* in the general population. The diagnostic validity of "adult ADHD" also has been confirmed by prospective studies in which children with ADHD have been followed into adulthood. In half of these individuals, symptoms have persisted into adulthood.

A conservative estimate of the prevalence of ADHD among school-age children is 3%–5%, although some studies have indicated rates as high as 10%. While ADHD once was believed to be more common in boys (with the sex ratio of boys to girls variously estimated at anywhere from 3:1 to 9:1), it now appears that ADHD simply is underdiagnosed in young girls, who are less likely to demonstrate hyperactivity, oppositionality, or delinquent behavior than boys and are more likely to present with inattention, impaired school performance, and underachievement. In adolescent and adult populations, ADHD is diagnosed as frequently in females as in males.

While the potential for overdiagnosing ADHD clearly is a concern, *underdiagnosing* it is perhaps a more relevant concern since children with unrecognized ADHD are at significantly greater risk of experiencing school failure and underachievement. Further, despite concerns that children treated with a stimulant medication will be-

come addicted either to the stimulant or to other substances, longitudinal studies suggest that in fact the opposite is the case. Preadolescents with ADHD treated with stimulant medication appear to have a significantly lower rate of substance abuse during their adolescent years (13%) than do preadolescents with ADHD who were not treated with stimulant medication (33%). Further, their rate of substance use during adolescence closely resembles the frequency of substance use in control subjects without ADHD (10%). Finally, it is important to recognize and treat ADHD because individuals with ADHD are at higher risk of developing other psychiatric illnesses in later childhood or adulthood. If a clinician doesn't recognize the underlying ADHD, these patients may appear to be "treatment refractory" when in fact the treatment for their comorbid conditions isn't addressing core ADHD symptoms such as inattention, impulsiveness, and disorganization.

The mainstay of treatment for ADHD is *stimulant medication*, although other treatments are important adjuncts. *Psychotherapy* plays an important role in treating comorbid disorders and in educating the patient and family about the disorder and its potentially disruptive effects on family and educational functioning. (This is especially important for parents who may have come to view their child as simply being "bad.") Many families find that a local chapter of the national organization Children and Adults with Attention-Deficit Hyperactivity Disorder (CHADD) can offer useful additional support and education. Instituting a *behavior plan* to manage disruptive behaviors can provide a framework for treatment and restore structure to the child's home and school life.

Children with ADHD also can benefit from *specialized educational planning*, with parents working in tandem with the child's teacher and ancillary support staff (such as school guidance counselors or psychologists.) Teaching plans usually emphasize structure, predictable routine, and the use of learning aids. Further, since about one-third of children with ADHD also have a comorbid *learning disorder*, testing for the latter should be conducted and the educational plan should be adapted accordingly when a learning disorder is uncovered. Adolescents can benefit from counseling about how to make use of *struc-*

tured study skills and time management techniques to improve their school and work performance. *Vocational guidance* also may be useful for older adolescents and adults with ADHD.

The major stimulant medications used to treat ADHD are dextroamphetamine (Dexedrine), a racemic mixture of amphetamine and dextroamphetamine (Adderall), and methylphenidate (Ritalin, others). All are schedule II controlled substances. All demonstrate a rapid onset of action but a short duration of clinical effects (only a few hours), so one must prescribe either several doses per day or a sustained-release preparation.

For example, **immediate-release (IR) methylphenidate**, the most commonly prescribed stimulant, must be taken about every 2.5–4 hours. Most younger children take it two or three times per day, but some older patients take methylphenidate as frequently as six times per day. (Two doses usually will get a child through the school day, but this still necessitates a daily trip to the school nurse for the second dose, which can be inconvenient to the school system and stigmatizing to the child.)

While methylphenidate has been marketed in a slower-release preparation (**RitalinSR**) that offers a slower onset of action and a longer half-life (about 4–6 hours), this formulation may be less effective than the IR preparation, perhaps due to what has been called the *ramp effect*: amphetamines and methylphenidate appear to be most effective at peak blood levels rather than at steady-state blood levels. Given this, several companies have introduced innovative extended-release delivery systems that closely mimic the pharmacokinetics of multiple daily doses of an IR preparation. These are rapidly gaining market share both due to their greater convenience and to their "smoother" effects over the course of the day.

Concerta is a methylphenidate preparation that utilizes osmotic pressure to deliver medication at a controlled rate through a semipermeable membrane over a 12 hour period, thereby simulating thrice-daily dosing. The whole tablet is surrounded by an outer layer of IR methylphenidate, thereby allowing for an initial drug peak during the first hour followed by gradual release of medication throughout the next 12 hours, thereby allowing for once-daily dosing

rather than three-times-daily dosing. **Metadate CD** and **Ritalin LA** are other methylphenidate preparations that use a different technology to achieve similar effects. Capsules contain a combination of immediate-release and extended-release coated beads. Plasma methylphenidate concentrations peak twice, first at about 1.5 hours (like immediate-release methylphenidate) and then at about 4.5 hours, with a total duration of about 8 hours, thereby simulating twice-daily dosing.

An alternative to methylphenidate is **dextroamphetamine (Dexedrine)**, which also is available in a shorter-acting form or a medium-acting form (**Dexedrine Spansules**). Dextroamphetamine is twice as potent as methylphenidate, and its duration of action is a bit longer. **Adderall** is a "mixed salt single-entity amphetamine product" containing a combination of dextroamphetamine (75%) and levoamphetamine (25%). It has a modestly longer half-life than dextroamphetamine, thereby allowing for twice daily dosing. **Adderall XR**, a delayed-release bead preparation of Adderall, allows for single daily dosing.

While as of this writing none of these agents has been directly compared against each other, one imagines that the longer duration of action associated with Concerta and Adderall XR would be advantageous for those children who require an afterschool dose of medication, but disadvantageous for those children who experience a loss of appetite at suppertime or insomnia at bedtime. For these latter children, the shorter-acting agents such as Metadate CD and Ritalin LA may be preferable. One other recently released methylphenidate formulation is **dexmethylphenidate (Focalin)**, which contains the active (d-isomer) form of methylphenidate but not the inactive (l-isomer) form. While this allows it to have double the potency on a per milligram basis over regular methylphenidate, whether this offers any advantages over methylphenidate in terms of greater efficacy or few side effects is unclear at this point.

Methylphenidate accounts for more than 90% of the use in ADHD in the United States. Perhaps it is so much more popular than the amphetamines because amphetamines were overused and abused in the 1960s when doctors prescribed them to treat obesity. While no stimulant has been shown to be more effective than any of the others in large studies, individual patients might respond better to one particular agent or another. One meta-analysis of studies directly comparing dextroamphetamine to methylphenidate found that 35% of subjects improved more on dextroamphetamine, 26% improved more on methylphenidate, and 38% did equally well with either agent. Other analyses have demonstrated that, overall, about 70% of child and adult patients respond to a trial of either methylphenidate or dextroamphetamine.

In refractory cases, one should ensure that dosage of stimulant being administered is high enough, especially when treating adults. Even when dosed on a milligram-per-kilogram basis, dosage requirements can vary widely between different patients. Since the symptoms of ADHD may not be pronounced when patients are seen in the clinical setting, the best way to assess the effectiveness of an ongoing course of treatment is through collateral information from parents and teachers, which can be facilitated by asking them to complete standardized rating scales such as the Parents' Rating Scale and the Wender Utah Rating Scale.

The most common side effects associated with the stimulants are decreased appetite (with the potential for a delay in gaining weight in children), insomnia, and tachycardia. Higher doses on occasion have been associated with sedation or psychotic symptoms (especially hallucinations). Some patients experience motor tics, and preexisting tics (e.g., in patients with Tourette's disorder) can be exacerbated. Stimulants also carry the potential for abuse, especially when they are taken in high doses, injected, snorted, or sniffed. However, it appears that the risk of addiction in patients who are prescribed stimulant medication for an appropriate medical indication has been overstated.

The Council on Scientific Affairs of the American Medical Association (Goldman et al., 1998) having reviewed all English language studies and Drug Enforcement Agency (DEA) data over a two-decade period pertaining to the treatment of ADHD, concluded:

ADHD is one of the best-researched disorders in medicine, and the overall data on its validity are far more compelling than for many medical conditions. . . . There have been more than 170 studies involving more than 6000 school-aged children using stimulant medication for ADHD. . . . Medications have been unequivocally shown (i.e., by double-blind, placebo-controlled studies) to reduce core symptoms of hyperactivity, impulsivity, and inattentiveness. They improve classroom behavior and academic performance; diminish oppositional and aggressive behaviors; promote increased interaction with teachers, family, and others; and increase participation in leisure time activities. Finally, stimulants have demonstrated improvement in irritability, anxiety, and nail biting. A recent meta-analysis found that the effect of stimulants on behavior and cognition may be severalfold greater than the effects on academic achievement. . . . [However, it] is important to emphasize that pharmacotherapy alone, while highly effective for short-term symptomatic improvement, has not yet been shown to improve the long-term outcome for any domain of functioning (classroom behavior, learning, impulsivity, etc.). This may be a function of several factors: most studies have been carried out only for a short term, there may have been inadequate dosage titration to maximize the number of responders, and dose–response relationships may be different for different domains.

A great deal of concern has been raised by the DEA and others about the potential for abuse or diversion of stimulant medication: production (and use) of methylphenidate in the United States has risen from less than 2000 kg in 1986 to 9000 kg in 1995, with a tripling between 1990 and 1995 alone. By contrast, amphetamine production rose from 400 to 1000 kg in the same period. More than 90% of US-produced methylphenidate is used in the United States. . . .

It is clear that there is a fair amount of use of stimulants by adolescents. The annual school survey of drug use conducted by the University of Michigan has shown an increase from 6.2% to 9.9% of eighth-graders reporting nonmedical stimulant use in the preceding year between 1991 and 1994. However, lifetime nonmedical methylphenidate use has remained essentially constant around 1% during the same period. Sixty percent of students who used any stimulants reported using them fewer than 6 times in their lifetime, and 80%, fewer than 20 times. Only 4% reported any injection use of stimulants. Thus, while nonmedical stimulant use may be somewhat more common among adolescents in recent years, little use is of methylphenidate itself, and the pattern of use for the vast majority appears to be experimental and not of the type (regular, heavy, injecting, etc) likely to lead to serious adverse consequences.

Drug Abuse Warning Network data on emergency

department visit monitoring show a 6-fold increase between 1990 and 1995 in mentions of methylphenidate. A "mention" simply indicates that the patient listed the drug as one taken: it is not necessarily the drug leading to the emergency department visit, nor is there any medical confirmation. The rate of cocaine mentions, by contrast, is 40 to 50 times higher. The methylphenidate cases are overwhelmingly young women, not the population (ie, male adolescents) felt to be at highest risk for abusing prescription methylphenidate. The DEA has had reports of thefts of methylphenidate, street sales, drug rings, illegal importation from outside the United States, and illegal sales by health professionals. There have also been reports of theft of school supplies of methylphenidate.

On the other hand, abuse of methylphenidate by patients with ADHD or their family members has been reported rarely. Only 2 cases of methylphenidate abuse by adolescents with ADHD have been described, and only 2 cases of methylphenidate abuse by parents of children taking it for ADHD have been reported. While there is no way to know how many cases may have been unrecognized or unreported, such a minimal published experience is quite remarkable in light of the population exposed. . . .

There is evidence to suggest that stimulants in ADHD populations are simply being used more broadly, for longer periods, and without interruptions in recent years than was done previously. Overall, there has been a 2.5-fold increase in the prevalence of child and adolescent methylphenidate treatment from 1990 to 1995, so that some 2.8% of US youth between the ages of 5 and 18 years were taking this medication in mid 1995. A recent national study found no evidence of overdiagnosis of ADHD or overprescription of methylphenidate. . . . There are several important clinical reasons for the increased diagnosis and stimulant treatment of ADHD. These include increased public and physician awareness and acceptance of the condition; acceptance of a broader case definition as appropriate; greater knowledge of the illness course, justifying lengthier treatment (e.g., of adolescents); fewer interruptions in treatment because of diminished concerns about growth retardation; and increased treatment of adults.

Since epidemiologic studies using standardized diagnostic criteria suggest that 3%–6% (or even higher) of the school-aged population may have ADHD, the percentage of American youth being prescribed stimulants is at the lower end of the prevalence range. Given this, while clinicians should be appropriately circumspect about prescribing stimulants, they shouldn't shy away from using them to treat patients who have ADHD. Before initiating a treatment plan, clinicians should take a careful history, attempting to distinguish symptoms of ADHD from normal developmental behavior and from symptoms of other psychiatric conditions. They also should design an individualized treatment plan for the patient that takes into account the patient's symptoms, the extent of social morbidity, any comorbid psychiatric conditions, and the preferences of the child and the child's family.

This treatment plan might involve a combination of medication, education, behavioral management strategies, and environmental interventions. There should be appropriate follow-up, including monitoring for efficacy of medications, for adverse effects, and for the ongoing need for treatment. This diagnostic assessment and treatment plan should be appropriately documented. Given the risk of abuse or diversion, the clinician should keep careful records of medication prescribed and should consider alternatives to stimulants in patients at high risk either because of comorbid substance use or conduct disorder or because of family members with substance abuse. The child should be reexamined periodically to assess the need for continued stimulant therapy.

Why is methylphenidate abuse so rare if—like amphetamine and cocaine—it targets the dopamine transporter and significantly raises synaptic dopamine levels? Why does cocaine cause a powerful "high" and trigger behavioral reinforcement and cravings while methylphenidate does not? Several positron emission tomography (PET) studies suggest an answer to this question. By measuring the levels of dopamine transporter occupancy achieved by various agents, PET has allow researchers to directly assess drug pharmacodynamics.

One such study demonstrated a correlation between the magnitude of cocaine-induced dopamine transporter blockade and the magnitude of subjects' self-reported "high." They also demonstrated a temporal correspondence between the pharmacokinetics of cocaine at the dopamine transporter and the perceived duration of the "high." For intravenous cocaine to consistently induce a "high," it had to block at least 60% of dopamine transporters. While one might speculate that methylphenidate simply doesn't achieve such high levels of transporter blockade when administered orally and in typically prescribed dosages, it turns out that this is not the case. Methylphenidate blocks the transporter to about the same extent as cocaine. However, even at 80% transporter occupancy, subjects who received methylphenidate did not report experiencing a "high."

However, while methylphenidate's *pharmacodynamic* profile resembles that of cocaine, its *pharmacokinetic* profile is quite different, reflecting its oral route of administration. The time to reach both peak blood levels (and, almost immediately paralleling this, peak brain levels) with orally administered methylphenidate is about 60 minutes. This time course also corresponds to the onset of clinical effects observed in treatment populations.

In contrast, with intravenously administered cocaine, brain level peaks in 4–6 minutes. Similarly, when methylphenidate is administered intravenously, brain levels peak in 8–10 minutes. This may explain why nonhuman primates offered either intravenous methylphenidate or cocaine self-administer either agent with comparable frequency. When humans do abuse methylphenidate, it is usually by an intravenous route. Therefore, it is likely that oral methylphenidate simply may be absorbed too slowly to cause a "high," despite having such powerful dopaminergic effects.

What alternatives are there to the traditional stimulants? **Pemoline (Cylert)** also is a stimulant, but it has a slower onset and a longer duration of effect. This allows for daily dosing, along with minimal wearing-off or "rebound" effects. It doesn't appear to have significant abuse potential due to its slow onset of action, and therefore is a schedule IV drug (allowing the clinician to prescribe refills and to telephone prescriptions in to the pharmacy). Unfortunately, pemoline rarely has been associated with hepatitis that has progressed to fatal liver failure in some cases. Given this, it now is prescribed far less frequently than previously. The lag between initiation of treatment and the onset of hepatic abnormalities has been as long as 6 months, suggesting the importance of obtaining liver enzyme assays at baseline and then every few months (although the optimal frequency of monitoring is uncertain).

Clonidine, an α-2 agonist, is helpful especially when ADHD accompanies a tic disorder and stimulant therapy has been associated with exacerbation of the tics. Unfortunately, it is highly sedating for some patients. **Guanfacine (Tenex)**, a related medication, is longer acting and less sedating.

Bupropion (Wellbutrin), which has mild dopaminergic effects, also has been used to treat ADHD, especially in cases where clinicians are concerned about the potential for stimulant abuse. TCAs have been used as well (desipramine may be the most effective), although they are less efficacious and carry a greater risk of causing anticholinergic effects (constipation, dry eyes, dry mouth), sedation, weight gain, and cardiotoxicity. They may be particularly useful in cases where the patient has failed more than one stimulant trial and when ADHD is complicated by oppositionality, anxiety, tics, or depressive symptoms. **Venlafaxine (Effexor)** also appears to be moderately beneficial in some cases and does not carry the risk of toxicity associated with the TCAs.

While **SSRIs** sometimes are useful in treating impulsiveness and aggressiveness in children and adults, they appear to have little or no effect on attention deficits associated with ADHD. However, they sometimes are prescribed in combination with a stimulant when ADHD is associated with comorbid major depressive or dysthymic disorder. **Lithium** also has been used in a similar manner, particularly in patients who demonstrate prominent emotional lability or aggressiveness or in patients also diagnosed with bipolar disorder.

THE DIMENSIONAL PERSPECTIVE

Mental retardation was discussed in Chapter 3. As noted in that chapter, intelligence is a broad construct that includes a variety of verbal and performance skills. Specific aspects of intelligence also may be impaired in children, whether due to genetic factors, environmental factors, or slower maturation of specific skills relative to their overall intelligence. *DSM-IV* recognizes three specific cognitive areas of potential impairment.

The **learning disorders** involve impairments in the *learning of academic skills*, especially reading, arithmetic, and expressive writing.

These impairments are measured using standardized achievement tests. A learning disorder is determined to be present when an individual's academic skills are substantially below that would be expected, taking into account that individual's chronological age, measured intelligence, and age-appropriate education. **Motor skills disorder** describes difficulty with *physical coordination*. The **communication disorders** involve problems with *speech and language*—specifically, expressive language, mixed receptive and expressive language, stuttering, and phonological production (articulation). Federal law mandates that specialized educational opportunities, including individualized educational plans, be devised for children with educational disabilities. These disorders are associated with significant psychiatric comorbidity, and often the presence of an academic skills disorder is only uncovered in the context of a psychiatric workup for conduct problems, anxiety, depression, or substance abuse.

We have discussed **personality disorders** in Chapter 10. According to *DSM-IV*, personality disorder categories should only be applied to children or adolescents in those relatively unusual instances where the individual's particular maladaptive personality traits appear to be pervasive, persistent, and unlikely to be solely attributable to the individual's developmental stage or to an Axis I condition (such as major depressive disorder). Since children's personalities are still subject to change at least into their young adulthoods, most clinicians are circumspect about diagnosing personality disorder in individuals under the age of 18. *DSM-IV* specifies that one should only assign a personality disorder diagnosis when the maladaptive traits have been present for at least 1 year. An exception to this rule is *antisocial personality disorder*, which *DSM-IV* specifies should not be diagnosed at all in individuals under age 18. In such cases, the diagnosis of *conduct disorder* would be assigned.

THE BEHAVIOR PERSPECTIVE

Conduct Disorder

In **conduct disorder** there is a repetitive and persistent pattern of behavior in which the basic rights of others or major age-appropriate socie-

tal norms or rules are violated. As can be seen in Table 19–5, individuals with conduct disorder exhibit four major types of behavior: *aggressive conduct that causes or threatens physical harm to other people or animals*, *nonaggressive conduct that causes property loss or damage*, *deceitfulness or theft*, and *serious violations of rules*. Three (or more) characteristic behaviors must have been present during the past 12 months, and at least one behavior must have been present during the past 6 months.

Individuals with conduct disorder may have little empathy or concern for the feelings, wishes, and well-being of others and may lack appropriate feelings of guilt or remorse. They may misperceive the intentions of others as more hostile and threatening than is the case, and they may respond with aggression that they feel is reasonable and justified. They frequently demonstrate low frustration tolerance, irritability, temper outbursts, and reckless behavior.

Conduct disorder is associated with an early onset of sexual behavior, alcohol and nicotine abuse, use of illegal substances, reckless and risk-taking acts, school suspensions or expulsions, problems in work adjustment, legal difficulties, sexually transmitted diseases, unplanned pregnancy, physical injury from accidents or fights, and suicidal ideation. With regard to the last, children and adolescents with conduct disorder have a higher rate of both suicide attempts and completed suicide.

Conduct disorder is more common in boys (up to 16% of boys) than girls (up to 9% of girls). Gender differences also are found with regard to the specific types of conduct problems that are exhibited. Males tend to engage in fighting, stealing and vandalism and to have school discipline problems. Females are more likely to engage in lying, truancy, running away, substance use, and prostitution. Males tend to engage in more confrontational acts of aggression, and females tend toward more nonconfrontational acts. In many individuals, the conduct disorder remits by adulthood, but almost half of them go on to ultimately develop an *antisocial personality disorder*. The prognosis is worse for individuals in whom the conduct disorder is associated with early childhood-onset comorbid ADHD, more severe interpersonal aggression, lower intelligence, and poorer social skills.

Table 19–5. *DSM-IV-TR* Criteria for Conduct Disorder

A. A repetitive and persistent pattern of behavior in which the basic rights of others or major age-appropriate societal norms or rules are violated, as manifested by the presence of three (or more) of the following criteria in the past 12 months, with at least one criterion present in the past 6 months:

AGGRESSION TO PEOPLE AND ANIMALS

1. Often bullies, threatens, or intimidates others
2. Often initiates physical fights
3. Has used a weapon that can cause serious physical harm to others (e.g., a bat, brick, broken bottle, knife, gun)
4. Has been physically cruel to people
5. Has been physically cruel to animals
6. Has stolen while confronting a victim (e.g., mugging, purse snatching, extortion, armed robbery)
7. Has forced someone into sexual activity

DESTRUCTION OF PROPERTY

8. Has deliberately engaged in fire setting with the intention of causing serious damage
9. Has deliberately destroyed others' property (other than by fire setting)

DECEITFULNESS OR THEFT

10. Has broken into someone else's house, building, or car
11. Often lies to obtain goods or favors or to avoid obligations (i.e., "cons" others)
12. Has stolen items of nontrivial value without confronting a victim (e.g., shoplifting, but without breaking and entering; forgery)

SERIOUS VIOLATIONS OF RULES

13. Often stays out at night despite parental prohibitions beginning before age 13 years
14. Has run away from home overnight at least twice while living in parental or parental surrogate home (or once without returning for a lengthy period)
15. Is often truant from school, beginning before age 13 years

B. The disturbance in behavior causes clinically significant impairment in social, academic, or occupational functioning
C. If the individual is age 18 years or older, criteria are not met for antisocial personality disorder

SPECIFY TYPE BASED ON AGE AT ONSET

Childhood-Onset Type

Onset of at least one criterion characteristic of conduct disorder prior to age 10 years

Adolescent-Onset Type

Absence of any criteria characteristic of conduct disorder prior to age 10 years

SPECIFY SEVERITY

Mild

Few if any conduct problems in excess of those required to make the diagnosis and conduct problems cause only minor harm to others

Moderate

Number of conduct problems and effect on others intermediate between "mild" and "severe"

Severe

Many conduct problems in excess of those required to make the diagnosis or conduct problems cause considerable harm to others

Source: Reprinted with permission from the *Diagnostic and Statistical Manual of Mental Disorders, Fourth Edition, Text Revision.* Copyright 2000 American Psychiatric Association.

Genetic and biological factors appear to play a predisposing role in the development of the disorder (as noted during the discussion of antisocial personality disorder in Chapter 10), as do learning disorders, communication disorders, and ADHD, all of which commonly predate the onset of conduct problems. Psychosocial predisposing factors include parental rejection and neglect, inconsistent child-rearing practices, harsh discipline, physical or sexual abuse, lack of supervision, early institutional living, frequent changes of caregivers, large family size, association with a delinquent peer group, and familial psychopathology.

The goal of treatment is to help parents and school officials set limits on the child's behavior, to treat comorbid psychiatric problems (especially ADHD, learning and communication disorders, mood disorders and substance-related disorders), and to use psychotherapy to attempt to teach the patient more appropriate and effective coping skills. Home-based behavioral management often is hindered by parental psychopathology or domestic conflict. In more severe cases, limit setting may require removal of the child from the home or arrest for illegal behaviors.

Oppositional–Defiant Disorder

Individuals with **oppositional–defiant disorder (ODD)** are negativistic, hostile, and defiant to an extent greater than typically would be observed in individuals at that developmental stage The diagnostic criteria for ODD are listed in Table 19–6. Since oppositional behavior also can represent transient developmental behavior (quite common both in preschool children and in adolescents), the criteria specify that these behaviors should have been present for at least 6 months and have led to significant impairment. The be-

haviors also shouldn't occur only in the setting of a mood or psychotic disorder. In contrast to individuals with conduct disorder, those with ODD don't engage in behavior that violates either the rights of others or societal norms. However, in some cases ODD in childhood ultimately progresses to conduct disorder by adolescence.

ODD occurs in about 6% of children. While ODD is more common in boys prior to puberty, its prevalence is equal in both sexes during adolescence. As with conduct disorder, learning and communication disorders and ADHD also are predisposing factors. In one community survey of boys aged 5–14, up to 93% of the children identified by teachers as having ODD also fulfilled the criteria for ADHD, as did almost 60% of those identified by parents as having ODD. Similarly 50% of the children identified as having ADHD also had ODD. ODD is more prevalent in families where child care has been disrupted by a succession of different caregivers and in families where child-rearing practices have been harsh, inconsistent, or neglectful. Treatment strategies are similar to those utilized in conduct disorder

Feeding and Elimination Disorders

Pica is the persistent eating of non-nutritive substances for at least 1 month. The substances ingested tend to vary with age: infants and younger children typically eat paint, plaster, string, hair, or cloth; older children may eat animal drop-

Table 19–6. *DSM-IV-TR* Criteria for Oppositional–Defiant Disorder

---

A. A pattern of negativistic, hostile, and defiant behavior lasting at least 6 months, during which four (or more) of the following are present:
  1. Often loses temper
  2. Often argues with adults
  3. Often actively defies or refuses to comply with adults' requests or rules
  4. Often deliberately annoys people
  5. Often blames others for his or her mistakes or misbehavior
  6. Is often touchy or easily annoyed by others
  7. Is often angry and resentful
  8. Is often spiteful or vindictive
  Note: consider a criterion met only if the behavior occurs more frequently than is typically observed in individuals of comparable age and developmental level
B. The disturbance in behavior causes clinically significant impairment in social, academic, or occupational functioning
C. The behaviors do not occur exclusively during the course of a psychotic or mood disorder
D. Criteria are not met for conduct disorder, and, if the individual is age 18 years or older, criteria are not met for antisocial personality disorder

---

Source: Reprinted with permission from the *Diagnostic and Statistical Manual of Mental Disorders, Fourth Edition, Text Revision.* Copyright 2000 American Psychiatric Association.

pings, sand, insects, leaves, or pebbles; adolescents and adults may consume clay or soil. Pica can be associated with mental retardation. Although vitamin or mineral deficiencies sometimes contribute to the development of pica, usually no specific biological abnormalities are found. Poverty, neglect, lack of parental supervision, and developmental delay all can increase the risk for developing the condition. Treatment typically involves attempting to address psychosocial stressors and medical complications of the behavior (e.g., lead toxicity due to having eaten lead-based paint). Behavior therapy sometimes helps in addressing the eating behavior itself.

Rumination disorder is the repeated regurgitation and rechewing of food by an infant or child. The food then is either ejected from the mouth or reswallowed. This disorder most commonly is observed in infants, but it also can be seen in older individuals, again particularly in individuals with mental retardation. Infants display a characteristic position of straining and arching their back with their head held back, make sucking movements with their tongues. They appear to enjoy the activity. Despite the ingestion of large amounts of food, the condition can lead to malnutrition and failure to thrive, and it is associated with a mortality of up to 25%. Lack of stimulation, neglect, stressful life situations, and problems in the parent–child relationship are risk factors for the condition to develop but are not invariably seen in all cases. Treatment involves treating any medical complications as well as evaluating the child for gastroesophageal reflux or hiatal hernia. Psychosocial stressors also should be addressed. Aversive behavioral therapy (squirting lemon juice into the infant's mouth whenever rumination occurs) often can be effective in addressing the rumination behavior itself.

Encopresis is the repeated passage of feces into inappropriate places (e.g., clothing or the floor), either involuntarily or intentionally. This must occur at least once a month for at least 3 months, and the chronological age of the child must be at least 4 years (or for children with developmental delay, a mental age of at least 4 years). When the passage of feces is involuntary (the most common presentation), it often is related to constipation, impaction, and retention, with subsequent fecal overflow around the im-

paction. This constipation may have developed for physiologic reasons (ineffective sphincter control, dehydration, or a medication side effect) and/or for psychological reasons (anxiety or oppositionality leading to an avoidance of defecation). Once constipation has developed, an anal fissure may develop which in turn makes defecating even more painful, thereby exacerbating the child's phobic avoidance of defecation and worsening the fecal retention. Treatment typically involves addressing the constipation (if present), family counseling, and behavioral skills training.

Enuresis is the repeated voiding of urine during the day or at night into the bed or one's clothing, either involuntarily or intentionally. This must occur at least twice per week for at least 3 months or else must cause clinically significant distress or impairment in social, academic (occupational), or other important areas of functioning. The individual must have reached an age at which continence is expected, and since this is usually by age 3 or 4, the *DSM* requires a chronological or mental age of at least 5 years for the condition to be diagnosed.

Enuresis often is self-limited, and its prevalence decreases with age: at age 5 years, it occurs in 7% of males and 3% of females; by age 10 years, it occurs in 3% of males and 2% of females; and by age 18 years, it occurs in 1% of males and very few females. The disorder is related to maturational delay and family and twin studies also suggest a strong genetic component. Insufficient nocturnal antidiuretic hormone secretion may be the cause of **nocturnal enuresis** (bed-wetting) in some patients who have never become continent. In cases where a previously continent child becomes enuretic, a psychosocial precipitant may be playing a role (e.g., the birth of a sibling, hospitalization, or parental divorce).

Treatment may not be necessary, as many children become continent in the course of time. Evaluation of enuresis (typically by a pediatrician) involves first assessing for a medical cause, especially urinary tract infection or obstruction (the latter most commonly being the result of repeated urinary infections). Behavioral strategies include restricting fluids before bedtime, waking the child to void before enuresis can occur, and rewarding the child for staying dry overnight. Using a bell or buzzer attached to a moisture-sensitive pad is successful in most cases. Relapse frequently occurs at a later date, but the system can be reinstated at that point. Some children and parents have difficulty complying with this system.

In more severe cases, pharmacotherapy might be indicated. TCAs have been used, especially imipramine, but relapse typically occurs once the drug is discontinued. Given the risk of side effects (including cardiac toxicity), the use of TCAs has become more rare. It isn't clear why TCAs are effective for enuresis: it doesn't appear to be due to their anticholinergic properties, since other anticholinergic agents aren't particularly effective in treating the condition.

A more commonly employed medication is **desmopressin (DDAVP)**, an analogue of the antidiuretic hormone vasopressin. It is available as a nasal spray. Only one quarter of patients who use DDAVP become completely "dry," but for children who wet the bed four nights per week or more there is about a one-third reduction in their wet nights. Relapse rates upon cessation of treatment are high. One treatment strategy involves combining DDAVP with behavior therapy (the bell or buzzer). Side effects of DDAVP tend to be mild (headache, abdominal pain, epistaxis, nasal stuffiness). However, there have been a few reports of hyponatremia and even hyponatremic seizures. Overall, the preferred treatment remains behavior therapy, although the use of desmopressin appears to be reasonable for older children who had failed to respond to these interventions or for occasional use in known responders—for example, on nights when they are sleeping away from home.

THE LIFE-STORY PERSPECTIVE

While a child or adolescent's life story hasn't progressed as far as that of an adult, both children and adults tend to present for treatment in a state of *demoralization*. This tends to be the case even for children with "externalizing" disorders such as conduct disorder and oppositional–defiant disorder (despite the difficulties that these children may have appreciating the relationship between their own attitudes and behavior and their current life difficulties). Psychotherapy can play an important role in the treatment of youths with psychiatric disorders, especially since the therapist may be intervening

so early in the patient's life that the psychotherapy may have a *preventive* and not simply a *reparative* function.

Complicating matters, however, many children only present for treatment because they have been forced to do so by their parents or by the school system. They may be angry and mistrustful, both due to this and due to past disappointing experiences with major attachment figures. Mental retardation, learning and communication disorders, and immaturity can further interfere with a child's receptiveness, willingness, and ability to engage in introspection and problem-solving.

Because of these factors, treatment tends to be more directive and less interpretive with children. Behavior plans and more interactive therapy (e.g., talking with a small child about drawings or fantasy play with dolls in the office) may be as important as more traditional psychotherapy techniques.

Similarly, while many parents become major allies in the treatment, even well-intentioned parents may turn out to be unwittingly reinforcing their child's problematic behavior and may be resistant to changing their own behavior. They also may be quite angry at the child by the time that they finally present for treatment, and they may become angry at the clinician when suggested behavioral interventions aren't initially successful. Some parents may feel that the clinician is "blaming them" for their child's problems. Oppositional children and angry parents may begin to try the patience of even the most compassionate clinician.

SUMMARY

In this chapter, we have approached psychiatric disorders that present during childhood by using the same conceptual framework that we applied earlier to disorders that present later in life. We have begun by examining clinical phenomenology and diagnostic reliability and then have shifted our attention to consideration of issues related to the underlying validity of these various disorders. As with adult psychopathology, psychiatric disorders presenting during childhood lend themselves to approaches from a variety of theoretical vantage points, including the perspectives of disease, dimensions, behaviors, and life stories. Approaching the childhood disorders from each of these different perspective helps us gain a better appreciation of some of the conceptual difficulties inherent in working with children.

The evaluation and treatment of children is complicated by several unavoidable factors. First, psychiatric disturbances in children present in the context of ongoing psychological and biological development. As a result, attitudes and behaviors that may be developmentally appropriate for youths at one stage of development (e.g., separation anxiety) may be maladaptive and disabling for children at later stages of development. It sometimes is difficult to distinguish a true "disorder" from a simple variation in normal development or from a developmental delay that will resolve over time without specific clinical intervention.

Second, the same psychiatric disorder can present differently in youths at different developmental levels, a difficulty not encountered in adults. Third, conflicts and tensions inherent in normal development may themselves precipitate or exacerbate an underlying psychiatric illness, even in the absence of other new or profound "life stressors."

Fourth, comorbidity is the rule in childhood disorders. This is an inevitable upshot of having defined these various disorders more on the basis of particular presenting cognitions and behaviors than on the basis of underlying neurobiologic predispositions. (For example, generalized anxiety disorder, social phobia, Separation-anxiety disorder, and avoidant personality disorder all share similar biological diatheses but are considered to be distinct clinical syndromes.) It also reflects the fact that difficulties in one aspect of functioning predispose toward difficulties in other aspects of functioning. (This likely accounts for the overlap between learning disorders, ADHD, and conduct disorder.)

Fifth, children are less able to reason abstractly and so have more difficulty introspecting and appreciating the relationship between their current circumstances, their thoughts, and their emotional states. Thus, clinicians often must obtain information indirectly: through interpretation of the child's drawings, stories, and games, through observation of the child's behavior, and through interviews with collateral informants such as parents and teachers.

Finally, since children's psychological states often reflect their surrounding circumstances (e.g., parental psychiatric disturbances, impaired family functioning, poverty, abuse, neglect, difficult peer relationships, etc.), it becomes essential when evaluating and treating children to assess (and to address, when possible) these circumstances. In some cases, doing so becomes the clinician's primary treatment intervention.

Chapter 20

Forensic Psychiatry

Forensic psychiatry is a subspecialty of psychiatry that deals with the interface between psychiatry and the law. Two types of interactions occur between psychiatry and the law: *psychiatry as applied to the law* and *the law as applied to psychiatry.*

With regard to the former, psychiatrists sometimes are asked to provide expert testimony in order to assist the court in making more informed decisions when an individual's mental state or treatment needs are at issue. Such psychiatric participation occurs in both the criminal and civil legal systems. Table 20–1 offers some examples.

With regard to the latter, the area of *mental health law* subsumes attempts by courts, legislatures, and regulatory agencies to resolve conflicts that sometimes arise between psychiatric patients, clinicians, and the state. The goals of these various parties sometimes are at odds with each other, especially in situations where patients' rights to refuse treatment are in conflict either with their potential need for treatment or with the community's interest in protecting public safety. Examples include laws regulating involuntary civil commitment to psychiatric hospitals, laws regulating the boundaries of patient confidentiality, and laws regulating when a patient's refusal of psychiatric treatment must be respected and when the patient can be treated over his objections.

In this chapter, we will briefly discuss these relationships and how forensic evaluation differs from general clinical evaluation. We then will focus on one example of forensic psychiatric assessment that *all* physicians implicitly perform during every clinical conversation with their patients (whether they realize that they are doing so or not): the assessment of patients' competence to participate in clinical decision-making and to provide valid informed consent.

HOW FORENSIC PSYCHIATRY DIFFERS FROM GENERAL PSYCHIATRY

Forensic psychiatry differs from general psychiatry in several key respects. These include the clinician's *agency*, the *purpose of the clinical examination* (which is to assess for specific types of functional impairment rather than to offer treatment), the *nature of "truth"* in forensic work, the *nature of the evaluee*, the *required level of diagnostic certainty*, and the need to work within an *adversarial model* rather than a collegial model.

Agency

"Agency" refers to the nature of the fiduciary relationship between the clinician and the individual that she is evaluating. In other words, the pri-

Table 20–1. Examples of Psychiatric Interaction with the Legal System

CRIMINAL

Pretrial evaluations (e.g., criminal responsibility [insanity], competence to stand trial), presentence evaluations (including capital sentencing cases involving the death penalty)

CIVIL

Competence to be a witness, testamentary capacity, child custody, competence to manage one's person or property (guardianship), personal injury, malpractice, disability

LEGISLATIVE

Assisting legislatures in crafting laws affecting psychiatric patients

---

mary question with regard to agency is: "For whom are you working?" Sometimes, even in general psychiatric practice, the answer to this question is not clear, as illustrated by the following three examples:

A psychiatrist providing psychotherapy to an adolescent with an eating disorder is asked by the child's mother for information about what her daughter is talking about in therapy. When the psychiatrist tells her that this information is confidential, the mother replies: "That's ridiculous. Aren't I paying the bill? You work for me. Besides, she's a minor and I'm her mother." The psychiatrist replies that, regardless of who is paying for the therapy, his primary fiduciary obligation is to the child.

A prison psychiatrist is evaluating an inmate for depression and anxiety. One day during a psychotherapy session, the patient states that he is especially anxious today, because several other inmates are planning to start a riot. He states: "I know I can tell you about this because it's all confidential, right?" The psychiatrist replies that in matters that threaten prison security, he is obligated to violate confidentiality and alert the prison administration.

A psychiatrist in a university student mental health clinic is treating a student referred by the dean of his college. Last semester the student received D's in most of his classes and then required acute psychiatric hospitalization when he became acutely psychotic. In the hospital, schizophrenia was diagnosed. The patient has been allowed to remain in school but this is contingent upon him remaining in psychiatric treatment and taking his

medications. He now informs the psychiatrist that he doesn't believe that he is mentally ill or needs medication, that he is tired of the sedation caused by the medication, and that he stopped taking the medication last week. He comments that he is willing to continue to see the psychiatrist for psychotherapy but he won't take the medication. He asks the psychiatrist to keep this information confidential, and specifically asks him not to discuss this with the dean of the college.

In all of these examples, the psychiatrist is faced with a situation that involves having divided loyalties (i.e., he has *dual agency*). These circumstances always have been there, but they are causing problems only now, because they now are coming into conflict with each other. Ethically, clinicians are best served by letting patients know from the outset of treatment about any potential limitations on the traditional doctor–patient relationship imposed by a particular treatment setting.

In forensic practice, these difficulties are further compounded by the fact that while forensic psychiatrists use clinical skills to conduct their forensic assessments, they usually have not entered into a traditional doctor–patient relationship with the evaluee. In other words, *their agency is usually to some outside party rather than to the evaluee.* For example, they may have been retained by the individual's attorney or by the prosecuting attorney to perform an assessment of his competence to stand trial or by a private insurance company to assess whether he meets their specific criteria for occupational disability.

An evaluee may not recognize this distinction, especially if he previously has received psychiatric treatment in the clinical setting. After all, the forensic psychiatrist is taking a history and asking typical questions about the individual's mental status. The forensic clinician therefore is ethically obligated to disclose at the outset of the evaluation the nature of his relationship with the evaluee and the purpose of the present evaluation. The clinician might even need to reiterate this information during the course of the evaluation if it appears to him that the evaluee is slipping into a "patient role."

For example, the forensic clinician might state: "I have been asked by the court to evaluate you. You need to understand that even though I'm a doctor,

I'm not working for you, I'm working for the court. Also, what you tell me will not be confidential, since I'm going to be submitting a report to the court that other people will read. So you should keep this in mind while you're talking to me. However, despite these limitations, I only can reach accurate conclusions if you're as honest and up front with me as you can be."

Some psychiatrists have argued that forensic work in general raises significant ethical questions since—while it is possible that one's evaluation and testimony might help the evaluee—it also is possible that they may harm the evaluee. In reply, other psychiatrists have noted that forensic psychiatric practice *is* rooted in the ethical principles of medical practice, but that at the heart of medical ethics is the weighing of competing interests. In forensic practice, while these principles remain intact, which principles are considered paramount changes. The forensic clinician's primary ethical obligation is to *conduct herself honestly and to strive for objectivity* rather than to represent the "best interests" of the individual that she is evaluating.

The U.S. legal process is adversarial in nature. Given this, when a psychiatrist is retained by one side or the other in either a civil or criminal matter, she risks developing an opinion that is subtly biased. Further, even when her opinion isn't biased, it still may be distorted by both parties. Forensic psychiatrists therefore strive to *carry out their responsibilities in an honest manner and to reach objective opinions*. They base their opinions on all of the data that is available to them rather than simply on what the evaluee (or other interested parties) may tell them; they attempt to distinguish facts from inferences; and they attempt to distinguish professional expert opinions from their own personal opinions. While they advocate for their opinions (it would be unethical not to do so), they avoid advocating for one side in a legal dispute. Regardless of who is paying their bill, their opinion should be the same, since they are being reimbursed for their time, not for their opinions.

When a physician assumes the "forensic role," he remains a physician but his *agency* is different. His primary obligation is to society rather than to the patient. He no longer is primarily concerned with doing what is best for the patient but with protecting the integrity of the system by offering opinions that are honest and objective. Therefore, treating physicians generally should avoid agreeing to act as expert witnesses for their patients or to perform evaluations of their own patients for legal purposes. First of all, conducting the forensic encounter usually will require that corroborative sources be interviewed, that information that they had obtained privately be exposed to public scrutiny, and that their patients (or their patients' disclosures) be subjected to potentially damaging cross-examination. All of these factors can adversely affect the doctor–patient relationship. Even the appearance of the treating clinician as a "fact" witness may lead to uncontrolled disclosure of private information or misinterpretation of testimony as "expert" opinion. Second of all, having been acting to date as the patient's treating physician likely will serve to bias the clinician and undermine the accuracy and utility of the forensic evaluation.

A psychiatrist who has been treating a woman with schizophrenia for the past two years is asked by her attorney, in the midst of divorce proceedings, to perform a child custody evaluation. Her husband currently is alleging that her two children might not be safe around her and he therefore is seeking sole custody of the children. The patient has been compliant with her medications for the past year and has not expressed any hallucinations or delusions. She does remain concrete in her thinking and distrustful of others. The psychiatrist has had no indications based on his interactions with the patient that she would be a danger to her children. On the other hand, he has never evaluated either of her two children, has never directly observed her interactions with her children, has never met her husband, and has not spoken to any collateral informants.

The psychiatrist therefore has several concerns about performing such an evaluation. He recognizes that he would be placed in a "double agent" role. Can he truly be a neutral, objective evaluator when he currently has a relationship with the patient, especially since the relationship has been based upon his working in her best interest? Second, his forensic conclusions might jeopardize his ability to treat the patient. What if his conclusions are unfavorable to her? Their relationship might never recover. She might even drop out of treatment and stop taking her medication. Even if his report is favorable to her, she might now be so indebted to him that she would be hindered from expressing negative feelings about him, and the latter also is an important part of psychotherapy. He therefore explains to the patient (and to her attorney) that he prefers to remain the patient's *treating* doctor, so that he can support her during this stressful period of her life. However, he does refer the patient to a colleague who has expertise in performing child custody evaluations.

Assessing Functional Impairment Rather Than Providing Treatment

In clinical practice, the primary goal is to elicit signs and symptoms of illness, to use these to determine the patient's diagnosis, and then—based on the diagnosis—to prescribe a particular treatment plan. In contrast, these matters are of little interest to the legal system, and judges and lawyers can become frustrated with clinicians who spend a great deal of time discussing the differential diagnosis of schizophrenia versus schizoaffective disorder versus bipolar disorder or the relative merits of prescribing a mood stabilizer versus an antipsychotic agent.

What the legal system *is* interested in is answering *specific legal questions*. These questions usually are defined either by statute or by legal precedent (i.e., by definitions offered by judges in previous cases in that jurisdiction). Therefore, the most important question for the forensic clinician to ask before initiating any evaluation is: "What's the legal question that I'm being asked to address?" The evaluation aimed at answering one particular legal question may not be sufficient to answer a different legal question.

For example, if the question is whether the evaluee is *competent to stand trial*, the clinician performing the clinician evaluation must first be aware of what specific tasks are required of individuals who are standing trial and how well individuals are expected to perform these tasks in order to be considered "competent." The requirements may be very different if one is assessing whether an evaluee is competent to manage his financial affairs or competent to draft a new version of his will. Similarly, if the question

tion is whether the evaluee was *insane at time of a criminal offense.* The clinician must know how "insanity" is defined in the evaluee's state. If the question is *disability*, the clinician must review the definition of disability, which varies in different settings (a private insurance policy, Social Security, or Workman's Compensation).

In addressing such legal questions, the clinical diagnosis in itself generally is of limited utility. The presence of a clinical diagnosis usually is necessary but not sufficient, in that the legal question typically hinges on whether the patient, as a *result* of their mental illness, is sufficiently impaired such that they *lack particular capacities*. Many patients who have symptoms of an illness still retain these capacities. Given this, the clinician must determine not only the evaluee's diagnosis and clinical symptoms but also the extent of any associated *functional impairment*—specifically, impairment in capacities required to perform a specific legal task. Functional impairment is not synonymous with any particular psychiatric diagnosis nor with any particular psychiatric symptom. The nature of these relationships is illustrated in Figure 20–1.

While the law is primarily concerned with the evaluee's degree of functional impairment, forensic clinicians still attempt to determine the evaluee's psychiatric diagnosis, for two reasons. First, the diagnosis links the evaluee's mental state to a larger database of scientific knowledge derived from clinical experience and empirical research. Thus, it informs the clinician's opinions about whether or not the evaluee is malingering, about whether the evaluee's behavior at the time of an offense is consistent with what commonly is observed in other individuals with the same diagnosis, and about whether particular illnesses impair particular mental abilities. It also helps the clinician predict whether the evaluee's condition is likely to respond to treatment (particularly important in disability evaluations, sentencing evaluations, and competence-to-stand-trial evaluations). Second, issues such as

Treatment ← Diagnosis ← **Signs and Symptoms** → Functional Capacity → Legal Question

Clinical Assessment   **Forensic Assessment**

Figure 20–1. Relationship between clinical assessment and forensic assessment.

insanity and civil commitment are predicated on the presence of a mental illness. Therefore, the clinician must address the "threshold" question, "Is a mental illness present?" before these other issues even can be considered.

A summary of some of the most common legal questions that require an assessment of functional capacity is provided in Table 20–2. Note that legal questions are always answered either "yes" or "no." They are therefore "all or nothing": a person is either committed to the hospital or released; a person is found incompetent to stand trial or is found competent to proceed to trial; a person is either insane or sane. In contrast, clinicians tend to assess a person's functional capacities along a *gradient*. For example, a person's degree of "dangerousness" can vary from a 0% likelihood of harming herself or others to a 100% likelihood. A person's capacity to understand legal charges against her also varies along a continuum; some individuals have no ability, other individuals have perfect ability, and most individuals fall somewhere in between these two extremes.

Where one draws the line when addressing such legal questions is a social rather than a clinical determination. Is a patient so dangerous as a result of mental illness that the state is justified in committing her to the hospital and depriving her of her freedom despite her having committed no crime? Was a person's understanding of the wrongfulness of her behavior so impaired at the time that she committed a legal offense that

Table 20–2. Various Legal Issues and Associated Functional Capacities

Legal Issue	Functional Capacity
Civil commitment	Capacity to refrain from "dangerous" behavior
Treatment over objection	Capacity to give informed consent
Testamentary capacity	Capacity to make a will
Guardianship	Capacity to make personal or financial decisions
Insanity	Capacity to understand right from wrong or control behavior
Trial competence	Capacity to understand trial and assist in defense
Disability	Capacity to work
Child custody	Capacity to parent

we should not consider her culpable? Generally, the courts draw the line near the extreme of severe impairment. For example, the overwhelming majority of individuals are determined by the court to be competent to stand trial provided that they can meet a minimal standard. Similarly, the overwhelming majority of criminal defendants are not found to have been insane at the time that they committed their offense. (Despite public misperceptions, the insanity defense is employed by defendants in only about 1% of felony cases and is successful in only a fraction of these cases.)

Example: Assessment of Disability

In disability assessments, the legal question is whether an individual is so impaired in his occupational functioning that he is unable to work and therefore is entitled to be relieved of work responsibilities. The first question that the clinician should ask is in such cases is: "What is the question?" A private disability policy may define disability as being unable to perform one specific job. For example, if a surgeon injures his hand and no longer can perform surgery, he might be considered to be disabled. In contrast, the Social Security Administration uses a much more restrictive definition. Under their definition, an individual is disabled only when he is "not only unable to do his previous work but cannot, considering his age, education and work experience, engage in any other kind of substantial gainful work which exists in the national economy regardless of whether such work exists in the immediate area in which he lives, or whether such a specific job vacancy exists for him, or whether he would be hired if he applied for work."

Studies involving patients with physical injuries have demonstrated that an individual's degree of functional impairment doesn't directly correlate with the severity of signs and symptoms of an associated illness. For example, some people with severe back pain can continue to work, while others with more "mild" pain are unable to do so. Similarly, some patients with schizophrenia function quite well on a social level despite having chronic psychotic symptoms. In other cases, a patient with schizophrenia whose psychotic symptoms have completely resolved following treatment with antipsychotic medica-

tion may remain unable to work due to occupational and social impairment related to subtle but
pervasive negative symptoms. Similarly, even
"mild" symptoms of a mood disorder (such as
difficulty with concentration, reading, or mental
stamina) can prevent formerly high-functioning
individuals (tax attorneys, nuclear physicists,
etc.) from being able to fulfill their occupational
responsibilities.

Clinicians often feel uncomfortable when their
patients ask them to assess functional capacity in
the context of a disability assessment, primarily
because it is difficult assess social or occupational functioning in the clinical setting. Is an individual with back pain able to return to work if
she only has to engage in "light lifting" or sitting at a desk? Can an individual with moderate
depression work as a cashier? In attempting to
answer such questions, the clinician's evaluation
needs to be specifically directed at the patient's
capacities to perform specific types of tasks.
What is the patient expected to be able to do on
a typical workday? How does her current functioning differ from past functioning? Review of
evaluations from supervisors or collateral information from peers can be helpful in this regard.

Example: Guardianship Assessment

A clinician sometimes is asked to assess whether
individuals with dementia no longer are capable
of managing their finances or living independently. If they are not, the court may need to ap-
point a legal guardian. Again, the *diagnosis* of
dementia in itself is not identical to an inability
to live independently. Further, even when the clinician has determined the degree of severity of
the individual's symptoms (in this case, cognitive deficits), she still may not have a clear sense
of whether the individual is capable of living independently. For example, if the clinician determines that the patient's Mini-Mental State Examination score is 23, this in itself tells her very
little about how the patient functions in the home
setting.

More relevant to an assessment of the patient's
ability to live independently would be questions
directed toward the patients current degree of
functional capacity in this particular domain. For
example, can the patient bathe, toilet, and dress
herself? Does she pay her own bills? Has she
ever left the oven on? The clinician then can

more directly assess the patient's capacities by
asking her questions specifically related to her
daily functioning. For example, he might ask her
how much money she has in her bank account,
how much money she spends on utilities each
month, etc. An even pertinent functional assessment might involve having an occupational therapist directly observe the patient performing various tasks, such as cooking a meal at the stove.
Does the patient remember to use oven mitts?
Does she remember to turn the oven off?

Note that this guardianship assessment does
not address any of the patient's other potential
capacities, such as her ability to revise her will
(i.e., her *testamentary capacity*) or her ability to
testify in court as a witness. If the clinician were
asked at some later point to offer opinions related to these other questions, he would need to
reexamine the patient, directing his attention toward capacities relevant to these specific areas.

Example: Assessment of Competence to Stand Trial and Sanity

A psychiatrist might be asked by the court to
"evaluate" an individual with schizophrenia accused of stabbing his daughter to death. Again,
the first question that she should ask is: "What
is the legal question that I am being asked to address?" She asks the defendant's attorney and is
informed that the court specifically is interested
in an assessment of both the defendant's competence to stand trial and his sanity at the time
of the alleged offense.

These two legal terms have different definitions in different states, so she will need to familiarize herself with the local definition. A common definition of competence to stand trial is that
the defendant—to be considered competent—
must have a "sufficient present ability to consult
with his lawyer with a reasonable degree of rational understanding, and must have a rational as
well as a factual understanding of the proceedings against him."

In essence, the defendant must be able to do
two things: assist his attorney and understand of
the charges against him. In order to do so, he
needs to have an appreciation of what people are
saying that he did, the range of possible sentences
should he be found guilty, and the roles of his
attorney, the prosecuting attorney, the judge, and
possibly a jury. He must be able to work with

his attorney. This potentially includes being able to disclose pertinent facts, assist in challenging the testimony of witnesses, and conduct himself appropriately in court. Since most criminal cases are disposed of via "plea bargains," the defendant also should have an understanding of what this process entails and what he would gain and lose by agreeing to a plea bargain.

A person would not be considered incompetent to stand trial simply by virtue of the fact that she has a diagnosis of schizophrenia. Even if she currently is experiencing active hallucinations or delusions, she still may be able to perform all of the above tasks. It is only when her symptoms substantially impair these specific capacities that she would be considered incompetent to stand trial. For example, if the patient has a persecutory delusion that her defense attorney, the judge, and the prosecuting attorney are all working together in a conspiracy against her, and that her only recourse is to refuse to speak to anybody (including her attorney), she might be adjudicated incompetent to stand trial. Note that the construct of trial competence refers to the defendant's *present capacity*. Most defendants who are judged incompetent due to psychosis do ultimately proceed to trial at some later date after receiving psychiatric treatment.

Sanity is a separate question from trial competence. It involves the defendant's capacities not at the present time but at a particular *point in the past*—that is, at the time of the offense. Usually the legal standard asks whether the patient—as a result of mental illness—either lacked substantial capacity to understand that his behavior was wrong or was unable to control his behavior at the time of the offense. For example, even if the defendant currently is incompetent to stand trial because of his delusions about the court system, this tells us little about whether he knew that it was wrong to kill his daughter at the time of the offense.

To answer that question, a forensic psychiatrist must attempt to reconstruct the defendant's mental status at the time of the offense. She does so based upon not only the defendant's retrospective reports but also any other available sources of data, such as interviews with family members or neighbors, police reports, records of previous hospitalizations (even the daughter's autopsy report).

Again, the fact that a defendant carries a diagnosis of schizophrenia says little about whether or not he was insane at the time of a legal offense. One cannot conclude, for example, "The defendant has schizophrenia, and therefore he was insane at the time of the offense." One cannot even move one step closer to the ultimate legal question, by saying, "The defendant has schizophrenia, was experiencing psychotic symptoms at the time of the offense, and therefore was insane." For example, what if a defendant was hearing voices telling him to kill himself, but his crime consisted of stealing a patient's wallet and using the money to buy illegal drugs? However, it would be appropriate for a forensic clinician to reach the following conclusion:

> The defendant has schizophrenia. At the time of his offense, he was experiencing delusional beliefs that his daughter was possessed by the devil. He also was experiencing hallucinations of voices telling him that the only way to save her eternal soul was to kill her. Psychiatric hospital records confirm that, prior to the offense, he repeatedly was admitted for treatment of similar delusions. I cannot discern an alternative, nonpsychotic motive for the stabbing, as his relationship with his daughter otherwise was without notable conflicts. He appears to have believed at the time of the offense that killing his daughter was a moral imperative. For example, he reports that as he stabbed his daughter repeatedly, he "knew" that her soul was ascending to heaven. All of these considerations argue for the defendant having lacked substantial capacity to distinguish right from wrong at the time of the offense.

The Nature of "Truth"

Treating clinicians generally are most interested in **narrative truth**—the "truth" as their patient perceives it. They may have little opportunity to corroborate whether the events that their patients describe actually transpired that way. However, since their primary goal is to help the patient, not to determine the "actual" truth or **historical truth**, in most cases they accept this degree of uncertainty.

Forensic clinicians, however, are asked to assess the historical truth of a situation. For example, in an insanity evaluation, the clinician is asked to reconstruct the defendant's state of mind at the time of the offense. Therefore, they routinely review not only on the defendant's recollections but also information obtained from interviews with witnesses and from reviews of police reports and medical records. It would be naive for the forensic clinician to "believe the defendant," whereas believing the patient is common in clinical work.

(Of course, this dichotomy is an oversimplification. Under some situations, treating clinicians do obtain extensive collateral information. They generally do so when the consequences of being wrong are greater or when the clinician suspects that the patient is not a reliable informant. For example, when a patient presents to an inpatient unit following a significant suicide attempt but denies having any symptoms of depression, denies having suicidal thoughts, and requests immediate hospital discharge, the treating clinician generally will attempt to obtain collateral information. In this case, the patient does not appear to be a reliable informant, and the consequences of releasing the patient prematurely might include another suicide attempt.)

The Nature of the Evaluee

Generally speaking, treating clinicians believe what their patients tell them, since these patients voluntarily present to the clinician seeking help and have little incentive to lie. In other words, the base rate for malingered mental illness is relatively low in the clinical treatment setting.

In contrast, forensic clinicians are not asked to assess individuals who are self-referred patients and seeking help but rather to assess individuals referred by outside parties for evaluation in the setting of ongoing criminal or civil litigation. In this context, the base rate for malingered or exaggerated psychiatric symptoms is much higher. Assessing for this therefore assumes greater importance.

Similarly, even the information obtained from collateral informants may be distorted, given the forensic context. For example, when conducting a child custody or testamentary capacity evaluation, "outside" informants sometimes are the same people who stand to gain or lose based upon the clinician's conclusions.

Finally, attorneys may be selective in the information or the materials that they provide to the clinician performing the forensic evaluation.

Therefore, forensic clinicians must temper their conclusions given the possibility that they may be predicated on a biased or distorted factual database.

The Required Level of Diagnostic Certainty

In clinical work, one's temptation is to "do what works." For example, a treating clinician might reason: "Perhaps this patient has a delusional disorder of the persecutory type, but perhaps he has paranoid personality disorder. Regardless, I will try prescribing an antipsychotic agent and will see if this helps." In forensic work, however, the clinician must specify the *degree of certainty* to which he holds his opinions and only should offer opinions that he holds to a reasonable degree of medical certainty. He also should be prepared to defend the *scientific basis* for each of his conclusions under cross-examination.

The Adversarial Model

Clinical work is based on *collaborative relationships* between physicians and their peers. Even when clinicians disagree, they recognize that they are striving to work together toward a common goal—that is, the patient's welfare. In contrast, the U.S. legal system is based on an *adversarial model*. In contrast to the medical system, which strives to determine the truth through collaboration, the legal system attempts to discover truth through a battle between diametrically opposed sides. In the criminal system, the battle is between the prosecution and the defense, while in the civil system, the battle is between the plaintiff and the defense.

Clinicians may be treated antagonistically or disrespectfully in court, and their opinions may be distorted by both sides. Such behavior is encouraged by the system itself, since lawyers representing each side are charged with zealously representing their side's point of view. However, the clinician's ethical obligation is to attempt to present her opinion to the finder of fact (the judge or jury) in an unbiased, undistorted form. If she is to do so, several "forensic" skills are required in addition to the usual "clinical" skills.

First, the clinician must present her opinion in a manner that is comprehensible to the layperson and that is relatively free of jargon but not overly simplistic. The clinician also must attempt to educate the judge or jury without appearing arrogant and must avoid becoming overly defensive when her views are challenged.

Second, the clinician must strive to avoid becoming overly invested in the outcomes of the legal proceedings. She must remember that she is only one small part of a much larger process. While the clinician may have spent hours conducting the clinical evaluation, researching the issues, formulating an opinion, and educating attorneys, the jury ultimately makes its decision based on factors well beyond the clinician's control.

Third, the clinician must attempt to avoid being manipulated by the attorney with whom she is working. While most attorneys are well intentioned, ethical practitioners, their primary goal is to obtain a good outcome for their client, not to accurately present the clinician's opinion. Similarly, they may not provide the clinician with all information relevant to the case, so the clinician must be amenable to modifying her opinion should further information later come to her attention that argues against her present conclusions.

Fourth, the clinician must attempt to avoid becoming enamored of the adversarial model—of the feeling that she only should present evidence that is favorable to "her side," leaving it to a clinician for the "other side" to present evidence that is less favorable to her opinion. Clinicians sometimes must step back and remind themselves that the goal in forensic work is not to win the case but to remain honest and objective.

Finally, the clinician must attempt to avoid making any statements or claims in her reports or testimony that she cannot fully defend, even when she strongly suspects that it likely is the truth. This is not a typical consideration in clinical practice.

EXAMPLE OF FORENSIC ASSESSMENT: EVALUATION OF DECISION-MAKING CAPACITY

Decision-making Capacity Versus Competence

All physicians routinely assess their patients' ability to make medical decisions, although they typically do so implicitly rather than explicitly. Psychiatric consultation tends to be requested only when an obvious question arises as to a patient's decision-making capacity or when the patient refuses an important procedure or medication. In many such cases, a psychiatrist may be asked to "declare the patient incompetent" so that treatment still can proceed. In other cases, the psychiatrist might be asked to "declare the patient competent" so that the primary treatment provider can feel more comfortable about allowing the patient to decline the recommended treatment (or even sign out of the hospital against medical advice).

"Competence" is a legal rather than a medical term and—technically speaking—only a judge can "declare a patient incompetent." All citizens are presumed competent unless they have been explicitly declared legally incompetent by the courts. This holds true even for grossly psychotic or severely demented patients who are refusing treatment.

While a psychiatrist can assess for the degree to which a patient's decision-making capacity is impaired along a dimensional continuum of severity, whether a given degree of impairment is so severe that the patient should no longer have the legal right to make certain decisions independently is more of a social determination than a medical one. However, while it is technically true that only a judge can declare a patient incompetent, in practice judges usually rely heavily on medical expert testimony when they make their determination and most often the judge ultimately agrees with the clinician's conclusions.

Competence Is Task-Specific

Any physician can perform an assessment of decision-making capacity. No state requires that such evaluations specifically be performed by a psychiatrist. For the moment, however, let us assume that you are a psychiatrist being requested by a primary care physician to assess whether a patient is "competent." Your first question should be: "Competent to do what?" There is no such thing as "global incompetence." Competence is task-specific. Patients may be competent to make some decisions and not others, depending on the level of complexity of the decision and of the related medical issues. Therefore, you need to find out from the person requesting the consultation exactly what decision they are asking the patient to make.

Think Clinically before Thinking Legally

Always think clinically before thinking legally. Many physicians, faced with a patient who is refusing a recommended treatment, immediately contact an attorney or risk manager to determine if they have a "right to proceed," even when they aren't sure *why* the patient is refusing a potentially beneficial treatment. Their first order of business *should* be to perform a detailed mental status examination in order to establish whether the refusal of treatment reflects the presence of an underlying psychiatric disturbance that might be amenable to relatively simple clinical intervention.

> A psychiatrist is asked to "declare a patient incompetent" because the patient is refusing a diagnostic test. He finds that the patient is delirious, likely due to sepsis and opioid intoxication. He recommends continuing to treat the patient with antibiotics (which were just initiated that morning) and holding all narcotic medication. He notes that in this particular case the diagnostic test likely can wait until the patient's delirium has been addressed. The following day, the patient is much more coherent, has no recall of the events of the previous day, and agrees to the test. Initiating legal measures to have the patient declared incompetent proves to have been unnecessary.

Similarly, some patients demand to sign out of the hospital against medical advice out of frustration with the medical system or fear of painful procedures. Counseling the patient or mediating between the patient and the primary treatment provider or hospital staff often leads to successful resolution of the conflict, again without having to resort to legal measures.

After you have completed the standard diagnostic portion of the clinical examination, you next need to direct your questioning specifically toward the patient's *functional capacities*. In this case, since the issue is the patient's capacity *to give or refuse informed consent*, you should go through each aspect of the informed consent with the patient: the *proposed procedure*, the *medical indication* for the procedure, the *potential risks* of the procedure, the *potential benefits* of the procedure, *alternatives to the procedure*, and the risks and benefits associated with each of these.

The patient should be able to paraphrase this information independently, not simply agree with the physician's statements. Obviously, it is important to know how this information already has been conveyed to the patient, since previous attempts to educate the patient may not have taken into account possible cognitive or emotional impairments. Even if the patient initially demonstrates a poor understanding of these elements, you should attempt to educate her and observe whether her performance subsequently improves.

> Psychiatric consultation is requested when a patient with amnestic (Korsakoff's) syndrome refuses amputation of gangrenous foot. The patient is unable to describe his illness or the proposed treatment, but displays a good understanding of these matters following a detailed explanation. In the short term, he is able to paraphrase the presented information and make an informed decision, and agrees to the procedure. The psychiatrist documents the patient's abilities and suggests that the patient might be capable of providing informed consent if the treatment team remains cognizant of his memory difficulties and offers the patient repeated education as needed over the course of treatment. However. 30 minutes later, the psychiatrist returns to the patient's room and finds that the patient again is refusing the amputation and has no recollection of their earlier discussion. The psychiatrist therefore modifies his opinion, noting that the patient's capacities likely are too impaired to be consistent with legal competence, since informed consent is an ongoing *process* that patients must engage in *throughout* the entire course of treatment and not simply an *isolated decision* that the patient makes at a single point in time.

Factors to Consider in Assessing Decision-making Capacity

At this point, you have performed a psychiatric history and mental status examination and have discussed the proposed medical treatment with the patient. As you attempt to assess the patient's decision-making capacity, what legal standard should you be keeping in mind? What is the legal definition of competence?

Unfortunately, there is no single legal standard. However, Appelbaum and Grisso, reviewing relevant case law and the scholarly literature, delineated four basic standards that courts traditionally have relied upon. These are *(1)* the ability to *communicate a choice, (2)* the ability to *understand the relevant facts, (3)* the ability to *appreciate one's circumstances* and how the facts apply to their particular case, and *(4)* the ability to *rationally manipulate information* in reaching a decision.

The first two standards have been universally accepted by all courts. The latter two standards are less "obvious" and may require more detailed explication in the patient's chart or in reports or expert testimony submitted to the a court. We will discuss each of these standards in turn.

Can the Patient Communicate a Choice?

The ability to communicate a choice is the least-debatable criterion for competence. All courts have accepted the idea that patients who are unable to communicate a choice about treatment are not competent. The patient may be comatose or aphasic or might speak a foreign language with no interpreter being available in the time frame in which an acute decision is required.

Note that some patients might understand what a clinician is explaining to them but still refuse to acknowledge this. For example, a patient with schizophrenia might lie in bed with blankets pulled over her head, refusing to speak or even to nod her head in response to various questions. The extent of her ability to understand therefore is unclear. One would have to presume that her decision-making is impaired, since—as a result of her illness—she appears to be unable to communicate a choice.

Even when a patient can say "yes" or "no," his decision should be *sufficiently stable*. If this isn't the case, the patient hasn't communicated a *consistent* choice, as in the example of the patient with amnestic syndrome. However, while the patient's choice should be stable, it does not necessarily have to be *fixed*. In other words, patients retain the right to change their minds. For example, patients have a right to change their mind about receiving antidepressant medication even if they are not experiencing any side effects and even if their depression is just beginning to improve provided that they understand and appreciate the issues that are involved.

Can the Patient Understand the Facts Relevant to the Proposed Decision?

Does the patient understand all of the elements of informed consent with respect to this particu-

lar medical decision? Is he able to paraphrase the information? While the determination that the patient does or does not understand specific information requires more clinical judgment than the determination that the patient is able to express a choice, the notion that a patient cannot truly give informed consent if he doesn't adequately understand the information being presented is not controversial.

Does the Patient Have an Appreciation of Her Current Circumstances?

Appreciation is a more abstract concept than simple factual understanding. In order to provide competent consent, patients must have an appreciation that they have an illness and that the information being provided is relevant to their circumstances. Patients who are delusional, who lack insight, who are nihilistically depressed, or who are grandiosely manic often lack an objective appreciation of their true circumstances. When this is the case, the patient also usually lacks an appreciation of the potential benefits of the treatments that treatment providers offer them.

> A psychiatrist proposes a trial of antipsychotic medication to a patient with schizophrenia who is experiencing paranoid delusions. The patient understands that the psychiatrist is saying that the patient has schizophrenia, that the psychiatrist would like to initiate treatment with antipsychotic medication, that these medications can help treat delusional thinking, and that the medications carry certain risks, such as parkinsonism and tardive dyskinesia. However, the patient still refuses the medication, stating: "I'm sure these medications are great for patients with schizophrenia. The only problem is, I don't have schizophrenia. And I'm not delusional."

In the above example, a focal deficit in insight (i.e., in the patient's *appreciation* of how the informed-consent information applies to his particular case) is enough to "short circuit" the entire informed-consent process despite his excellent *understanding* of the facts that have been presented to him.

> A depressed patient on the oncology floor understands all of the risks and benefits and alternatives to a proposed chemotherapy regimen but then refuses to give consent due to a severe sense of hopelessness. She says, "I know I'll be in the 10% who don't respond." The patient then adds that she "de-

serves to die" given the awful things that she has done throughout her life. Further evaluation fails to reveal evidence of delusional thinking.

In this example, while the patient is not clearly delusional, it still appears that her depressive state is influencing her decision making to a significant degree. While she understands that 90% of people respond to the proposed chemotherapy regimen, because of her pervasive nihilistic, hopeless attitude, she doesn't believe that this statistic *applies to her.*

In both of the above cases, since the patients appear to "understand" the basic facts, a psychiatric report that attempts to argue for "incompetence" will need to clearly document both the nature of the patient's psychiatric illness and the manner in which it is influencing the patient's thinking. Otherwise, a judge might at some point ask the patient a few basic questions and come away satisfied that the patient "appears to understand the situation and is making a clear choice to refuse treatment."

Does the Patient Have the Ability to Rationally Manipulate Information?

Patients also should be able to rationally manipulate information. Can the patient weigh several potentially competing interests in a rational manner? For example, can the patient being offered information about cancer treatments rationally weigh the potential to become cancer-free against the potential for experiencing postoperative pain or chemotherapy-related nausea and hair loss? Some patients, either due to psychiatric illness or intellectual limitations, are unable to *(1)* consider multiple factors, *(2)* reflect on the impact of these factors on their short-term and long-term interests, and *(3)* make a reasoned decision.

The clinician must not confuse assessing whether a patient can rationally manipulate information with assessing whether or not he agrees with the patient's *ultimate decision.* He is merely attempting to assess the *process* by which the patient reaches that decision. The clinician might disagree with a patient's decision but still respect the decision, provided that he can understand how the decision relates to the patient's lifestyle, values, or preferences.

A patient with a history of recurrent episodes of severe depression, who now is in a state of remis-

sion, informs his psychiatrist that he wishes to discontinue his antidepressant medication. He recognizes that to do so will increase his risk of experiencing a relapse, but states, "I just don't like the way that the medication makes me feel. I just feel . . . medicated, sluggish." His psychiatrist suggests alternative medications but the patient adamantly reiterates that he wishes to be medication-free. The psychiatrist suggests that follow-up visits with him will become that much more important if the patient discontinues his medication, given the need to monitor closely for depressive relapse. He also comments that they will have to discuss this issue further should the patient appear to be relapsing. The patient readily agrees to this plan.

Proceeding after the Assessment

How you proceed at this point will depend on whether the situation is nonemergent or emergent, on whether you assess the patient as having adequate decision-making capacity or not, and on whether the patient is agreeing to the procedure or refusing the procedure.

Nonemergent Situations

Let us assume that you are called to the inpatient medical unit because the treating physician wants the patient to consent to a treatment but the patient is refusing. Refusal of the treatment will not result in immediate harm to the patient. The key point here is that *competent patients have the right to refuse any treatment.*

Your evaluation can have two possible outcomes. If after your exam you feel the patient *is able to give (or refuse to give) informed consent* to the specific nonemergency procedure, you should say so to the treating physician. You should educate the physician that competent adult patients have the right to refuse treatment. However, this doesn't mean that you should not attempt to help the physician involve the patient's family, the nursing staff, or any other available resources to try to persuade the patient to change his mind. You can also suggest to the physician that if the patient continues to refuse the recommended treatment that he reevaluate the necessity of the procedure, consider alternative treatments that might be more palatable to the patient, or discharge the patient.

A patient is furious about having received three intravenous lines over a 2-day period, as well as about having suffered through multiple failed at-

tempts to start these lines. She therefore is refusing further antibiotic treatment. Psychiatric consultation is requested in order to "assess her competency." The psychiatrist asks the patient if she
would agree to oral antibiotics and she replies that
she would have absolutely no problem with this.
The internist says that he hadn't planned to switch
to oral antibiotics for another 24 hours, but he
would be willing to do this provided that the patient agree to resume intravenous therapy if she becomes febrile over the next 2 days. The patient
agrees to this plan.

If, however, you believe that because of a mental
disorder the patient *is unable to give informed consent* to a particular nonemergency procedure, you
should explain to the treating physician that merely
because *you* feel that the patient possibly is not
competent, this does not give the treating physician the right to proceed. Consent must be obtained
from some surrogate decision-maker. At this point,
the next question is whether the patient is agreeing to the procedure (i.e., he is *assenting* to the procedure but is unable to give true informed consent)
or whether he is refusing the procedure.

If the impaired patient is *agreeing to or is not
protesting the procedure, consent should be so-
licited from an appropriate surrogate decision-
maker.* Since the patient isn't protesting, judicial
intervention may not be necessary. However, for
the patient's protection, somebody other than the
patient needs to be given clinical information in
order for a decision to be made as to what is in
the patient's best interests. For example, when a
patient is in a coma after having suffered a traumatic brain injury during a car accident, physicians in the intensive care unit typically obtain
surrogate consent to proceed with treatment from
a spouse, parent, adult child, or sibling. Clinicians should familiarize themselves with local
laws that relate to such situations.

However, if the impaired patient is *protesting
the procedure*, and if the procedure is felt to be
clinically indicated and in the best interest of the
patient, the treating physician will need to pursue *judicial authorization*. Consent from a family member alone is insufficient, since every patient is presumed to be competent to refuse
treatment unless a court has declared her to be
incompetent and has appointed a legal guardian.
Family members can't "overrule" an individual
who is legally presumed to be competent.

In any of the above scenarios, it is essential
that you document that in your opinion the patient has a specific psychiatric diagnosis (which
you should name) and that the diagnosis is associated with specific symptoms that you believe
to be responsible for the patient's impaired decision-making. For example, you might write:

> The patient has vascular dementia, characterized
> by memory loss, confabulation, irritability, and ag-
> gressive behavior. As a result, his decision-making
> capacity is impaired in several important areas. He
> is extremely impaired in his ability to manage his
> personal affairs and make medical decisions. He
> denies that he has memory problems. He believes
> that his wife is at home and manages his finances
> when in fact his wife died 2 years ago. He was
> found lying in feces yet has no memory of this be-
> ing the case. His daughter reports that he has started
> several fires due to carelessness with cigarettes.
> When we discussed his decubitus ulcers, he denied
> that he had any, and he was unaware that he was
> in a hospital. He denies that he has hypertension.
> He is unable to understand the need for nursing
> home placement. Given all of the above, I recom-
> mend that you obtain substituted consent from his
> daughter to treat his decubitus ulcers and to treat
> his hypertension and aggression. He likely will re-
> quire nursing home placement, and his daughter
> can consent to this if the patient is not objecting to
> this. However, in the long run, she probably still
> should pursue formal guardianship both for per-
> sonal and medical decisions, and this will be nec-
> essary should he refuse nursing home placement.

Emergent Situations

Let us assume that a patient is brought into the
emergency room with a life-threatening illness.
However, she is refusing treatment. Without the
treatment, she will almost certainly die within
hours. The treating physician calls you to "declare the patient incompetent." The patient refuses a detailed mental status examination, repeatedly yelling, "Go away!" However, time is
of the essence. What should you do?

First, try to figure out why the patient is refusing a potentially life-saving procedure and try
to explain to her that she will die without it. Attempt to convince the patient to change her mind.
If the patient still refuses, you should inform the
primary physician that in your opinion the patient is not acting rationally since she is refusing
a life-saving procedure. Advise the physician

that, although he has to be the one to ultimately decide whether to proceed, in your opinion he should go ahead and proceed. Although technically the physician could later be sued for civil assault, it is extremely unlikely that a physician will be found negligent for attempting an emergency, life-saving procedure in good faith.

Obviously, you should document: (1) your mental status examination, (2) that you clearly told the patient that she would die without the procedure, and that the patient still refused, (3) the immediate, life-threatening nature of the patient's illness, and (4) that a reasonable, competent person would not refuse under such circumstance.

Overall, then, you should think clinically first. *Why* is a particular patient refusing a treatment that his physicians feel is important? You should always begin with the history and mental status examination. When possible, try to turn an adversarial "competency issue" into a therapeutic "process issue" involving the patient, the physician, the family, friends, or relevant other parties.

SUMMARY

Forensic psychiatry is a subspecialty of psychiatry that deals with the interface between psychiatry and law. While forensic psychiatrists are clinicians who apply medical *expertise* to legal issues, they are not acting as treating clinicians. Often, a traditional doctor–patient relationship is not established, and the fundamental ethical principles are to strive for honesty and objectivity

rather than to necessarily act in an evaluee's best interest.

Working in the legal arena presents other challenges not commonly encountered in the clinical arena. These include attempting to assess various capacities that are related only indirectly to clinical diagnoses and symptoms, having to review extensive records and interview multiple informants in order to reach more objective conclusions, dealing with a population of individuals who may be motivated to exaggerate or fabricate clinical symptoms, and working within a system that is inherently adversarial in nature.

One example of a forensic psychiatric assessment that all physicians routinely engage in is the assessment of patients' capacity to make medical decisions. While informed consent has become a cornerstone of clinical care, the informed-consent process requires not only that detailed clinical information be presented to patients in the absence of coercion but also that the patient be capable of understanding, appreciating, and weighing this clinical information and then expressing a choice. A variety of factors can interfere with each of these requirements, thereby preventing some patients from adequately engaging in the consent process. Physicians need to be aware of how to screen for such factors. They also should have a basic understanding of which factors are potentially amenable to clinical remedies that might improve patients' capacities. Psychiatric consultation may be useful in more complex cases.

References

Chapter 1

Chalmers DJ: The Conscious Mind: In Search of a Fundamental Theory. London, Oxford University Press, 1997.

Cooper JE, Kendell RE, Gurland BJ, et al: Psychiatric Diagnosis in New York and London: A Comparative Study of Mental Hospital Admissions. London, Oxford University Press, 1972.

Costa PT, McCrae RR: Theories of personality and psychopathology: approaches derived from philosophy and psychology, in Comprehensive Textbook of Psychiatry/VII, 7th Edition. Edited by Kaplan HI, Sadock BJ. Baltimore, Williams & Wilkins, 2000.

Dennett D: Consciousness Explained. Boston, Little, Brown, 1992.

Engel GL: The clinical application of the biopsychosocial model. Am J Psychiatry 137:535–544, 1980.

Freedman, DX: The search: body, mind, and human purpose. Am J Psychiatry 149:858–866, 1992.

Gabbard GO: Mind and brain in psychiatric treatment, in Treatment of Psychiatric Disorders, 2nd edition. Edited by Gabbard GO. Washington, DC, American Psychiatric Press, 1995.

Kandel ER: A new intellectual framework for psychiatry. Am J Psychiatry 155:457–469, 1998.

Kandel ER: Biology and the future of psychoanalysis: a new intellectual framework for psychiatry revisited. Am J Psychiatry 4:505, 1999.

Kleinman A: Re-Thinking Psychiatry: From Cultural Category to Personal Experience. New York, Free Press, 1988.

McHugh PR, Slavney PR: The Perspectives of Psychiatry. Baltimore, Johns Hopkins University Press, 1986.

McHugh PR, Slavney PR: The Perspectives of Psychiatry, 2nd Edition. Baltimore, Johns Hopkins University Press, 1998.

Searle, JR: The Rediscovery of the Mind. Boston, MIT Press, 1992.

Sims A: Symptoms In the Mind. Philadelphia, WB Saunders Co., 1988.

Szasz TS: Ideology and Insanity. New York, Doubleday, 1970.

Szasz TS: The Myth of Mental Illness. St. Albans, UK, Paladin, 1972.

Verhulst J, Tucker GJ: Medical and narrative approaches in psychiatry. Psychiatr Serv 46:513–514, 1995.

Williams, JB: Psychiatric classification, in Treatment of Psychiatric Disorders, 2nd edition. Edited by Gabbard GO. Washington, DC, American Psychiatric Press, 1995.

Chapter 2

Amador XF, Strauss DH, Yale SA, et al: Assessment of insight in psychosis. Am J Psychiatry 150:873–879, 1993.

American Psychiatric Association: Diagnostic and Statistical Manual of Mental Disorders, 4th Edition. Washington, DC, American Psychiatric Association, 1994.

American Psychiatric Association: Practice Guideline for Psychiatric Evaluation of Adults. Am J Psychiatry 152(suppl 11):1–14, 1995.

Andreasen NC: Thought, language, and communication disorders. I: Clinical assessment, definition of terms, and evaluation of their reliability. Arch Gen Psychiatry 36:1315–1321, 1979.

Crum RM, Anthony JC, Bassett SS, et al: Population-based norms for the Mini-Mental State Examination by age and educational level. JAMA 1993; 269:2386–2391.

Cummings JL: Mini-Mental State Examination: norms, normals, and numbers (editorial Comment). JAMA 269:2420–2421, 1993.

Ewing JA: Detecting alcoholism: the CAGE questionnaire. JAMA 252:1905–1907, 1984.

Folstein MF, Folstein SE, McHugh PR: "Mini-Mental State": a practical method for grading the cognitive state of patients for the clinician. J Psychiatr Res 12:189–198, 1975.

Jaspers K: General Psychopathology, translated by Hoenig J, Hamilton MW. Chicago, IL, University of Chicago Press, 1963.

Malloy PF, Cummings JL, Coffey CE, et al: Cognitive screening instruments in neuropsychiatry: a report of the committee on research of the American Neuropsychiatric Association. J Neuropsychiatry Clin Neurosci 9:189–197, 1997.

McEvoy JP, Apperson LJ, Appelbaum PS, et al: Insight in schizophrenia: its relationship to acute psychopathology. J Nerv Ment Dis 177:43–47, 1989.

McEvoy JP, Freter S, Everett G, Geller JL, Appelbaum PS, Apperson LJ, Roth L: Insight and the clinical outcome of schizophrenic patients. J Nerv Ment Dis 177:48–51, 1989.

MacKinnon RA, Yudofsky SC: The Psychiatric Evaluation in Clinical Practice. Philadelphia, JB Lippincott, 1986.

Ovsiew F: Bedside neuropsychiatry: eliciting the clinical phenomena of neuropsychiatric illness, in American Psychiatric Press Textbook of Neuropsychiatry, 3rd Edition. Edited by Yudofsky SC, Hales RE. Washington, DC, American Psychiatric Press, 1997.

Sims A: Symptoms in the Mind, 2nd Edition. Philadelphia, WB Saunders Co., 1995.

Spitzer RL, Williams JBW: Instruction Manual for the Structured Clinical Interview for DSM-III (SCID). New York, Biometrics Research Department, New York State Psychiatric Institute, 1984.

Chapter 3

McHugh PR, Slavney PR: The Perspectives of Psychiatry, 2nd Edition. Baltimore, Johns Hopkins University Press, 1998.

Slavney PR, McHugh PR: Psychiatric Polarities: Methodology and Practice. Baltimore, Johns Hopkins University Press, 1987.

Chapter 4

Bechara A: Neurobiology of decision-making: risk and reward. Semin Clin Neuropsychiatry 6:205–216, 2001.

Cravchik A, Goldman D: Neurochemical individuality: genetic diversity among human dopamine and serotonin receptors and transporters. Arch Gen Psychiatry 57:1105–1114, 2000.

Charney DS, Bremner JD: The neurobiology of anxiety disorders, in Neurobiology of Mental Illness. Edited by Charney DS, Nestler EJ, Bunney BS. New York, Oxford University Press, 1999.

Duman RS, Heninger GR, Nestler EJ: A molecular and cellular theory of depression. Arch Gen Psychiatry 54:597–60, 1997.

Edelman GM: Neural Darwinism: The Theory of Neuronal Group Selection. New York, Basic Books, 1987.

Johnson JG, Cohen P, Skodol AE, et al: Personality disorders in adolescence and risk of major mental disorders and suicidality during adulthood. Arch Gen Psychiatry 56:805–811, 1999.

Lang PJ, Bradley MM, Cuthbert BN: Emotion, motivation, and anxiety: brain mechanisms and psychophysiology. Biological Psychiatry 44:1248–1263, 1998.

Leckman JF, Mayes AL: Understanding developmental psychopathology: how useful are evolutionary accounts? J Am Acad Child Adolesc Psychiatry 37:1011–1021, 1998.

Liggan DY, Kay J: Some neurobiological aspects of psychotherapy: a review. J Psychother Pract Res 8:103–114, 1999.

McQuade R, Young AH: Future therapeutic targets in mood disorders: the glucocorticoid receptor. Br J Psychiatry 177:390–395, 2000.

Nestler EJ, Hyman SE, Malenka RC: Molecular Neuropharmacology: a Foundation for Clinical Neuroscience. New York, NY, McGraw-Hill, 2001.

Sapolsky RM: Glucocorticoids and hippocampal atrophy in neuropsychiatric disorders. Arch Gen Psychiatry 57:925–935, 2000.

Siever LJ, Davis KL; A psychobiological perspective on the personality disorders. Am J Psychiatry 148:1647–1658, 1991.

Chapter 5

Armstrong SC, Cozza KL, Attanabe KS: The misdiagnosis of delirium. Psychosomatics 38:433–439, 1997.

Levkoff S, Liptzin B, Evans D, et al: Progression and resolution of delirium in elderly patients hospitalized for acute care. Am J Geriatr Psychiatry 2:230–238, 1994.

Levkoff, SE, Liptzin, B, Cleary, PD, et al: Subsyndromal delirium. Am J Geriatr Psychiatry 4:320–329, 1996.

Lipowski ZJ: Delirium: Acute Confusional States. New York, Oxford University Press, 1990.

Liptzin B, Levkoff SE, Gottlieb GL, et al: Delirium. J Neuropsychiatry Clin Neurosci 5:154–160, 1993.

Margolis RL: Nonpsychiatrist house staff frequently misdiagnose psychiatric disorders in general hospital inpatients. Psychosomatics 35:485–491, 1994.

Rabins PV, Folstein MF: Delirium and dementia: diagnostic criteria and fatality rates. Br J Psychiatry 140:149–153, 1982.

Tune L, Carr S, Hoag E, et al: Anticholinergic effects of drugs commonly prescribed for the elderly: potential means for assessing risk of delirium. Am J Psychiatry 149:1393–1394, 1992.

Trzepacz PT, Wise MG: Neuropsychiatric aspects of delirium, in American Psychiatric Press Textbook of Neuropsychiatry, 3rd Edition. Edited by Yudofsky SC, Hales RE. Washington, DC, American Psychiatric Press, 1997.

Wise MG: Delirium due to a general medical condition, delirium due to multiple etiologies, and delirium not otherwise specified, in Treatment of Psychiatric Disorders, 2nd edition. Edited by Gabbard GO. Washington, DC, American Psychiatric Press, 1995.

Wise MG, Brandt GT: Delirium, in American Psychiatric Press Textbook of Neuropsychiatry, 2nd edition. Edited by Yudofsky SC, Hales RE. Washington, DC, American Psychiatric Press, 1992.

Chapter 6

Aisen PS, Davis KL: Inflammatory mechanisms in Alzheimer's disease: implications for therapy. Am J Psychiatry 151:1105–1113, 1994.

American Psychiatric Association: Practice guideline for the treatment of patients with Alzheimer's disease and other dementias of late life. Am J Psychiatry 154(suppl 5):1–39, 1997.

Alexopoulos G, Meyers BS, Young RC, et al: The course of geriatric depression with "reversible dementia": a controlled study. Am J Psychiatry 150:1693–1699, 1993.

Cummings JL, Benson DF: Dementia: A Clinical Approach, 2nd Edition. Boston, Butterworths, 1992.

Cummings JL: Amnesia and memory disturbances in neurologic disorders, in American Psychiatric Press Review of Psychiatry, Vol 12. Edited by Oldham JM, Riba MB, Tasman A. Washington, DC, American Psychiatric Press, 1993.

Doody RS, Stevens JC, Beck C, et al: Practice parameter: management of dementia (an evidence

based review). Report of the Quality Standards Subcommittee of the American Academy of Neurology. Neurology 56:1154–1166, 2001.

Knopman DS, DeKosky ST, Cummings JL, et al: Practice parameter: diagnosis of dementia (an evidence based review). Report of the Quality Standards Subcommittee of the American Academy of Neurology. Neurology 56:1143–1153, 2001.

Mandell AM, Albert ML: History of subcortical dementia, in Subcortical Dementia. Edited by Cummings JL, New York, Oxford University Press, 1990.

Masterman DL, Craig AL, Cummings JL: Alzheimer's disease, in Treatment of Psychiatric Disorders, 2nd edition. Edited by Gabbard GO. Washington, DC, American Psychiatric Press, 1995.

Mega MS, Cummings JL, Fiorello T, Gornbein J: The spectrum of behavioral changes in Alzheimer's disease. Neurology 46:130–135, 1996.

National Institute on Aging/Alzheimer's Association Working Group: Apolipoprotein E genotyping in Alzheimer's disease. Lancet 347:1091–1095, 1996.

Peterson RC, Smith GE, Waring SC, et al: Mild cognitive impairment: clinical characterization and outcome. Arch Neurol 55:303–308, 1999.

Peterson RC, Stevens JC, Ganguli M, et al: Practice parameter: early detection of dementia: mild cognitive impairment (an evidence based review). Report of the Quality Standards Subcommittee of the American Academy of Neurology. Neurology 56:1133–1142, 2001.

Rubin EH, Morris JC, Grant EA, et al: Very mild senile dementia of the Alzheimer's type. I. Clinical assessment. Arch Neurol 46:379–382, 1989.

Small GW, Rabins PV, Barry PP, et al: Diagnosis and treatment of Alzheimer disease and related disorders: consensus statement of the American Association for Geriatric Psychiatry, the Alzheimer's Association, and the American Geriatrics Society. JAMA 278:1363–1371, 1997.

Stahl SM: Essential Psychopharmacology: Neuroscientific Basis and Practical Applications, 2nd edition. New York, Cambridge University Press, 2000.

Tariot PN: Treatment strategies for agitation and psychosis in dementia. J Clin Psychiatry 57(suppl 14):21–29, 1996.

Weihl CC, Roos RP: Creutzfeldt-Jakob disease, new variant Creutzfeldt-Jakob disease, and bovine spongiform encephalopathy. Neurol Clin 17:835–59, 1999.

Chapter 7

Akiskal HS: Mood disorders: introduction and overview, in Comprehensive Textbook of Psychiatry/VII, 7th Edition. Edited by Kaplan HI, Sadock BJ. Baltimore, Williams & Wilkins, 2000.

Akiskal HS, Mallya G: Criteria for the "soft" bipolar spectrum: treatment implications. Psychopharmacol Bull 23:68–73, 1987.

American Academy of Child and Adolescent Psychiatry: Practice parameters for the assessment and treatment of children and adolescents with bipolar disorder. J Am Acad Child Adolesc Psychiatry 36(suppl):157S–176S, 1997.

American Psychiatric Association: Practice guideline for major depressive disorder in adults. Am J Psychiatry 150(suppl 1):1–26, 1993.

American Psychiatric Association: Practice guideline for bipolar disorders. Am J Psychiatry 151(suppl 12):1–36, 1994.

Beck AT, Rush AJ, Shaw BF, et al: Cognitive Therapy of Depression. New York, Guilford, 1979.

Biederman J, Faraone S, Milberger S, et al: A prospective four-year follow-up study of attention deficit hyperactivity and related disorders. Arch Gen Psychiatry 53:437–446, 1996.

Blazer DG: Is depression more frequent in late life? An honest look at the evidence. Am J Geriatr Psychiatry 2:193–199, 1994.

Bostwick JM, Pankratz VS: Affective disorders and suicide risk: a reexamination. Am J Psychiatry 157:1925–1932, 2000.

Crismon ML, Trivedi M, Pigott TA, et al: The Texas Medication Algorithm Project: report of the Texas Consensus Conference Panel on medication treatment of major depressive disorder. J Clin Psychiatry 60:142–56, 1999.

DeVane CL: Differential pharmacology of newer antidepressants. J Clin Psychiatry 59(suppl 20):85–93, 1998.

Frances A, Docherty JP, Kahn DA: The expert consensus guidelines for the treatment of bipolar disorder. J Clin Psychiatry 57(suppl 12A):20, 1996.

Frasure-Smith N, Lesperance F, Talajic M: Depression following myocardial infarction: impact on six-month survival. JAMA 270:1819–1825, 1993.

Gardner DM, Shulman KI, Walker SE, et al: The making of a user friendly MAOI diet. J Clin Psychiatry 57:99–104, 1996.

Glassman AH, Shapiro PA: Depression and the course of coronary artery disease. Am J Psychiatry 155:4–11, 1998.

Goodwin FK, Jamison KR: Manic-Depressive Illness. Oxford University Press, New York, 1990.

Hyman SE, Nestler EJ: Initiation and adaptation: a paradigm for understanding psychotropic drug action. Am J Psychiatry 153:151–162, 1996.

Katon W, Von Korff M, Lin E, et al: Distressed high utilizers of medical care: DSM-III-R diagnoses and treatment needs. Gen Hosp Psychiatry 12:355–362, 1990.

Klerman GL, Weissman MM, Rounsaville BJ, et al: Interpersonal Psychotherapy of Depression. New York, Basic Books, 1984.

Kupfer DJ: Long-term treatment of depression. J Clin Psychiatry 52(suppl 5):28–34, 1991.

Luborsky L: Principles of Psychoanalytic Psychotherapy: A Manual for Supportive-Expressive Treatment. New York, Basic Books, 1984.

Manji HK, Moore GJ, Chen G: Bipolar disorder: leads from the molecular and cellular mechanisms of action of mood stabilizers. Br J Psychiatry 178(suppl 4):s107–s119.

Mayberg HS: Frontal lobe dysfunction in secondary depression. J Neuropsychiatry Clin Neurosci 6:428–442, 1994.

Murphy DL, Andrews AM, Wichems CH, et al: Brain serotonin neurotransmission: an overview and update with an emphasis on serotonin subsystem heterogeneity, multiple receptors, interactions with other neurotransmitter systems, and consequent implications for understanding the actions of serotonergic drugs. J Clin Psychiatry 59(suppl 15):4–12, 1998.

Nemeroff CB, DeVane CL, Pollock BG: Newer antidepressants and the cytochrome P450 system. Am J Psychiatry 153:311–320, 1996.

Nestler EJ, Hyman SE, Malenka RC: Molecular Neuropharmacology: a Foundation for Clinical Neuroscience. New York, NY, McGraw-Hill, 2001.

Paternak RE, Reynolds CF, Miller MD, et al: The symptom profile and two-year course of subsyndromal depression in spousally bereaved elders. Am J Geriatr Psychiatry 2:210–219, 1994.

Paternak RE, Reynolds CF, Miller MD, et al: Spousally bereaved elders with subsyndromal depression: a descriptive analysis and comparison with major depression. Am J Geriatr Psychiatry 4:61–68, 1996.

Post RM: Transduction of psychosocial stress into the neurobiology of recurrent affective disorder. Am J Psychiatry 149:999–1010, 1992.

Preskorn SH: Selection of an antidepressant: mirtazapine. J Clin Psychiatry 58(suppl 6):3–8, 1997.

Prigerson HG, Frank E, Kasl SV: Complicated grief and bereavement-related depression as distinct disorders: preliminary empirical validation in elderly bereaved spouses. Am J Psychiatry 152:22–30, 1995.

Public Health Service Agency for Health Care Policy and Research. Depression in Primary Care: Detection and Diagnosis. Rockville, MD, US Dept of Health and Human Services. AHCPR publication 93–0551, 1993.

Reid IC, Stewart AC: How antidepressants work: new perspectives on the pathophysiology of depressive disorder. Br J Pschiatry 178:299–303, 2001.

Shelton RC, Tomarken AJ: Can recovery from depression be achieved? Psychiatr Services 52: 1469–1478, 2001.

Stahl SM: Essential Psychopharmacology: Neuroscientific Basis and Practical Applications, 2nd edition. New York, Cambridge University Press, 2000.

Stahl, SM: Basic psychopharmacology of antidepressants, part 1: antidepressants have seven distinct mechanism of action. J Clin Psychiatry 59(suppl 4):5–14, 1998.

Stahl, SM: Selecting an antidepressant by using mechanism of action to enhance efficacy and avoid side effects. J Clin Psychiatry 59(suppl 18):23–29, 1998.

Stoudemire A, Hill CD, Morris R, et al: Improvement in depression-related cognitive dysfunction following ECT. J Neuropsychiatry Clin Neurosci 7:31–34, 1995.

Weissman MM, Livingston B, Leaf FJ, et al: Affective Disorders, in Psychiatric Disorders in America: The Epidemiologic Catchment Area Study. Edited by Robins LN, Regier DA. Free Press, New York, 1991.

Wells KB, Stewart A, Hays RD, et al: The functioning and well-being of depressed patients: results from the Medical Outcomes Study. JAMA 262:914–919,1989.

Wright JH, Beck AT: Cognitive therapy, in American Psychiatric Press Textbook of Psychiatry, 3rd Edition. Edited by Hales, RE, Yudofsky SC, Talbott JA. Washington, DC, American Psychiatric Press, 1999.

Zisook S, Shuchter SR: Depression through the first year of life after the death of a spouse. Am J Psychiatry 148:1346–1352, 1991.

Zisook S, Shuchter SR, Sledge PA. et al: The spectrum of depressive phenomena after spousal bereavement. J Clin Psychiatry 55(suppl 4):29–36, 1994.

Chapter 8

Abi-Dargham A, Laruelle M, Aghajanian, GK, et al: The role of serotonin in the pathophysiology and treatment of schizophrenia. J Neuropsychiatry Clin Neurosci 9:1–17, 1997.

American Psychiatric Association: Practice guideline for the treatment of patients with schizophrenia. Am J Psychiatry 154(suppl 4):1–63, 1997.

Andreason NC: A unitary model of schizophrenia: Bleuler's "fragmented phrene" as schizencephaly. Arch Gen Psychiatry 56:781–787, 1999.

Buckley PF, Meltzer HY: Treatment of schizophrenia, in American Psychiatric Textbook of Psychopharmacology. Edited by Schazberg AF, Nemeroff CB, Washington, DC, American Psychiatric Press, 1995.

Bustillo JR, Lauriello J, Horan WP, et al: The psychosocial treatment of schizophrenia: an update. Am J Psychiatry 158:163–175, 2001.

Carpenter W, Strauss J, Muleh S: Are there pathognomonic symptoms in schizophrenia? Arch Gen Psychiatry 28:847–852, 1973.

Crow TJ: Molecular pathology of schizophrenia: more than one disease process? Br Med J 280:66–68, 1980.

Davidson M, Reichenberg MA, Rabinowitz J, et al: Behavioral and intellectual markers for schizophrenia in apparently healthy male adolescents. Am J Psychiatry 156:1328–1335, 1999.

Feltner DE, Hertzman M: Progress in the treatment of tardive dyskinesia: theory and practice. Hosp Community Psychiatry 44:25–34, 1993.

Fenton WS, Wyatt RJ, McGlashan TH: Risk factors for spontaneous dyskinesia in schizophrenia. Arch Gen Psychiatry. 51:643–650, 1994.

Goldman D, Hier DA, Haas DL, et al: Bizarre delusions and DSM-III-R schizophrenia. Am J Psychiatry 149:494–499, 1992.

Goff DC, Coyle JT: The emerging role of glutamate in the pathophysiology and treatment of schizophrenia. Am J Psychiatry 158:1367–1377, 2001.

Hegarty JD, Baldessarini RJ, Tohen M, et al: One hundred years of schizophrenia: a meta-analysis of the outcome literature. Am J Psychiatry 151:1409–1416, 1994.

Kapur S, Remington G: Serotonin-dopamine interaction and its relevance to schizophrenia. Am J Psychiatry 153:466–476, 1996.

Kavanaugh DJ: Recent developments in expressed emotion and schizophrenia. Br J Psychiatry 160: 601–620, 1992.

Keck PE, Caroff SN, McElroy SL: Neuroleptic malignant syndrome and malignant hyperthermia: end of a controversy? J Neuropsychiatry Clin Neurosci 7:135–144, 1995.

Koehler K, Seminario I: "First-rank" schizophrenia and research diagnosable schizophrenic and affective illness. Compr Psychiatry 19:401–407, 1978.

McEvoy JP, Scheifler PL, Frances A, eds: The Expert Consensus Guideline Series: Treatment of Schizophrenia 1999. J Clin Psychiatry 60(suppl 11):1–80, 1999.

McGlashan TH, Hoffman, RE: Schizophrenia as a disorder of developmentally reduced synaptic connectivity. Arch Gen Psychiatry 57:637–648, 2000.

McGlashan TH, Krystal JH: Schizophrenia-Related

Disorders and Dual Diagnosis, in Treatment of Psychiatric Disorders, 2nd edition. Edited by Gabbard GO. Washington, DC, American Psychiatric Press, 1995.

Mellor CS: First rank symptoms in schizophrenia. Br J Psychiatry 117:15–23, 1970.

Miller AL, Chiles JA, Chiles JK, et al: The Texas Medication Algorithm Project (TMAP) schizophrenia algorithms. J Clin Psychiatry 60:649–657, 1999.

Nestler EJ, Hyman SE, Malenka RC: Molecular Neuropharmacology: a Foundation for Clinical Neuroscience. New York, McGraw-Hill, 2001.

Owens MJ, Risch C: Atypical antipsychotics, in American Psychiatric Textbook of Psychopharmacology. Edited by Schazberg AF, Nemeroff CB. Washington, DC, American Psychiatric Press, 1995.

Philbrick KL, Rummans TA: Malignant catatonia. J Neuropsychiatry Clin Neurosci 6:1–13, 1994.

Seeman P, Lee T, Chau-Wong M, et al: Antipsychotic drug doses and neuroleptic/dopamine receptors. Nature 261:717–719, 1976.

Stahl SM: Essential Psychopharmacology: Neuroscientific Basis and Practical Applications, 2nd edition. New York, Cambridge University Press, 2000.

Taminga CA: Neuropsychiatric aspects of schizophrenia, in American Psychiatric Press Textbook of Neuropsychiatry, 3rd Edition. Edited by Yudofsky SC, Hales RE. Washington, DC, American Psychiatric Press, 1997.

Taylor MA: Are schizophrenia and affective disorder related? A selective literature review. Am J Psychiatry 149:22–32, 1992.

Tsuang, MT, Stone WS, Faraone SV: Toward reformulating the diagnosis of schizophrenia. Am J Psychiatry 157:1041–1050, 2000.

Weinberger DR: Implications of normal brain development for the pathogenesis of schizophrenia. Arch Gen Psychiatry 44:660–669, 1987.

Woods BT: Is schizophrenia a progressive neurodevelopmental disorder? Toward a unitary pathogenetic mechanism. Am J Psychiatry 155:1661–1670, 1998.

Yamamoto BK, Meltzer HY: Basic neuropharmacology of antipsychotic drugs, in Treatment of Psychiatric Disorders, 2nd edition. Edited by Gabbard GO. Washington, DC, American Psychiatric Press, 1995.

Chapter 9

Barlow DH, Craske MG: Mastery of Your Anxiety and Panic. 2nd Edition. Albany, NY, Graywind Publications, 1994.

Ballenger JC: Panic disorder in the medical setting. J Clin Psychiatry 58(suppl 2):13–17, 1997.

Bremner JD, Davis M, Southwick SM, et al: Neurobiology of posttraumatic stress disorder, in American Psychiatric Press Review of Psychiatry, Vol 12. Edited by Oldham JM, Riba MB, Tasman A. Washington, DC, American Psychiatric Press, 1993.

Brown TA, Barlow DH, Liebowitz MR: The empirical basis of generalized anxiety disorder. Am J Psychiatry 151:1272–1280, 1994.

Goddard AW, Charney DS: Toward an integrated neurobiology of panic disorder. J Clin Psychiatry 58(suppl 2):4–11, 1997.

Gorman JM, Kent, JM, Sullivan GM, et al: Neuroanatomical hypothesis of panic disorder, revised. Am J Psychiatry 157:493–505, 2000.

Greist JH, Jefferson JW: Obsessive-compulsive disorder, in Treatment of Psychiatric Disorders, 2nd edition. Edited by Gabbard GO. Washington, DC, American Psychiatric Press, 1995.

Hollander, E, Simeon D, Gorman JM: Anxiety disorders, in American Psychiatric Press Textbook of Psychiatry, 3rd Edition. Edited by Hales, RE, Yudofsky SC, Talbott JA. Washington, DC, American Psychiatric Press, 1999.

Katon W: Panic disorder and somatization: a review of 55 cases. Am J Med 77:101–106, 1984.

Klein, DF: False suffocation alarms, spontaneous panics, and related conditions: an integrative hypothesis. Arch Gen Psychiatry 50:306–317, 1993.

Marmar CR, Foy D, Kagan B, et al: An integrated approach for treating posttraumatic stress disorder, in American Psychiatric Press Review of Psychiatry, Vol 12. Edited by Oldham JM, Riba MB, Tasman A. Washington, DC, American Psychiatric Press,1993.

Mathew SJ, Coplan JD, Gorman JM: Neurobiological mechanisms of social anxiety disorder. Am J Psychiatry 158:1558–1567, 2001.

Mindus P, Rasmussen SA, Lindquist C: Neurosurgical treatment for refractory obsessive-compulsive disorder: implications for understanding frontal lobe function. J Neuropsychiatry Clin Neurosci 6:467–477, 1994.

Nutt DJ, Malizia AL: New insights into the role of GABAA-benzodiazepine receptor in psychiatric disorder. Br J Psychiatry 179:390–396, 2001.

Rauch SL, Jenike MA: Neurobiological models of obsessive-compulsive disorder. Psychosomatics 34:20–32, 1993.

Schwartz JM, Stoessel PQ, Baxter LR, et al: Systematic changes in cerebral glucose metabolic rate after successful behavior modification treatment of obsessive-compulsive disorder. Arch Gen Psychiatry 53:109–113, 1996.

Shear KS, Cooper AM, Klerman GL, et al: A psychodynamic model of panic disorder. Am J Psychiatry 150:859–866, 1993.

Sheehan DV, Ballenger JC, Jacobsen G: Treatment of endogenous anxiety with phobic, hysterical, and hypochondriacal symptoms. Arch Gen Psychiatry 37:51–59, 1980.

Stahl SM: Essential Psychopharmacology: Neuroscientific Basis and Practical Applications, 2nd edition. New York, Cambridge University Press, 2000.

Stein MB, Uhde, TW: Biology of anxiety disorders, in American Psychiatric Press Textbook of Psychopharmacology. Edited by Schazberg AF, Nemeroff CB. Washington, DC, American Psychiatric Press, 1995.

Stone AA: Post-traumatic stress disorder and the law: critical review of the new frontier. Bull Am Acad Psychiatry Law 21:23–36, 1993.

Taylor CB: Treatment of anxiety disorders, in American Psychiatric Press Textbook of Psychopharmacology. Edited by Schazberg AF, Nemeroff CB. Washington, DC, American Psychiatric Press, 1995.

Yehuda, R, McFarlane, AC: Conflict between current knowledge about posttraumatic stress disorder and its original conceptual basis; Am J Psychiatry 152:1705–1713, 1995.

Zorumski CF, Isenberg KE: Insights into the structure and function of GABA-benzodiazepine receptors: ion channels and psychiatry. Am J Psychiatry 148:162–173, 1991.

Chapter 10

Bolton S, Gunderson JG: Distinguishing borderline personality disorder from bipolar disorder: differential diagnosis and implications (clinical case conference). Am J Psychiatry 153:1202–1207 1996.

Bouchard TJ, Lykken DT, McGue M, et al: Sources of human psychological differences: the Minnesota study of twins reared apart. Science 250: 223–228, 1990.

Chess S, Thomas A: Origins and Evolution of Behavior Disorders From Infancy to Early Adult Life. New York, Brunner/Mazel, 1984.

Cleckley H: The Mask of Sanity, 4th Edition. St. Louis, CV Mosby, 1964.

Cohen BJ, Nestadt G, Samuels JF, et al: Personality disorder in later life: a community study. Br J Psychiatry 165:493–499, 1994.

Costa PT, McCrae RR: Theories of personality and psychopathology: approaches derived from philosophy and psychology, in Comprehensive Textbook of Psychiatry/VII, 7th Edition. Edited by Kaplan HI, Sadock BJ. Baltimore, Williams & Wilkins, 2000.

Gabbard GO: Theories of personality and psychopathology: psychoanalysis, in Comprehensive Textbook of Psychiatry/VII. 7th Edition. Edited by Kaplan HI, Sadock BJ. Baltimore, Williams & Wilkins, 2000.

Gunderson JG, Links P: Borderline personality disorder, in Treatment of Psychiatric Disorders, 2nd edition. Edited by Gabbard GO. Washington, DC, American Psychiatric Press, 1995.

Hirshfeld DR, Rosenbaum JF, Biederman J, et al: Stable behavioral inhibition and its association with anxiety disorder. J Am Acad Child Adolesc Psychiatry 31:103–111, 1992.

Kagan J, Reznick JS, Gibbons J: Inhibited and uninhibited types of children. Child Dev 60:838–845, 1989.

Kernberg OF: Borderline Conditions and Pathological Narcissism. New York, Jason Aronson, 1975.

Kohut H: The Restoration of the Self. New York, International Universities Press, 1977.

Mahler MS, Pine F, Bergman A: The Psychological Birth of the Human Infant: Symbiosis and Individuation. New York, Basic Books, 1975.

Nestadt G, Romanoski AJ, Brown CH, et al: DSM-III obsessive-compulsive disorder: an epidemiological survey. Psychol Med 21:461–471, 1991.

Phillips KA, Gunderson JG: Personality disorders, in American Psychiatric Press Textbook of Psychiatry, 3nd Edition. Edited by Hales RE, Yudofsky SC, Talbott JA. Washington, DC, American Psychiatric Press, 1999.

Siever LJ, Davis KL: A psychobiological perspective on the personality disorders. Am J Psychiatry 148:1647–1658, 1991.

Vaillant GE: Adaptation to Life. Boston, Little, Brown, 1977.

Winchel RM, Stanley M: Self-injurious behavior: a review of the behavior and biology of self-mutilation. Am J Psychiatry 148:306–317, 1991.

Chapter 11

American Psychiatric Association: Practice guideline for the treatment of patients with eating disorders (revision). Am J Psychiatry 157(suppl 1):1–39, 2000.

Andersen AE: Practical Comprehensive Treatment of Anorexia Nervosa and Bulimia. Baltimore, Johns Hopkins University Press, 1985.

Aronne LJ: Obesity. Med Clin North Am 82:161–81, 1998.

Carlat, DJ, Camargo CA, Herzog DB: Eating disorders in males: a report on 135 patients. Am J Psychiatry 154 1127–1132, 1997.

Carney CP, Andersen AE: Eating disorders. Guide to medical evaluation and complications. Psychiatr Clin North Am 19:657–79, 1996.

Comerci, GD: Medical complications of anorexia nervosa and bulimia nervosa. Med Clin North Am
74:1293–310, 1990.

Garner DM, Garfinkel PE, Rockert W, et al: A
prospective study of eating disturbances in the ballet. Psychother Psychosom 48:170–175, 1987.

Habermas T: The psychiatric history of anorexia nervosa and bulimia nervosa: weight concerns and
bulimic symptoms in early case reports. Int J Eat
Disord 8:259–273, 1989.

Hall RCW, Beresford TP: Medical complications of
anorexia and bulimia. Psychiatr Med 7:165–192,
1989.

Heatherton TF, Nichols P, Mahamedi F, et al: Body
weight, dieting, and eating disorder symptoms
among college students, 1982 to 1992. Am J Psychiatry 152:1623–1629, 1995.

Hsu, G: Epidemiology of the eating disorders. Psychiatr Clin North Am 19:681–700, 1996.

Kaye WH, Gendall K, Kye C: The role of the central
nervous system in the psychoneuroendocrine disturbances of anorexia and bulimia nervosa. Psychiatr Clin North Am 21:381–396, 1998.

Kreipe RE, Harris JP: Myocardial impairment resulting from eating disorders. Pediatr Ann 21:760–
768, 1992.

Mitchell JE, Raymond N, Specker S: A review of the
controlled trials of pharmacotherapy and psychotherapy in the treatment of bulimia nervosa.
Int J Eat Disord 14:229–247, 1993.

Rigotti NA, Neer RM, Skates SJ, et al: The clinical
course of osteoporosis in anorexia nervosa. A longitudinal study of cortical bone mass. JAMA
265:1133–1138, 1991.

Yates A: Current perspectives on the eating disorders:
I. History, psychological and biological aspects. J
Am Acad Child Adolesc Psychiatry 28:813–828,
1989.

Yates A: Current perspectives on the eating disorders:
II. Treatment, outcome, and research directions. J
Am Acad Child Adolesc Psychiatry 29:1–9, 1990.

Chapter 12

American Psychiatric Association: Practice guideline
for the treatment of patients with substance use
disorders: alcohol, cocaine, opioids. Am J Psychiatry 152(suppl 11):1–80, 1995.

American Psychiatric Association: Practice guideline
for the treatment of patients with nicotine dependence. Am J Psychiatry 153(suppl 10):1–31, 1996.

Cornelius JR, Salloum IM, Ehler JG: Fluoxetine in depressed alcoholics, a double-blind, placebo-controlled study. Arch Gen Psychiatry 54:700–705,
1997.

Cornish JW, McNicholas LF, O'Brien CP: Treatment

of substance-related disorders, in American Psychiatric Press Textbook of Psychopharmacology.
Edited by Schazberg AF, Nemeroff CB, Washington, DC, American Psychiatric Press, 1995.

Covey L, Glassman AH, Stetner F: Cigarette smoking
and major depression. J Addict Disord 17:35–46,
1998.

Dixon L, McNary S, Lehman A: One-year follow-up
of secondary versus primary mental disorder in
persons with comorbid substance use disorders.
Am J Psychiatry 154:1610–1612, 1997.

Jaffe JH: Substance-related disorders: introduction
and overview, in Comprehensive Textbook of
Psychiatry/VII, 7th Edition. Edited by Kaplan HI,
Sadock BJ. Baltimore, Williams & Wilkins, 2000.

Koob GF: Drug addiction, dysregulation of reward,
and allostasis. Neuropsychopharmacology 24:97–
129, 2001.

Meyer, RE: Biology of psychoactive substance dependence disorders: opiates, cocaine, and ethanol,
in American Psychiatric Press Textbook of Psychopharmacology. Edited by Schazberg AF, Nemeroff CB. Washington, DC, American Psychiatric Press, 1995.

Nestler EJ: Molecular basis of long-term plasticity underlying addiction. Nat Rev Neurosci 2:119–128,
2001.

Nestler EJ, Hyman SE, Malenka RC: Molecular Neuropharmacology: a Foundation for Clinical Neuroscience. New York, NY, McGraw-Hill, 2001.

O'Connor PG, Kosten TR: Rapid and ultrarapid detoxification techniques. JAMA, 279:229–234, 1998.

Watson, SJ, Benson JA, Joy JE: Marijuana and medicine: assessing the science base: a summary of
the 1999 Institute of Medicine report. Arch Gen
Psychiatry 57:547–552, 2000.

Chapter 13

Bach M, Bach D, Zwaan MD: Independency of alexithymia and somatization: a factor analytic study.
Psychosomatics 37:451–458, 1996.

Barsky AJ: Amplification, somatization, and the somatoform disorders. Psychosomatics 33:28–34,
1992.

Barsky AJ: Hypochondriasis. Psychosomatics 37:48–
56, 1996.

Costa P, McCrae R: Neuroticism, somatic complaints,
and disease: is the bark worse than the bite? J Pers
55:299–316, 1987.

Feighner, JP, Robins E, Guze SB, et al: Diagnostic criteria for use in psychiatric research. Arch Gen Psychiatry 26:57–63, 1972.

Ford CV: The somatizing disorders. Psychosomatics
27:327–337, 1986.

Ford, CV: Conversion disorder and somatoform disorder not otherwise specified, in Treatment of Psychiatric Disorders, 2nd edition. Edited by Gabbard GO. Washington, DC, American Psychiatric Press, 1995.

Groves JE: Management of the borderline patient on a medical or surgical ward: the psychiatric consultant's roles. Int J Psychiatry Med 6:337–348, 1975.

Groves JE: Taking care of the hateful patient. N Engl J Med 298:883–887, 1978.

Mechanic D: The concept of illness behavior. J Chronic Dis 15:189–194, 1962.

Merskey H: The importance of hysteria. Br J Psychiatry 149:23–28, 1986.

Parsons T: Social Structure and Personality. Free Press, New York, 1964.

Pilowsky I: Abnormal illness behavior. Br J Med Psychol 42:347–351, 1969.

Pilowsky I: A general classification of abnormal illness behaviors. Br J Med Psychol 51:131–137, 1978.

Pribor EF, Yutzy SH, Dean JT, et al: Briquet's syndrome, dissociation. and abuse. Am J Psychiatry 150:1507–1511, 1993.

Russo J, Katon W, Sullivan M, et al: Severity of somatization and its relationship to psychiatric disorders and personality. Psychosomatics 35:546–556, 1994.

Slavney PR: Perspectives on "Hysteria." Baltimore, MD, Johns Hopkins University Press, 1990.

Smith GR: Toward more effective recognition and management of somatization disorder. J Fam Pract 25:551–552, 1987.

Smith GR: The course of somatization and its effects on utilization of health care resources. Psychosomatics 35:263–267. 1994.

Yutzy SH, Cloninger CR, Guze SB, et al: DSM-IV field trial: testing a new proposal for somatization disorder, Am J Psychiatry 152:97–101, 1995.

Chapter 14

American Academy of Child and Adolescent Psychiatry: Practice parameters for the forensic evaluation of children and adolescents who may have been physically or sexually abused. J Am Acad Child Adolesc Psychiatry 36:423–442, 1997.

Bernet W: False statements and the differential diagnosis of abuse allegations. J Am Acad Child Adolesc Psychiatry 32:903–910, 1993.

Dinwiddie SH, North CS, Yutzy SH: Multiple personality disorder: scientific and medicolegal issues. Bull Am Acad Psychiatry Law 21:69–79, 1993.

Frankel FH: Adult reconstruction of childhood events in the multiple personality literature. Am J Psychiatry 150:954–958, 1993.

Freinkel A, Koopman C, Speigel D: Dissociative

symptoms in media eyewitnesses of an execution Am J Psychiatry 151:1335–1339, 1994.

Loewenstein RJ: Dissociative amnesia and dissociative fugue, in Treatment of Psychiatric Disorders, 2nd edition. Edited by Gabbard GO. Washington, DC, American Psychiatric Press, 1995.

Loftus EF: The reality of repressed memories. Am Psychol 48:518–537, 1993.

McHugh PR, Putnam FW: Resolved: multiple personality disorder is an individually and socially created artifact. J Am Acad Child Adolesc Psychiatry 34:957–963, 1995.

Merskey H: The manufacture of personalities. Br J Psychiatry 160:327–340, 1992.

Ofshe R, Watters E: Making Monsters: False Memories, Psychotherapy, and Sexual Hysteria. New York, Charles Scribner's Sons, 1994.

Putnam FW: The Diagnosis and Treatment of Multiple Personality Disorder. New York, Guilford Press, 1989.

Ross CA: Multiple Personality Disorder: Diagnosis, Clinical Features, and Treatment. New York, John Wiley & Sons, 1989.

Shearer SL: Dissociative phenomena in women with borderline personality disorder. Am J Psychiatry 151:1324–1328. 1994.

Siegel DJ: Memory, trauma, and psychotherapy. J Psychotherapy Practice Res 4:93–122, 1995.

Simon D, Gross S, Guralnik O, et al: Feeling unreal: 30 cases of DSM-III-R depersonalization disorder. Am J Psychiatry 154:1107–1113, 1997.

Spence DP: Narrative Truth and Historical Truth. New York, WW Norton, 1982.

Steinberg M: Depersonalization, in Treatment of Psychiatric Disorders, 2nd edition. Edited by Gabbard GO. Washington, DC, American Psychiatric Press, 1995.

Spiegel D, Maldonado JR: Dissociative disorders, in American Psychiatric Press Textbook of Psychiatry, 3rd Edition. Edited by Hales RE, Yudofsky SC, Talbott JA. Washington. DC, American Psychiatric Press, 1999.

Spiegel D, Maldonado JR: Hypnosis, in American Psychiatric Press Textbook of Psychiatry, 3rd Edition. Edited by Hales, RE, Yudofsky SC, Talbott JA. Washington. DC, American Psychiatric Press, 1999.

Squire LR: Mechanisms of memory. Science 232: 1612–1619, 1986.

Squire LR, Zola-Morgan S: Memory: brain systems and behavior. Trends Neurosci 22:170–175, 1988.

Chapter 15

Anderson, KE: Pharmacology of penile erection. Pharmacol Rev 53:417–450, 2001.

Becker JV, Johnson BR, Kavoussi RJ: Sexual and gender identity disorder, in American Psychiatric Press Textbook of Psychiatry, 3rd Edition. Edited by Hales, RE, Yudofsky SC, Talbott JA. Washington, DC, American Psychiatric Press, 1999.

Berlin FS, Malin M, Thomas K: Nonpedophiliac and nontransvestic paraphilias, in Treatment of Psychiatric Disorders, 2nd edition. Edited by Gabbard GO. Washington, DC, American Psychiatric Press, 1995.

Bradford JM, Pawlak A: Double-blind placebo crossover study of cyproterone acetate in the treatment of the paraphilias. Arch Sex Behav 22:383, 1993.

Bradford JM: Pharmacological treatment of the paraphilias, in American Psychiatric Press Review of Psychiatry, Vol 14. Edited by Oldham JM, Riba MB. Washington, DC, American Psychiatric Press, 1995.

Diamond M, Sigmundson HK: Sex reassignment at birth: long-term review and clinical implications. Arch Pediatr Adolesc Med 151:298–304, 1997.

Evans C: The use of penile prostheses in the treatment of impotence. Br J Urology 81:591–598, 1998.

Fagan P, Wise T, Schmidt C Jr, Ponticas Y, Marshall R, Costa P: A comparison of five-factor personality dimensions in males with sexual dysfunction and males with paraphilia. J Pers Assess 57:434, 1991.

Friedman RC, Downey J: Neurobiology and sexual orientation: current relationships. J Neuropsychiatry Clin Neurosci 5:131–153, 1993.

Furby LU, Weinrott ML, Blackshaw L: Sex offender recidivism: a review. Psychol Bull 105:3–30, 1989.

Kaplan HS: Sexual desire disorders (hypoactive sexual desire and sexual aversion), in Treatment of Psychiatric Disorders, 2nd edition. Edited by Gabbard GO. Washington, DC, American Psychiatric Press, 1995.

Laughman E, Gagnon J, Michael R, Michaels S: Sex in America. Chicago, University of Chicago Press, 1994.

Leiblum SR, Segraves RT: Sex and aging, in American Psychiatric Press Review of Psychiatry, Vol 14. Edited by Oldham JM, Riba MB. Washington, DC, American Psychiatric Press, 1995.

Lue TF: Erectile dysfunction. New Engl J Med 342:1802–1813, 2000.

Mate-Kole C, Freschi M, Robin A: A controlled study of psychological and social change after surgical gender reassignment in selected male transsexuals. Br J Psychiatry 157:261, 1990.

McWhirter DP: Biological theories of sexual orientation, in American Psychiatric Press Review of Psychiatry, Vol 12. Edited by Oldham JM, Riba MB, Tasman A. Washington, DC, American Psychiatric Press, 1993.

Pinker S: Boys will be boys. The New Yorker, February 9, 1998, pp. 30–31.

Ponticas Y: Sexual aversion versus hypoactive sexual desire: a diagnostic challenge. Psychiatr Med 10: 273–281, 1992.

Rosenbaum, M: Female sexual arousal disorder and female orgasmic disorder, in Treatment of Psychiatric Disorders, 2nd edition. Edited by Gabbard GO. Washington, DC, American Psychiatric Press, 1995.

Rubinow DR, Schmidt PJ: Androgens, brain, and behavior. Am J Psychiatry 153:974–984, 1996.

Seidman SN, Rieder RO: A review of sexual behavior in the United States. Am J Psychiatry 51:330–341, 1994.

Chapter 16

Brown JH, Henteleff P, Barakat S, et al: Is it normal for terminally ill patients to desire death? Am J Psychiatry 143:208–211, 1986.

Chochinov HM, Wilson KG, Enns M, et al: Desire for death in the terminally ill. Am J Psychiatry 152:1185–1191, 1995.

DuRand CJ, Burtka GJ, Federman EJ, et al: A quarter century of suicide in a major urban jail: implications for community psychiatry; Am J Psychiatry 152:1077–1080, 1995.

Goldstein RB, Black DW, Nasrallah MA, et al: The prediction of suicide. Arch Gen Psychiatry 48: 418–422, 1991.

Hendin H, Kerman G: Physician-assisted suicide: the dangers of legalization. Am J Psychiatry 150:143–145, 1993.

Hollis C: Depression, family environment, and adolescent suicidal behavior J Am Acad Child Adolesc Psychiatry 35:622–630, 1996.

Hughes DH: Can the clinician predict suicide? Psychiatric Services 46:449–451, 1995.

Isometsä ET, Henriksson MM, Heikkinen ME, et al: Suicide among subjects with personality disorders. Am J Psychiatry 153:667–673, 1996.

Jacobs, D: The Harvard Medical School Guide to Suicide Assessment and Intervention. San Francisco, Jossey-Bass, 1999.

Kellermann AL, Rivara FP, Somes G, et al: Suicide in the home in relation to gun ownership. N Engl J Med 327:467–472, 1992.

Malone KM, Szanto K, Corbitt EM, et al: Clinical assessment versus research methods in the assessment of suicidal behavior. Am J Psychiatry 152:1601–1607, 1995.

Mann JJ, Waternaux C, Haas GL, et al: Toward a clinical model of suicidal behavior in psychiatric patients. Am J Psychiatry 156:181–189, 1999.

Mann JJ: A current perspective of suicide and attempted suicide. Ann Intern Med 136:302–311, 2002.

Perr IN: Suicide litigation and risk management: a review of 32 cases. Bull Am Acad Psychiatry Law 13:209–219, 1985

Pokorny AD: Prediction of suicide in psychiatric patients: report of a prospective study. Arch Gen Psychiatry 40:249–257, 1983.

Simon RI: Clinical Psychiatry and the Law, 2nd Edition. Washington, DC, American Psychiatric Press, 1992.

Soloff PH, George A, Nathan RS, et al: Paradoxical effects of amitriptyline on borderline patients. Am J Psychiatry 143:1603–1605, 1986.

Sweig RA, Hinrichsen GA: Factors associated with suicide attempts by depressed older adults a prospective study. Am J Psychiatry 150:1687–1692, 1993.

Young MA, Fogg LF, Scheftner WA, et al: Interactions of risk factors in predicting suicide. Am J Psychiatry 151:434–435, 1994.

Weisman AD, Worden JW: Risk-rescue rating in suicide assessment. Arch Gen Psychiatry 26:553–560, 1972.

Chapter 17

Aggleton JP, ed: The Amygdala: Neurobiological Aspects of Emotion, Memory, and Mental Dysfunction. New York, Wiley, 1992.

Appelbaum PS, Robbins PC, Monahan J: Violence and delusions: data from the MacArthur Violence Risk Assessment Study. Am J Psychiatry 157:566–572, 2000.

Coccaro EF, Siever LJ, Klar H, et al: Serotonergic studies in affective and personality disorder patients: correlates with suicidal and impulsive aggressive behavior. Arch Gen Psychiatry 46:587–599, 1989.

Davidson RJ, Putnam KM, Larson CL: Dysfunction in the neural circuitry of emotion regulation—a possible prelude to violence. Science 289:591–594, 2000.

Hellerstein, D, Frosch W, Koenigsberg HW: The clinical significance of command hallucinations. Am J Psychiatry 144:219–21, 1987.

Lidz CW, Mulvey EP, Gardner W: The accuracy of predictions of violence to others. JAMA 269:1007–1011, 1993.

Link BG, Stueve GA: Psychotic symptoms and the violent/illegal behavior of mental patients compared to community controls, in Violence and Mental Disorders: Developments in Risk Assessment. Edited by Monahan J, Steadman HJ. Chicago, University of Chicago Press, 1994.

McNiel, DE: Hallucinations and violence, in Violence and Mental Disorders: Developments in Risk Assessment. Edited by Monahan J, Steadman HJ. Chicago, University of Chicago Press, 1994.

McNeil DE, Eisner JP, Binder RL The relationship between command hallucinations and violence. Psychiatr Serv 51:1288–1292, 2000.

Monahan J: Mental disorder and violent behavior: perceptions and evidence. Am Psychol 47:511–521, 1992.

Monahan J, Steadman HJ: Toward a rejuvenation of risk assessment research, in Violence and Mental Disorder: Developments in Risk Assessment. Edited by Monahan J, Steadman H. Chicago, University of Chicago Press, 1994.

Monahan J, Steadman HJ, Appelbaum PS, et al: Developing a clinically useful tool for assessing violence risk. Br J Psychiatry 176:312–319, 2000.

Monahan J, Steadman HJ, Silver E, et al: Rethinking Risk Assessment: The MacArthur Study of Mental Disorder and Violence. New York, Oxford University Press, 2001.

Mulvey EP: Assessing the evidence of a link between mental illness and violence. Hosp Community Psychiatry 45:663–668, 1994.

Murdoch D, Pihl RO, Ross D: Alcohol and crimes of violence: present issues. Int J Addictions. 25:1065–1081, 1990.

Murray GB: Limbic music. Psychosomatics 33:16–23, 1992.

Newhill CE, Mulvey EP, Lidz CW: Characteristics of violence in the community by female patients seen in a psychiatric emergency service. Psychiatric Services 46:785–789, 1995.

Steadman HJ, Mulvey EP, Monahan J et al: Violence by people discharged from acute psychiatric inpatient facilities and by others in the same neighborhoods. Arch Gen Psychiatry 55:393–401, 1998.

Stein DJ, Hollander E, Liebowitz MR: Neurobiology of impulsivity and the impulse control disorders. J Neuropsychiatry Clin Neurosci 5:9–17, 1993.

Swanson JW, Holzer CE, Ganju VK, et al: Violence and psychiatric disorder in the community: evidence from the Epidemiologic Catchment Area surveys. Hospital and Community Psychiatry 41:761–770, 1990.

Tardiff K: Violence, in American Psychiatric Press Textbook of Psychiatry, 3rd Edition. Edited by Hales RE, Yudofsky SC, Talbott JA. Washington, DC, American Psychiatric Press, 1999.

Volavka J: Neurobiology of Violence. Washington, DC, American Psychiatric Press, 1995.

Volavka J: The neurobiology of violence: an update. J Neuropsychiatry Clin Neurosci 11:307–314, 1999.

Chapter 18

Barber JP: Efficacy of short-term dynamic psychotherapy. J Psychotherapy Practice Res 3:108–121, 1994.

Bennet MJ: The catalytic function in psychotherapy. Psychiatry 52:351–364, 1989.

Blackwell B, Bloomfield SS, Buncher CR: Demonstration to medical students of placebo responses and nondrug factors. Lancet 1:1279–1282, 1972.

Buckalew LW, Coffield KE: An investigation of drug expectancy as a function of capsule color and size and preparation form. J Clin Psychopharmacol 2:245–248, 1982.

Cobb LA, Thomas GI, Dillard DH, et al: An evaluation of internal mammary artery ligation by a double-blind technique. N Engl J Med 260:1115–1118, 1959.

Docherty JP, Streeter MJ: Progress and limitations in psychotherapy research. J Psychotherapy Practice Res 2:100–118, 1993.

Frank JD, Frank JB: Persuasion and Healing: A Comparative Study of Psychotherapy, 3rd edition. Baltimore, Johns Hopkins University Press, 1991.

Gabbard G: Psychodynamic Psychiatry in Clinical Practice: The DSM-IV Edition. Washington, DC, American Psychiatric Press, 1994.

Gabbard GO: Psychodynamic Psychotherapies, in Treatment of Psychiatric Disorders, 2nd edition. Edited by Gabbard GO. Washington, DC, American Psychiatric Press, 1995.

Kleijnen J, de Craen AJM, Everdingen JV, et al: Placebo effect in double-blind clinical trials: a review of interactions with medications. Lancet 344:1347–1349, 1994.

Lambert MJ, Anderson EM: Assessment for the time-limited psychotherapies, in American Psychiatric Press Review of Psychiatry, Vol 15. Edited by Dickstein LJ, Riba MB, Oldham JM. Washington, DC, American Psychiatric Press, 1996.

Lasagna L, Laties VG, Dohan JL: Further studies on the "pharmacology" of placebo administration. J Clin Invest 37:533–537, 1958.

Lazar SG, Gabbard GO: The cost-effectiveness of psychotherapy. J Psychotherapy Practice Res 6:307–314, 1997.

Luborsky L, Singer B, Luborsky L: Comparative studies of psychotherapies: is it true that "everyone has won and all must have prizes"? Arch Gen Psychiatry 32:995–1008, 1975.

MacKenzie KR: The time-limited psychotherapies: An overview, in American Psychiatric Press Review of Psychiatry, Vol 15. Edited by Dickstein LJ, Riba MB, Oldham JM. Washington, DC, American Psychiatric Press, 1996.

Omer H, London P: Signal and noise in psychotherapy: the role and control of nonspecific factors. Br J Psychiatry 155:239–245, 1989.

Peabody FW: The care of the patient. JAMA 88:877–882, 1927.

Piper WE: Psychodynamic psychotherapy, in American Psychiatric Press Review of Psychiatry, Vol 15. Edited by Dickstein LJ, Riba MB, Oldham JM. Washington, DC, American Psychiatric Press, 1996.

Rockland LH: A review of supportive psychotherapy, 1986–1992. Hosp Community Psychiatry 44:1053–1060, 1993.

Rosenthal R: Interpersonal expectations: effects of the experimenter's hypothesis, in Artifact in Behavioral Research. Edited by Rosenthal R, Rosnow RL. New York, Academic Press, 1969.

Rosenzweig S: Some implicit common factors in diverse methods of psychotherapy. Am J Orthopsychiatry 6:412–415, 1936.

Seligman MEP: The effectiveness of psychotherapy: the Consumer Reports study. Am Psychol 50:965–974, 1995.

Schapira K, McClelland HA, Griffiths NR, et al: Study of the effects of tablet colour in the treatment of anxiety states. BMJ 2:446–449, 1970.

Shapiro AK: The placebo effect in the history of medical treatment: implications for psychiatry. Am J Psychiatry 116:298–304, 1959.

Shapiro AK: A contribution to a history of the placebo effect. Behav Sci 5:398–430, 1960.

Shapiro AK: Factors contributing to the placebo effect: their implications for psychotherapy. Am J Psychotherapy 18:73–81, 1964.

Smith TC, Thompson TL: The inherent, powerful therapeutic value of a good physician-patient relationship. Psychosomatics 3:166–170, 1993.

Straus JL, Cavanaugh SVA: Placebo effects: issues for clinical practice in psychiatry and medicine. Psychosomatics 37:315–326, 1996.

Thomson R: Side effects and placebo amplification. Br J Psychiatry 140:64–68, 1982.

Winston A, Muran JC: Common factors in the time-limited psychotherapies, in American Psychiatric Press Review of Psychiatry, Vol 15. Edited by Dickstein LJ, Riba MB, Oldham JM. Washington, DC, American Psychiatric Press, 1996.

Wolf S: Effects of suggestion and conditioning on the action of chemical agents in human subjects: the pharmacology of placebos. J Clin Invest 29:100, 1950.

Yalom ID: Theory and Practice of Group Psychotherapy, 4th edition. New York, Basic Books, 1994.

Chapter 19

Allen AJ, Leonard H, Swedo SE: Current knowledge of medications for the treatment of childhood anxiety disorders J Am Acad Child Adolesc Psychiatry 34:976–986, 1995.

Ambrosini PJ: A review of pharmacotherapy of major depression in children and adolescents. Psychiatr Serv 51:627–633, 2000.

American Academy of Child and Adolescent Psychiatry: practice parameters for the assessment and treatment of children, adolescents, and adults with attention-deficit/hyperactivity disorder. J Am Acad Child Adolesc Psychiatry 36(suppl 10):085S–121S, 1997.

American Academy of Child and Adolescent Psychiatry: Practice parameters for the assessment and treatment of children and adolescents with conduct disorder. J Am Acad Child Adolesc Psychiatry 36(suppl):122S–139S, 1997.

American Academy of Pediatrics: Clinical practice guideline: diagnosis and evaluation of the child with attention-deficit/hyperactivity disorder. Pediatrics 105:1158–1170, 2000.

American Academy of Pediatrics: Clinical practice guideline: treatment of the school-age child with attention-deficit/hyperactivity disorder. Pediatrics 108:1033–1044, 2001.

Berenson CK: Anxiety and the developing child, in American Psychiatric Press Review of Psychiatry, Vol 15. Edited by Dickstein LJ, Riba MB, Oldham JM. Washington, DC, American Psychiatric Press, 1996.

Black B, Uhde TW: Psychiatric characteristics of children with selective mutism: A pilot study. J Am Acad Child Adolesc Psychiatry 34:847–856, 1995.

Black B: Social anxiety and selective mutism, in American Psychiatric Press Review of Psychiatry, Vol 15. Edited by Dickstein LJ, Riba MB, Oldham JM. Washington, DC, American Psychiatric Press, 1996.

Carlson GA: Identifying prepubertal mania. J Am Acad Child Adolesc Psychiatry 34:750–753, 1995.

Dow SP, Sonies BC, Scheib D, et al: Practical guidelines for the assessment and treatment of selective mutism. J Am Acad Child Adolesc Psychiatry 34:836–846, 1995.

Goldman LS, Genel M, Bezman RJ, et al: Diagnosis and treatment of attention-deficit/hyperactivity disorder in children and adolescents: report of the Council on Scientific Affairs, American Medical Association. JAMA 279:1100–1107, 1998.

Greenhill LL: Practice parameter for the use of stimulant medications in the treatment of children, adolescents, and adults. J Am Acad Child Adolesc Psychiatry 41(2 suppl):26S–49S, 2002.

Filipek PA, Accardo PJ, Ashwal S, et al: Practice parameter: screening and diagnosis of autism: report of the Quality Standards Subcommittee of the American Academy of Neurology and the Child Neurology Society. Neurology 55:468–479, 2000.

Harrington R, Whittaker J, Shoebridge P: Psycholog-

ical treatment of depression in children and adolescents: a review of treatment research. Br J Psychiatry 173:291–298, 1998.

Kafantaris V: Treatment of bipolar disorder in children and adolescents. J Am Acad Child Adolesc Psychiatry 34:732–741, 1995.

Kovacs M: Presentation and course of major depressive disorder during childhood and later years of the life span. J Am Acad Child Adolesc Psychiatry 35:705–715, 1996.

Lawless MR, McElderry DH: Nocturnal enuresis: current concepts. Pediatr Rev 22:339–407, 2001.

McKenna K, Gordon CT, Lenane M, et al: Looking for childhood-onset schizophrenia: the first 71 cases screened. Am Acad Child Adolesc Psychiatry 33:636–644, 1994.

Mikkelsen EJ: Enuresis and encopresis: ten years of progress. J Am Acad Child Adolesc Psychiatry 40:1146–1158, 2001.

Moreau D, Weissman M: Panic disorder in children and adolescents: a review. Am J Psychiatry 149:1306–1314, 1992.

Naylor MW, Staskowski M, Kenney MC, et al: Language disorders and learning disabilities in school-refusing adolescents. J Am Acad Child Adolesc Psychiatry 33:1331–1337, 1994.

Popper CW, West SA: Disorders usually first diagnosed in infancy, childhood, or adolescence, in American Psychiatric Press Textbook of Psychiatry, 3rd Edition. Edited by Hales RE, Yudofsky SC, Talbott JA. Washington, DC, American Psychiatric Press, 1999.

Posey DJ, McDougle CJ: The pharmacotherapy of target symptoms associated with autistic disorder and other pervasive developmental disorders. Harvard Rev Psychiatry 8:45–63, 2000.

Putnam FW: Posttraumatic stress disorder in children and adolescents, in American Psychiatric Press Review of Psychiatry, Vol 15. Edited by Dickstein LJ, Riba MB, Oldham JM. Washington, DC, American Psychiatric Press, 1996.

Rapoport, JL, Giedd J, Blumenthal J et al: Progressive cortical change during adolescence in childhood-onset schizophrenia. Arch Gen Psychiatry 54:649–654, 1999.

Richters MM, Volkmar FR: Reactive attachment disorder of infancy or early childhood. J Am Acad Child Adolesc Psychiatry 33:328–332, 1994.

Steinhausen H: Elective mutism: an analysis of 100 cases J Am Acad Child Adolesc Psychiatry 35:606–614, 1996.

Tanguay PE: Pervasive developmental disorders: a 10-year review. J Am Acad Child Adolesc Psychiatry 39:1079–1095, 2000.

Thompson S, Rey JM: Functional enuresis: is desmopressin the answer? J Am Acad Child Adolesc Psychiatry 34:266–271, 1995.

Volkow ND, Wang GJ, Fowler JS, et al: Dopamine transporter occupancies in the human brain induced by therapeutic doses of oral methylphenidate. Am J Psychiatry 155:1325–1331, 1998.

Weller E, Weller R, Fristad M: Bipolar disorder in children: misdiagnosis, underdiagnosis, and future directions. J Am Acad Child Adolesc Psychiatry 34:709–714, 1995.

Wender PH: Attention-deficit hyperactivity disorder in adults. Psychiatr Clin North Am 21:761–774, 1998.

Zametkin AJ, Nordahl TE, Gross M, et al: Cerebral glucose metabolism in adults with hyperactivity of childhood onset. New Engl J Med 323:1361–1366, 1990.

Chapter 20

Appelbaum PS, Gutheil TG: Clinical Handbook of Psychiatry and the Law, 3rd Edition. Baltimore, Williams & Wilkins, 2000.

Appelbaum PS, Lidz CW, Meisel A: Informed Consent: Legal Theory and Clinical Practice. New York, Oxford University Press, 1987.

Grisso T, Appelbaum PS: Assessing Competence to Consent to Treatment: A Guide for Physicians and Other Health Professionals. New York, Oxford University Press, 1998.

Grisso T, Appelbaum PS: Comparison of standards for assessing patients' capacities to make treatment decisions. Am J Psychiatry 152:1033–1037, 1995.

Grisso T, Appelbaum PS: The MacArthur Treatment Competence Study. III: Abilities of patients to consent to psychiatric and medical treatments. Law and Human Behavior 19:149–174, 1995.

Melton GB, Petrila J, Poythress NG, et al: Psychological Evaluations for the Courts: A Handbook for Mental Health Professionals and Lawyers. 2nd Edition. New York, Guilford, 1997.

Simon RI: Clinical Psychiatry and the Law, 2nd Edition. Washington, DC, American Psychiatric Press, 1992.

Index